P9-CLH-532

TRANSVAGINAL ULTRASOUND

SECOND EDITION

TRANSVAGINAL ULTRASOUND

SECOND EDITION

Edited by

MELVIN G. DODSON, M.D., Ph.D.

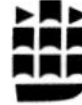

CHURCHILL LIVINGSTONE
New York, Edinburgh, London, Madrid, Melbourne, Milan, Tokyo

Library of Congress Cataloging-in-Publication Data

Transvaginal ultrasound / edited by Melvin G. Dodson.
p. cm.
Rev. ed. of: Transvaginal ultrasound / Melvin G. Dodson. date.
Includes bibliographical references and index.
ISBN 0-443-08953-1
1. Transvaginal ultrasonography. I. Dodson, Melvin G.
II. Dodson, Melvin G. Transvaginal ultrasound.
[DNLM: 1. Genital Diseases, Female—ultrasonography. WP 141
T7723 1995]
RG107.5.T73T73 1995
618′.047543—dc20
DNLM/DLC
for Library of Congress 94-36305
CIP

Distributed in the United Kingdom by Churchill Livingstone, Robert Stevenson House, 1–3 Baxter's Place, Leith Walk, Edinburgh EH1 3AF, and by associated companies, branches, and representatives throughout the world.

Acquisitions Editor: *Jennifer Mitchell*
Assistant Editor: *Shireen Dunwoody*
Copy Editor: *Donna C. Balopole*
Production Supervisor: *Sharon Tuder*
Cover Design: *Jeannette Jacobs*

Production services provided by Bermedica Production, Ltd.
Printed in the United States of America

First published in 1995 7 6 5 4 3 2 1

To my wife, Laura,
and to my children,
Diana, Melvin, and Melanie

Contributors

Michael J. Gast, M.D., Ph.D.

Associate Professor, Division of Reproductive Endocrinology and Infertility, Department of Obstetrics and Gynecology, Washington University School of Medicine, St. Louis, Missouri; Vice-President, Ob/Gyn Clinical Research and Development, Wyeth-Ayerst Research, Radnor, Pennsylvania

Sanja Kupesic, M.D, Ph.D.

Assistant Professor, Department of Obstetrics and Gynecology, Ultrasonic Institute, Medical School, University of Zagreb; Consultant, Department of Obstetrics and Gynecology, Sveti Duh Hospital, Zagreb, Croatia

Asim Kurjak, M.D., Ph.D.

Professor and Chairman, Department of Obstetrics and Gynecology, Ultrasonic Institute, Medical School, University of Zagreb, Zagreb, Croatia

Gregory S. Neal, M.D.

Fellow, Reproductive Endocrinology, The Center for Reproductive Medicine and Infertility, The New York Hospital-Cornell Medical Center, New York, New York

Thierry D. Pache, M.D, Ph.D.

Chef de Clinique, Clinic for Infertility and Gynecologic Endocrinology, WHO Collaborating Centre for Research in Human Reproduction, Department of Obstetrics and Gynecology, University Cantonal Hospital; Geneva University School of Medicine, Geneva Switzerland

Mladen Predanic, M.D, M.Sc.

Research Fellow, Department of Obstetrics and Gynecology, State University of New York Health Science Center at Brooklyn College of Medicine and The Brookdale Hospital Medical Center, Brooklyn, New York

Zev Rosenwaks, M.D.

Professor, Department of Obstetrics and Gynecology, Cornell University Medical College; Director, The Center for Reproductive Medicine and Infertility, Program of In Vitro Fertilization, The New York Hospital-Cornell Medical Center, New York, New York

Rudy E. Sabbagha, M.D.

Professor, Department of Obstetrics and Gynecology, Northwestern University Medical School; Director, Diagnostic Ultrasound Center, Department of Obstetrics and Gynecology, Prentice Women's Hospital and Maternity Center, Northwestern Memorial Hospital, Chicago, Illinois

Ivica Zalud, M.D., Ph.D.

Research Fellow, Department of Obstetrics and Gynecology, State University of New York at Stony Brook Health Sciences Center School of Medicine, Stony Brook, New York; Research Fellow, Department of Obstetrics and Gynecology, Winthrop University Hospital, Mineola, New York

Preface to the Second Edition

Since the publication of the first edition of *Transvaginal Ultrasound*, the number of ultrasound texts has increased due to continuing development in this area. This book is intended primarily as an introductory text for gynecologists and gynecology residents who are interested in learning how to apply ultrasound techniques and for radiologists who are interested in the specific application of ultrasound to gynecologic problems.

Transvaginal Ultrasound does not try to be the definitive reference for ultrasound but does provide a good, solid background in a practical format for individuals who are either not very familiar with gynecologic diseases or not familiar with the techniques of ultrasound. This book not only focuses on technique but includes anatomy, physiology, and the disease process and summarizes practical clinical information needed in everyday practice. For example, ultrasound reports often describe multiple ovarian cysts in patients, when in fact these "cysts" are nothing more than the normal immature follicles noted in a normal ovary throughout the menstrual cycle. In fact, the absence of such immature follicles is suggestive evidence that the patient is anovulatory, perimenopausal, or postmenopausal.

Likewise, "normal" ultrasound reports for patients with abnormal vaginal bleeding include detailed measurements, for example, of the ovary and uterus but no mention of the endometrium. It is this type of report that has made many clinicians feel that they have not gained any new diagnostic information from an ultrasound scan that they did not know from the history and physical examination. However, an astute ultrasonographer will recognize that the patient has a thin (single-line) endometrium with very little endometrial tissue and that such an endometrium is unlikely to respond to progesterone therapy (a common form of therapy by gynecologists for abnormal bleeding). Recognizing this very simple pattern will give the clinician significant additional information that can be useful in management of the bleeding. Ultrasound can be a very valuable technique, but only if one understands both the tool and the clinical problems to which the tool can be applied.

The basic concepts of transvaginal ultrasound are updated from the first edition. The text has been expanded to include additional techniques in clinical areas such as color flow Doppler, invasive techniques, the application of ultrasound to menometrorrhagia and urogynecology, and the diagnosis of congenital anomalies.

In this edition a group of internationally recognized sonologists and clinicians have contributed to the text. Dr. Thierry Pache contributed to some of the initial chapters involving the general concepts and application of ultrasound. Dr. Rudy Sabbagha summarized the information that a practitioner of ultrasound should know regarding the diagnosis of common congenital anomalies. Drs. Asim Kurjak, Ivica Zalud, Sanja Kupesic, and Mladen Predanic reviewed the use of transvaginal color Doppler and have included color illustrations demonstrating this technology. Drs. Gregory Neal and Zev Rosenwaks revised the chapter on the application of ultrasound techniques to assisted reproductive technologies. Dr. Michael Gast assisted me in revising the chapter on early pregnancy.

Overall, I hope the reader will find the second edition a practical introductory text to the application of ultrasound technology to gynecology.

Melvin G. Dodson, M.D., Ph.D.

Preface to the First Edition

The development of high-frequency transvaginal probes is literally producing a diagnostic revolution in gynecology. Those who think this is an overstatement have either not used the technique or have not invested the time to become proficient enough with the technique to appreciate its real potential. Gynecologic ultrasound (or at least the use of ultrasound to image pelvic structures) has been in use for 20 years. In the past, however, ultrasound has had a minimal impact on the day to day practice of gynecology. A gynecologist who receives an ultrasound report noting a 6-cm adnexal mass with internal echoes after referring a patient for a pelvic ultrasound because of an adnexal mass noted on pelvic examination has really learned no new diagnostic information. In fact, the gynecologist could interpret the internal echo in the cyst as consistent with a possible indication of a neoplasm. On the other hand, a careful transvaginal ultrasound examination by a skilled sonographer who recognizes a luteal phase endometrium and the internal echo in the cyst as a hemorrhagic corpus luteum will have gained important diagnostic information that would affect patient management. However, despite the example cited, the revolution in diagnostic gynecology will not occur because of the ability to differentiate a neoplastic from a functional cyst or of any single sonographic diagnostic advancement. The important contribution of transvaginal ultrasound in the practice of gynecology will be in the day to day use of sonography for such a variety of problems that the technique will become as much a part of the routine office visit as the pelvic examination. In fact, I can envision the day when a transvaginal ultrasound examination will be as common a procedure and as much a routine part of gynecology as the Pap smear.

Transvaginal ultrasound adds information on the size, location, physiology, and possible pathology of every organ system in the pelvis. It allows the gynecologist to see into the pelvis and even into the interior of the ovary and uterus where once we could only grasp and feel. I now use transvaginal ultrasound to evaluate pelvic pain, abnormal bleeding, missed periods and amenorrhea, adnexal masses, infertility, and early pregnancy; to monitor ovulation induction; to diagnose anovulation; to rule out ectopic pregnancy; and so on. The list of indications continues to grow. If you think that I am exaggerating, use this technique for a year and become familiar with its potential. You may find that you will not be able to practice without it.

Melvin G. Dodson, M.D., Ph.D.

Contents

Section I ***Basic Considerations***

1. *Clinical Uses* 1
   Melvin G. Dodson and Thierry D. Pache

2. *Basic Principles and Equipment* 17
   Melvin G. Dodson and Thierry D. Pache

3. *The Pelvic Ultrasound Examination and Pelvic Anatomy* 25
   Melvin G. Dodson and Thierry D. Pache

4. *Artifacts in Ultrasound* 43
   Melvin G. Dodson

Section II ***Regional Approaches***

5. *The Uterus* 51
   Melvin G. Dodson and Thierry D. Pache

6. *The Endometrium* 73
   Melvin G. Dodson

7. *The Ovary* 105
   Melvin G. Dodson

8. *Small Bowel, Sigmoid Colon, and Rectum* 133
   Melvin G. Dodson

Section III ***Disease Processes***

9. *Acute Pelvic Inflammatory Disease* 147
   Melvin G. Dodson

10. *Infertility* 157
    Melvin G. Dodson

11. *Amenorrhea and Menometrorrhagia* *163*
Melvin G. Dodson

12. *Other Clinical Problems* *179*
Melvin G. Dodson

Section IV ***Pregnancy and Complications of Pregnancy***

13. *Early Pregnancy* *187*
Melvin G. Dodson and Michael Gast

14. *Congenital Anomalies* *219*
Rudy E. Sabbagha

15. *Ectopic Pregnancy* *237*
Melvin G. Dodson

Section V ***Techniques***

16. *Urogynecology* *249*
Melvin G. Dodson

17. *Invasive Techniques* *271*
Melvin G. Dodson

18. *Ovulation Induction* *279*
Melvin G. Dodson

19. *Follicular Aspiration and In Vitro Fertilization* *311*
Gregory S. Neal, Zev Rosenwaks, and Melvin G. Dodson

20. *Transvaginal Color Doppler* *325*
Asim Kurjak, Ivica Zalud, Sanja Kupesic, and Mladen Predanic

Index *341*

Color plates for Chapter 20 follow pages 326 and 330.

1

Clinical Uses

Melvin G. Dodson
Thierry D. Pache

Ultrasonography has become a very important diagnostic tool in obstetrics and is now used extensively to determine anatomic parameters, such as location of the placenta and fetal presentation and lie, and biometric measurements of the fetus to date the gestation. Ultrasonography is also used to assess fetal growth and to diagnose congenital anomalies. In fact, the indications for ultrasound in obstetrics have become so numerous and the information obtained so valuable that ultrasonographic equipment has moved from the radiology department to the delivery floor and into the obstetrician's office.

Until recently, ultrasonography has had much less of an impact on the practice of gynecology. However, the introduction of high frequency transvaginal ultrasound for use in gynecology and early pregnancy (and occasionally even advanced pregnancy) has had a profound effect on the diagnosis and management of adnexal masses, abnormal bleeding, pelvic pain, uterine enlargement, ectopic pregnancy, threatened abortion, and a continually growing list of important clinical situations and problems. In addition, transvaginal ultrasound has become an invaluable tool for the care of the infertility patient. It is used to diagnose anovulation or confirm ovulation, monitor ovulation induction, diagnose congenital anomalies or leiomyoma, and evaluate the endometrium. Currently, most in vitro fertilization (IVF) oocyte retrievals are done by the ultrasound guided transvaginal technique. We cannot overstate the considerable amount of diagnostic information gained from the use of transvaginal ultrasound to the clinician just beginning to learn the technique. The comparative lack of utilization of ultrasound in gynecology probably is due to technical, economic, and educational considerations.

TECHNICAL ADVANTAGES OF HIGH FREQUENCY TRANSVAGINAL ULTRASONOGRAPHY

In the past, the use of a 1.6- to 3.5-MHz transducer and the full bladder imaging technique with transabdominal sonography did not produce adequate resolution of the fine structures of the ovary, adnexa, and endometrium to allow the diagnosis of many gynecologic conditions or early pregnancy complications that were not already obvious to the gynecologist by history and physical examination. In fact, some gynecologists legitimately complained that the pelvic ultrasound examination often gave little or no new diagnostic information and sometimes even confused the diagnosis and management. In obstetrics, the fetus and placenta are much larger structures surrounded by fluid compared to the smaller non-pregnant uterus and ovaries, and as a consequence, sonographic imaging and biometric measurements using lower frequency transducers have been at least adequate for obstetrics. However, imaging smaller structures, such as the ovary, the endometrium, the nonpregnant uterus, or an early pregnancy, with lower frequency transducers is less than optimal. Improved resolution using high frequency transvaginal transducers now allows better imaging of smaller pelvic structure, and the diagnosis of many pathologic pelvic conditions that were difficult or impossible to see only a few years ago. In addition, a detailed transvaginal ultrasonographic examination gives valuable information on the physiologic status of the ovary and endometrium that can be very helpful in the diagnosis and treatment of infertility, menometrorrhagia, amenorrhea, evaluation of bleeding in early pregnancy, and many other conditions.

Axial resolution—that is, the ability to distinguish two separate points in the direct line of the ultrasound beam—is a function of the transducer's frequency. Axial resolution improves with increased frequency. Unfortunately, the higher the frequency of the sound, the greater the attenuation or loss of sound intensity as it passes through tissue. This rapid attenuation limits the depths at which structures can be imaged with higher frequency sound. Therefore, using the standard transabdominal technique, lower frequencies with poorer axial resolution must be used to image structures deeper in the body, such as the pelvic organs. The development of the transvaginal probe has allowed the use of higher frequencies, since the pelvic structures are near the ultrasound probe. Because the structures being imaged are closer to the transducer, the problem of tissue attenuation is not as critical. This has resulted in much better resolution of pelvic structures. Using a 5- or 7.5-MHz transvaginal probe has allowed accurate resolution of even small follicles or cysts within the ovary and of small leiomyomas, better visualization of the endometrium, and very early diagnosis of normal or abnormal pregnancies (see Ch. 14).

In addition to its properties that depend on the physics of sound, there are anatomic and physiologic advantages to the use of transvaginal ultrasound. Bowel loops adjacent to the pelvic organs may interfere with the sound beam or produce shadow effects that may obscure an area of interest. Using transabdominal ultrasonography, Hull noted that it was impossible to evaluate adequately the ovarian architecture in as many as 42 percent of cases.[1] The use of transvaginal ultrasound often avoids such problems because the transducer is approximated close to the organ being evaluated.

New techniques, such as sonosalpingography, endouterine scanning with enhanced contrast ultrasound, tridimensional ultrasound, color flow, and the use of ultrasound in surgery, will continue to expand the horizons of ultrasound in the future. Three-dimensional sonography is just one example of what is right around the corner in new sonographic techniques.[2]

ECONOMICS OF TRANSVAGINAL ULTRASONOGRAPHY

Another factor limiting the use of ultrasound in gynecology has been economic. The cost of high quality ultrasonographic equipment has, in the past, generally been beyond the reach of the average gynecologist for office use. Since most gynecologists did not have ultrasonographic equipment in their offices, patients with gynecologic indications for an ultrasound examination were generally referred to a hospital or radiologist, just as are patients referred for an intravenous pyelogram or barium enema. However, more recently, smaller and less expensive office equipment has become available for the obstetrician-gynecologist's office. Despite the decrease in cost, most currently available ultrasonographic office equipment gives better images than were obtained only a few years ago with equipment normally only found in hospitals. Another important factor that has made office gynecologic ultrasonographic equipment economically feasible is that the same basic machine, with some variation in the transducers, can be used for both obstetrics and gynecology. Many obstetricians have found that ultrasound equipment is almost a necessity for the practice of obstetrics. The same equipment can be used for the gynecologic examination with the addition of a 5- or 7.5-MHz transvaginal probe. In fact, the combined use of the same equipment for both obstetrics and gynecology, the introduction of less expensive office equipment, and the increasing number of clinical indications have made the equipment more cost effective. Since the patient does not have to be referred out, the diagnostic information is immediately available when the ultrasound examination is performed in the office by the gynecologist. The office transvaginal pelvic ultrasound examination is much more convenient and economical for both the patient and the physician.

The use of the empty bladder technique in transvaginal ultrasound has resulted in considerable time savings, which has an economic impact in a busy clinical practice. This technique is also much better accepted by patients. Those who have not lived through the "agonies" of the use of the full bladder technique necessary with the transabdominal ultrasound approach will not truly appreciate the considerable time saved and the much improved patient comfort of the transvaginal approach.

Although concerns regarding the cost of an ultrasound examination are often expressed, ultrasound may be used effectively to decrease cost in some clinical settings. For example, about 15 percent of pregnancies end in spontaneous abortions. A frequent clinical scenario is an early pregnant patient presenting in the emergency room with bleeding and the passage of tissue. If a complete abortion cannot be confirmed, the most common clinical approach is to treat the patient using a suction curettage. However, ultrasound may be used to determine whether any significant amount of tissue remains within the uterine cavity. Many such patients do not need a suction curettage. Other patients thought to have a complete abortion may in fact need a suction curettage.[3] The use of ultrasound may be 20 to 30 times as cost effective as curettage and will save many patients the discomfort and inconvenience of surgery (anesthesia) when there is very little tissue remaining in the uterus (and very little advantage to the surgery had the physician known that there was a minimal amount of tissue remaining).

Likewise, ultrasound has had a dramatic effect on the diagnosis of ectopic pregnancy. In the past, many patients underwent a diagnostic laparoscopy to diagnose or rule out an ectopic pregnancy. Currently, many, if not most, patients are diagnosed by ultrasound, and in many patients an early intrauterine pregnancy is confirmed by ultrasound, which eliminates the expense, discomfort, and risks of surgery and anesthesia to rule out an ectopic pregnancy. In addition, some patients with an ectopic pregnancy are now being treated on an outpatient basis with methotrexate after sonographic diagnosis.

Some have suggested that the transvaginal ultrasound examination become a part of the routine pelvic examination.[4–6] Although this suggestion might seem overzealous to the uninitiated, the fact is that the routine application of transvaginal ultrasound is almost inevitable. The demand for excellence in care will require it, and the routine application will decrease the cost of utilization. It is simply a matter of time.

PHYSICIAN TRAINING

An important factor that has limited the use of ultrasound has been lack of physician training. Most gynecologists were not trained in the use of ultrasonography during their residency. More recently, residents in obstetrics and gynecology are receiving training in obstetric ultrasound, but unfortunately, training in gynecological ultrasound is still quite limited. As with other new techniques, this problem will undoubtedly be solved by continuing medical education courses, practical experience, and wider availability of textbooks and reviews on gynecological ultrasound. Learning ultrasound is not difficult; it simply requires some basic knowledge, some hands-on experience, and a little persistence. The rewards in terms of diagnostic information are considerable.

The clinician must become accustomed to the fact that sound echoes are being visualized. Ultrasound can give the clinician a new "sense organ" that can be just as valuable as one's eyes when one learns to see with echoes and when one appreciates fully the capabilities and the limitations of the technique.

Two additional properties of the ultrasound image to which some individuals learning sonography have difficulty adjusting are that a plain or slice of tissue is being imaged and the field of view (particularly with magnification) can be very narrow. The ultrasound image literally consists of the surface of the tissue or object being imaged (the way we are used to seeing an object), but it is only a one dimensional slice of the surface while, at the same time, the inside of the object (organ) and even structures beneath the object are all being imaged together. With a narrow field of view it is easy to become disoriented. The sonographer must reconstruct a three dimensional view from the two dimensional ultrasound image and appreciate what is inside from the surface of an object and orient this "view" to the pelvic structures as a whole.

With the development of transvaginal real-time ultrasonography and the use of the higher frequency 5- and 7.5-MHz probes with better resolution, with the smaller and less expensive office equipment that many obstetrician-gynecologists now have available in their offices for their obstetric practice, and as gynecologists gain experience with this valuable technique, gynecological office ultrasonography is coming of age (Table 1-1).

Table 1-1. Reasons for Increased Use of Ultrasound in Gynecology

Technical
Improved resolution (high frequency probes)
Decreased attenuation (transvaginal probes)
Economic
Cheaper equipment
Use of the same equipment for obstetrics and gynecology
Increased number of indications for pelvic sonography
Decrease in some common surgical procedures
Educational
Increased training and experience of gynecologists in pelvic sonography
Increasing clinical research and reports dramatically expanding the knowledge base of pelvic sonography

Table 1-2. Clinical Uses for Transvaginal Ultrasonography

Evaluation of gynecologic complaints
- Amenorrhea
- Menometrorrhagia
- Postmenopausal bleeding
- Vaginal bleeding in early pregnancy
- Pelvic pain
- Evaluation of pelvic mass noted on physical examination
- Pelvic evaluation in the obese patient

Oncology
- Screening of postmenopausal patients for ovarian and uterine cancer
- Screening of the ovary for small neoplasms or cancer in menstruating patients
- Screening for bladder cancer

Infertility
- General evaluation of pelvic anatomy
- Confirmation of ovulation
- Diagnosis of anovulation
- Ovulation monitoring during clomiphene citrate or human menopausal gonadotropin (Pergonal) therapy
- Diagnosis and follow-up of endometriomas of the ovary
- IVF follicular aspiration
- Diagnosis of polycystic ovary syndrome
- Diagnosis of LUF syndrome
- Diagnosis of congenital anomalies of the uterus

Evaluation of the fallopian tubes
- Diagnosis of hydrosalpinx
- Water tubal hydrotubation

Pregnancy
- Early pregnancy evaluation, including gestational dating, congenital anomalies, location of the gestation, threatened abortion, prognosis of bleeding
- Diagnosis of ectopic pregnancy
- Diagnosis of hydatidiform mole
- Evaluation and localization of placenta previa (late pregnancy)
- Evaluation for incompetent cervix

Other indications
- Evaluation for pelvic adhesions
- Localization of intrauterine device (IUD)

Uses in conjunction with the pelvic examination
- Evaluation of the internal character of ovarian cysts
- Diagnosis, location, and size measurement of uterine fibroids
- Evaluation of pelvic infection for development of hydrosalpinx or tubo-ovarian abscess

CLINICAL INDICATIONS FOR TRANSVAGINAL ULTRASOUND

Ultrasonography, and particularly the use of the transvaginal probe, has resulted in a significant change in our clinical practice of gynecology. The indications and use of ultrasound have continued to expand. Table 1-2 is a partial list of indications in which ultrasonography may be of benefit. Most of the diagnostic indications are discussed under the appropriate anatomic organ system or specific clinical indications or techniques in this text.

Transvaginal pelvic ultrasonography can also be used in screening of the asymptomatic patient and as an adjunct to the pelvic examination. It is not infrequent to make a diagnosis using ultrasound that would not generally be made from the history and pelvic examination. For example, congenital anomalies can be diagnosed, as noted in Figure 1-1 showing a bicornuate uterus, and Figure 1-2 showing a hematometrium in an 18-year-old patient with pain. The etiology of postmenopausal bleeding can also be diagnosed; Figure 1-3 shows a patient with bleeding from cystic hyperplasia of the endometrium, whereas Figure 1-4 shows an intracervical polyp. Sonography can be used to confirm a suspected diagnosis, as for example the pyosalpinx noted in a patient with signs and symptoms of pelvic inflammatory disease (Fig. 1-5). Pelvic sonography can even be used to diagnose bladder conditions, such as tumors or polyps (Fig. 1-6).

Transvaginal Ultrasound and the Pelvic Examination

The development of real-time transvaginal sector scanning has literally enabled gynecologists to "see" where we could once only grope and feel. In addition, ultrasonography allows an examination of the internal structure and sometimes even the physiologic status of the pelvic organs, rather than just the gross evaluation of the anatomic size and general contour that is gained from the pelvic examination. Frequently, during the ultrasound examination, information is obtained about the internal anatomy and physiology of the ovary or uterus that would not even be evident by direct visualization of the pelvic organs at laparoscopy or laparotomy. It is quite probable, as more gynecologists become familiar with the newer technique of transvaginal ultrasound, that a sonographic examination will eventually become a routine part of every gynecologic examination.

Although the relative value of the patient's chief complaint and history versus the physical examination varies with different disease processes, it is a clear diagnostic principle that both techniques should be utilized and the information integrated into the

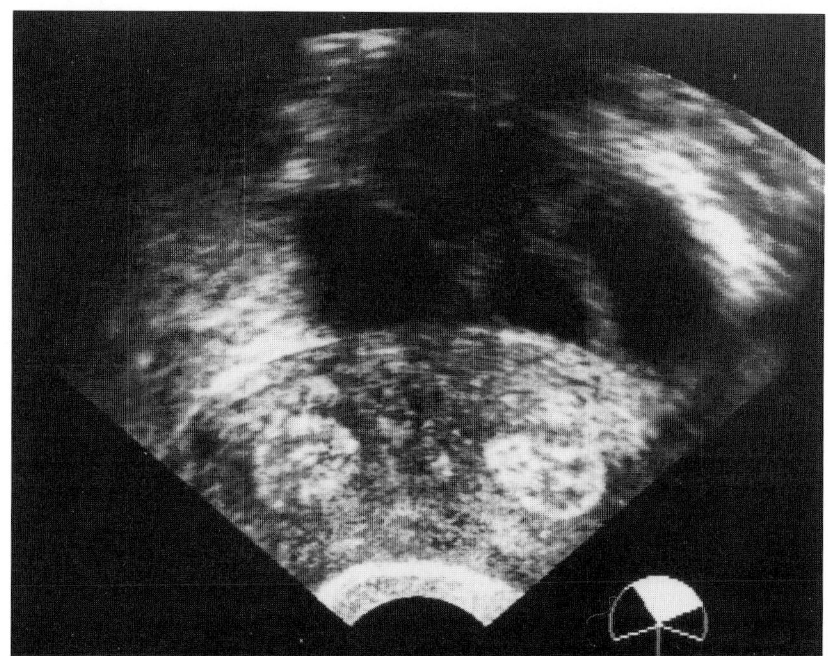

Fig. 1-1. Transverse view of a bicornual uterus pictured in a 30-year-old white woman, undergoing hMG treatment in an IVF program. In this respect, note the stimulated aspect of the ovary above the uterus featuring four large follicles. Endometrium of the two horns can be distinctly observed, thickened under the effect of ovarian stimulation (Courtesy of I. Vial, M.D., Department of Obstetrics and Gynecology, CHUV, Lausanne, Switzerland).

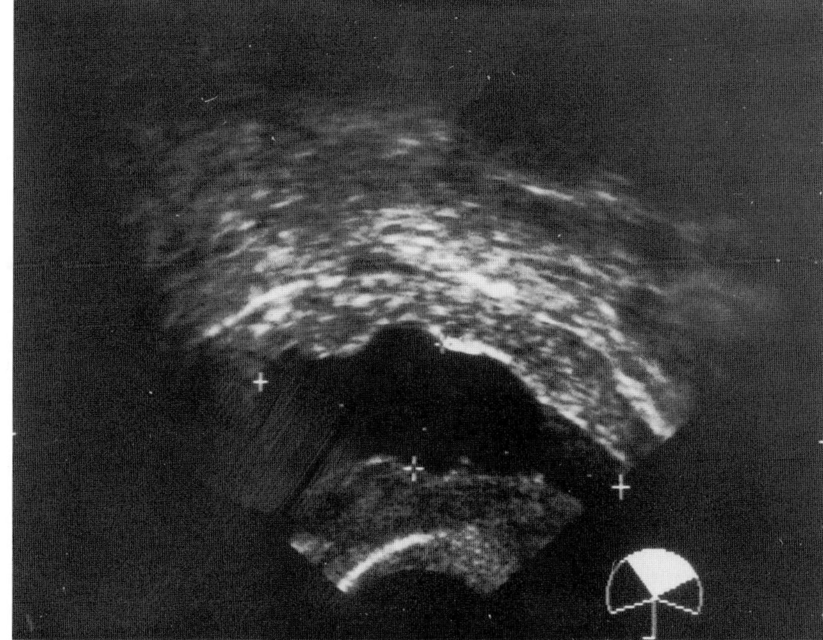

Fig. 1-2. Sagittal view of an hematometrium, sized 44 mm (L) by 15 mm (AP). This was found in a 18-year-old white woman presenting with abdominal pain. Ultrasound examination was followed by hysterosalpingography and laparoscopy. A pseudo-unicornuate uterus was diagnosed. Note contrast between the dilatation of the endometrial cavity and decreased thickness of the myometrial walls. Eventually, laparotomy was performed for resection of the pseudohorn (Courtesy of I. Vial, M.D., Department of Obstetrics and Gynecology, CHUV, Lausanne, Switzerland).

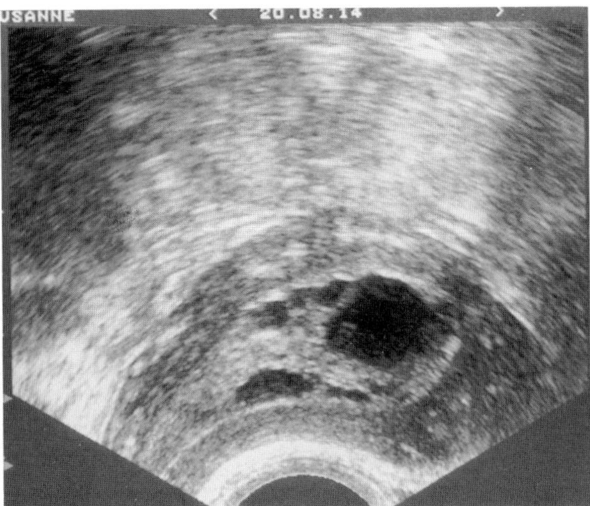

Fig. 1-3. Cystic hyperplasia of the endometrium (sagittal view). Note the endometrial thickness above 20 mm and the marked heterogeneity of endometrial tissues. This 79-year-old white woman complained of metrorrhagia. She was initially diagnosed with breast cancer, and mastectomy had been performed. Tamoxifen treatment, 20 mg daily, was initiated 18 months before the endovaginal ultrasound examination. Diagnosis was confirmed by curettage (Courtesy of I. Vial, M.D., Department of Obstetrics and Gynecology, CHUV, Lausanne, Switzerland).

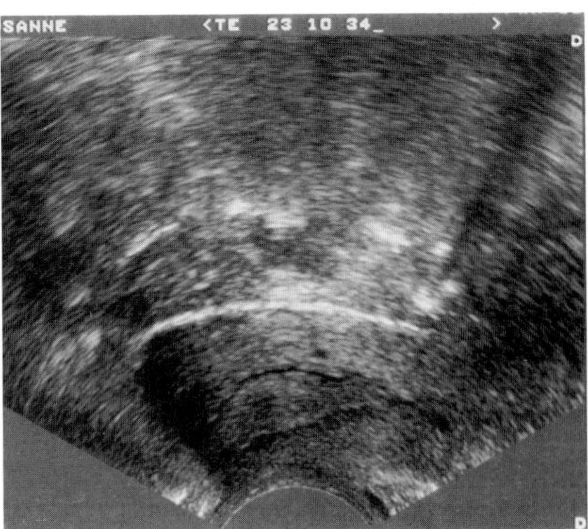

Fig. 1-4. Sagittal view of an intracervical polyp in a 60-year-old postmenopausal patient with bleeding who was receiving hormonal replacement therapy (Courtesy of I. Vial, M.D., Department of Obstetrics and Gynecology, CHUV, Lausanne, Switzerland).

diagnostic process. Few cardiologists would consider a physical examination complete without auscultation of the heart. The stethoscope is a rcognized and invaluable clinical tool that has become an integral part of routine patient evaluation. However, even though the stethoscope is very valuable in the physical examination of the heart and lungs, it offers little aid in the gynecologic examination. The transvaginal probe has perhaps made diagnostic office ultrasound the stethoscope for gynecologists. Pelvic sonography can almost be viewed as a form of physical examination using sound in which organ size, internal consistency, location, and other anatomic parameters and physiologic changes are appreciated. However, pelvic sonography does not replace the pelvic examination or the patient history, just as auscultation of the heart by a cardiologist does not replace a complete history and physical examination when evaluating a patient with cardiac complaints.

In some clinical circumstances, the ultrasound examination is invaluable. For example, the evaluation of an obese patient is a clinical situation in which the transvaginal sonographic examination is generally superior to the pelvic examination (Fig. 1-7). There is little argument that the amount of diagnostic information and anatomic detail obtained by a gynecologist during a pelvic examination is inversely related to the weight of the patient. In the patient over 200 pounds, the pelvic examination gives, at best, only a vague appreciation of the pelvic organs. Likewise, transabdominal sonography is seriously compromised in the obese patient. However, it is generally possible to obtain detailed anatomic information including measurements of ovarian and uterine size and evaluation of their position and internal anatomy even in the obese patient. Transvaginal ultrasonography is also of value in the young athletic woman with very strong abdominal muscles that frequently compromise the pelvic examination.

Andolf and Jorgensen[7] evaluated 194 patients by ultrasound the day before surgery and compared the sonographic findings with the pelvic examination. All findings were verified by surgical exploration. Ultrasound had a specificity of 96.3 percent compared to the pelvic examination's specificity of 94 percent. Ultrasound was also superior in sensitivity to the pelvic examination in detecting pelvic pathology (83 percent versus 67 percent, respectively). Small solid lesions were more commonly missed by ultrasound, and larger cystic lesions were missed more often by pelvic examination. The authors thought that ultrasound

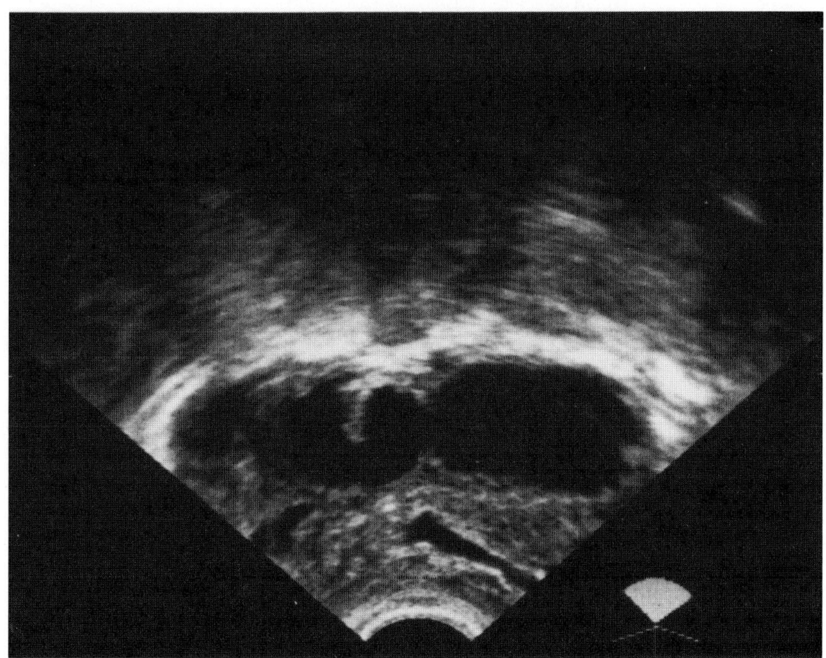

Fig. 1-5. Left adnexal pyosalpinx (transverse/oblique view), diagnosed in a 20-year-old white woman presenting with signs and symptoms of acute pelvic inflammatory disease (PID). Note the impressive dilatation and considerable thickening of the fallopian tube walls (Courtesy of I. Vial, M.D., Department of Obstetrics and Gynecology, CHUV, Lausanne, Switzerland).

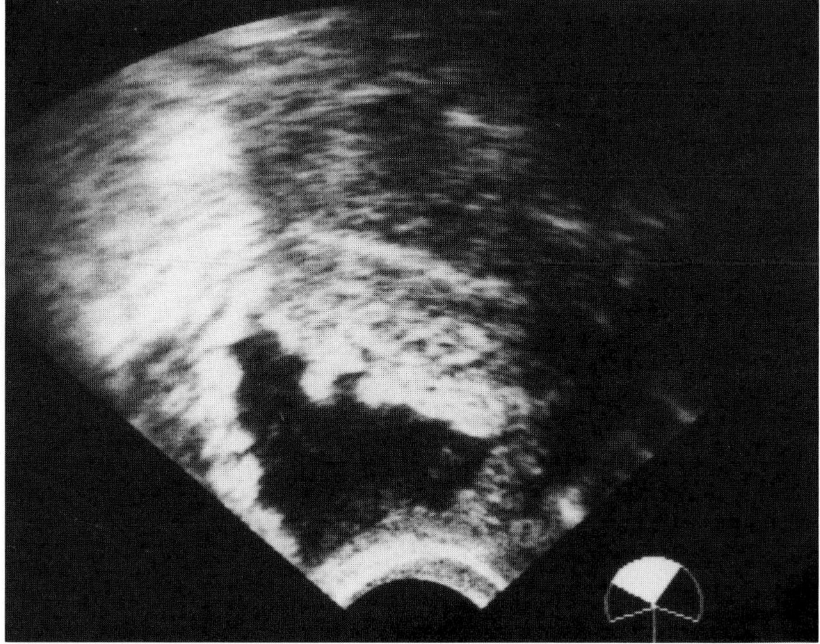

Fig. 1-6. Sagittal view of multiple polyps of the bladder. The patient was a postmenopausal woman presenting with bleeding. Endovaginal examination of internal genital organs disclosed a small, regularly echogenic uterus, with a normal thin endometrial line. Polyps of the bladder were noted (Courtesy of I. Vial, M.D., Department of Obstetrics and Gynecology, CHUV, Lausanne, Switzerland).

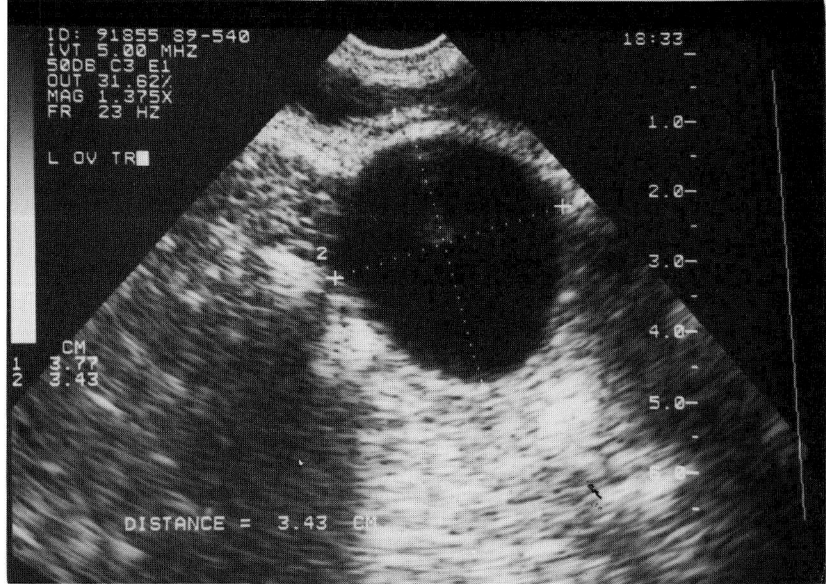

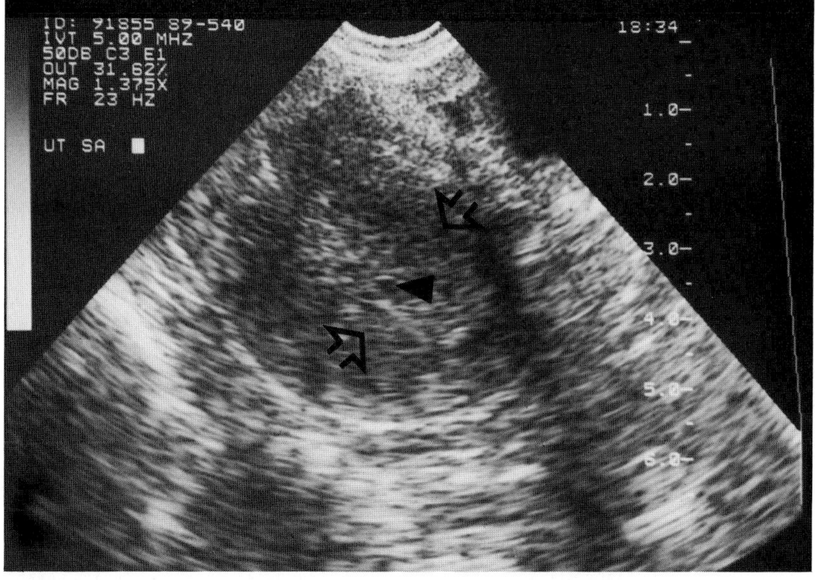

Fig. 1-7. **(A)** A 40-year-old obese (210 pounds) woman with a chief complaint of having missed her last period. She reported regular periods before missing her last period. Her pregnancy test was negative. She was using barrier contraceptive methods. The physical examination was less than optimal. Because of her weight, neither the uterus or ovaries could be palpated. The transvaginal sonographic examination revealed a 3.8- by 3.4-cm left ovarian cyst. The walls were smooth with no internal echoes. (The small echoes noted in the superior and middle of the cyst are due to artifacts; see Ch. 4.) **(B)** The endometrium (open arrows) was not characteristic of either the follicular or luteal phase. This type of endometrium is frequently seen after chronic low level estrogen stimulation. The serum estradiol level was 58 pg/ml, and the serum progesterone level was 0.4 ng/ml. There were some small (1 mm) anechoic areas in the endometrium (arrowhead) suggesting early breakdown of the endometrium. The patient was told that her missed period was probably due to the cyst. Since the sonographic image of the endometrium was atypical, with multiple small anechoic areas suggesting early endometrial breakdown, the patient was told that she would probably begin her mensutral period within the next week. The patient began bleeding 4 days later.

was superior in overall performance and a useful complement to the pelvic examination. These studies used a 3.5-MHz transducer and the full bladder transabdominal sonographic technique, which is much less sensitive than transvaginal sonography. Similar well-controlled studies using high frequency transvaginal ultrasound are not currently available. However, considering the improved images obtained with the transvaginal technique, the diagnostic capability would be expected to be at least as good, if not better, in experienced hands.

Interestingly, not all studies in the past have agreed on the value of the sonographic evaluation of the pelvis or pelvic masses. Reeves et al.,[8] working at The National Naval Medical Center, reported a 90 percent diagnostic accuracy by both pelvic examination and ultrasonography. Ultrasonography had a 5.6 percent false-negative rate and a 4.4 percent false-positive rate. Ultrasound was reported to be significantly more accurate in determining the cystic or solid nature of a mass than a pelvic examination. The authors concluded that preoperative ultrasound evaluation of a pelvic mass was not necessary.

This study, done in the mid-1970s, was not inconsistent with the beliefs of many gynecologists, including ourselves, at that time. Information obtained from ultrasound examinations frequently offered little additional diagnostic information and occasionally was misleading. However, as noted previously, we must recognize both the limitations of the equipment used in the 1970s and the learning curve involved in the medical application of a new technique. The high false-negative rate using ultrasonography reported in this study probably reflects the limitation of imaging using 1.6- to 3.5-MHz transducers and the transabdominal full bladder technique. Four of the 72 patients in this study had pelvic masses 5 to 10 cm in size that were missed by ultrasound examination, but were noted on pelvic examination. It is difficult to imagine missing a 5- to 10-cm pelvic mass using transvaginal ultrasonography unless the cyst or mass is completely out of the pelvis and beyond the range of the transvaginal probe. Current transvaginal ultrasonography technique can visualize 4- to 8-mm anechoic immature follicules in the ovary. A 400 to 500 mm cyst in the pelvis on transvaginal ultrasound is a massive structure.

In another more recent study, reported by O'Brien et al.,[9] a technician performed pelvic sonographic studies that were interpreted by a staff radiologist who was not informed of the clinical diagnosis or physical findings of the patient. Again, the ultrasound examinations were performed using the transabdominal full bladder approach. The investigators concluded that the overall performance of sonography was inferior to clinical examination, and there was a high number of false-positive diagnoses using sonography. Interestingly, this study defined an ovarian cyst as a "fluid-filled area greater than 1.5 cm in diameter." Since a normally developing follicle is generally 1.8 to 2.5 cm in diameter before ovulation, it is probable that all ovulating women scanned during the late follicular phase of their cycle were diagnosed as having an ovarian cyst in this study. Not surprisingly, incorrect sonographic diagnoses were made in 58 percent of patients in this study. Six of 13 false-positive diagnoses involved ovarian cysts 1.5 to 2.5 cm in size. This study illustrates the problem of the learning curve associated with the use of a new technology and, more specifically, the importance of knowing what constitutes an ovarian cyst versus a normally developing follicle. The problem of defining an ovarian cyst is discussed in Chapter 7.

Although earlier reports noted that pelvic ultrasonography added little to the pelvic examination, these studies were done using the transabdominal full bladder technique and lower frequency probes (less than 5 MHz) and sometimes reflected the limited knowledge base that is probably inevitable with the introduction of new technology or the application of technology in areas where it has not previously been utilized.[8,9] The new enthusiasts of sonography should be aware of the limitations of many of these earlier studies, as discussed above, since they are still sometimes quoted in the literature or at gynecologic meetings. Such studies reflect the historical development of pelvic ultrasound, rather than the state of the art.

REAL-TIME SONOGRAPHY

The real-time transvaginal ultrasound examination involves interpretation of tens of thousands of images with evaluation of literally thousands of slices of pelvic anatomy and of the relationship of organs during the examination. Unfortunately, in some centers, a technician performs an ultrasound examination with interpretation of the results at a later time by a physician looking at a few films taken in certain planes. This approach negates most of the advantages of real-time pelvic sonography. Although a technician can be of considerable aid, having a technician do the entire examination, with interpretation later of a few Polaroids, thermal photographs, or radiographic films by a physician, is a less than optimal evaluation. Photographs or radiographs are of value in recording and documenting pathology and anatomy, but the use of only a few such images for diagnostic purposes provides at best a limited examination. The transvaginal pelvic ultrasound examination cannot be treated like a chest radiograph. The accuracy and thoroughness of diagnosis using real-time transvaginal ultrasonography are no better than the knowledge of anatomy, physiology, and potential pathology of the individual holding the transducer and watching the monitor screen. During the real-time pelvic sonographic examination, the physician should try to mentally construct a three dimensional image of the organ being scanned and the anatomic relationship among the different pelvic organs, such as the uterus and ovaries.

TRANSABDOMINAL VERSUS TRANSVAGINAL ULTRASOUND IMAGING

Since a very full bladder is not required, the transvaginal sonographic examination is generally preferred by patients to the transabdominal sonographic examination. Many patients are quite uncomfortable with the very distended bladder required for an adequate transabdominal examination. A full bladder not only is not necessary for the transvaginal examination, but an empty or minimally filled bladder is generally preferred. Although this may seem like a matter of minor importance, from a practical perspective the fact that a full bladder is not required for the examination is a very real consideration for both the patient and the physician. In addition to the discomfort for the patient caused by the full bladder, invariably many patients arrive for their transabdominal ultrasound examination without an adequately prepared bladder. These patients then have to drink water and be scanned again in 30 to 45 minutes. The continued delays and loss of time in repeatedly scanning the patient with an inadequately prepared bladder and waiting for the patient to drink more fluid to fill her bladder, as well as the need to move the patient in and out of the examination room, can play havoc on a busy physician's office schedule. These repeated delays will rapidly dampen, if not destroy, any initial enthusiasm of the average gynecologist for the transabdominal ultrasound scanning, except for the more pressing indications. This is particularly true when the last patient of the afternoon has a poorly prepared bladder, and the office staff and physician must wait an hour until she is prepared properly. The problems of bladder discomfort, office scheduling, and wasted office time are eliminated by using the transvaginal approach.

Transvaginal ultrasonography is well tolerated. The authors has only rarely had a patient refuse an examination. Complaints of significant discomfort have been uncommon in over several thousand transvaginal examinations. Vilaro et al.[10] questioned patients undergoing both transabdominal and transvaginal ultrasound examinations, and 89 percent preferred the transvaginal approach. Schats performed both transabdominal and transvaginal ultrasound in 100 patients to determine the acceptability of the technique.[11] The resemblance between the ultrasound transducer and the speculum was noted, and only 3 percent of patients felt some discomfort when the transducer was introduced into the vagina. Most patients preferred the transvaginal approach to the transabdominal approach mainly because of the discomfort of the full bladder when using the latter approach. Only one patient preferred the transabdominal approach. The patient who complains of pain or discomfort with a transvaginal sonographic examination should be evaluated for severe vaginitis, vaginismus, pelvic inflammatory disease, ectopic pregnancy, or painful adnexal masses. In this respect, the transvaginal examination gives information similar to the pelvic examination regarding pelvic tenderness. However, there is considerable variability in the transvaginal probe design and shape of different manufacturers. Some transvaginal probes are less well tolerated than others.

Mendelson et al.[12] compared the image quality of transabdominal and transvaginal ultrasonography in 200 patients in terms of resolution, contrast, and anatomic detail. The use of the transvaginal approach for visualizing the endometrium, myometrium, and ovaries was superior in 85, 79, and 87 percent of images and equal in 10, 18, and 10 percent, respectively. In the studies of Mendelson et al.,[12] additional diagnostic information was gained in 15 to 37 percent of patients with the transvaginal approach compared with the transabdominal approach. Equal information was noted in 60 to 84 percent of cases. The transabdominal approach gave added diagnostic information not noted during the transvaginal sonograms in only 1 to 3 percent of cases.

In comparing pathologic lesions in gynecologic patients, adnexal masses and pelvic inflammatory disease were the most common finding in 30 percent of patients reported by Mendelson et al.,[12] and were better imaged by transvaginal ultrasonography in 78 percent of cases. Transvaginal and transabdominal sonography were equivalent in 8 percent of patients. Transabdominal sonography was found to be superior in 14 percent of patients. Transabdominal scanning is superior when the ovaries are located high in the pelvis out of the range of the transvaginal probe.

Uterine leiomyomas were noted in 26 percent of Mendelson's series and were better imaged in 74 percent of patients with the transvaginal ultrasound technique.[12] Leiomyomas were better imaged in 18 percent of patients by the transabdominal technique (see Ch. 5). Generally, large fibroids are better seen by the transabdominal technique because of the large field of view.

Cul-de-sac fluid was noted in 20 percent of patients and again was imaged better by the transvaginal technique in 64 percent of these patients.[12]

Leibman et al.[13] compared transabdominal and transvaginal ultrasonography in evaluating pelvic masses in 67 women. More information was obtained and the internal architecture of the mass was delineated better in 76 percent of patients with transvaginal ultrasound than with the transabdominal examination. The transabdominal approach did not provide more diagnostic information in any patient in their series. Vilaro et al.[10] also reported increased diagnostic accuracy in 62 percent of cases, with additional information obtained in 55 percent of cases by the transvaginal approach compared with the transabdominal approach.

Ovarian follicles are much better visualized by the transvaginal technique. In a series of 41 studies reported by Andreotti et al.,[14] follicular margins were sharply defined in 90 percent of the studies using transvaginal ultrasonography compared with 40 percent of the studies using the transabdominal technique. More follicles were seen using transvaginal sonography, and there was a much more accurate calculation of the size of the dominant follicle and serum estradiol levels compared with the transabdominal technique.

Lande et al.[15] reported that transvaginal ultrasound added useful information in 25 of 28 patients (89 percent) with cystic adnexal masses and in all of 7 patients with cul-de-sac disease. Transvaginal ultrasound may also be particularly useful in patients with bowel ileus and abdominal sutures or drains, in some patients with a retroverted uterus, and in obese patients.

These studies quantitated the superiority of transvaginal ultrasonography to the transabdominal approach. Even the novice sonographer will rapidly appreciate the greater anatomic details in evaluating the pelvic organs obtained using the transvaginal approach. However, the transabdominal approach is superior for evaluating large masses that extend out of the pelvis and for giving a more panoramic view. Therefore, it is generally advisable to have a transabdominal sector probe available as well. If an ovary is not imaged clearly by transvaginal ultrasound, a transabdominal scan should be performed to ensure that an ovarian tumor out of the pelvis is not missed. The authors use transabdominal ultrasound in less than 5 percent of scans.

TRANSVAGINAL ULTRASOUND SCREENING

Transvaginal ultrasonography as a screening tool in the asymptomatic patient is currently being evaluated. Andolf et al.[16] noted pelvic pathology in 6 percent of asymptomatic patients undergoing sonographic screening. The pelvic examination detected pathology in only 23 percent of these patients. All pathology was confirmed surgically. This preliminary experience suggests that screening ultrasonography may, in fact, be of value. Considering the data of Andolf et al.,[16] ultrasound was almost four times more sensitive in detecting ovarian or adnexal pathology in the asymptomatic patient than was a pelvic examination. This is particularly true in the obese patient (see Fig. 1-7).

Screening for ovarian cancer in asymptomatic postmenopausal patients is an area in which ultrasound might have an important impact. Ovarian cancer is the leading cause of gynecologic cancer deaths in the United States. The cure rate for early ovarian cancer (stage 1) is as high as 90 percent. Unfortunately two thirds of ovarian cancers are not diagnosed until an advanced stage, in which the survival rates are only 15 to 20 percent. There have been no dramatic or even moderately effective new treatments for advanced ovarian cancer in the past 30 years. The only current technique known to significantly improve prognosis is early diagnosis.

Critics of ovarian cancer screening note the low incidence of ovarian cancer and the cost of screening. Unfortunately, there is no other accurate screening technique for this very serious and frequently fatal problem. In addition, the cost of ultrasound for ovarian cancer screening should be measured not only by the number of early ovarian cancers detected but also by the total consideration of the health care of the patient. The detection of ovarian abnormalities in 2.5 percent of screened patients is therefore quite impressive. It should also be appreciated that screening for ovarian cancer is not the only diagnostic information gleaned from the ultrasound examination. The endometrium and uterus should be evaluated, as well as the bladder, space of Retzius, and pelvis in general. The value of transvaginal ultrasound for evaluating the postmenopausal patient with bleeding is becoming increasingly clear (see Ch. 11).[17–20] When the ultrasound examination is viewed as an integral part of the patient evaluation, rather than as only a screening evaluation of one organ, such as the ovary, its cost effectiveness is much more apparent.

THE ACCURACY OF TRANSVAGINAL ULTRASOUND MEASUREMENTS

The validity of transabdominal ultrasound measurements of uterine size, endometrial thickness, and ovarian volume has previously been demonstrated by comparing ultrasound measurements with caliper measurements of the pelvic organs made at the time of hysterectomy and salpingo-oophorectomy.[21] Accuracy of the transabdominal ultrasound measurements of the number and size of uterine leiomyomas has also been reported. Transvaginal ultrasound measurements of pelvic structures using the 5- and 7-MHz endovaginal transducer have also been demonstrated to be accurate (Pache et al., unpublished data). Rodriquez and colleagues investigated the use of transvaginal sonography to evaluate the ovaries in postmenopausal women who were planning abdominal surgery unrelated to adnexal disease.[22] Ultrasonographic observations in 52 patients were compared to the findings at surgery and the pathologic evaluation of the ovaries. The correlation coefficient between ultrasound and surgical measurements was 0.78 in normal ovaries and 0.99 in abnormal ovaries. Eighty-five of 104 ovaries were visualized by ultrasound (82 percent). Ovaries that could not be visualized by ultrasound were atrophic at the time of surgery, and none of the nonvisualized ovaries was abnormal. Among the 85 ovaries that were visualized, 10 were found to be histologically abnormal. Nine of these abnormal findings had been suspected by the endovaginal ultrasound examination. Sensitivity and specificity of endovaginal ultrasound in evaluating abnormal ovarian morphology were 90 and 100 percent, respectively.

PELVIC PLANES

The use of transvaginal ultrasonography has resulted in some confusion regarding the anatomic planes being imaged. The terms coronal, transverse, sagittal, and longitudinal do not apply correctly to the planes being imaged during transvaginal ultrasonography. During the transvaginal pelvic sonographic examination, the sound beam is being directed through the vagina, which runs superiorly and posteriorly. In addition, the pelvis is tilted at a 30 degree angle to the long axis of the body. The range of motion of the transducer is also limited by the introitus and vagina. Although the term transverse plane is commonly used, no true transverse plane is imaged during transvaginal sonography. Anatomically, a transverse plane is at right angles to the long axis of the body. Some sonographers prefer the term coronal instead of transverse. A true coronal plane runs through the coronal sutures and is parallel to the long axis of the body (Fig. 1-8). However, almost all the planes imaged during a pelvic ultrasonographic examination are at an oblique angle to the long axis. The sound beam is generally being directed posteriorly, as well as superiorly. Dodson and Deter[23] have suggested the term trans-pelvic (T-pelvic) for this plane. *Trans-* refers to through or across. Since the sound beam is being directed across and through the pelvis, T-pelvic would be an appropriate term for such a plane. In fact, the term T-pelvic is relatively self-descriptive (Fig. 1-9).

There is a similar problem with the use of such terms as longitudinal and sagittal when applied to transvaginal sonography. When the sound beam is directed in an anterior posterior manner in the pelvis, the plane imaged is not longitudinal and is sagittal in only one central plane. Because movement of the transducer is restricted at the introitus, parasagittal planes are never obtained. The term anterior posterior-pelvic (AP-pelvic) has been suggested instead (Figs. 1-10).[23] The AP-pelvic plane refers to any pelvic plane where the sound beam is directed from anterior to posterior, and the T-pelvic plane refers to any plane imaged when the sound beam is directed across or from side to side in the pelvis. Each term can be subdivided further to give more precise anatomic localization of images by referring to a right or left AP-pelvic or T-pelvic when the transducer tip is di-

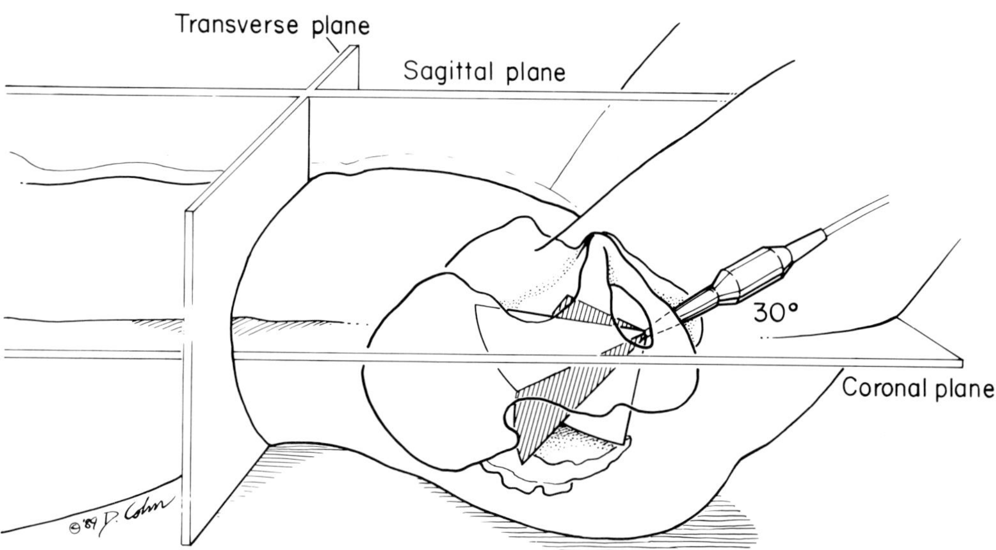

Fig. 1-8. Demonstration of the transverse, sagittal, and coronal planes in a female figure in the lithotomy position. These true anatomic planes can be compared with pelvic imaging planes when the sound beam is being diverted from side to side in the pelvis (lined plane in the pelvis) and when the sound beam is directed anteriorly and posteriorly in the pelvis (clear plane in the pelvis). The pelvic planes can vary considerably by manipulating the transducer. However, the pelvic plane never corresponds to a true anatomic transverse plane, and rarely are true sagittal or coronal planes imaged. (Illustration by Delilah R. Cohn, Nashville, TN.)

Fig. 1-9. Projection showing the bony pelvis with a transducer oriented in such a way as to project the sound beam from side to side in the pelvis. Multiple different T-pelvic planes can be imaged by moving the transducer handle up or down or right or left, projecting the sound beam in different T-pelvic planes. (Illustration by Delilah R. Cohn, Nashville, TN.)

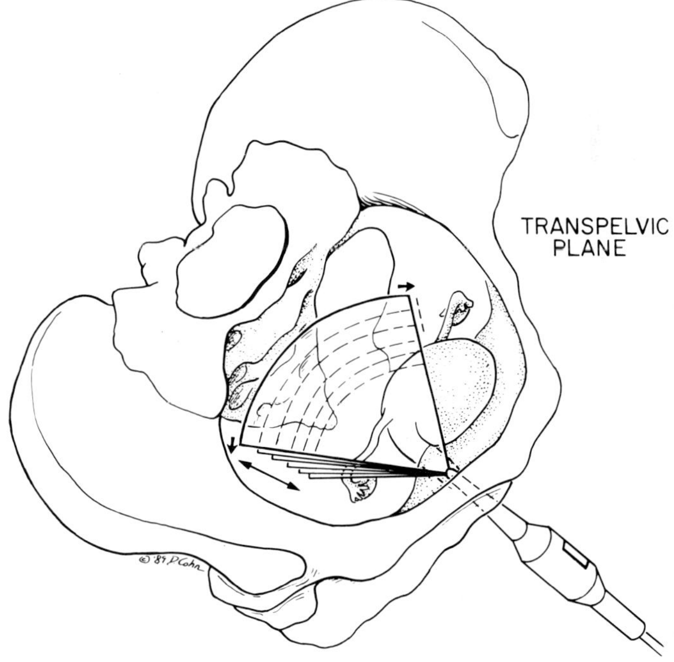

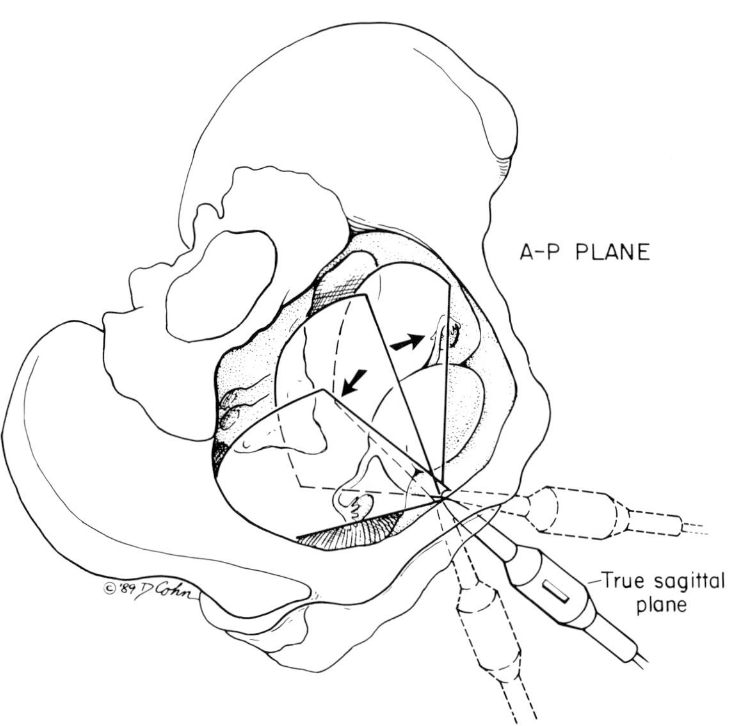

Fig. 1-10. Projection of the bony pelvis showing several AP-pelvic planes obtained by moving the transducer from side to side. Only the central AP-pelvic planes correspond to the anatomic sagittal plane. (Illustration by Delilah R. Cohn, Nashville, TN.)

rected to the right or left. When a T-pelvic view is being imaged with the sound beam directed from side to side in the pelvis and the transducer tip is tilted either further anteriorly or posteriorly, such an image can be defined further as an anterior trans-pelvic image or posterior trans-pelvic image. The terms *T-pelvic* and *AP-pelvic* are used to delineate image planes in this text.

IMAGE DISPLAY ORIENTATION

Just as with anatomic planes, there continues to be confusion regarding image displays using transvaginal ultrasonography. The majority of texts and publications orient the image display in such a way that the sound beam (initial sound bang) projects from the top of the display screen. However, Bernaschek and Deutinger[24] have recommended that transvaginal images be displayed projecting from the bottom of the display screen to differentiate clearly transvaginal sonographic images from transabdominal images. They also recommend that the left side of the screen should correspond to the dorsal and right side of the patient and the right side of the screen to the ventral and left side of the patient (Fig. 1-11). Unfortunately, there is no currently accepted standard for display of transvaginal images. This text continues to use the more common display method with the sound beam projected from the top of the screen. Generally in this text, the patient's right side is displayed on the left side of the screen just as when viewing a chest or abdominal radiograph. This right-left orientation of images in which the patient's left side is on the right side of the screen in the T-pelvic plane is one of the few display orientations that most sonographers agree upon and use, probably because it agrees with display methods of radiographs with which most physicians are familiar. It also agrees with the orientation that gynecologists are familiar with during a pelvic examination, with the patient's right to the physician's left.

This text generally displays dorsal to the left and ventral to the right, as suggested by Bernaschek and Deutinger.[24] However, because the projection is from the top of the screen, the orientation is quite different. Currently, there is no agreed standard for screen orientation using transvaginal sonography.

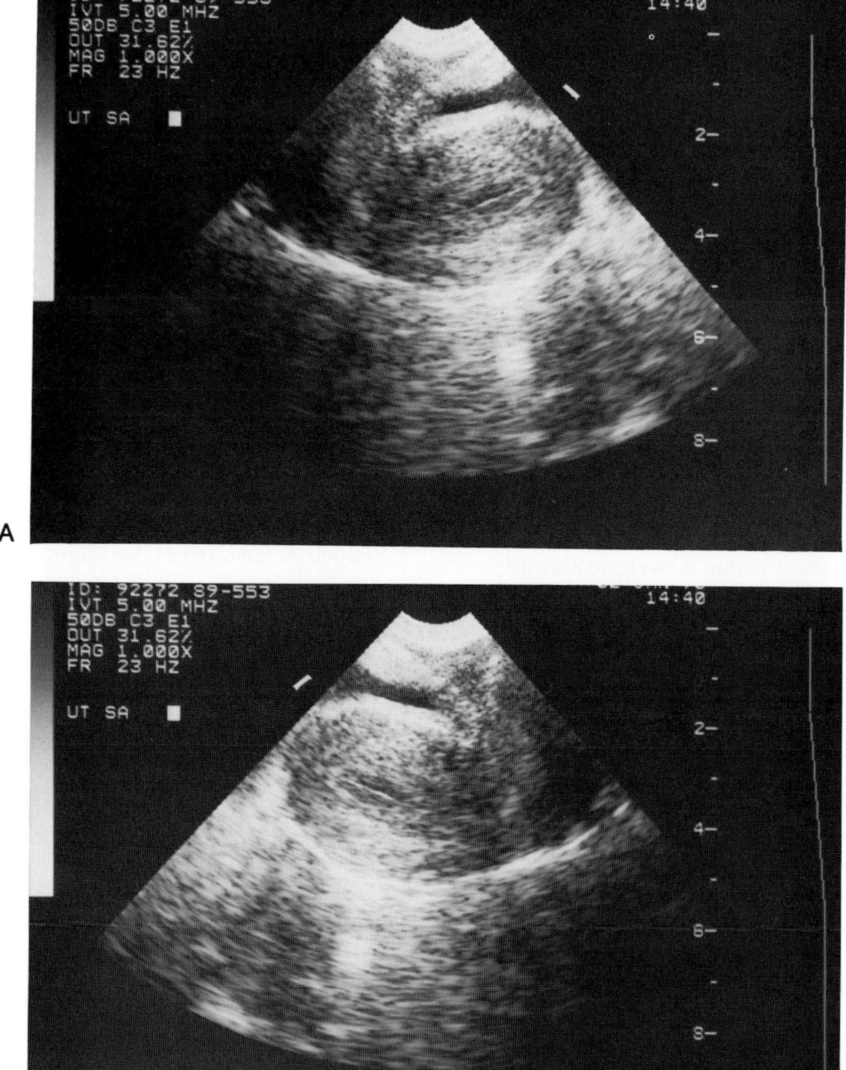

Fig. 1-11. **(A)** Initial sound bang displayed from the top of the screen with the bladder to the top and right. The ventral (abdomen) portion of the patient is to the right, and the dorsal surface of the patient is to the left. **(B)** Same view of the uterus with the image reversed. The initial sound bang is at the top, and the bladder is to the top and left. The uterus is antiverted.

CONCLUSION

Transvaginal ultrasonography is a powerful new technique that provides considerable diagnostic information to the gynecologist willing to invest the time to learn how to use it. Gaining expertise in this new and rapidly developing area requires knowledge of the technique and equipment, the characteristic ultrasound images of the normal pelvic anatomy, the physiologic changes occurring through the menstrual cycle, and also pathologic variants. In addition, just as with other techniques, a detailed knowledge of the subject must be integrated with hands-on experience to gain real expertise.

REFERENCES

1. Hull MGR: Polycystic ovarian disease: clinical aspects and prevalence. Res Clin Forums 11:21, 1989
2. Hanna MD, Chizen DR, Pierson RA: Characteristics of follicular evacuation during human ovulation. Abstract 0-78 of the 1993 Meeting of the American Fertility Society, Montreal, Canada. S37, 1993
3. Rulin MC, Bornstein SG, Campbell JD: The reliability of ultrasonography in the management of spontaneous abortion, clinically thought to be complete: a prospective study. Am J Obstet Gynecol 168:12, 1993
4. Goldstein SR: Incorporating endovaginal ultrasonography into the overall gynecologic examination. Am J Gynecol Obstet 162:652, 1990
5. Schiller VL, Tessler FN, Gambone JC et al: Endovaginal pelvic sonography as the primary method of examination of the pelvis. J Obstet Gynecol 12:121, 1992
6. Nasri MN, Sheperd JH, Setchell ME et al: Transvaginal ultrasound. A reliable basis for clinical management? Br J Obstet Gynecol 98:485, 1991
7. Andolf E, Jorgensen C: A prospective comparison of clinical ultrasound and operative examination of the female pelvis. J Ultrasound Med 7:617, 1988
8. Reeves RD, Drake TS, O'Brien WF: Ultrasonographic versus clinical evaluation of a pelvic mass. Obstet Gynecol 55:551, 1980
9. O'Brien WF, Buck DR, Nash JD: Evaluation of sonography in the initial assessment of the gynecologic patient. Am J Obstet Gynecol 149:598, 1984
10. Vilaro MM, Rifkin MD, Pennell RG et al: Endovaginal ultrasound: a technique for evaluation of nonfollicular pelvic masses. J Ultrasound Med 6:697, 1987
11. Schats R: Acceptability of transvaginal sonography. In Pasmans (ed): Transvaginal Sonography in Early Human Pregnancy. Ph.D. Thesis, Erasmus University, The Hague, 1991
12. Mendelson EB, Bohm-Velez M, Joseph N, Neiman HL: Gynecologic imaging: comparison of transabdominal and transvaginal sonography. Radiology 166:321, 1988
13. Leibman AJ, Kruse B, McSweeney MB: Transvaginal sonography: comparison with transabdominal sonography in the diagnosis of pelvic masses. AJR 151:89, 1988
14. Andreotti RF, Thompson GH, Janowitz W et al: Endovaginal and transabdominal sonography of ovarian follicles. J Ultrasound Med 8:555, 1989
15. Lande IM, Hill MC, Cosco FE, Kator NN: Adnexal and cul-de-sac abnormalities: transvaginal sonography. Radiology 166:325, 1988
16. Andolf E, Svalenius E, Astedt B: Ultrasonography for early detection of ovarian carcinoma. Br J Obstet Gynaecol 93:1286, 1986
17. Osmers R, Volksen M, Schauer A: Vaginosonography for early detection of endometrial carcinoma. Lancet 335:1569, 1990
18. Goldstein SR, Nachtigall M, Snyder JR, Nachtigall L: Endometrial assessment by vaginal ultrasonography before endometrial sampling in patients with postmenopausal sampling. Am J Obstet Gynecol 163:119, 1990
19. Granberg S, Wikland M, Karisson B et al: Endometrial thickness as measured by endovaginal ultrasonography for identifying endometrial abnormality. Am J Obstet Gynecol 164:47, 1991
20. Nasri M, Sheperd J: The role of vaginal scan in measurement of endometrial thickness in postmenopausal women. Br J Obstet Gynecol 98:470, 1991
21. Saxton DW, Farquhar CM, Rae T et al: Accuracy of ultrasound measurements of female pelvic organs. Br J Obstet Gynecol 97:695, 1990
22. Rodriquez MH, Platt LD, Medearis AL et al: The use of transvaginal sonography for evaluation of postmenopausal ovarian size and morphology. Am J Obstet Gynecol 159:810, 1988
23. Dodson MG, Deter RL: Definition of anatomical planes for use in transvaginal sonography. J Clin Ultrasound 18:239, 1990
24. Bernaschek G, Deutinger J: Endosonography in obstetrics and gynecology: the importance of standardized image display. Obstet Gynecol 74:817, 1989

2

Basic Principles and Equipment

Melvin G. Dodson
Thierry D. Pache

The use of ultrasonography in clinical medicine requires a detailed knowledge of the anatomy being imaged, physiology, and potential disease processes that might alter or distort the anatomy. However, it should be appreciated that we are visualizing sound reflections, rather than seeing with light. This appreciation is not trivial. Although it may be possible to utilize ultrasonographic imaging quite effectively as a diagnostic tool without understanding the physics involved, an understanding of the basics of ultrasound can be of real value in enhancing its use as a diagnostic tool. A basic appreciation of the physics involved helps in recognizing and understanding ultrasonographic artifacts and the advantages and limitations of the equipment.

PHYSICS OF SOUND

Galileo suggested that sound was a wave motion "produced by vibration of a sonorous body." A more recent concept characterized sound as a longitudinal wave traveling through a compressible medium. Sound is generally produced by a vibrating object, such as a tuning fork, a speaker diaphragm, or our vocal cords. The vibrations disturb the surrounding air, producing (1) a compression or a region of higher than normal density where air molecules are pushed or forced closer together and (2) a region of rarefaction where the air molecules are spread apart. A sound wave is a series of such compressions and rarefactions producing a longitudinal propagating wave. Energy is transferred through the medium in which the sound is traveling without the particles or atoms themselves moving through the medium. A medium is essential for sound transmission. There is no sound in a vacuum. Several basic characteristics of a longitudinal propagating wave are its frequency, intensity, amplitude, wavelength, and velocity or speed.

Frequency is the number of waves per second and is expressed in hertz (Hz). One hertz is one wave cycle per second (Fig. 2-1). A megahertz (MHz) is 1,000,000 Hz. Audible sound can be heard by the human ear in the range of 16 to 20,000 Hz. Ultrasound refers to those frequencies above the range of human hearing. Frequencies used in diagnostic ultrasound range from 1 to 10 MHz. The more common frequencies currently used in gynecologic and obstetric ultrasound are 3.5 to 7.5 MHz.

The *period* is the time of one cycle. It varies inversely with the frequency: $f(\text{MHz}) = 1/\text{period}$ (microsecond).

The *wavelength* is the linear measure of one complete wave or compression-rarefaction cycle expressed in meters or millimeters. The *velocity* or *speed of sound* depends on the medium through which it is moving. Sound travels through sea water at a velocity of about 1,500 m/s. In air, sound travels at a speed of about 350 m/s. The average speed of sound in soft tissue is 1,540 m/s. Sound travels faster in a solid. The speed of sound in steel is about 5,000 m/s, and in bone it is 2,000 to 4,000 m/s.[1,2] Sound will not travel through a vacuum.

The *wavelength* (λ) is equal to the velocity (V) of sound in a given medium divided by the frequency (f): $\lambda = V/f$. A frequency of 5 MHz, often used in diagnostic ultrasound, traveling through soft tissue with a speed of 1.54 mm/μs, will have a wavelength of 0.31 mm.

The *amplitude* is related to the pressure variation of

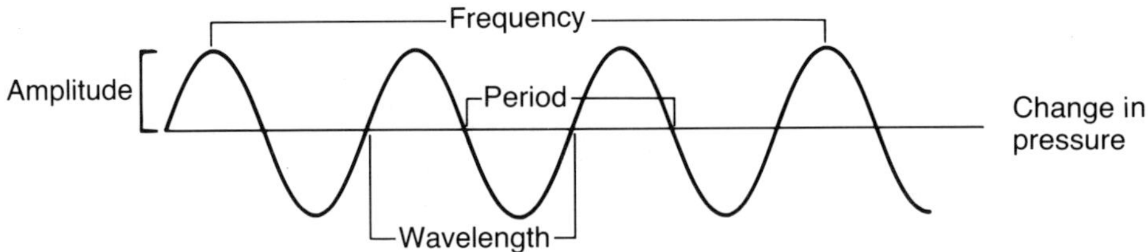

Fig. 2-1. Diagram of a sound wave showing changes in amplitude, wavelength, period, and frequency.

the sound wave. The *intensity* of sound is the power of the sound, generally expressed in watts, divided by the area over which the power is spread. The intensity of sound varies as the square of the amplitude. The intensity of the Ultramark 4 (Advanced Technology Laboratories, Inc., Bothell, WA) transvaginal 5-MHz real-time transducer varies from 1 to 50 $\mu W/cm^2$ depending on the power setting chosen.

There are several ways to measure or express the intensity of diagnostic ultrasound. It may be expressed as the temporal peak or the temporal average. Since ultrasound energy is emitted intermittently, the sound pulse generally lasts only a microsecond, but is repeated every millisecond. The intensity of sound expressed as the temporal peak energy or maximum energy in the pulse is 2,000 to 10,000 times greater than the same sound energy when expressed as the temporal average, with the energy of the sound pulse averaged over the time between pulses. Likewise, sound intensity may be expressed as a spatial peak or spatial average. The spatial peak intensity is the greatest intensity value in the plane. The spatial average intensity averages the sound intensity over a definite area, usually the sound beam's cross-sectional area. Spatial peak intensities can be two to four times greater than spatial average rates found in unfocused ultrasonic fields and up to 50 times greater in focused fields.[3]

The resistance that a given medium has to the transmission of sound is expressed as *impedance*. Impedance is independent of the frequency and is equal to the product of the density of the medium and the velocity of the sound in the medium. The unit of impedance is the RAYL: Impedance = density (kg/m^3) × sound velocity (m/s).

A relative scale used to express sound intensity is the bel, named after Alexander Graham Bell. It is generally expressed in decibels (dB) or 1/10th of a bel. The *decibel* is not an absolute measure of amplitude or sound intensity, but is a relative or comparative scale: $dB = 10 \log_{10} > (I_2/I)$, where I_2 and I_1 are the power or intensity of two different sounds. When the amplitude is used, $dB = 20 \log (A_2/A_1)$ when A_2 and A_1 are the amplitudes of two sound waves. The zero point of the scale is the threshold of hearing or 10^{-16} W/m^2 of sound power.[2] Ten decibels are therefore ten times the intensity of 0 dB, and 30 dB are 1,000 times the intensity of 0 dB.

Sound waves have all the basic characteristics of waves, including the property of reflection, in which a sound wave bounces back from an interface or boundary, producing an echo. Echoes are the basis of ultrasound imaging. The angle of reflection of a sound wave hitting a reflector is equal to the angle of incidence (Fig. 2-2). In addition to reflection, some of the sound may be transmitted and pass through the reflecting boundary.

The transmitted sound waves may be refracted or bent, as described by Snell's law. When passing from one medium into another in which the sound travels

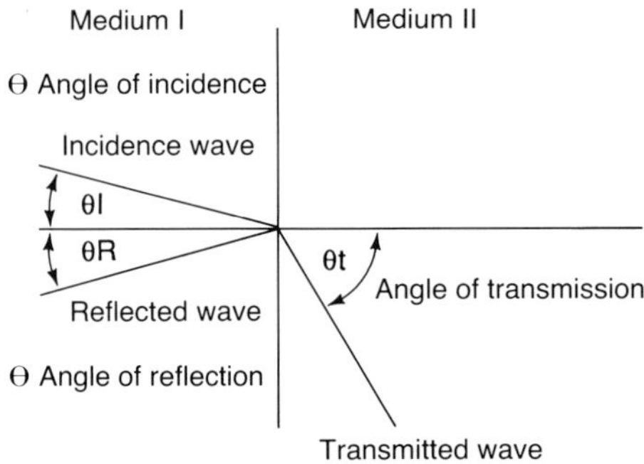

Fig. 2-2. Diagram showing an incidence sound wave with the angle of incidence (θI) to the reflector and the reflected wave and angle of reflection (θR). Some sound energy is transmitted through the reflecting body. The angle of transmission (θT) is a function of Snell's law. The transmission angle is greater than the incidence angle if the velocity of the sound in the second medium is greater than in the first medium.

at a different speed, the sound is refracted or bent. The transmission angle is greater than the incidence angle if the velocity of the sound in the second medium is greater than in the first medium. The transmission angle is less when sound passes into a medium in which the velocity is slower.

When a sound wave travels through a medium, such as the human body, its intensity is attenuated or decreased. *Attenuation* results from absorption of the sound, in which the acoustic energy is converted into heat or is reflected or scattered. *Scatter* occurs when a sound wave encounters a surface with a reflecting area that is smaller than the wavelength of the sound, such as a rough surface. The sound is radiated away from the object in all directions. The amount of attenuation is a function of the distance the sound travels in a medium, as well as the characteristics of the medium. The higher the frequency, the greater the attenuation per unit length of medium. Sound attenuation can be estimated as 1 dB of decrease per cm of tissue penetrated per MHz. For example, 80 percent of the sound intensity from a 7.0-MHz transducer is attenuated after traveling through only 1 cm of tissue, and 90 percent of the energy from a 10-MHz transducer is attenuated after traveling the same distance. This is why higher frequencies, such as 7.0 or 10 MHz, cannot be used to image structures deep in the body. The *half-value layer* is the distance the sound wave travels before the intensity is reduced by one-half.

THE ULTRASOUND TRANSDUCER

The use of diagnostic ultrasound is based on the piezoelectric effect, which was discovered by Pierre and Jacques Curie in 1880. Some materials, such as ceramics or quartz, deform when a voltage is applied to them. The application of a pulse of electric charge to a piezoelectric transducer element produces a change in the thickness of the element. Repeated application of voltage results in the generation of pressure or sound waves.

A transducer converts one form of energy into another form. An ultrasound transducer converts electricity into mechanical energy in the form of vibrations by using the piezoelectric effect. This conversion occurs only in certain types of crystals that display the piezoelectric effect. The waves produced in diagnostic ultrasound are generated in short pulses often lasting only about 1 μs, but the pulses are repeated 1,000 times a second. After sending a sound pulse, the transducer listens for a returning echo or reflected sound wave. Therefore, 99.9 percent of the time the transducer is listening. A reflected sound wave distorts the transducer crystal, resulting in the generation of an electrical pulse, or a reverse piezoelectric effect. The returning sound wave vibrates the crystal, producing an electric pulse, the reverse of the phenomenon or mechanism used to generate the sound wave with an applied voltage. The piezoelectric crystal is mounted in a transducer probe consisting of the transducer crystal itself, the mechanical housing, electrical connections, damping material used to decrease the number of cycles of vibration resulting from an excitation pulse, and a matching layer over the face of the probe used to reduce sound reflection at the transducer surface. The transducer pulse is produced by an electrical pulse generator that delivers a short burst of voltage to the transducer. This results in multiple vibrations or sound waves in a single transducer pulse. When listening, the voltage produced by distortion of the piezoelectric crystal is then electrically amplified and processed to be displayed on a cathode ray tube (Fig. 2-3).

THE ULTRASOUND MACHINE

An ultrasound machine basically consists of a pulse generator sending an electrical pulse to the transducer. The transducer itself houses a transducer crystal, damping material, and electrical connections as noted above. An amplifier amplifies the returning echo signal. The returning echo signals are then electronically processed for display on a cathode ray tube (television tube). As the technology has developed, signal processing and control have become more sophisticated. Computers have been added to process data, with cameras and videocassette recorders added to record images and data (Fig. 2-4).

Different methods are used to process and display the echo information. In the amplitude or A-mode (amplitude mode), a vertical deflection of a single oscillographic line is used to display a reflected echo. The amplitude of the deflection is proportional to the reflected sound energy. Distance or biometric measurements, such as the biparietal diameter, can be measured using the A-mode, since the horizontal distance between two displayed deflections is proportional to the distance between the two reflections. The displayed deflections are a fraction of the time

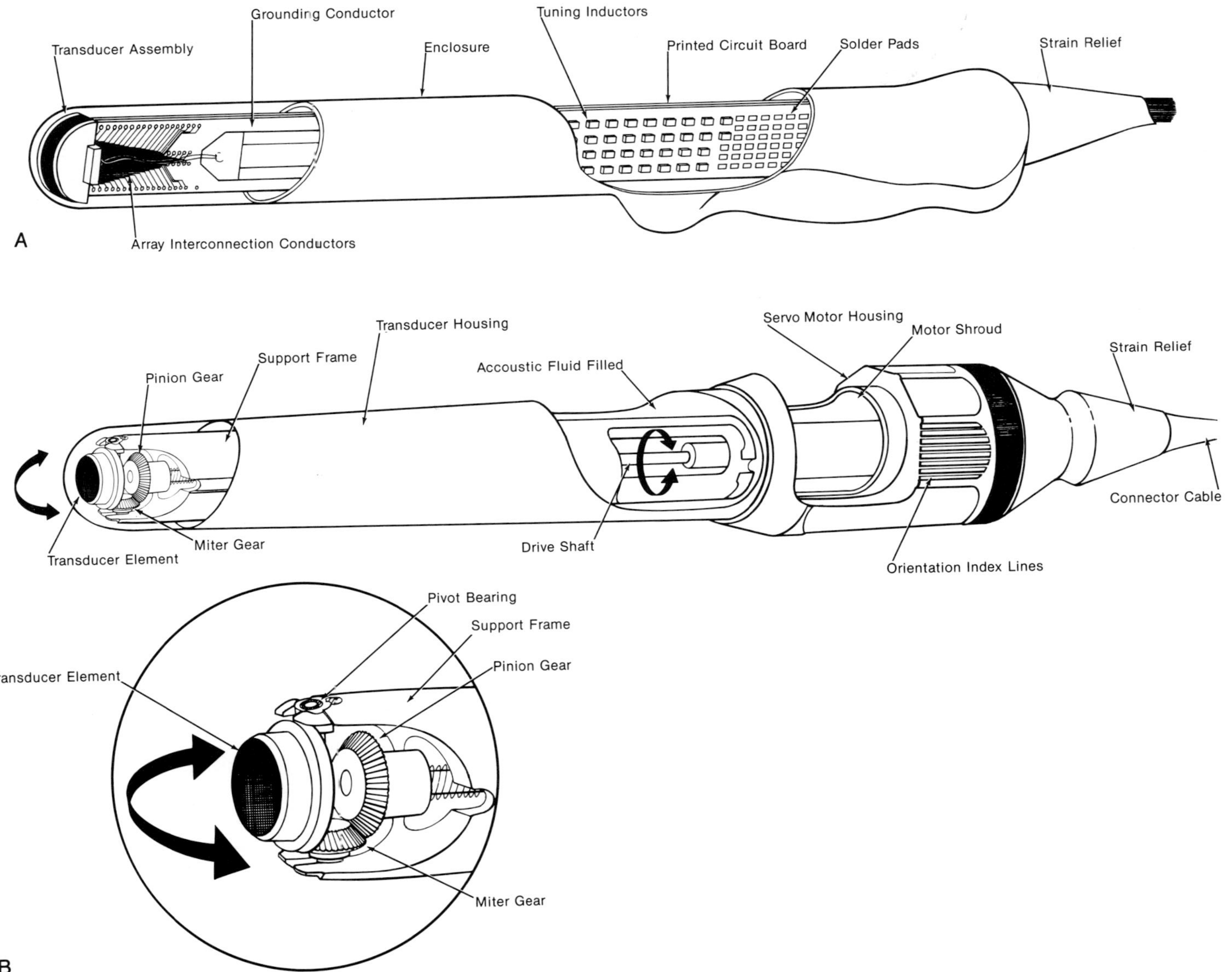

Fig. 2-3. **(A)** Cut-away view of a typical solid state sector transvaginal probe. The transducer ultrasound beam is steered electronically. There are no moving parts in the probe. **(B)** Cut-away view of a typical mechanical sector transvaginal probe showing the transducer element and mechanical drive, and housing. (Courtesy of Advanced Technology Laboratories, Inc., Bothell, WA.)

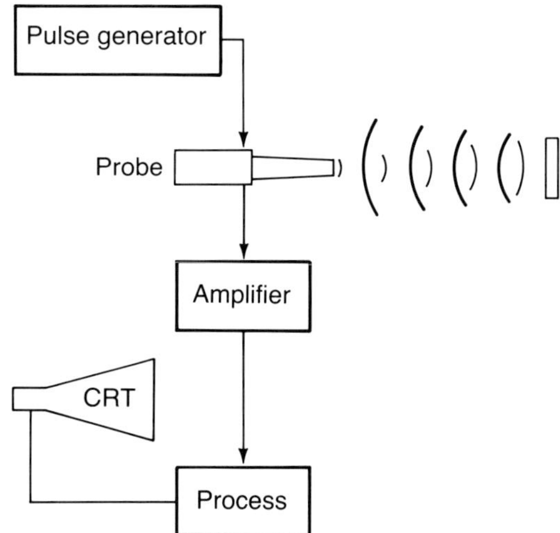

Fig. 2-4. Simplified diagram of an ultrasound machine showing a pulse generator, transducer and housing (transvaginal probe), sound amplifier, electrical processing, and display screen (cathode ray tube). Data processing and other more sophisticated components are frequently added.

the sound pulse is required to travel to the reflector and return.

In brightness or B-mode, the intensity of the reflection is displayed by variations in brightness. In B-mode scannings, repeated B-mode echoes build a two-dimensional image that is displayed on the cathode ray tube.

In motion or M-mode, the motion of a reflector is displayed so that a B-mode tracing is moved across the cathode ray tube like a strip chart recording. When the multiple B-mode scan images produced each second (10 to 60 frames per second) are displayed as they are produced, a real-time image is produced.

IMAGE RESOLUTION

Resolution is the minimum distance between two target reflectors required to distinguish them as separate entities. Several factors influence the resolution of the ultrasound images. In ultrasound there are two different components to resolution: (1) axial resolution, or the resolution of objects along the path of the sound beam, and (2) lateral resolution, or the ability to separate objects perpendicular to the sound beam.

Axial resolution is the minimum reflector separation required along the directions of sound travel so that separate reflections will be produced.[3] It depends on the pulse length, which is equal to the number of cycles in a pulse multiplied by the wavelength. The relationship between axial resolution and pulse length can be described by the following equation: axial resolution = spatial pulse length/2. Therefore, the shorter the wavelength, the better the axial resolution. Also, the fewer the number of cycles in a pulse, the better the axial resolution. Accordingly, to improve axial resolution, either the frequency has to be increased or the number of cycles per pulse has to be decreased. To reduce the number of cycles in any given pulse, a damping material is generally placed in the transducer adjacent to the transducer crystal. Since the wavelength is equal to the velocity of sound in a given medium divided by the frequency, axial resolution is also a function of the frequency. Therefore, a 7.5-MHz transducer gives better axial resolution than a 3.5-MHz transducer. However, as noted earlier, as the frequency increases, the absorption of the sound also increases and the depth of sound penetration decreases. Therefore, the depth that the structures can be imaged in the body is limited, which is particularly relevant to the pelvic ultrasound examination, since the uterus and ovaries lie deep in the pelvis. Therefore, the frequency of the transducer selected is generally a compromise between axial resolution and the depth of tissue penetration needed. This is why transvaginal probes are particularly well suited for visualizing the pelvic organs in the female. By placing the transducer against one of the vaginal fornices, the ovaries, uterus, and other pelvic structures are close enough to allow adequate penetration and give excellent axial resolution using a 5- to 7.5-MHz probe. In contrast, using the bladder as an acoustic window in transabdominal sonography, the 7.5-MHz and sometimes even the 5.0-MHz transducer will not give adequate penetration. Structures deep in the pelvis often cannot be imaged.

Lateral resolution is the minimum separation in the direction perpendicular to the course of the ultrasonic beam. This is the minimal distance between two reflectors that will produce two separate reflections when the beam is scanned across them.[3] Lateral resolution is a function of the sound beam diameter, e.g., lateral resolution is directly proportional to the beam width. The smaller the sound beam diameter, the better the lateral resolution. Beam diameter varies along the sound path from the transducer (Fig. 2-5), and can be reduced by increasing the frequency.

A focused sound beam, similar to a focused light beam, may be obtained by using an acoustic lens in

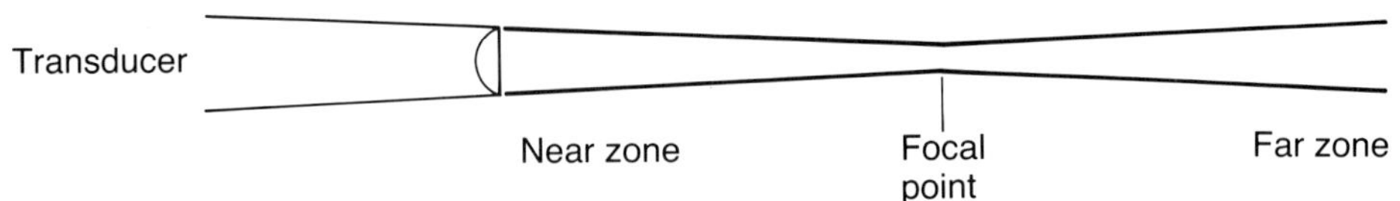

Fig. 2-5. Lateral resolution is a function of the sound beam diameter. The sound beam narrows to the focal point and then widens beyond the focal point. The sound beam between the transducer and the focal point is referred to as the near zone, and beyond the focal point it is referred to as the far zone. Lateral resolution is greatest at the focal point, but rapidly degenerates in the far zone.

the transducer or a curved transducer element. The beam diameter decreases to the focal point (the narrowest point in the sound beam) and then widens beyond the focal point. The higher the frequency (for a given transducer element diameter), the longer the focal length. Likewise, the larger the transducer element diameter (for a given frequency), the longer the focal length. The lateral resolution is best at the focal point where the beam diameter is smallest. A transducer element with a small diameter has a shorter focal point and better resolution near the transducer but poorer resolution as the sound beam diameter widens beyond the focal point. Therefore, a small diameter transducer crystal narrows the sound beam and increases resolution in the near field (to the focal point). However, there is an increase in divergence in the far field, and lateral resolution decreases rapidly in the far field. From a practical standpoint, to solve in part the "problem of a fixed focal point" of a transducer, several of the newer probes available on the market have been equipped with focusing acoustic lenses that allow for electronic variation of focusing, generally between 5.0 and 7.5 MHz.

In summary, the main advantage of the vaginal transducer over the transabdominal transducer is the possibility of placing the probe closer to pelvic organs that generally lie within 6 to 8 cm of the vaginal fornices. The closer the probe is approximated to the organ to be scanned, the higher the frequency that can be used. High ultrasonic frequencies allow for significantly improved lateral and axial resolutions. As compared to resolution obtained with 2.5- to 5.0-MHz transabdominal imaging, it has been estimated that axial resolution is improved by up to 50 percent by using a 7.5-MHz probe.[3]

BIOLOGIC EFFECTS OF SOUND

Four mechanisms of biologic effects of ultrasound are recognized: (1) heat, (2) cavitation, (3) mechanical distortion, and (4) radiation force. When ultrasound energy propagates through biologic tissue, heat is produced due to absorption of the sound wave. The higher the frequency and/or intensity of ultrasound, the higher the absorption and consequently a higher conversion into heat. However, it has to be appreciated that tissue temperature must reach 42 degrees Celsius before detrimental biologic effects of the ultrasound wave can be observed. To the best of our knowledge, a significant elevation in temperature has never been demonstrated in mammalian tissues exposed to diagnostic ultrasound intensity levels. Cavitation is a general term applied to the generation and behavior of gas bubbles that may be generated in media from dissolved gases by intense sound. When a continuous ultrasound wave is generated, enlargement of gas bubbles may result. Enlargement of a gas bubble may cause a resonance phenomenon called stable cavitation. A continuous wave intensity between 150 and 500 mW/cm^2 may lead to stable cavitation in vivo[4]. The generation of a pulsed ultrasound wave may cause implosion of gas bubbles, eventually leading to very high temperatures and pressures. This phenomenon is called transient cavitation and is thought not to occur in vivo below a peak ultrasound intensity of 1500 W/cm^2[5]. In this regard, it is noteworthy that intensities used in diagnostic ultrasound are 1/100 to 1/1,000th the intensities that have generally been associated with tissue damage.[2] In respect to mechanical distortion, a phenomenon called *radiation torque* can be induced by the ultrasound wave. It consists of a rotating movement either of the cells or of their intracellular elements that may damage the walls of the cell. Radiation forces are generated by ultrasound on the interface between two tissues and possibly inside the cells, producing aggregation.

The effect of sound beams on tissues depends on the sound intensity at the target level and on the distance between the probe and the target together with probe frequency. Therefore, it is important to know the characteristics of the transducers being used. Since many ultrasound systems are available, three different definitions of sound intensity have been proposed (Table 2-1). These three definitions take

Table 2-1. Three Definitions of Sound Intensity That May Be Used to Characterize Intensities of the Tranducers

SATA Intensity:	Temporal mean intensity averaged over the beam cross-sectional area in Watt/cm². This intensity is often reported by manufacturers. SATA means Spatial Average, Temporal Average.
SPTA Intensity:	The local maximal and temporal average intensity in Watt/cm². SPTA means Spatial Peak, Temporal Average.
SPTP Intensity:	The local maximal and temporal peak intensity in Watt/cm². This intensity is of course higher than the SPTA. SPTP means Spatial Peak, Temporal Peak.

(From Schats,[3] with permission.)

into account the notion that acoustic dosage is dependent on which area in a certain period of time is covered, the determination of intensity by pulse frequency and duration, the intensity peak value during the pulse, and the intensity mean value in time.[6] The intensity (I) of the ultrasound systems that are generally used in pulse/echo imaging is between 0.01 and 15 mW/cm² (I_{-SATA}), or between 0.5 and 200 mW/cm² (I_{-SPTA}).[6]

Although a variety of biologic effects have been noted after ultrasound exposure, the Consensus Development Conference sponsored by the National Institute of Child Health and Human Development noted no significant evidence linking ultrasound exposure to the production of genetic effects.[7] There have been three reports noting increased sister chromatid exchange frequency after ultrasound exposure. However, 11 other reports have not confirmed such an effect.[7] Studies on animals and particularly pregnant mice have been conflicting.[7] Some studies reporting a biologic effect from ultrasound have used sound intensities much higher than encountered in medical diagnostic ultrasound. Most studies have not shown an increased incidence of congenital anomalies or any effect on litter size or resorption rate.[7] However, an occasional study has reported an adverse effect, and several studies have noted a reduction in fetal weight in animals.[7] However, there are at this point no reliable data linking ultrasound even in early pregnancy to fetal congenital anomalies or other adverse effects in humans.

It is likely that abdominal and transvaginal ultrasound scanning procedures have different implications in terms of safety. In other words, the vaginal ultrasound approach has problems specific to it. For example, the distance from the tip of the probe to the target is shorter, and the embryo is studied as a whole and at earlier stages than with the transabdominal approach. The seventh newsletter published by the European Federation of Societies for Ultrasound in Medicine and Biology (EFSUMB) in 1993,[8] clearly reports that the exposure conditions are not the same for transvaginal and transabdominal ultrasound. However, since the path lengths for both transmitted and received beams are shorter, lower output intensities can be used for the endovaginal route. In addition, higher frequencies allow for both better image resolution and increased absorption between the transducer and the target tissue. The EFSUMB has nevertheless estimated that exposure levels (at the embryo level) are similar using either transvaginal or transabdominal ultrasound. It has also postulated that better visualization may result in a shorter examination time. In this respect, a shorter exposure time of the target to the ultrasound beam should be beneficial and should increase the safety of the transvaginal procedure.[8]

In 1980 the Federal Republic of Germany was the first country to recommend the routine use of an ultrasound examination in pregnancy.[7] The Royal College of Obstetrics and Gynaecology in Great Britain has also recommended a single screening ultrasound examination in early pregnancy to estimate gestational age.[7] Although early pregnancy and complications of early pregnancy are important indications for a transvaginal ultrasonographic examination, there are a large and growing number of purely gynecologic indications (see Ch. 1). Currently, there are few reliable data indicating any harmful effect of gynecologic ultrasound.

Official statements on the biologic effects of ultrasound have been issued by two major associations involved in its use: the American Institute for Ultrasound in Medicine (AIUM) and the above-mentioned EFSUMB. The AIUM March 1993 declaration on effect on patients resulting from the usage of ultrasound since the 1950s has ever been demonstrated.[9] Notwithstanding, carrying out ultrasound examinations for other purposes than direct medical benefit of the patient requires informed consent[9]. Recommendations on the safety of transvaginal scanning by the EFSUMB provide clear indications for daily practice:

> "Information available at present, either from acoustic output data from commercial equipment, or from calculations of embryonic exposures, do not provide any contra-indication for transvaginal ultrasound safety of ultrasound notes that no adverse biologic scanning when clinically indicated, or for early pregnancy screening where there are firm clinical

> grounds. The absence of long-term, large scale follow-up studies following first trimester ultrasound exposures, means that care is required in the application of transvaginal ultrasound in early pregnancy. It should only be performed for pure medical reasons that are to the benefit of the mother and/or of the embryo. The power setting and the exposure times should be kept as low as possible whilst still giving the desired clinical answer.[8]

Most importantly, the EFSUMB has drawn attention to the fact that routine examination by pulsed Doppler and color flow mapping of every woman during pregnancy should not be considered at present because of the potential for increased temperatures in utero.

Altogether, there seems to be general agreement that ultrasound scanning procedures are safe, whatever the route of scanning. It is nevertheless advisable that output parameters of the ultrasound beam should always be kept to a minimum and exposure time of the target should be limited as much as possible. One of the most accurate statements regarding the safety of ultrasound scanning was suggested by Ter Haar: "probably the greatest risk associated with a pulse-echo diagnostic field come from misdiagnosis and lack of user education."[10]

REFERENCES

1. Goss SA, Johnston RL, Dunn F: Comprehensive compilation of empirical ultrasonic properties of mammalian tissues. J Acoust Soc Am 64:423, 1978
2. Ziskin MC: Basic principles. p. 1. In Goldberg BB, Kotler MN, Ziskin MC, Waxham RD (eds): Diagnostic Uses of Ultrasound. Grune & Stratton, Orlando, 1975
3. Schats R: Technical and methodological aspects of transvaginal sonography. p. 11-21. In Pasmans (ed): Transvaginal Sonography in Early Human Pregnancy. Ph.D. Thesis. Erasmus University, Rotterdam. The Hague, 1991
4. Ter Haar GR, Daniels S, Eastaugh K, Hill CR: Ultrasonically induced cavitation in-vivo. Br J Cancer 45:151, 1982
5. Gross DR, Miller DL, Williams AR: A search for ultrasonic cavitation within the canine cardiovascular system. Ultrasound Med Biol 11:85, 1985
6. Schats R: The safety of diagnostic ultrasound with particular reference to the transvaginal application. p. 23. In Pasmans (ed): Transvaginal Sonography in Early Human Pregnancy. Ph.D. Thesis, Erasmus University, Rotterdam. The Hague, 1991
7. Diagnostic Ultrasound Imaging in Pregnancy: Report of a Consensus Development Conference. U.S. Department of Health and Human Services, National Institutes of Health, NIH Publication No. 84-667, 1984
8. European Federation of Societies for Ultrasound in Medicine and Biology: Transvaginal sonography—safety aspects. Newsletter 7:10, 1993
9. American Institute of Ultrasound in Medicine: Safety of diagnostic ultrasound in training and research. AIUM Reporter, November 1993
10. Ter Haar GR: Safety of routine ultrasound. Ultrasound Obstet Gynecol 2:237, 1992

3

The Pelvic Ultrasound Examination and Pelvic Anatomy

Melvin G. Dodson
Thierry D. Pache

The patient should be given a brief explanation of the ultrasonographic procedure. The pelvic ultrasonographic examination is generally performed in an examination room or a specific ultrasound room equipped with a standard gynecologic examining table. The patient is allowed to undress from the waist down in private with adequate clothes hooks or clothes hangers for clothing. She is prepared by a nursing assistant in the lithotomy position in stirrups and draped with a sheet as for a standard pelvic examination. A gurney or bed may be used instead of the standard examination table with stirrups. However, doing so generally limits the sonographer's ability to move the probe and particularly to scan the anterior pelvis, which requires the transducer handle to be pressed down toward the floor so that the transducer tip is projected upward, directing the sound beam into the anterior pelvis. The vaginal probe is covered with a condom or glove. A sonic coupler is placed in the condom or glove, and an additional sonic coupler is added on the outside. The transducer is gently placed into the vagina and advanced to the level of the vaginal fornix and the examination begins. Most patients are very interested in what is being imaged, and we usually allow them to see the screen. Important pelvic structures are pointed out to the patient during the procedure. This generally informs the patient of the findings and increases her cooperation during the procedure.

SONIC COUPLING AND PREVENTION OF PROBE CONTAMINATION

A sonic coupler is needed to decrease the acoustic impedance as sound leaves the transducer and enters the body. Even a small layer of air between the transducer and the body will result in marked sound attenuation and artifacts. To acoustically couple the transducer to the vaginal mucosa, jelly is placed into a condom or one finger of a rubber examination glove. We prefer to use a rubber glove because it is thicker, and tearing or holes occur less frequently when a glove is used. The use of a condom or glove is essential to protect the patient and the transducer from contamination. The glove or condom should always be checked for a leak. This is generally easier to do with an examination glove since it is dry, and any gel on the outside of the glove indicates a small hole and is quickly noted. After checking for a hole and placing the transducer in the glove finger containing a sonic coupler, additional lubricant is placed on the surface of the glove to serve as an acoustic coupler between the glove and the patient. The same type of lubricant used for the pelvic examination can be used.

In addition to protecting the probe from contamination with a glove or condom, the probe should be decontaminated between patients. It is neither prac-

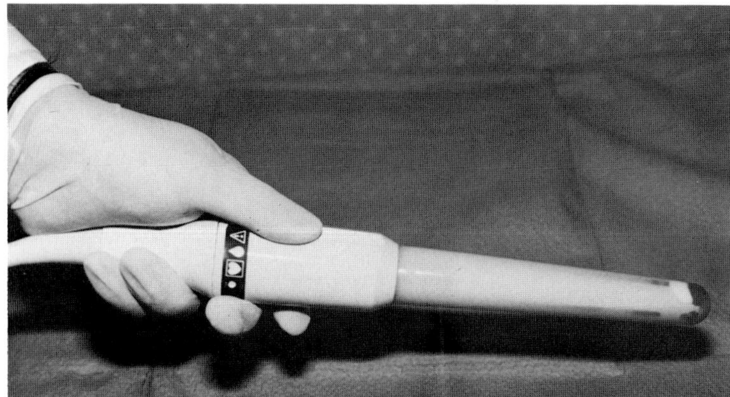

A

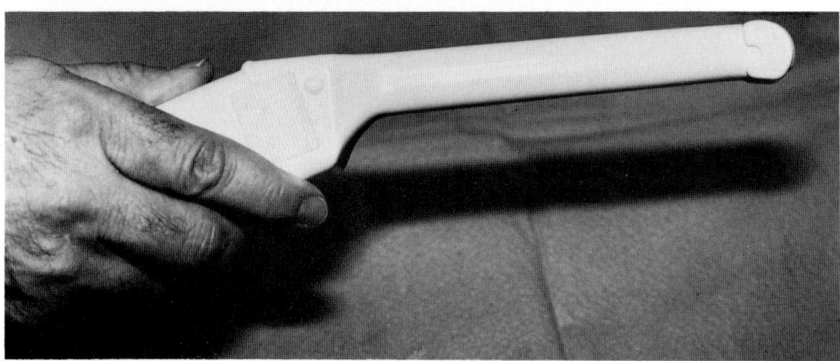

B

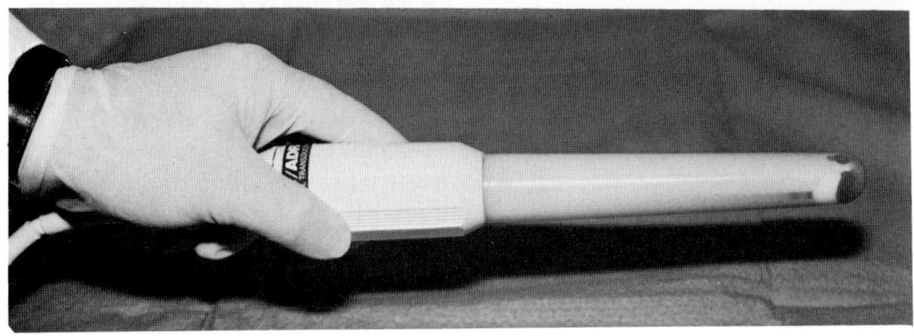

C

Fig. 3-1. (**A**) Photograph of ATL transvaginal probe (Advanced Technology Laboratories [ATL], Inc., Bothell, WA) oriented to give an AP-pelvic image plane. The thumb is on the transducer markings used for orientation. (**B**) Photograph of Hitachi probe (Hitachi Medical Corporation, Tokyo,Japan) turned 90 degrees to give a T-pelvic image plane. (**C**) Photograph of ATL transvaginal probe oriented to give a T-pelvic image plane.

tical nor possible to sterilize transvaginal probes using operating room techniques, such as heat or gas sterilization. However, a variety of liquid solutions for decontamination are available. Each transvaginal probe is different, and the recommendation of the manufacturer for decontamination should be followed meticulously. Some probes may be soaked in povidone-iodine (Betadine). Others require different decontaminating liquids and may not be immersed totally.

Most transvaginal transducers are marked to help orient the probe (Fig. 3-1). When the transducer is oriented or held so that the sound beam is being directed across the pelvis from side to side, a trans-pelvic (T-pelvic) plane is being imaged (see discussion in Ch. 1 on pelvic planes). Rotating the transducer 90 degrees will direct the sound beam anteriorly and posteriorly in the pelvis, giving an anterior posterior-pelvic (AP-pelvic) plane image. A T-pelvic image and an AP-pelvic image of the uterus and ovaries are obtained and recorded with biometric measurements during each examination. Oblique images can also be obtained, as needed, by rotating the probes. The orientation of the initial sound bang (top versus bottom)

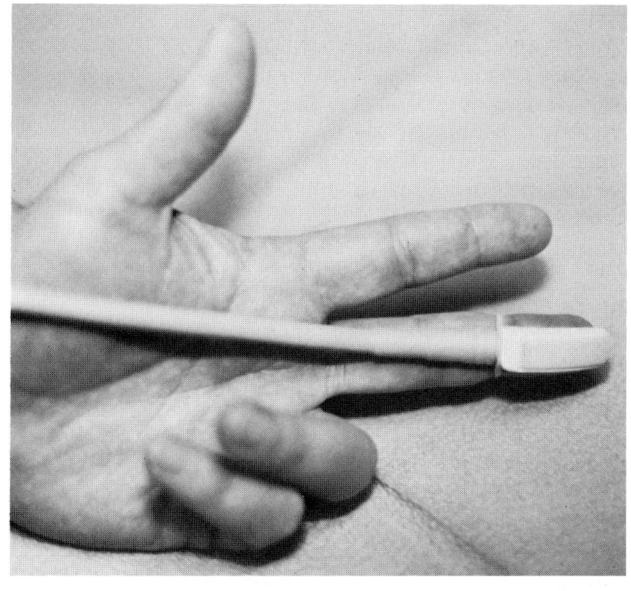

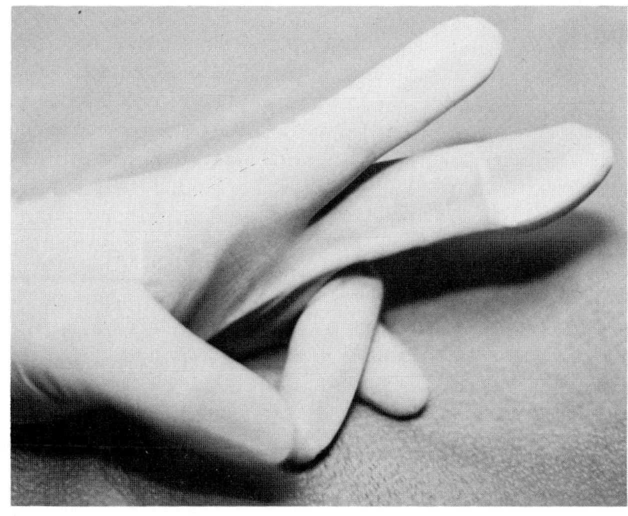

Fig. 3-2. (**A**) Photograph of 5-MHz Hitachi transvaginal finger probe attached by a rubber band to the middle finger. (**B**) Photograph of a finger probe covered by an examination glove. Ultrasound gel is used as a sonic coupler in the gloved finger and is also used on the glove for a lubricant and as a sonic coupler.

and the right-left orientation of the screen must also be set. Interestingly, finger probes can be used that allow for imaging of pelvic structures at the same time as the pelvic examination (Fig. 3-2). However, they offer no definite advantage as compared to the regular endovaginal probes.

PELVIC ANATOMY USING THE TRANSVAGINAL PROBE

Although the clinical indications for any given transvaginal ultrasound study will often focus the sonographer's attention on a given anatomic structure, such as the endometrium when trying to confirm an early intrauterine pregnancy or the ovary when the ultrasound is being done to evaluate an ovarian mass, all pelvic structures should be reviewed systematically before completing a pelvic sonographic study. A systematic review is best performed in the same manner in each scan so that the regimen becomes routine for the physician just as is a physical examination. All anatomic structures of the pelvis should be imaged. We use the following image routine:

1. Uterus
2. Myometrium and endometrium
3. Bladder and anterior pelvic structures
4. Right ovary
5. Right ovarian follicles and stroma echogenicity
6. Right adnexa
7. Right pelvic wall
8. Left ovary
9. Left ovarian follicles and stroma echogenicity
10. Left adnexa
11. Left pelvic wall
12. Cul-de-sac
13. Rectum
14. Small bowel
15. Posterior pelvis

The examination is generally done in two planes, T-pelvic and AP-pelvic, with an oblique view if necessary to fully appreciate the organs being imaged and to mentally construct a three dimensional image of the anatomy. Measurements of the uterus and ovaries in the T-pelvic and AP-pelvic planes are generally recorded.

During the ultrasound examination of each area or organ system, consideration should be given to both the anatomic and physiologic findings and any evidence of variations that might suggest pathology (Tables 3-1 and 3-2). Anatomic considerations should include the location, size, and texture and recording of biometric measurements as indicated. Physiologic changes occurring through the menstrual cycle result in anatomic changes in the uterus and ovaries. The size and location of the dominant follicle, the number and size of cohort follicles in the ovaries, and the thickness and textural changes in the endometrium are particularly relevant to reproductive functions and vary considerably with the physiologic changes through the menstrual cycle. Pathologic conditions should be diagnosed and quantitated, as, for example, the location, size, texture, and characteristics of ovarian cysts or uterine leiomyomas.

Table 3-1. Anatomy and Physiology

Organ or Area	*Anatomy and Physiology*
Uterus	Size, shape, contour, position, texture
Bladder	Size, shape
Endometrium	Thickness, texture, menstrual phase, intrauterine device, hormonal status
Ovaries	Size, position, follicular development
Adnexa	Thickness, vessels
Pelvic side walls	Identification of muscles and blood vessels
Cul-de-sac	Fluid, bowel

Table 3-2. Pathology

Organ	*Pathology*
Uterus	Leiomyomas, adenomyosis, congenital anomalies
Endometrium	Anovulation, polyps, submucosal or pedunculated leiomyomas, carcinomas, pregnancy, bleeding, hematocolpos, hormonal status
Ovaries	Ovulation, neoplasms, cysts, carcinomas, polycystic ovarian disease, postmenopausal screening
Adnexa	Hydrosalpinx, ectopic pregnancy
Cul-de-sac	Ascites, blood, blood clots
Bladder	Stones
Other	Adhesions, pelvic thrombosis, endometriosis, acute pelvic inflammatory disease

Uterus

The uterus is visualized first because it is generally the largest and most centrally placed midline structure in the pelvis. It is also the easiest pelvic organ to image. In addition, localization of the uterus orients the sonographer. The myometrium should have a homogeneous echo density. The gain of the ultrasound machine should be adjusted to give an appropriate echo texture to the myometrium and it should be used as a reference for average echogenicity (see the section, *Time-Gain Compensation,* below). The bladder should be anechoic. The width and thickness of the uterus should be measured in the T-pelvic plane. It is sometimes difficult to delineate the lateral borders of the uterus when measuring the width, since it blends into the broad ligament, and parametrial vasculariza-

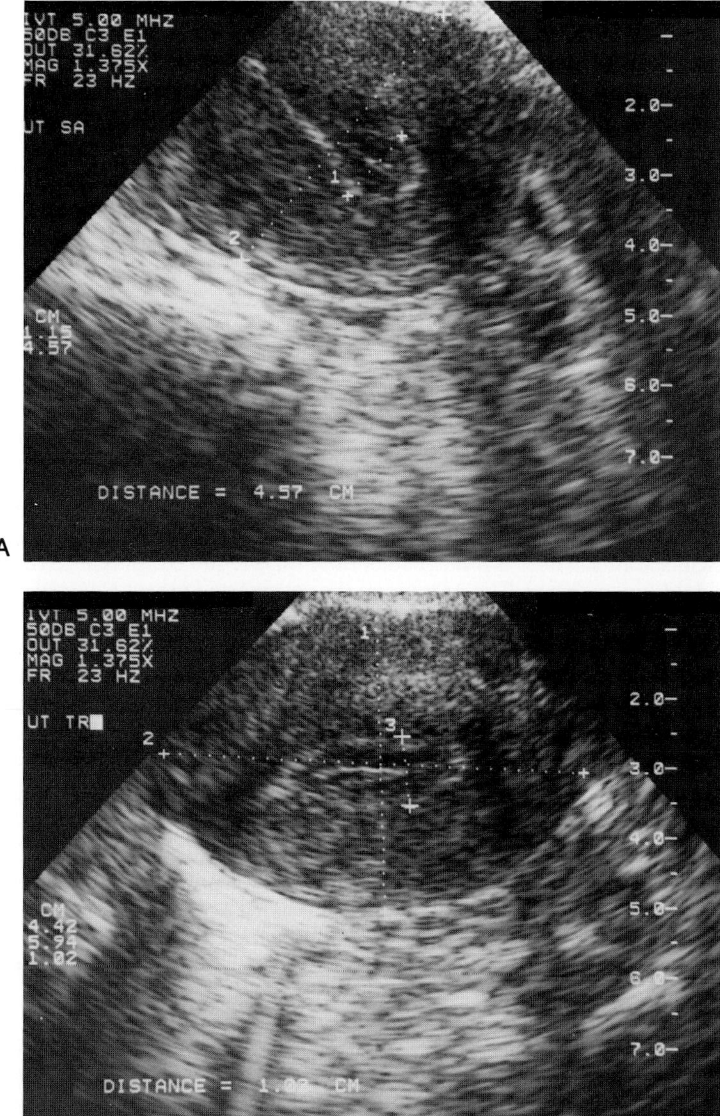

Fig. 3-3. (**A**) AP-pelvic view of the uterus shows a follicular endometrium 11.5 mm thick on day 16 of a menstrual cycle. The anterior posterior diameter of the uterus is 4.57 cm. (**B**) T-pelvic view of the same patient gives an anterior posterior uterine measurement of 4.42 cm and an endometrial thickness of 10.2 mm. The 1-mm difference in measurements is within the accuracy expected in biometric measurements or may also be due to measurements being taken in slightly different planes or in different areas of the uterine fundus. Frequently, greater differences in the anterior posterior measurements (thickness) of the uterus are noted between the T-pelvic and AP-pelvic planes because of the position of the uterus and the fact that measurements may be made in an oblique plane.

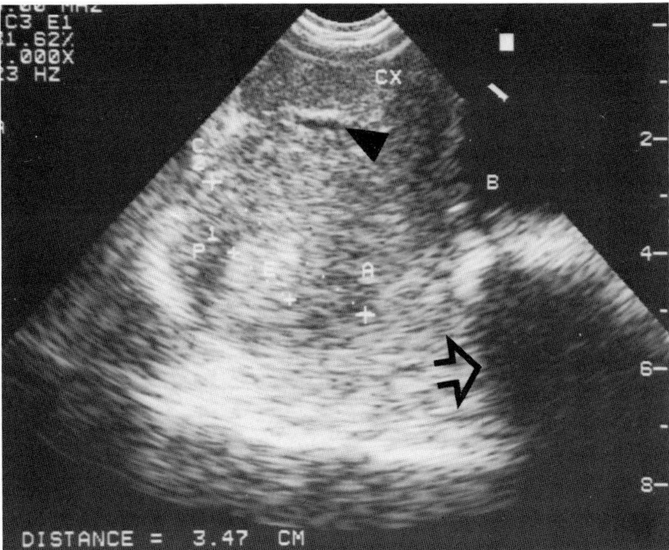

Fig. 3-4. Sagittal view of a retroverted uterus with bladder (B) on the right and cervix (CX) on the left. Note that the uterus is bent backward in relationship to the cervix. A, anterior wall of the uterus; P, posterior wall; E, endometrium; C, cul-de-sac area. There is a small amount of fluid in the cul-de-sac (arrowhead). Note a bladder angle shadow on the right (open arrow). The position of the retroverted uterus can be compared with that of the anteverted uterus shown in Figure 3-3A.

tion is highly variable. The thickness is also measured in the AP-pelvic plane. The upper limits of size of a normal nongravid uterus are 5 cm in width and 4 cm in thickness in the premenopausal adult woman (Fig. 3-3).

Measurement of the cervical-fundal length during the transvaginal ultrasound examination generally requires that the transvaginal probe be withdrawn partially from the vagina to allow imaging of the cervix. It is often a difficult measurement to obtain using the transvaginal technique. Care must be taken to ensure that the ultrasound transducer tip has not been placed in the anterior or posterior vaginal fornix, in essence cutting off the cervix. The cervical-fundal uterine length is more easily measured using the transabdominal full bladder technique. The upper cervical-fundal length of a normal uterus is 8 cm in the premenopausal adult woman.[1,2]

The consistency of the myometrium and contour of the uterus should be evaluated. Areas of hyper- or hypoechogenicity should be noted. The position of the uterus, anteverted or retroverted, should be noted (Fig. 3-4). Sometimes veins can be imaged within the myometrium.

Endometrium

The endometrium can be visualized within the uterus as a central echo on both T-pelvic and AP-pelvic scans. The echogenic character of the endometrium varies through the menstrual cycle and in the postmenopausal patient. The accuracy of pelvic sonography examination to assess the endometrium has been demonstrated in transabdominal[3-5] and transvaginal[6,7] ultrasound studies.[8] Recent modifications of transvaginal sonography transducers that offer a shorter probe-to-target distance allow use of high frequency (5 to 7-MHz) transducers,[9] which in turn result in significant improvements in sonographic depiction of the endometrium (see Ch. 6).[10]

Cervix

The cervix is generally routinely visualized using the transabdominal full bladder imaging technique. When the transvaginal approach is used, the transducer usually rests in the anterior cul-de-sac area and

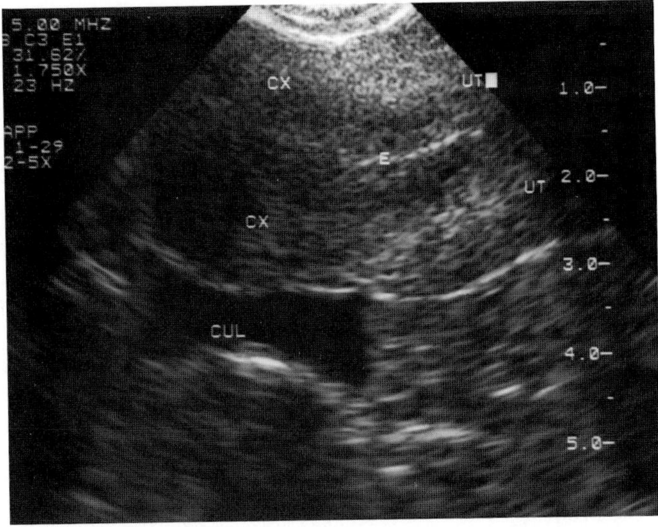

Fig. 3-5. AP-pelvic view of the cervix obtained by inserting the transducer only a short distance into the vagina. The cervix (CX) and endometrial canal are imaged clearly. The vagina is to the left, and the body of the uterus is to the right (UT). There is a small amount of fluid in the cul-de-sac (CUL).

the cervix, per se is not imaged. However, the cervix can be imaged by placing the transducer in the vagina without applying it against the upper vaginal mucosa (Fig. 3-5).

Sometimes, poor contact between the transducer and vagina gives a poor image quality or results in reverberation artifact if air has been introduced into the vagina during insertion of the transducer. Poor contact can generally be corrected by additional lubricating jelly or by placing a small amount of water in the vagina.

Bladder

If there is urine in the bladder, the bladder will be easily recognized as an anechoic area anterior to the uterus. Gain settings are adjusted to produce a black

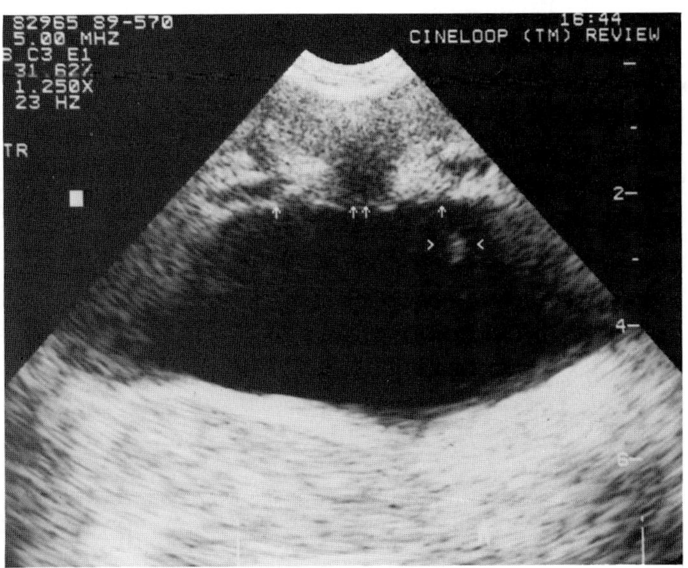

Fig. 3-6. T-pelvic view of bladder showing the urethra (two arrows) and both ureteral orifices (single arrow). A urine jet is noted coming from the left ureter (between double arrowheads). Additional portions of the ureter can be seen on both sides above the orifices. The ureters and urethra are anterior on transvaginal ultrasound since the probe is in the anterior cul-de-sac.

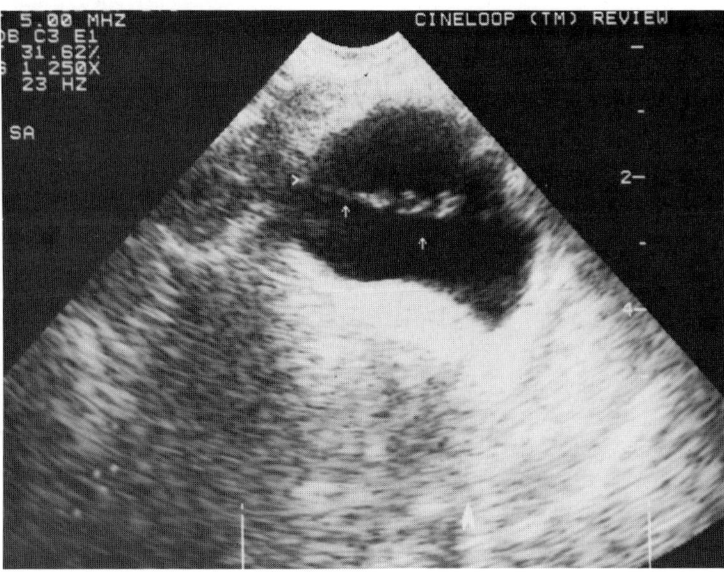

Fig. 3-7. AP-pelvic view of bladder showing a urine jet. The ureteral orifice is marked by an arrowhead. The urine jet entering the bladder is marked by arrows.

or anechoic bladder. It may be necessary to push the handle of the transducer downward to direct the probe tip and sound beam anteriorly to visualize the bladder better. If a standard gynecologic examination table with stirrups is not used, it may be necessary to have the patient lift her pelvis off the table or place a pillow under her buttocks to visualize the anterior pelvis adequately. The ureteral orifices are generally visualized in a T-pelvic plane at the top of the display screen (when the initial sound bang is oriented at the top of the screen). The urethra can generally also be imaged in the midline. Sometimes, with angulation of the transducer, the urethra and ureter are imaged as if they are in the same plane (Fig. 3-6). Urine can be noted entering the bladder from the ureters (Fig. 3-7). If a Foley catheter is in place, it can readily be visualized by ultrasound, thereby demonstrating the location of the urethra. The mucosa of the bladder

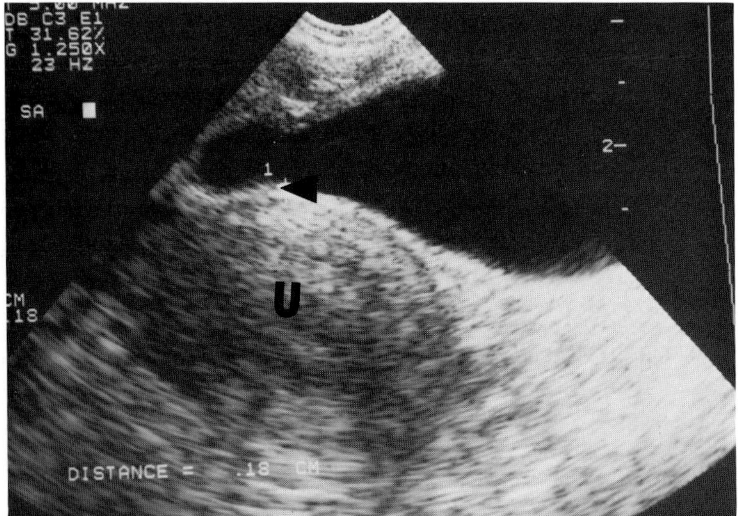

Fig. 3-8. AP-pelvic view of the bladder and uterus. The bladder wall is 1.8 mm thick (number 1 and arrowhead). The uterus is below the bladder (U). There is usually acoustic enhancement of the posterior bladder wall adjacent to the uterus.

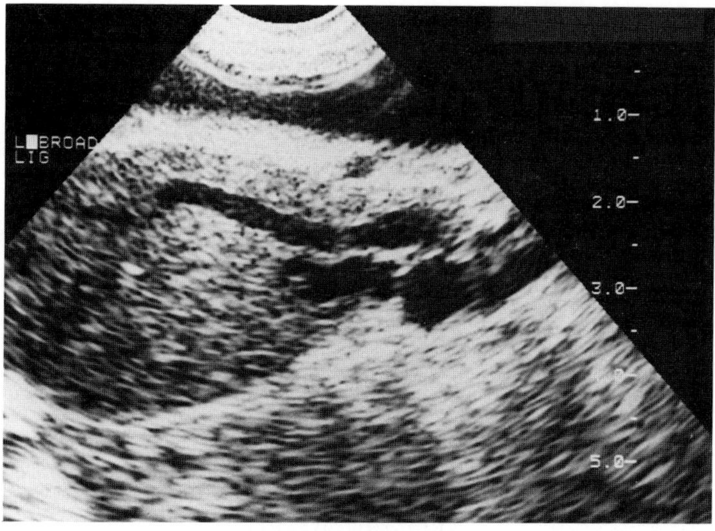

Fig. 3-9. T-pelvic view of the uterus showing a large dorsal fundal vein draining into the venous complex of the left ovarian vein in the infundibulopelvic ligament. A venous complex consisting of the ovarian and other veins are consistently imaged in the cornual area of the broad ligament.

should be noted for papillar or polypoid projections. The thickness of the bladder should also be noted. It is generally 3 to 6 cm thick (Fig. 3-8).

Broad Ligament and Arcuate Vessels

The arcuate uterine blood vessels comprise the vascular bed of the uterus and can frequently be imaged. They are best seen 1 to 3 weeks from the last menses and are more difficult to visualize just before and during menses.[11] DuBose et al.[11] have suggested that this difficulty results from normally mediated vasoconstriction during the late luteal phase, with vasodilatation during the follicular phase and midcycle resulting from estrogen. A full bladder may decrease blood vessel size owing to compression. Two major complexes of veins are generally noted. One complex is in the infundibulopelvic ligament and is imaged adjacent to the cornual area of the uterus and often adjacent to the ovary (Fig. 3-9). The other complex is imaged lateral to the cervix and lower uterine segment at the level of the internal cervical os (Fig. 3-10). Such vessels are normal and should not be confused with follicles, hydrosalpinx, or pelvic pathology. However, markedly dilated or varicose veins may also be noted.

Ovary

The ovaries are generally easily recognized as homogeneous echo densities located lateral to the uterus with the transducer in the T-pelvic plane. However, not uncommonly, the vaginal transducer handle will have to be angled anteriorly or posteriorly (by flexing or extending the sonographer's hand holding the transducer) to image out of the plane of the uterus in order to visualize the ovaries when they are located in the cul-de-sac or high in the pelvis. A very limited number of studies have tried to establish the aspect of "normal" ovaries[12,13] in regularly cycling volunteers. Using a 5-MHz endovaginal probe, one single observer performed scans between the 4th and 11th day of the follicular phase of the menstrual cycle.[13] Accuracy and reproducibility of ovarian measurements were checked.[12] After localization of the ovaries in relation to the iliac vessels, the number of follicles, appearing as anechoic, round, or ovoid structures, was established by scanning each ovary from the inner to the outer margin in longitudinal cross-sections. Follicle size was determined from two dimensions (longitudinal and anterior posterior) or from three dimensions (longitudinal, anterior posterior, and transverse) depending on the longitudinal diameter of the follicle (less than 6.0 mm or more than 6.0 mm respectively). From the longitudinal (A), anterior posterior (B), and transverse (C) dimension of the ovary, its volume was calculated according to the formula ½X (A X B X C). Echogenicity of the ovarian stroma was scored as normal (= 1), moderately increased (= 2), or markedly increased (= 3). In these premenopausal volunteers with normal weight and regular cycles, no more than 11 follicles could be observed in any one normal ovary. Normal ovaries were never

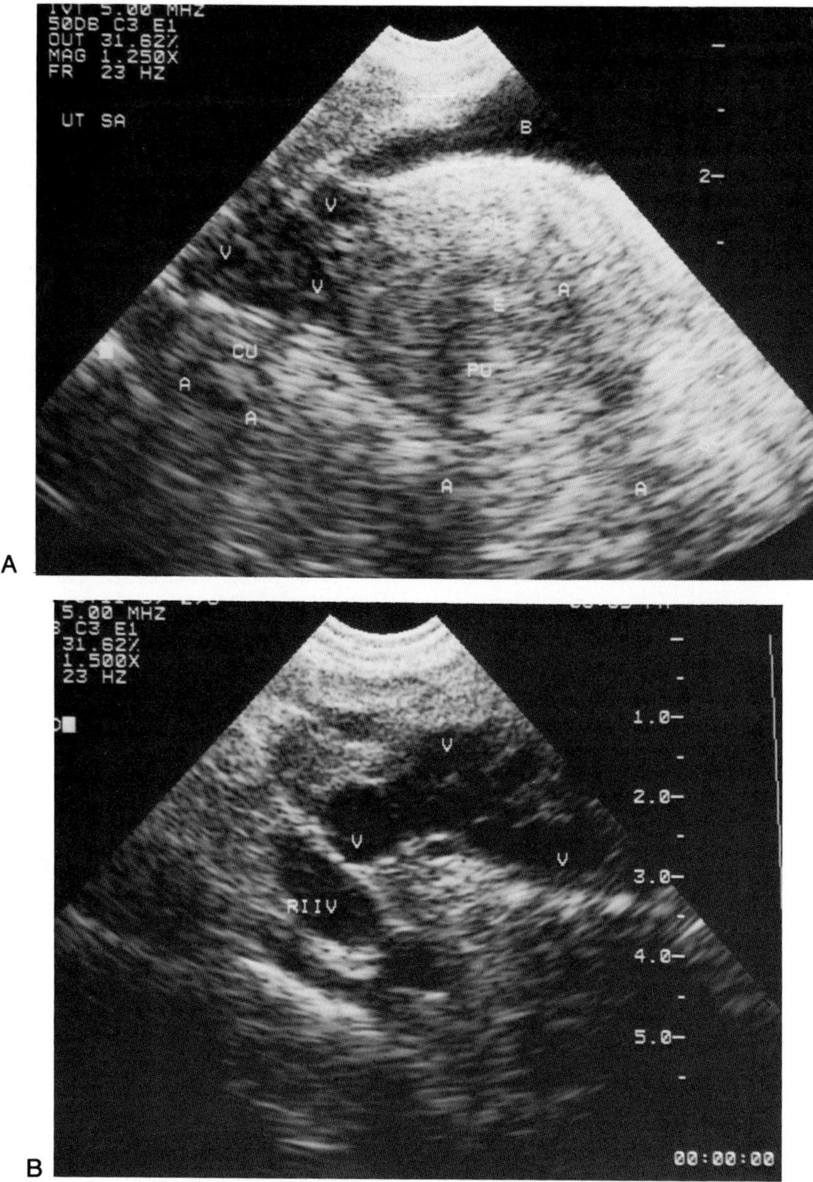

Fig. 3-10. (**A**) AP-pelvic view of the uterus lateral to the midline showing a complex of veins in the broad ligament at the level of the internal os. V, vein; B, bladder; CU, cul-de-sac; E, endometrium; PU, posterior uterine wall; A, artifact shadow. (**B**) T-pelvic view of the broad ligament showing a complex of veins (V) and the right internal iliac vein (RIIV). The venous complex could be seen emptying into the right internal iliac vein in a different plane.

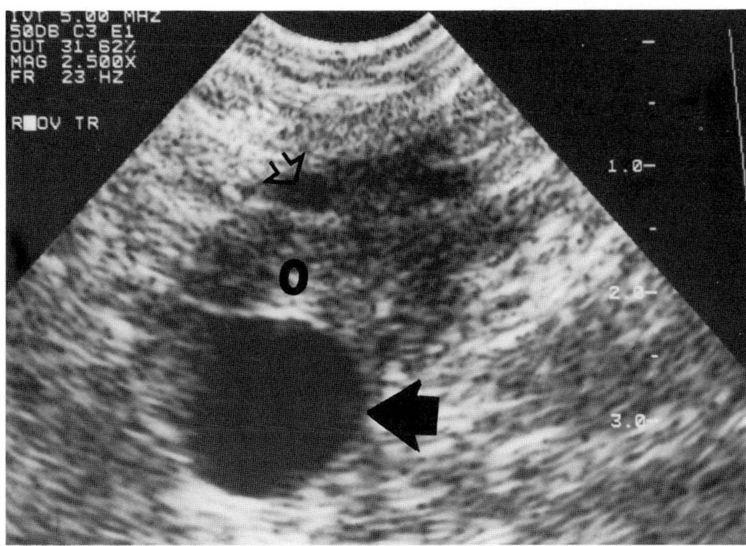

Fig. 3-11. T-pelvic view of the right ovary (O) showing a 1.4-cm follicle (arrow). One or two small preovulatory follicles are also present (open arrows).

found to exhibit a volume above 8.0 ml. The median values of mean follicle size and number were 5.1 mm and 5.0, whereas the median value of mean ovarian volume was 5.9 ml. Echogenicity of the ovarian stroma was normal in 90 percent and only moderately increased in 10 percent of the cases.

Localization of the postmenopausal ovaries can occasionally be difficult because of their small size (average, about 1.5 cm^3) and because of the lack of anechoic follicles that generally make identification easy (Fig. 3-11). Identification of the hypogastric vein may be helpful in localizing the small postmenopausal ovary in difficult cases. The ovary is frequently adjacent to the hypogastric vein and peritoneum defining the lateral pelvic wall, or in the space between the hypogastric vein and the uterus (Fig. 3-12). The hypogastric vessels also help delineate the lateral pelvic wall. Care must be taken not to mistake the hypogas-

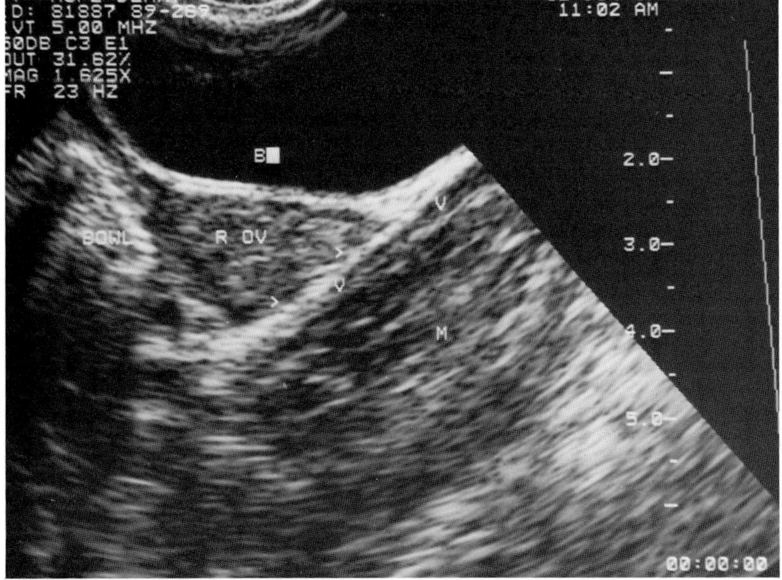

Fig. 3-12. T-pelvic view of the right ovary (ROV). Bowel with air (BOWL) is present to the left of the ovary. The bladder (B) is above. The internal iliac vein (V) is only partially seen in this plane. The obturator muscle (M) is noted. The peritoneum gives a hyperechoic reflection (small white arrows).

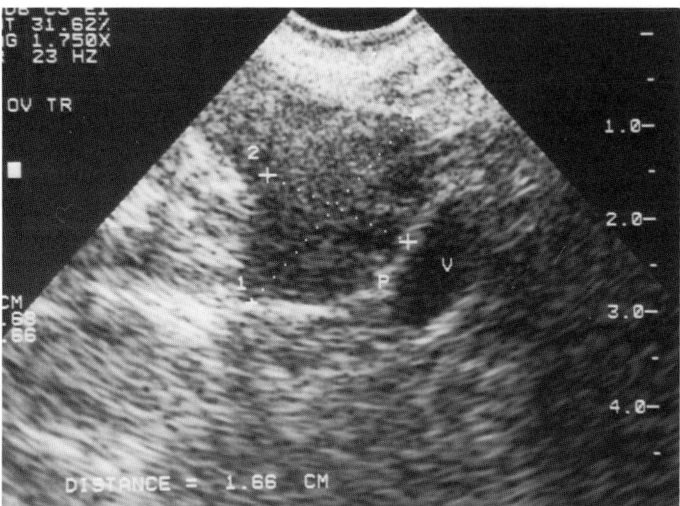

Fig. 3-13. T-pelvic view of the left ovary. The internal iliac vein (V) is imaged on the right side of the photograph. The peritoneum (P) is noted medial to the vein. Although there are no follicles in the ovary, it is easily identified adjacent to the internal iliac vein and lateral pelvic side wall. The limits of the ovary are defined by cursor lines 1 and 2. The ovary measures 2.7 by 1.7 cm.

tric vessels for an ovarian follicle. In some planes the hypogastric vein appears circular, and its proximity to the ovary may suggest a follicle. When the vaginal transducer is moved, the anechoic area representing the hypogastric vein will spread out into a cylinder and can be traced along the pelvic wall and correctly identified as the internal iliac vein (Fig. 3-13). The internal iliac vein is an important pelvic landmark that can almost always be imaged. The artery may be seen as a smaller structure adjacent to the vein. However, misidentification is rarely a problem with experience. The peritoneum along the pelvic side walls, which separates the peritoneal cavity from the underlying vessels and muscles, can generally be visualized as a hyperechoic line. By moving the transducer, the peritoneal hyperechoic echo can be visualized from the area of the psoas muscle down toward the sacrum. Fluid in loops of small bowel adjacent to the ovary can also be mistaken for a follicle. However, generally, a little patience in observation will result in recognition of peristalsis, and the fluid in the bowel will shift. The circular anechoic area can then be correctly identified as bowel. In fact, sometimes active peristalsis of the small bowel delineates the boundaries of the broad ligament, adnexal structures, and ovaries and aids in identification of these structures.

Fallopian Tubes

Generally, the fallopian tubes cannot be visualized by transabdominal sonography, but can sometimes be seen using the transvaginal probe when sufficient cul-de-sac fluid is present (Fig. 3-14). When there is even a mild degree of hydrosalpinx, visualization of the tubes is relatively easy.

Cul-de-Sac

Cul-de-sac fluid may be present during any phase of the menstrual cycle. However, Davis and Gosink[14] most frequently noted fluid during the 5 days preceding the onset of menses (Fig. 3-15). This was true for both users and nonusers of oral contraceptives. The second most common time to note cul-de-sac fluid was between day 13 and day 21 in nonusers of oral contraceptives. The percentage of patients with identifiable cul-de-sac fluid varied from 12 percent (days 8 to 12) to 30 percent (before menses). Patients taking oral contraceptives only occasionally (5 percent) had midcycle cul-de-sac fluid. At least some midcycle cul-de-sac fluid probably reflected follicular fluid released into the pelvic cavity after ovulation. Some increased cul-de-sac fluid may also result from estrogen-induced capillary permeability.

Increased cul-de-sac fluid may be associated with acute pelvic inflammatory disease, ruptured ectopic pregnancies, ovarian hyperstimulation syndrome following the use of clomiphene citrate (Clomid) or human menopausal gonadotropin (Pergonal), ovarian cysts, or other gynecologic pathology. Nongynecologic causes of increased cul-de-sac fluid include appendicitis, abdominal infections, nongynecologic intra-abdominal cancers, or intra-abdominal bleeding from trauma, such as rupture of the spleen.

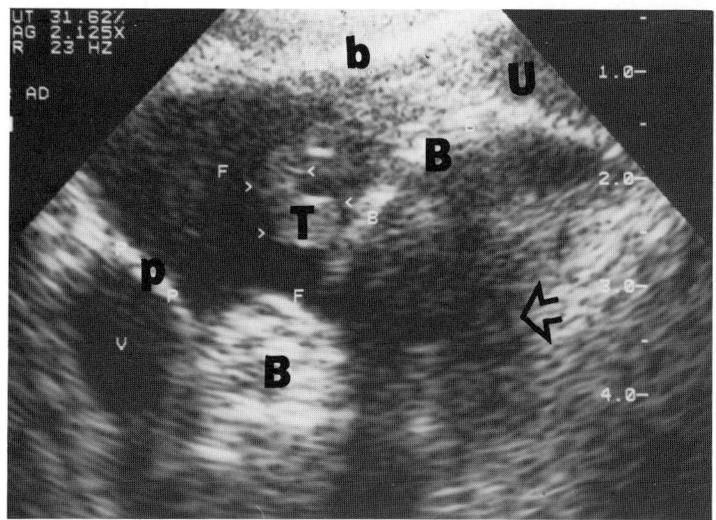

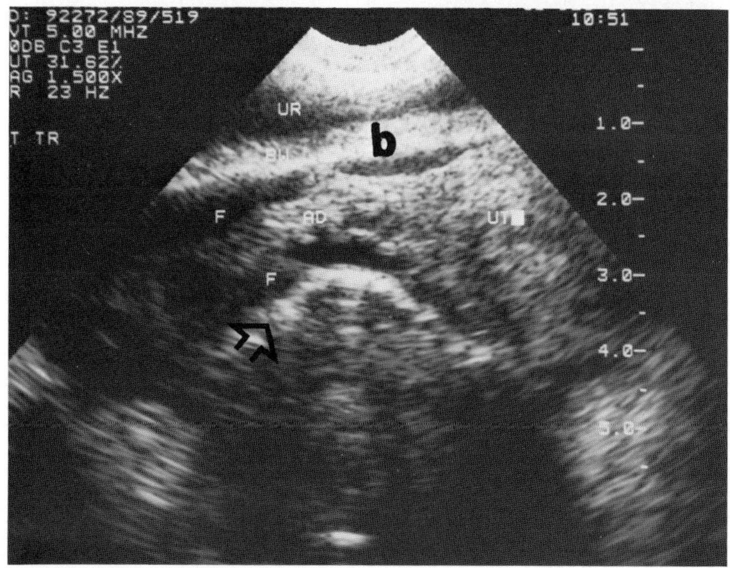

Fig. 3-14. **(A)** T-pelvic image of the right adnexa in a patient with increased peritoneal fluid (F). The right tube (T) is outlined (small white arrows) and is normal in size. The internal iliac vein (V) with overlying peritoneum (small white Ps and large black P) defines the pelvic wall. Hyperechoic bowel and a portion of bowel wall (B) are seen. An artifact shadow is present below the bowel (open arrow). Fluid (F) surrounds the tube. The adnexa and cornual area of the uterus are seen on the right. The bladder wall is at the top of the photograph (b). **(B)** The right adnexa is easily imaged because of increased peritoneal fluid. The uterus is to the right of the photograph (UT). The bladder wall (small white BW and black b)with urine (UR) in the bladder are seen at the top of the photograph. The adnexa (AD) and tube can be seen as a continuation of the cornual areas of the uterus. A loop of small bowel lies below the adnexa (open arrow) with some reverberation artifact (see Ch. 8).

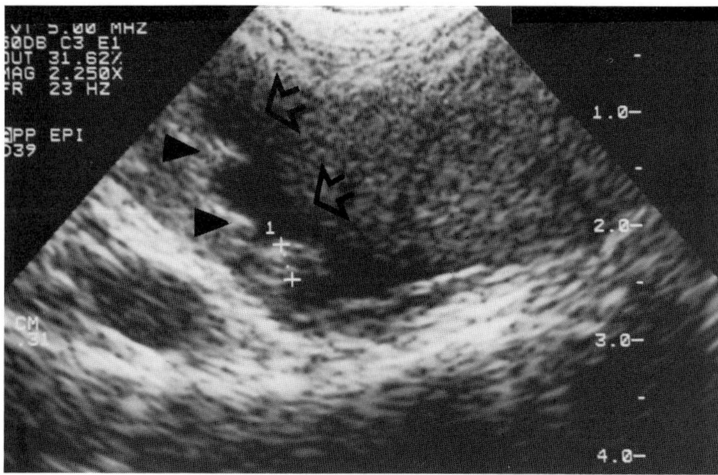

Fig. 3-15. Small amount of fluid in the cul-de-sac (open arrows) outlining several appendices epiploicae (arrowhead) on the sigmoid colon. The appendices measured 3.1 mm in thickness (cursor line 1).

Timor-Tritsch et al.[15] introduced fluid into the pelvis at the time of surgery and reported that 25 ml coated the lower portion of the uterus and ovaries and 50 ml produced a clear picture of all pelvic organs floating freely in the fluid. Rosen and colleagues have quantitated pelvic fluid preoperatively in ten healthy women using a 6.5-MHz transducer.[16] When the volume of fluid in the cul-de-sac was below 35 to 40 ml, it could not be detected by endovaginal ultrasound examination. Between 35 ml and 100 ml of fluid, there was a good correlation between the estimated volume of fluid and the corresponding echoscopic image.

Pelvic Muscle and Pelvic Sidewall

The levator and obturator muscles of the pelvis can be visualized as well as the iliopsoas muscles (Figs. 3-16 and 3-17). The sacrum can generally be visualized as a hyperechoic structure posterior to the uterus.

Sigmoid Colon and Small Bowel

The sigmoid colon is frequently visualized between the posterior aspect of the uterus and the sacrum. Stools and air may often be seen in the sigmoid colon. The small bowel can be visualized filling the pelvis (Figs. 3-18 and 3-19) and small bowel peristalsis is often seen. The small bowel is frequently filled by anechoic areas of fluid, hyperechoic areas of gas with shadowing and reverberation artifacts, and solid material generally with a mixed echo pattern (see Ch. 8).

Blood Clots

Echogenicity of blood clots depends on the amount of time that elapsed between the bleeding episode and scanning of the pelvis. Fresh pelvic blood clots generally produce irregular hypoechoic masses often associated with increased cul-de-sac fluid, whereas older clots present as grayish, more irregular echogenic structures.

Pelvic Adhesions

Ultrasound cannot image pelvic adhesions. However, the motility of the ovaries in relationship to the uterus has been used as a suggestive test for pelvic adhesions. Simultaneously applying pressure to the pelvic organs with both the transvaginal probe and transabdominally with the examiner's free hand has been suggested as a potential means of evaluation for pelvic adhesions by Lande et al.[17] En bloc motion of contiguous viscera rather than independent motion of the uterus, ovaries, and tubes suggests pelvic adhesions.

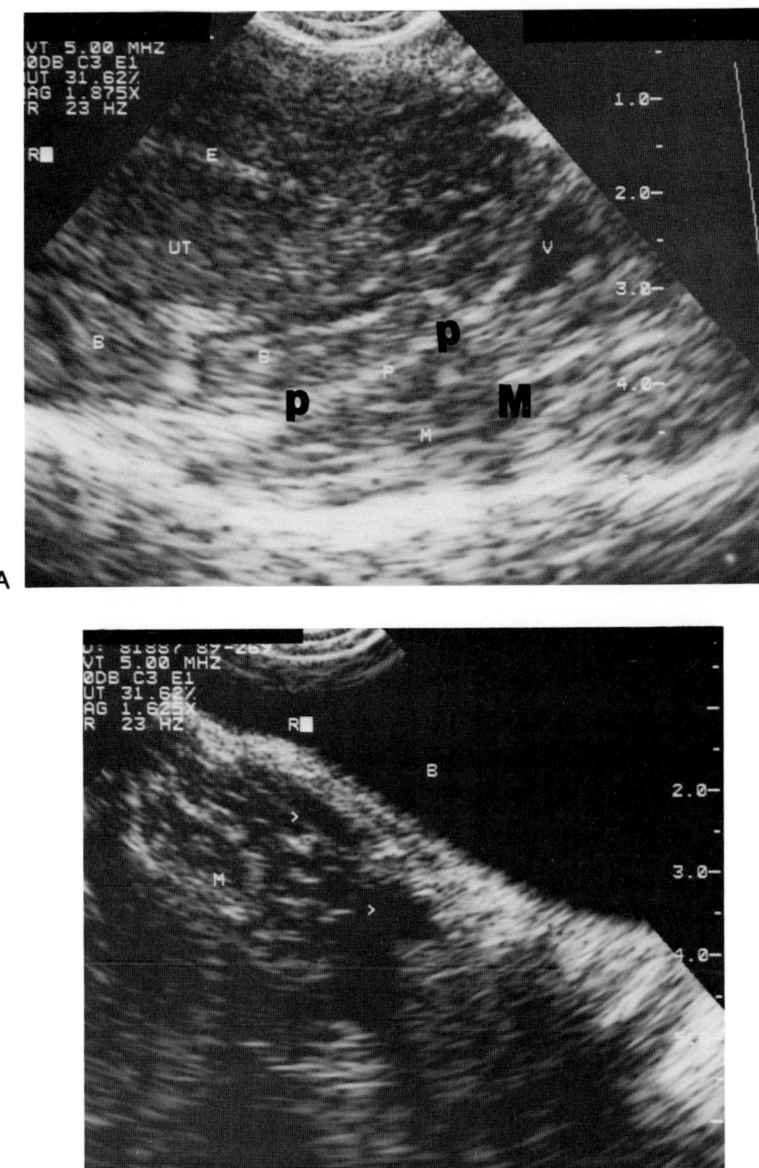

Fig. 3-16. **(A)** T-pelvic view showing uterus (UT) and single line endometrium (E) with bowel (B) in the cul-de-sac. Levator muscle (small white M and large black M) is noted along the left pelvic side wall. A branch of the hypogastric vein (V) is seen running beneath the pelvic peritoneum (small white P and large black P). **(B)** Image of psoas muscle (M) with iliac vein (white arrowheads) and right anterior pelvis and bladder (B) obtained by directing the transducer tip to the right and anteriorly.

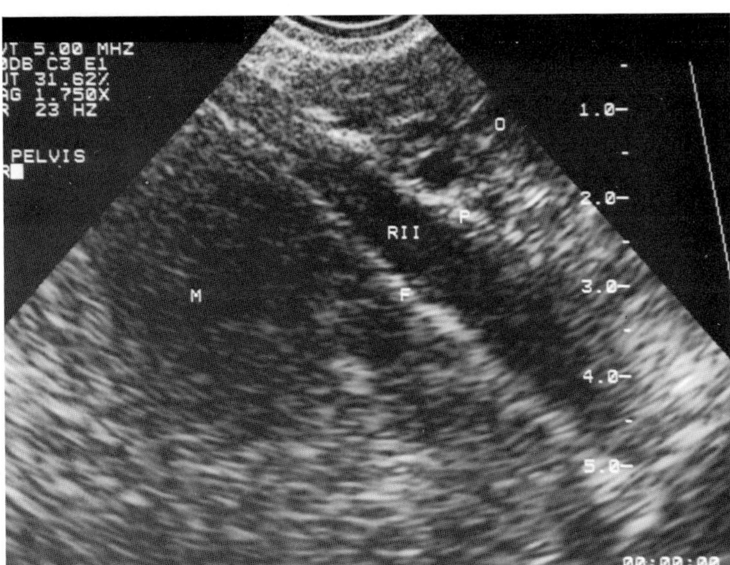

Fig. 3-17. Pelvic side wall showing the right internal iliac vein (RII). The obturator muscle (M) is imaged as a mixed echo pattern beneath the vein. The edge of the right ovary is seen (O). Note the hyperechoic reflection of the peritoneum and fat over the vein (P) and the fascia overlying the muscle (F).

GAIN

One point of confusion to the new sonographer is the gain setting and the concept of anechoic, isoechoic, and hyperechoic or hypoechoic echogenicity (Table 3-3).

The gain controls the amount of amplification applied to the reflected signal or echo. The gain setting may be expressed in decibels or as a ratio of the output to input signals. When the gain setting is turned up, almost any structure can be made to appear hyperechogenic or white on the display screen; when the gain is turned down, anechoic or dark cystlike structures can be produced in any pelvic organ.

Baltarowich et al.[18] have suggested that the uterine myometrium should be used as a marker of average echogenicity and used for comparison with other pelvic structures. Pelvic structures can then be judged as hyperechogenic or hypoechogenic compared with

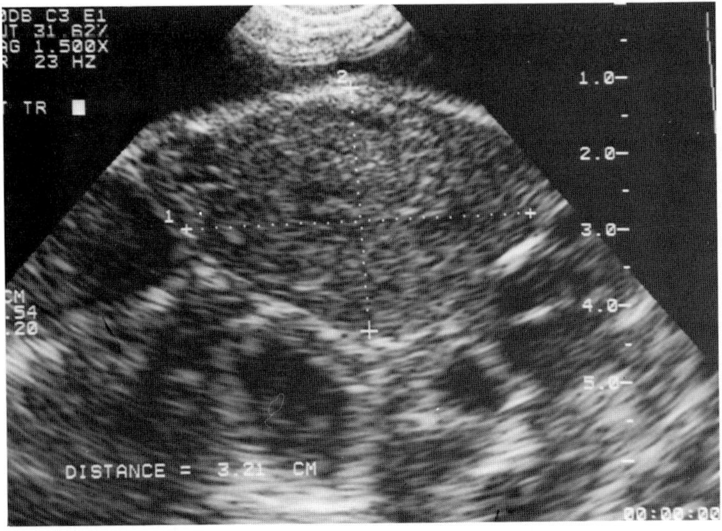

Fig. 3-18. T-pelvic view of the uterus with multiple fluid-filled loops of small bowel below the uterus.

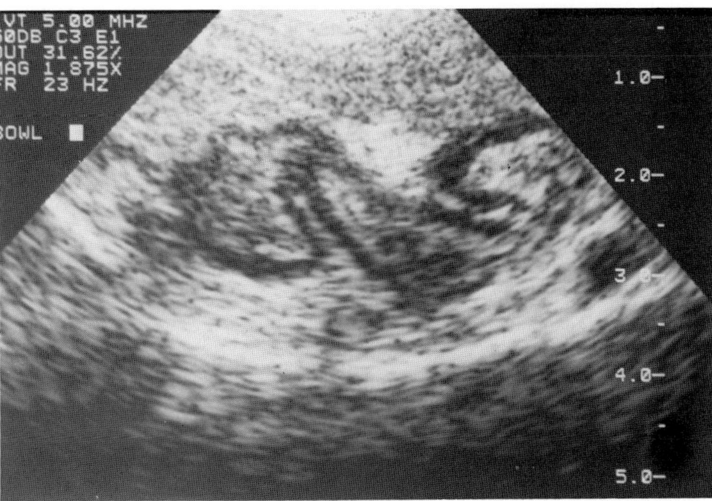

Fig. 3-19. Small bowel with some solid bowel contents.

Table 3-3. Ultrasound Terms as Applied to Transvaginal Ultrasound

Hyperechoic	Increased echogenicity; appears white on the screen. In pelvic sonography, the echogenicity is generally compared with that of the myometrium and bladder.
Hypoechoic	Decreased echogenicity; appears darker than the myometrium.
Anechoic	No echo; appears black, similar to the bladder.
Isoechoic	Has the same echo texture as the myometrium.

the uterus. A pelvic structure with the same echogenicity as the uterus would be considered isoechogenic. Gain settings are adjusted to produce an anechoic (dark) bladder without internal echoes and to give the uterus a consistent and homogeneous echogenicity. It may be made brighter or darker by adjusting the gain setting as the sonographer desires. The related echogenicity and distal acoustic properties of other structures can be compared with those of the uterus and bladder using the terms hyperechoic, hypoechoic, or anechoic.

TIME-GAIN COMPENSATION

The time-gain compensation (TGC) allows structures of equal echogenicity to be displayed with equal brightness regardless of their depth within the body. The TGC compensates for sound beam attenuation with increased tissue depth. It consists of a near gain that controls the amount of amplification in the near field, a slope delay that determines the depth at which the TGC slope begins, and the slope rate or rate at which returning echo signals are amplified with respect to depth. By adjusting the TGC, structures deep in the pelvis can be given the same display brightness as structures nearer the transducer.

DOCUMENTATION

A vital part of every ultrasound examination is a formal report and hard copy documentation, usually in the form of photographs, radiograph films, or videotape recordings. The busy clinician who does a quick ultrasound with a report consisting of only a few lines in the chart or a note stating the pelvic ultrasonographic examination was normal with no formal documentation may find this type of practice a medicolegal trap. More important, it is less than ideal medical practice. Third-party payers tend to look on such a practice as inadequate and may refuse to pay for such an ultrasound examination. A printed form can be very helpful in providing a format for an organized ultrasound report.

There are several ways to make hard copy prints, including Polaroid pictures and matrix cameras that give the typical radiographic film images; more recently, thermal printers have become a popular and relatively inexpensive mechanism of preserving images. Such photographs may be attached to the ultrasound report or filed in some organized manner. Videotapes are also a popular method of preserving images. A formal interpretation or written summary should be given.

REFERENCES

1. Callen PW: Ultrasonographic evaluation of pelvic disease. p. 209. In Goldberg HI (ed): International Radiology and Diagnostic Imaging Modalities. Department of Radiology, University of California, San Francisco, 1982
2. Fleischer AC, James AE, Jr, Millis JB, Julian C: Differential diagnosis of pelvic masses by gray scale sonography. AJR 131:469, 1978
3. Sakamoto C, Nakano H: The echogenic endometrium and alterations during the menstrual cycle. Int J Gynaecol Obstet 20:255, 1982
4. Fleischer AC, Kalemeris GC, Entman SS, James AE: Sonographic depiction of normal and abnormal endometrium with histopathologic correlation. J Ultrasound Med 5:445, 1986
5. Lenz S, Lindenberg S: Ultrasonic evaluation of endometrial growth in women with normal cycles during spontaneous and stimulated cycles. Hum Reprod 5:377, 1990
6. Randal JM, Fisk NM, McTavish A, Templeton AA: Transvaginal ultrasonic assessment of endometrial growth in spontaneous and hyperstimulated cycles. Br J Obstet Gynaecol 96:954, 1989
7. Grunfeld L, Walker B, Bergh PA et al: High-resolution endovaginal ultrasonography of the endometrium: a noninvasive test for endometrial adequacy. Obstet Gynecol 78:200, 1991
8. Li TC, Nuttall L, Klentzeris L, Cooke ID: How well does ultrasonographic measurement of endometrial thickness predict the results of histological dating? Hum Reprod 7:1, 1992
9. Fleischer AC, Gordon AN, Entman SS, Kepple DM: Transvaginal sonography of the endometrium: current and potential clinical applications. p. 583. In Fleischer AC, Romero R, Manning F et al (eds): The Principles and Practice of Ultrasonography in Obstetrics and Gynecology. 4th Ed. Appleton & Lange, Norwalk, CT, 1991
10. Thaler I, Bruck A: Transvaginal sonography and dopplear measurements-physical considerations. p. 1. In Timor-Tritsch IE, Rottem S (eds): Transvaginal Sonography. 2nd Ed. Elsevier, New York, 1991
11. DuBose TJ, Hill LW, Hennigan HW, Jr et al: Sonography of arcuate uterine blood vessels. J Ultrasound Med 4:229, 1985
12. Pache TD, Wladimiroff JW, de Jong FH et al: Growth patterns of nondominant ovarian follicles during the normal menstrual cycle. Fertil Steril 54:638, 1990
13. Pache TD, Wladimiroff JW, Hop WCJ, Fauser BCJM: How to discriminate between normal and polycystic ovaries. A transvaginal ultrasound study. Radiology 183:421, 1992
14. Davis JA, Gosink BB: Fluid in the female pelvis: cyclic patterns. J Ultrasound Med 5:75, 1986
15. Timor-Tritsch IE, Bar-Yam Y, Elgali S, Rottem S: The technique of transvaginal sonography with the use of a 6.5-MHz probe. Am J Obstet Gynecol 158:1019, 1988
16. Rosen DJD, Ben-Nun I, Arvel Y et al: Transvaginal ultrasonography quantitative assessment of accumulated cul-de-sac fluid. Am J Obstet Gynecol 166:542, 1992
17. Lande IM, Hill MC, Cosco FE, Kator NN: Adnexal and cul-de-sac abnormalities: transvaginal sonography. Radiology 166:325, 1988
18. Baltarowich OH, Kurtz AB, Pasto ME et al: The spectrum of sonographic findings in hemorrhagic ovarian cysts. AJR 148:901, 1987

4

Artifacts in Ultrasound

Melvin G. Dodson

ACOUSTIC ARTIFACTS

Recognizing sonic artifacts in ultrasound is important in order to interpret images correctly and to minimize errors. Image artifacts may result from the basic physical properties of sound, from the interaction of sound with body structures, from the processing of ultrasound data, or from the equipment used. Artifacts can produce images of masses or structures that do not really exist in the patient or may distort or misplace real masses or organ structures. As noted by Goldstein and Madrazo,[1] ultrasound equipment makes three assumptions in processing acoustic data that may not be true and may lead to artifacts.

1. The equipment assumes a uniform acoustic velocity of 1,540 m/s through all tissues; therefore, variations in the velocity of sound through different tissues will produce a distance measurement error, and the image will be placed improperly in relationship to surrounding structures.
2. The ultrasound equipment assumes that the sound waves travel in a straight line; bending of the sound wave secondary to refraction or reflection as it passes from one acoustic medium into another will also result in artifactual placement of the reflected sound in the ultrasound image; for example, when the reflecting surface is perpendicular to the beam axis, multiple reflections (specular reflections) may result and give a tissue density distal to the reflection that is not present.
3. All detected reflections are on the central ray of the transducer beam.[1] This assumption may lead to lateral resolution difficulties or lateral image degeneration.

Commonly encountered ultrasound artifacts are due to absorption, reverberation, refraction, and reflection. Shadowing results from the reduced amplitude of echoes after passage through a structure with high reflectivity or absorption, as when a gallstone or calcified mass is imaged. The weak echoes distal to the object appear dark, giving an acoustic shadow.[2] Shadows frequently occur from bowel gas (Fig. 4-1). Acoustic shadows distal to calculi or solid objects, such as an intrauterine device (IUD), contain significantly fewer echoes, and the margins are defined more sharply than shadows distal to gas collections (Fig. 4-2). Acoustic shadows distal to calcified masses are referred to as clean shadows. Shadows distal to gas collections have been called dirty shadows and generally have low level echoes in the shadow with less distinct borders.

Shadowing may also occur at the edge of a curved object as a result of refraction of sound, rather than absorption. This type of shadow has also been called the critical angle phenomenon (Fig. 4-3).[3] Critical angle acoustic shadowing or edge shadows may occur when sound passes from one medium into a medium of higher acoustic velocity. At the critical angle, total reflection occurs and a shadow is noted. Refraction shadows may also occur when sound passes from a medium with higher velocity into a medium with a lower velocity (Figs. 4-4 to 4-6).[4]

Reverberation artifact results from multiple reflection of the same sound wave. When sound waves are reflected from a tissue-gas interface with a high acoustic impedance, the strong returning echo may again be reflected by the transducer face and re-enter the patient (Figs. 4-7 and 4-8; also see Fig. 4-1).[5] When the echo is reflected at the tissue-gas interface a second time and detected by the transducer, the signal will be incorrectly registered as an echo twice as deep as the original soft tissue-air interface. Multiple reflections result in multiple echoes of the same reflection, producing reverberation artifacts.[4]

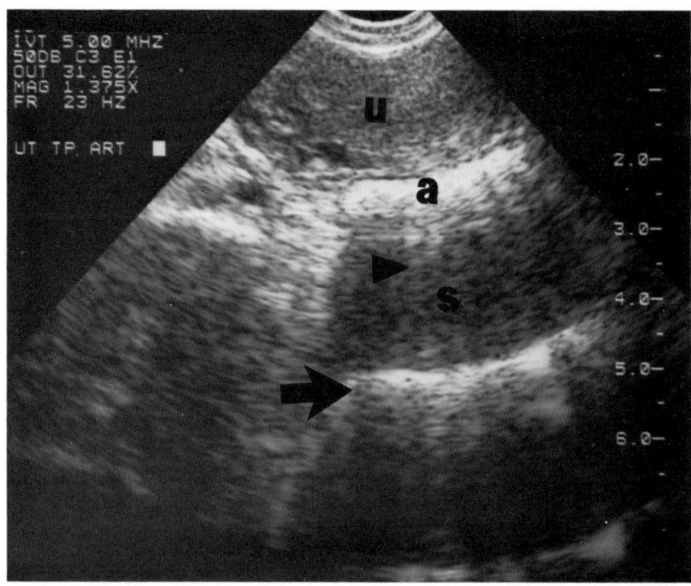

Fig. 4-1. Trans-pelvic (T-pelvic) image of the uterus (u) with air (a) in bowel in the cul-de-sac. Note the hyperechoic air in bowel with shadowing (s). A reverberation artifact is also present (arrow). There are also some smaller reverberation artifacts (arrowhead). There is a third reverberation artifact at the bottom of the image. Note that the distances between the artifact are the same.

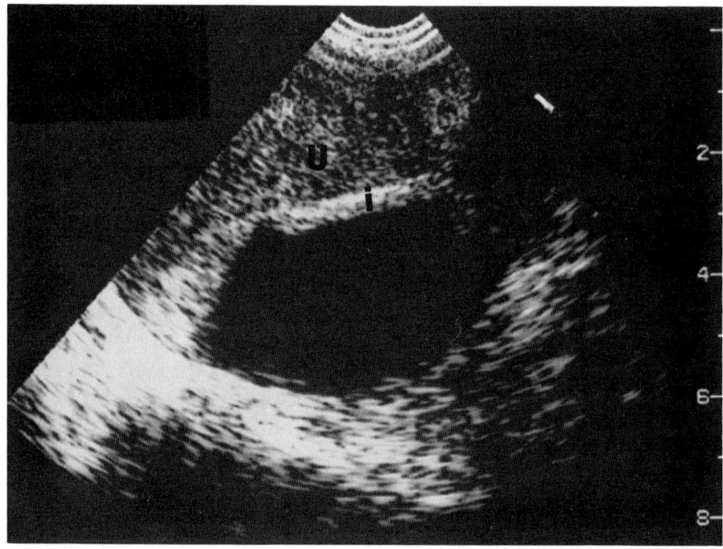

Fig. 4-2. Hyperechoic Progestasert IUD in the endometrial cavity with a posterior clean shadow, uterus (U), and IUD (i).

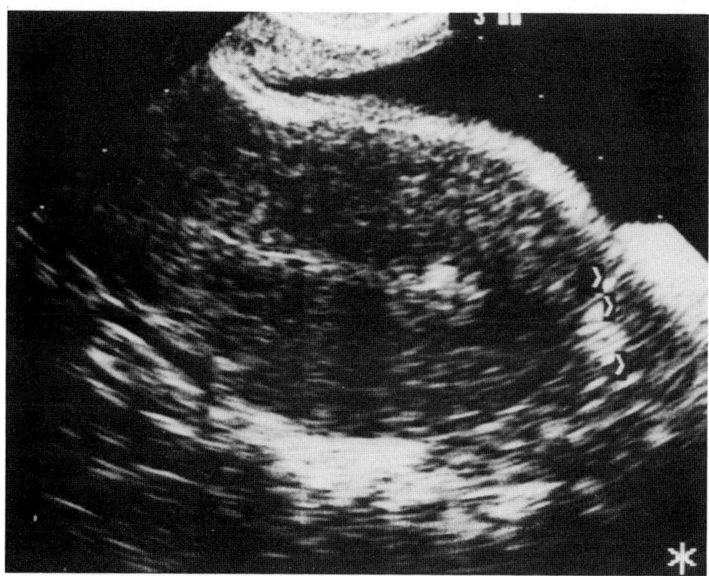

Fig. 4-3. AP-pelvic view of the uterus with critical angle shadow. Bladder is noted anteriorly. The endometrium is in the early follicular (day 10) phase. The critical angle shadow is outlined by arrows.

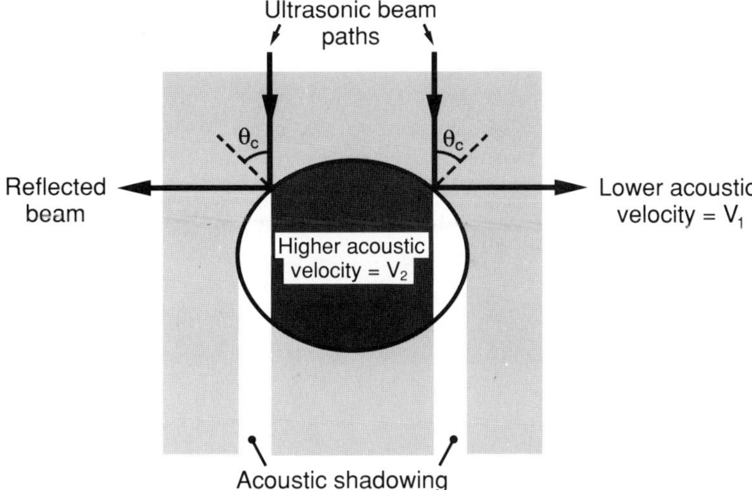

Fig. 4-4. Acoustic shadowing distal to a rounded region of an object with higher acoustic velocity that may occur when the critical angle, θ_c, of the incidence sound wave is exceeded, resulting in total reflection of the incident sound. (From Sommer et al,[4] with permission.)

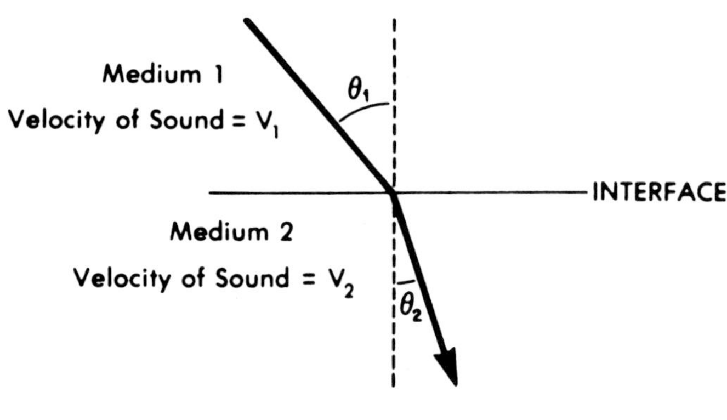

Fig. 4-5. Snell's law of refraction applied to ultrasound. Ratio of sinc of angle of incidence to sine of angle or refraction equals the ratio of velocities of sound in two media. (From Sommer et al,[4] with permission.)

The distance between each line or reverberation artifact corresponds to the distance between the transducer and the gas interface (Figs. 4-1 and 4-8). Each reverberation is generally smaller or weaker than the preceding artifact. Reverberation artifacts appear as a series of parallel lines with diminished intensity occurring at regular intervals and have been described as originating from gas-filled structures.[5] Prominent reverberation artifacts may occur because of poor contact between the vaginal transducer and the vagina (Fig. 4-9). Reverberation (multiple reflections of sound) within an anechoic mass may also occur. When reverberations are produced by a metal object or foreign body, a comet tail artifact may result (Fig. 4-10).

Reverberation artifacts may be noted in association with shadow artifacts distal to gas, such as air bubbles in the bowel (see Figs. 4-1 and 4-8). In contrast, as noted above, calcified stones produce high level echoes with anechoic, well-defined, clean shadows without reverberation artifacts. Most of the sound energy is absorbed by a stone, with only 20 to 30 percent being reflected. Therefore, the shadow is mainly due to absorption. Reverberation artifacts distal to stones are uncommon.[6]

When there are large impedance differences be-

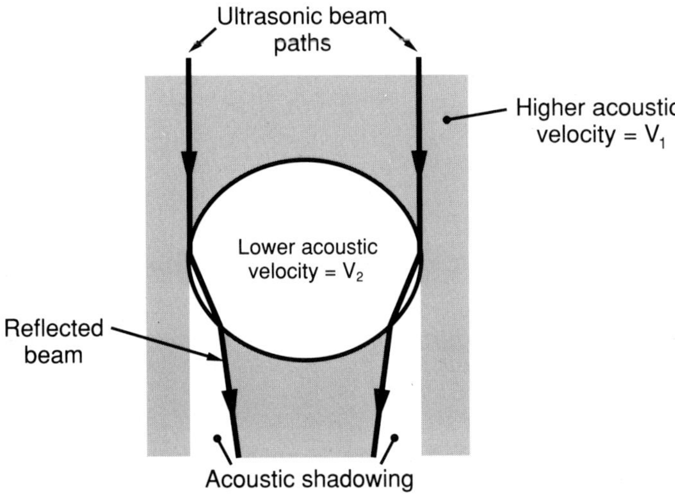

Fig. 4-6. Acoustic shadowing may occur as a result of refraction at the interface between two media of different acoustic velocities. (From Sommer et al,[4] with permission.)

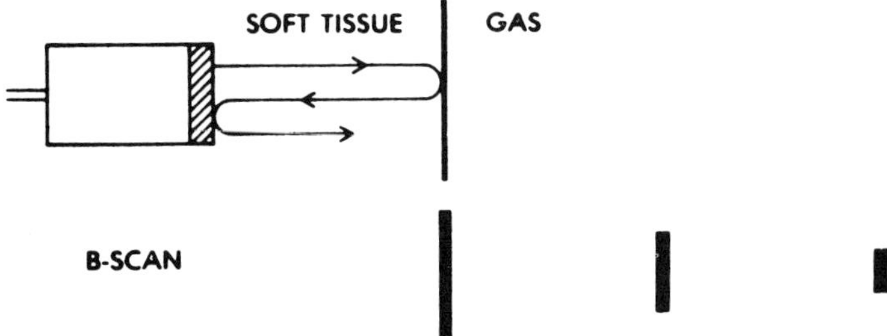

Fig. 4-7. Reverberations are due to complete sound reflection at a soft tissue-gas interface. When the sound beam returns to the transducer, it is reflected from the transducer and re-enters the patient. The B-scan reveals a series of parallel equidistant lines. The distance between each line corresponds to the distance between the transducer and the gas interface. Each reverbation is weaker than the preceding one. (From Laing,[5] with permission.)

tween tissue, most of the sound will be reflected and transmission will be small. Acoustic impedance is a product of the density of the tissue and the speed of the sound in that tissue. A soft tissue-gas boundary is an example of a large impedance difference with almost complete sound reflection. Reverberation artifacts and acoustic shadowing commonly result from such a boundary. Therefore, the character of an acoustic shadow depends on the object casting the shadow and whether the shadow results from absorption, reflection, or refraction.

Ring-down artifacts are the solid streaks or series of parallel bands resulting from reverberation associated with a collection of gas that is often found within the gastrointestinal tract.[7] In vivo experiments have shown that a single layer or a single large bubble will not produce ring-down artifacts. Two layers of bubbles are required. The term ring-down has also been used to describe a mist or diffuse-appearing echoes between or following each reverberation artifact (see Fig. 4-9).[3,5] The term ring-down is also applied to the process by which a transducer loses energy. Each cycle of vibration decreases, and the system rings down. The comet tail is a reverberation artifact similar in appearance to ring-down but results from foreign bodies, particularly metal, and the reverberations are close together and short.

When the ultrasound signal takes a different path to and from a reflection, a position error or mirror image artifacts may occur. These artifacts may result in phantom images and split, double, or mirror images.

A split image artifact with widening or even dou-

A
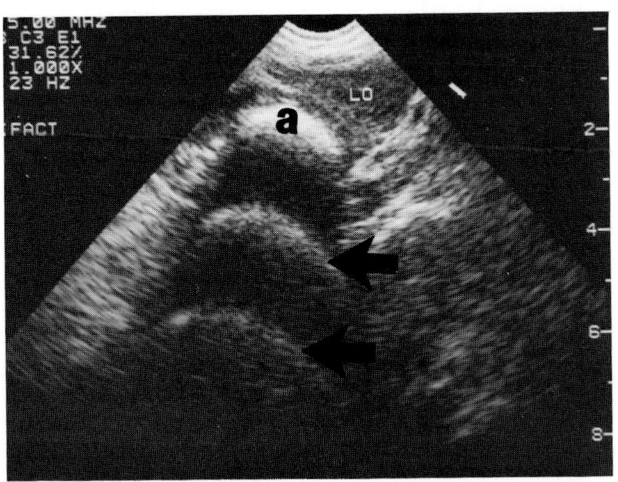

B
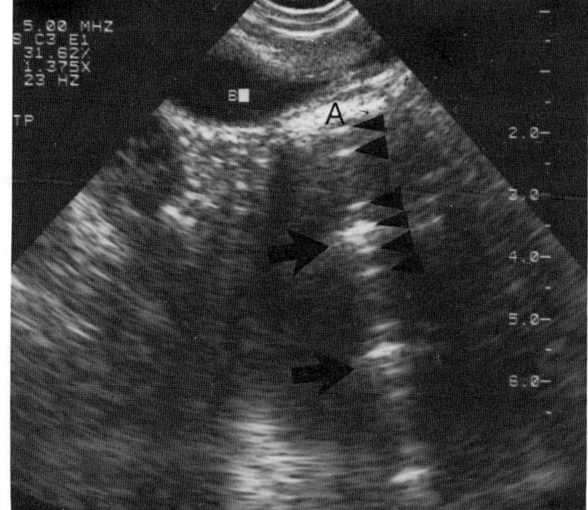

Fig. 4-8. **(A)** T-pelvic view of the left ovary (LO) with air (a) in the sigmoid colon below the ovary. Note the reverbation artifact (arrows) and shadowing. **(B)** Small bowel with hyperechoic air (a) with shadowing and reverberation artifact (arrow). Note that repeat reverberations become smaller. There are small reverberations in addition to the larger ones (arrowhead). The bladder (B) is at the top of the photo.

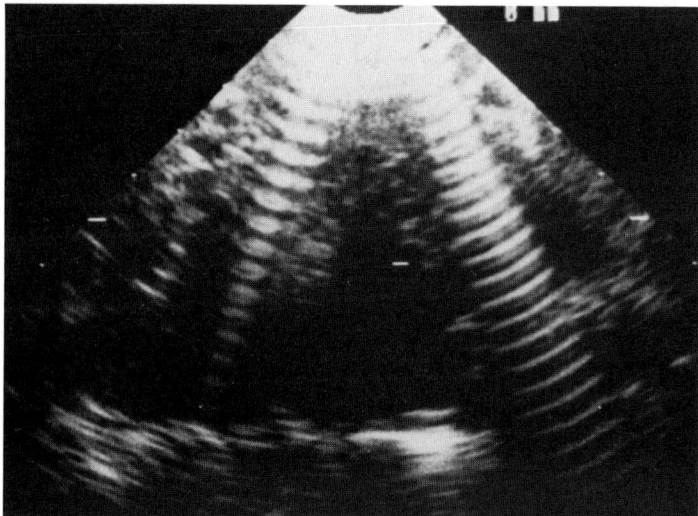

Fig. 4-9. Reverberation artifact secondary to poor contact between the transvaginal probe and the vagina.

bling of an image has been reported using a sector or linear array transducer placed in the midline during a transabdominal scan.[2] The artifact results from refraction of sound waves by the muscle-fat interface in the abdominal wall. The best means of recognizing such an artifact is to scan the patient in several planes. The sonographer should be very suspicious of any areas or lesions that cannot be seen in more than one plane. Real-time scanning is particularly suited for detecting and evaluating such artifacts.

Refraction occurs when sound crosses a boundary where a speed change occurs. Refraction of sound can cause a reflector to be placed improperly on the display.

Enhancement results from an increase in the relative amplitude of echoes after passage through structures with little attenuation.[2] Edge enhancement may also occur.

Acoustic speckling is a common cause of image degradation and results from construction and destruction interferences of returning echoes that give a scattered distribution suggesting a tissue texture.

Side-lobe artifacts result from transducer side-lobe beams that are 1/100th the intensity of the main beam, but are still strong enough to produce images from stray reflections situated well off the central axis of the sound beam. These side-lobe artifacts are frequently noted when scanning the urinary bladder. Diffuse side-lobe artifacts may result from structures adjacent to cystic structures, as, for example, specular reflection in the bladder from side-lobe reflections from bowel gas lying beneath the bladder wall. Such artifacts may be eliminated or reduced by repositioning the patient so the gas-filled bowel falls away from the area where the artifact is being generated and by reducing the machine's output or changing the transducer angulation.

An artifact termed slice-thickness artifact results in

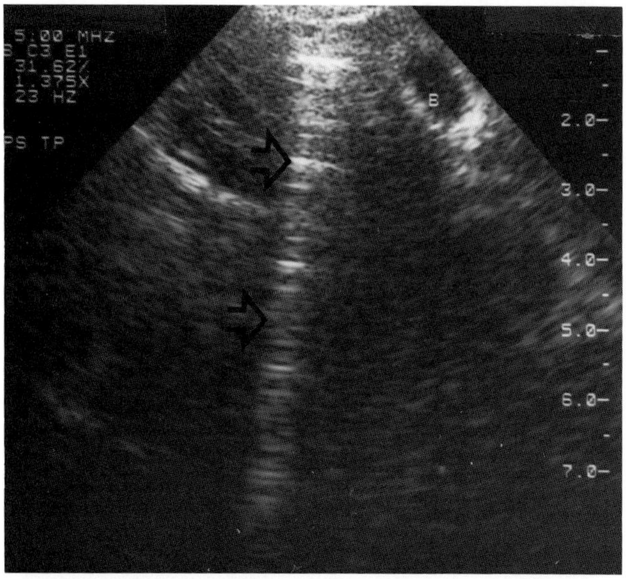

Fig. 4-10. Several metal clips along the left pelvic wall placed during a previous surgery. Note the reverberation artifact sometimes referred to as a comet tail artifact (open arrows). There is misting or ring-down between stronger reverberation echoes. Note the small bowel (B) next to the pelvic side wall.

lateral resolution blurring of the image owing to the equipment's interpretation of a thin scan plane while, in fact, reflections lateral to the central sound ray are registered. A strong reflection located laterally to the central beam will be imaged as if in the central beam. Slice-thickness artifacts widen the image with increased receiver gain, transducer beam width, and slice plane tilt. Although this type of artifact is more commonly seen in static B-scanners, misalignment in scan plane consistency of sector scanners can also result in slice-thickness artifacts.[1]

REFERENCES

1. Goldstein A, Madrazo BL: Slice-thickness artifacts in gray-scale ultrasound. J Clin Ultrasound 9:365, 1981
2. Kremkau FW, Taylor KJW: Artifacts in ultrasound imaging. J Ultrasound Med 5:227, 1988
3. Sample WF, Erikson K: Basic principles of diagnostic ultrasound. p. 365. In Sarti DA, Sample DF (eds): Diagnostic Ultrasound—Text and Cases. GK Hall Medical Publishers, Boston, 1980
4. Sommer FG, Filly RA, Minton MJ: Acoustic shadowing due to refractive and reflective effects. AJR 132:973, 1979
5. Laing FC: Commonly encountered artifacts in clinical ultrasound. Semin Ultrasound 4:27, 1983
6. Sommer FG, Taylor KJW: Differentiation of acoustic shadowing due to calculi and gas collections. Radiology 135:399, 1980
7. Avruch L, Cooperberg PL: The ring-down artifact. J Ultrasound Med 4:21, 1985

5

The Uterus

Melvin G. Dodson
Thierry D. Pache

Transvaginal ultrasound examination of the uterus allows evaluation of uterine position, size, and shape and a detailed view of the myometrium. Uterine enlargement, leiomyomas, and congenital anomalies of the uterus can be diagnosed. Vessels coursing through the myometrium can be readily visualized.

SIZE AND SHAPE OF THE UTERUS

One of the problems with current estimates of normal uterine size is that there is still no large ultrasound study evaluating the biometry of the uterus in the living state that takes into consideration such variables as age, parity, and phase of the menstrual cycle, all of which are known to affect uterine size. The use of autopsy data as a reference for normal uterine size is based on measurements of morbid organs not being perfused with blood. Also, such measurements do not consider the variation in the menstrual cycles. In addition, when autopsy or hysterectomy specimens are used, there are clearly fewer measurements of uterine size in younger patients for obvious reasons.

Any biometric measurements, such as height, weight, or measurement of the uterus or ovaries, that take a mean value of a population and utilize two standard deviations (SDs) as the limits of normal automatically label 5 percent of the population as abnormal. Using these types of measurements, most professional basketball players would be labeled abnormal in terms of their height. Clearly, we know the approximate size of the uterus. Callen[1] considered the upper limits of the normal nongravid uterus to be 4 cm in anterior posterior diameter (thickness), 7 cm in length, and 4 cm in diameter in the transverse plane (width). Fleischer et al.[2] suggested a normal uterine size of 3 cm anterior posterior with a length of 8 cm. *Gray's Anatomy* notes the normal uterus to be 7.5 cm in length, 5 cm in breadth, and 2.75 cm in thickness.[3] However, again, the data from *Gray's Anatomy* do not take into consideration the age, parity, and hormonal status of the patient.[3] In our ultrasound experience, these normal values are reasonable except that the thickness of the in situ uterus as measured by ultrasound is more commonly in the range of 4 cm.

From the clinician's perspective, more important issues than the average size of the uterus are the upper limits of normal and the significance of a measurement above those limits. We use uterine measurements of 5 cm in width, 4 cm in the anterior posterior plane in thickness, and 8 cm in length as the general upper limits of a normal uterus. Measurements above these limits do not necessarily indicate pathology, but do require a detailed search for an explanation, such as leiomyomas, congenital anomalies, adenomyosis, pregnancy or complications of pregnancy, an enlarged endometrium secondary to a polyp or cancer, or adherence of adjacent structures, such as the ovary, that might be mistakenly imaged as a part of the uterus, giving an artifactual uterine enlargement. However, small leiomyomas may still be found in uteri with biometric measurements well within the limits of normal.

Ultrasound biometric measurement may be inaccurate when taken in the wrong plane. The width and thickness of the uterine fundus should be taken in the largest imaged plane in the uterine fundus. Measurements of the uterus taken in the trans-pelvic plane are sometimes inaccurate because the lateral limits of the uterus blend into the broad ligament, and the exact lateral boundaries may be difficult to determine accurately (Table 5-1). Likewise, measurements of the an-

Table 5-1. Factors Causing Variation or Inaccuracies in Uterine Measurement

Oblique plane imaged.
Lateral border of the uterus indistinct from the broad ligament, measuring the posterior bladder wall as a part of the uterus
Hormonal changes during the menstrual cycle, including adjacent structures, such as the ovaries or bowel in the uterine measurement

terior posterior diameter of the uterus in a trans-pelvic (T-pelvic) plane may produce an organ plane that does not truly represent the thickness in the anterior posterior dimensions, but represents a conical slice. This is particularly common when measuring the uterus, since the uterus may be bent and retroverted or anteverted.

One indication that an inaccurate oblique plane has been imaged is a significant discrepancy between the thickness of the anterior and posterior wall that is noted in only one plane; for example, an increase in the posterior wall thickness in the T-pelvic plane, but not in the anterior posterior-pelvic (AP-pelvic) plane measurements. However, consistent differences in the thickness of the anterior or posterior wall that are noted on both the AP-pelvic and T-pelvic planes may occur secondary to a leiomyoma or adenomyosis. Thickening of the posterior uterine wall has been reported to be particularly common with adenomyosis. There is frequently enhancement of the posterior bladder wall that makes it appear thicker. Imaging the posterior bladder wall as a part of the uterus will result in an inaccurate anterior posterior uterine measurement.

Weiner et al[4] compared ultrasonographic measurements of uterine volume with measurements using water displacement after hysterectomy. The uterine volume was calculated by ultrasound using the formula for a prolate ellipsoid: V = 0.5236 · length (external cervical os to fundus) · largest anterior posterior diameter · largest transverse diameter. There was a large potential discrepancy relative to the typical size of the uterus (−33.6 to +37.6 percent). Weiner et al[4] and Goldstein and colleagues[5] noted the clinical practice of expressing uterine size by palpation in terms of "menstural weeks" of a comparable gravid uterus and stated that it would be more precise to measure uterine size sonographically and equate the corresponding volume to the gravid uterus. Goldstein et al[5] have estimated the total uterine volume in normal pregnancies as noted in Table 5-2. The use of the volume measurements of the uterus by the prolate

Table 5-2. Total Uterine Volume in the Gravid Uterus

Menstrual Weeks	*Uterine Volume (ml)*	*Standard Deviation*
5	79	16
6	109	21
8	190	17
10	296	12
12	383	29
14	494	31

(Data from Goldstein et al.[5])

ellipsoid is not precise enough to determine true uterine size to within one gestational week.[4]

The myometrium increases in size by about 3.2 percent per day during the follicular phase and 1.8 percent per day during the luteal phase, but abruptly returns to its unstimulated size during menses.[7] Therefore, some variation in size when measured at different times is real and results from hormonal changes during the menstrual cycle.

POSTMENOPAUSAL UTERUS

It is important not to apply normal values for the biometric measurements of uterine size of the menstruating patient to the postmenopausal patient or child. The upper size limit of the postmenopausal uterus has been suggested to be 3 cm in the anterior posterior diameter, with a cervical-fundal length of 8 cm. There is generally a homogeneous echo pattern, and the uterine cavity frequently is not imaged. A normal sized uterus in a postmenopausal woman may be abnormal or reflect continued estrogen stimulation. The patient who is only 1 to 3 years postmenopausal who still has significant endogenous estrogen production by the ovaries will have a larger uterus than the patient who is 10 to 15 years postmenopausal. Clinical judgment is needed in interpreting normality of uterine size in the postmenopausal patient.

Endometrial and myometrial thickness in postmenopausal women have recently been assessed by Zalud and colleagues.[7] One hundred and nine women aged 45 to 72 years volunteered for pelvic cancer screening and were scanned by using 5-MHz transvaginal ultrasound examination. Twenty (18 percent) had been using hormonal replacement therapy (HRT), either from 1 to 5 years or for longer than 5 years. The

Table 5-3. Myometrium Thickness Visualized by Vaginal Sonography in 109 Women with or without Hormonal Replacement Therapy

Subgroups According to Duration of Menopause	*One-Half Myometrial Thickness (mm)*[a]
1 to 5 years	1.16 ± 0.29 cm
6 to 10 years	1.19 ± 0.22 cm
11 to 15 years	1.18 ± 0.35 cm
More than 15 years	0.93 ± 0.13 cm
1 to 5 years, with HRT	1.13 ± 0.25 cm
More than 5 years, with HRT	1.17 ± 0.15 cm

[a] As measured from the anterior outer uterus to the anterior inner myometrium-endometrium border.

(Adapted from Zalud et al.[7], with permission.)

89 patients who were not receiving HRT (82 percent) were subdivided into four subgroups: a first group that was 1 to 5 years postmenopausal, a second group that was 6 to 10 years postmenopausal, a third group that was 11 to 15 years postmenopausal, and a fourth group that was more than 15 years postmenopausal (Table 5-3). Myometrial thickness in all four groups of patients without HRT did not change significantly over the years after menopause. Comparing myometrial thickness between the two groups with HRT and the four groups without HRT, no statistically significant difference could be demonstrated. Zalud and his collaborators[7] concluded that continuous HRT does not influence myometrial thickness. They also suggested that uterine involution is a slow process.

THE UTERUS IN CHILDREN

Transvaginal ultrasound is almost never used in newborns and young children because of their small vaginal size. Instead, because of their small overall size, transabdominal ultrasound can be done with high frequency probes giving good image resolution.

Nussbaum et al.[8] used transabdominal ultrasound to image the neonatal uterus (newborn, days 1 to 7). The mean uterine length was 3.4 cm (range, 2.3 to 4.6 cm). The uterus was tubular in 58 percent, and the anterior posterior diameter of the cervix was equal to the anterior posterior diameter of the fundus. The anterior posterior diameter of the fundus ranged from 0.8 to 2.1 cm with a mean of 1.26 ± 0.29 cm. The anterior posterior diameter of the cervix ranged from 0.8 to 2.2 cm with a mean of 1.41 ± 0.32 cm. The endometrial cavity was visualized as a thin echogenic line in 97 percent of cases, and the myometrial anechoic halo surrounding the endometrium was noted in 29 percent of cases. The length of the uterus correlated with birth weight. Because of maternal estrogen stimulation during intrauterine life, the neonate's uterus is much larger than the uterus during early childhood. After delivery, when the neonate is no longer exposed to maternal estrogen, estrogen levels drop rapidly and the uterus becomes smaller.

Table 5-4. Uterine Length in Children

	Range (cm)	*Mean (cm)*
Neonates[8]	2.3–4.6	3.4
Children (> 1 yr)[10]	2.0–3.3	2.8
Age 2–7[11,12]	2.0–4.2	2.5–3.3
Age 10[12]	2.2–4.8	3.5
Age 11[11]		3.5–4.2

(Data from Nussbaum et al,[8] Sample et al,[10] Orsini et al,[11] and Ivarsson et al.[12])

After the postnatal regression in uterine size in the newborn that occurs following removal of the infant from the estrogen environment of the uterus, the average uterine length at 1 month of age is 2.5 cm and the greatest average width is 1 cm.[9] The cervix accounts for two-thirds to five-sixths of the total uterine length, and the uterine corpus is one-half the diameter of the cervix.

In girls older than 1 year, uterine length has been reported to range from 2.0 to 3.3 cm with a mean of 2.8 cm.[10] Orsini et al[11] reported a mean uterine length of 3.3 cm from 2 to 7 years of age and of 3.5 to 4.2 cm by age 11. Ivarsson et al[12] noted a mean uterine length of 2.5 cm with a range from 2.0 to 3.5 cm at age 7 years, and 3.5 cm with a range from 2.2 to 4.8 cm at 10 years (Table 5-4).

UTERINE POSITION

When the bladder is empty, the uterus is the largest normal structure in the pelvis, and because of its central location it is generally the first structure visualized. However, it is not uncommon for the uterus to be deviated to one side. By definition, lateral deviation of the uterus takes place around the axis of the

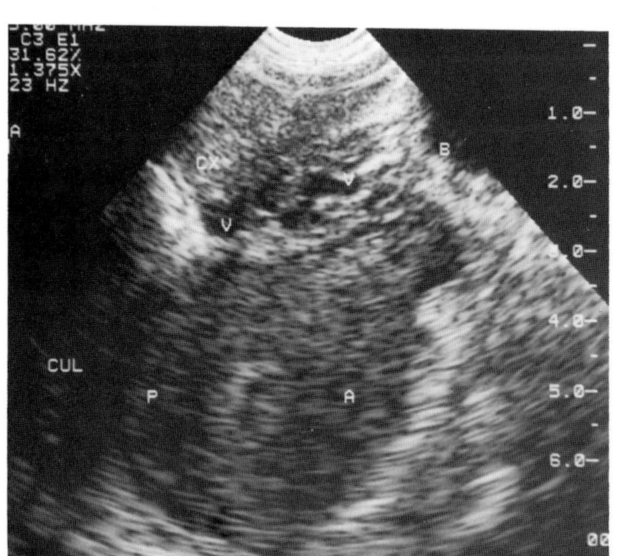

A

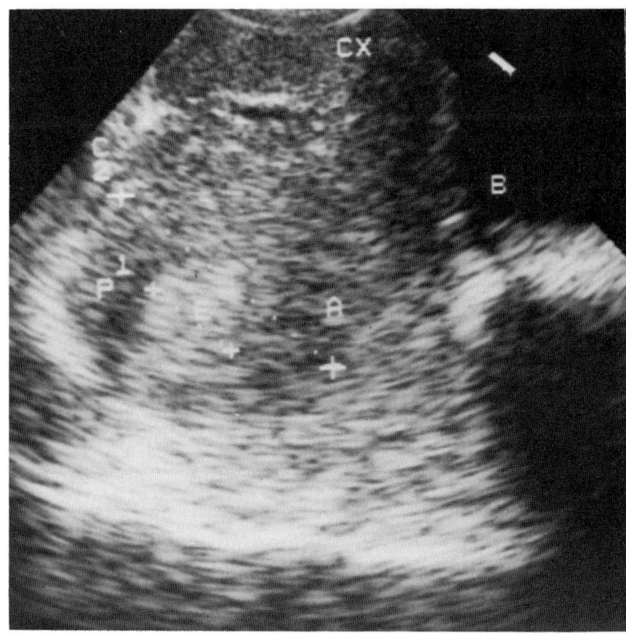

B

C

Fig. 5-1. (**A**) AP-pelvic view of a retroverted uterus. Note the tip of the bladder at the upper right (**B**). The cervix is at the left (CX). The uterus is acutely bent backward. Note the veins at the level of the internal os (V). There is a small amount of fluid in the cul-de-sac (CUL). The posterior wall of the uterus is on the left (P) and the anterior wall is on the right (A). (**B**) Retroverted uterus. CX, cervix; **B**, bladder; A, anterior wall of uterus; P, posterior wall of uterus; E, endometrium. The initial sound bang is at the top of the photograph. (**C**) Same image turned 90 degrees. The initial sound bang is now to the left of the photograph. This orientation and the image would compare to the patient's head to the right and feet to the left. The bladder and anterior adnexal wall are at the top and the buttocks and back are at the bottom of the photograph. Using this orientation, it is easy to appreciate the retroverted uterus.

uterine isthmus. It may occur as a normal variant or secondary to pelvic adhesions. The uterus may also be pushed to one side because of ovarian enlargement. The anterior posterior position of the uterus varies considerably. The uterus may be anteverted, midposition, or retroverted (Fig. 5-1A); the "version" of the uterus describes the organ position according to the angle between the uterine body and axis of the pelvis. The "flexion" of the uterus can be described as the angle that is observed between the axis of the uterine body and the axis of the cervix. Most commonly, in 85 percent of the cases the uterus is anteverted and anteflexed.

In addition, the position of the uterus may change depending on whether the bladder is full or empty. An acutely anteverted uterus may be pushed backward to a midposition by a full bladder. Interestingly, a retroverted uterus may be pulled forward by a very full bladder.

The position of the uterus may be confusing when using the transvaginal probe. One must recall that the image is being viewed rotated 90 degrees to the patient when the sound beam display originates at either the top or bottom of the cathode ray tube screen. An anteverted uterus may appear midposition or retroverted, and a truly retroverted uterus may actually appear to be facing in an opposite direction (Fig. 5-1B & C). Looking at the endometrial cavity of an acutely retroverted uterus, the sonographer may think that the image reverse has been changed when, in fact, the uterus is retroverted. One way to appreciate better the true position of the uterus is to rotate the AP-pelvic image 90 degrees.

LEIOMYOMAS

Leiomyomas are one of the most common benign neoplasms in women and have been reported to occur in up to 40 percent of women over the age of 35.[13] A leiomyoma may be suggested by generalized enlargement of the uterus, irregularities in the surface contour, distortion of the endometrial echo, or areas of hyper- or hypoechogenicity compared with the surrounding normal myometrium (Fig. 5-2, Table 5-5).

Calcifications or shadows may suggest areas for detailed evaluation for the presence of leiomyomas. Small leiomyomas (less than 3 cm) may be difficult to diagnose using ultrasound unless they are subserosal (Figs. 5-3 and 5-4). Since leiomyomas are composed of smooth muscle cells with acoustic characteristics similar to the surrounding normal uterine tissue, they may not be imaged as a separate entity. Uterine leiomyomas do not have a true capsule, and there may not be an acoustic interface and therefore no echo resulting from a structural boundary. Diagnosis may be suggested by indirect evidence, such as uterine enlargement or distortion of the endometrial or uterine contour, calcification, or degeneration within the leiomyomas.

Bowie[14] has described an indefinite uterus pattern in which the outline of the uterus or the uterus per se cannot be defined clearly. This pattern is most commonly caused by uterine leiomyomas or pelvic inflammatory disease (Figs. 5-5).

A submucosal leiomyoma within the uterine cavity

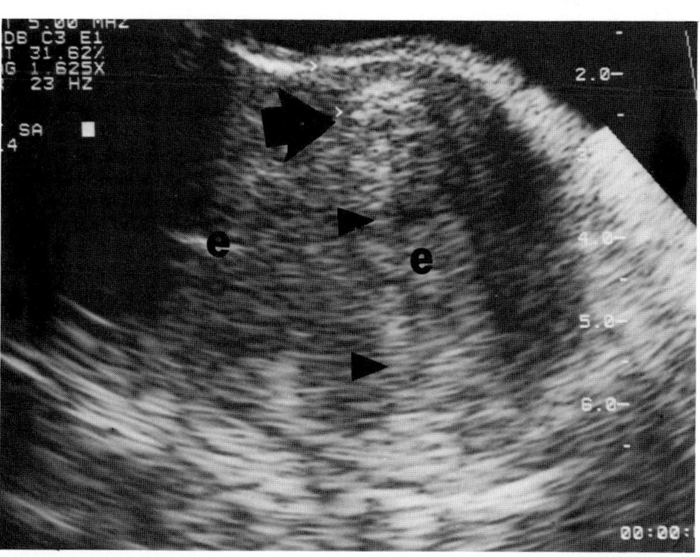

Fig. 5-2. AP-pelvic view of the uterus showing an enlarged uterus with an anterior posterior diameter of 5.1 cm (normal is 4 cm or less). There is an irregularity of the anterior uterine wall with a hyperechoic area (large arrow) with posterior enhancement (arrowheads), indicating a small uterine leiomyoma. The endometrium (e) is not well visualized because of the enhancement and shadows.

Table 5-5. Sonographic Signs of Leiomyoma

Contour irregularity
Altered echo texture
Diffuse uterine enlargement
Localized uterine enlargement
Calcification with shadowing
Indefinite uterus

may be imaged as an area of increased echogenicity and may be mistaken initially for blood, mucus, or a polyp in the uterine cavity. Submucosal leiomyomas may later prolapse through the cervix.[15]

Dudiak et al[16] used a systematic approach to evaluate the uterus. This approach may be helpful in diagnosing leiomyomas. The uterus is divided into multiple anatomic areas. Each area is evaluated separately: fundus; right and left cornu; anterior, posterior, right, and left corpus; and anterior, posterior, right, and left isthmus (Fig. 5-6). Using this technique of evaluating separated areas of the uterus, Dudiak et al[16] noted an ultrasound sensitivity in diagnosing leiomyomas of 60 percent, a specificity of 99 percent, and an overall accuracy of 87 percent. However, myomas as large as 3 cm were missed.

Using ultrasound Gross et al[17] noted a sensitivity in detecting leiomyomas of 60 percent. The most frequent sonographic finding of a leiomyoma, noted in 76 percent of cases, was an irregular uterine contour. An altered echo texture was noted in 68 percent, and uterine enlargement was present in 66 percent of cases (Fig. 5-7). The irregular uterine contour may be manifested by a bulbous fundus, lobularity of the uterus, or a focal mass. Anterior contour irregularity can be seen easily in Figure 5-8 in a patient with a full bladder (also see Figs. 5-3 and 5-4).

Hypoechoic or hyperechoic changes in echo texture may be seen in association with leiomyomas (Figs. 5-5 and 5-7). Cystic degeneration may also be noted. Increased attenuation of sound and calcification are occasionally noted. Calcification may appear as a hyperechoic focus with acoustic shadowing. Two or more abnormal sonographic findings were noted in 94 percent of patients in the series of Gross et al.[17] However, even using a retrospective review, no abnormalities were noted in 22 percent of patients with proven leiomyomas. Uterine size greater than 8 by 5 by 4 cm ($l \cdot w \cdot h$) in the multiparous patient should be considered suspicious for leiomyomas or other pathology.[17]

ADENOMYOSIS

The incidence of adenomyosis has been reported in autopsy data to vary from 10 to 50 percent and in surgical specimens to vary from 5.6 to 61.5 percent.[18] The wide variations in incidence probably reflect the number of histologic sections reviewed and the intensity of the search for adenomyosis. The symptoms generally attributed to adenomyosis include dysmenorrhea, pelvic pain, and menometrorrhagia. However, these symptoms are common gynecologic complaints that may be due to a variety of other pelvic pathology or may even be present without discernible

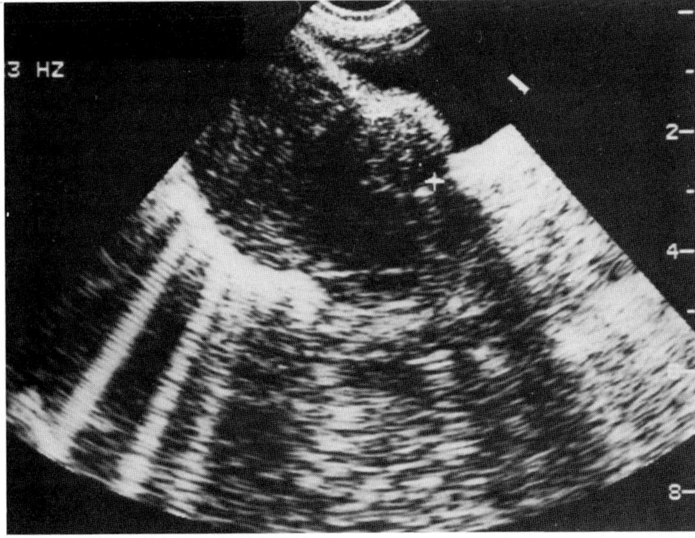

Fig. 5-3. AP-pelvic view of uterus shows a small 1.48-cm anterior subserosal leiomyoma distorting the anterior contour of the uterus and casting several acoustic shadows. There is an additional fundal fibroid. There are multiple reverberation artifacts probably secondary to air in the small bowel posterior to the uterus. Small fibroids are difficult to diagnose unless they are subserosal and distort the uterine contour or have an altered echo texture.

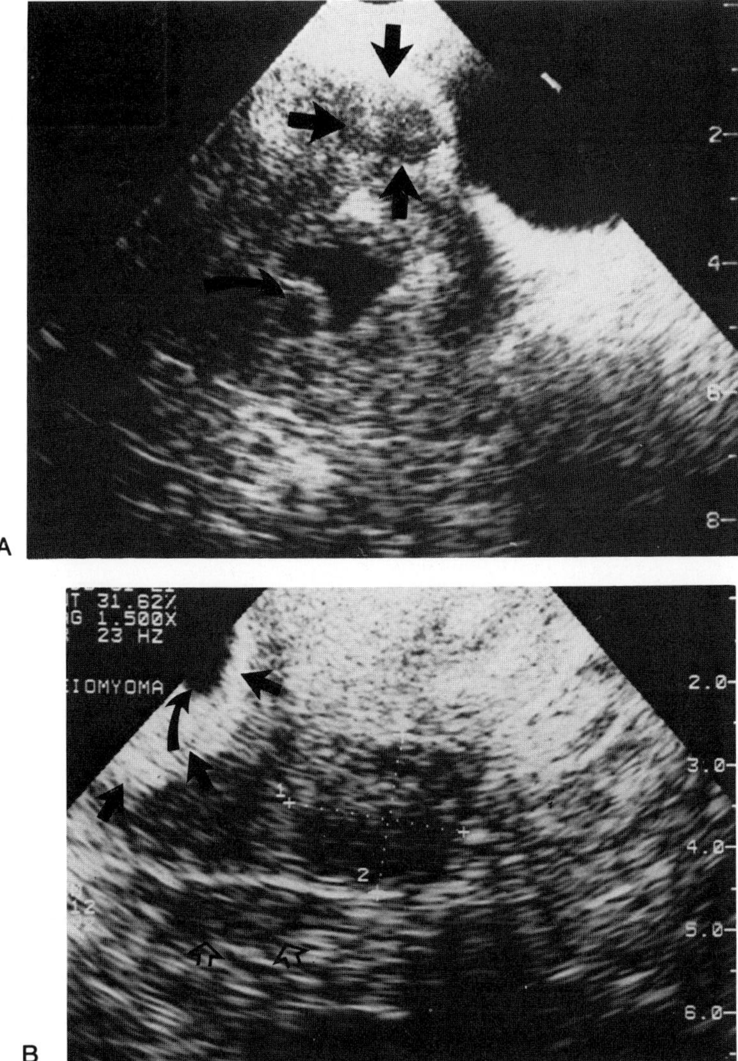

Fig. 5-4. (A) AP-pelvic view of the uterus at 6.5 weeks gestation showing an intrauterine pregnancy with an irregular endometrial cavity and an anterior leiomyoma bulging into the bladder (arrows). Fetus with fetal heart beat and yolk sac was noted out of the plane of this photograph. A small circular anechoic area could represent a twin or a small area of subchorionic hemorrhage (curved arrow). (B) The same patient 6 weeks later. Magnified AP-pelvic view of the uterus (fundus outlined by open arrows) with a well-developed gestational reaction at 12.6 weeks (black arrows pointing to gestational reaction of the endometrium). Note the gestational sac (curved black arrow) in the upper left. The small leiomyoma (1.9 by 2.1 cm, defined by cursors) is still noted subserosal on the anterior fundal uterus. The previous separate small anechoic area is no longer present.

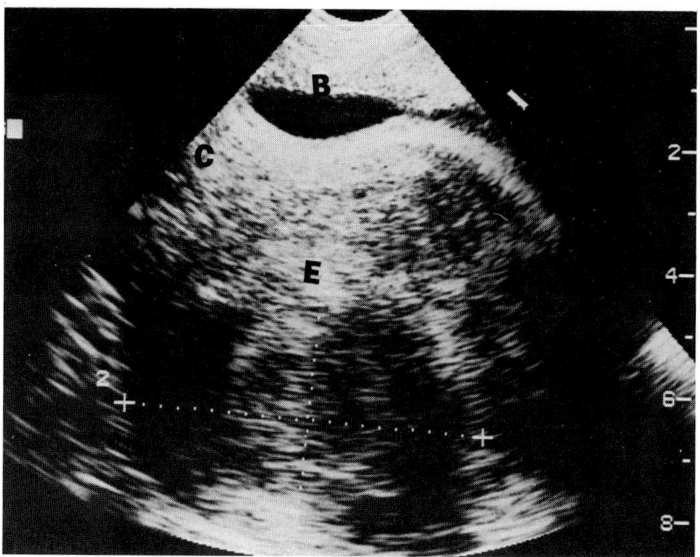

Fig. 5-5. Sagittal view of a 4.5 by 5.9 cm posterior uterine fibroid (cursor lines 1 and 2) impinging on the endometrium (E). The patient was complaining of menometrorrhagia. The posterior contour of the uterus is difficult to define because of the distortion of the echo pattern by the leiomyoma. The bladder is at the top (B), and the cervix is toward the left (C).

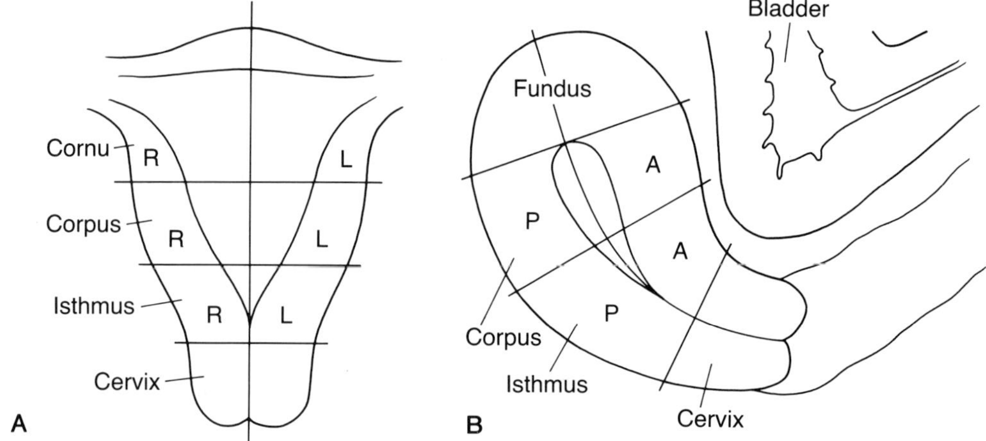

Fig. 5-6. (**A**) Diagram of the uterus in a longitudinal plane showing the fundus, right and left cornu, corpus and isthmus uterine area, and cervix. (**B**) Diagram of the uterus in a sagittal plane showing the fundus and anterior and posterior corpus, isthmus, and cervical areas. By carefully evaluating each uterine area, greater accuracy may be obtained in diagnosing small uterine leiomyomas.

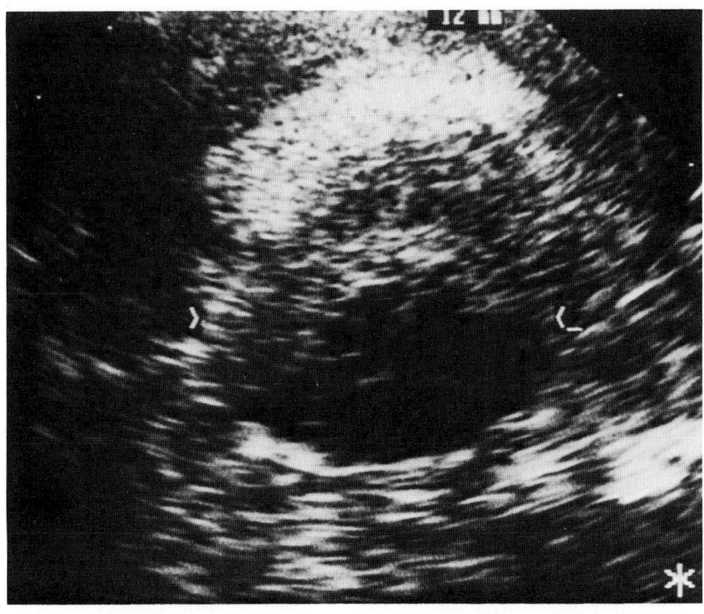

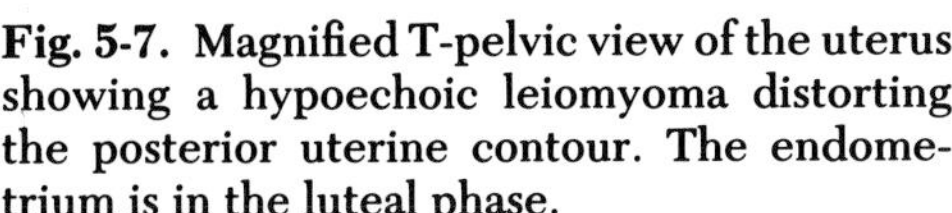

Fig. 5-7. Magnified T-pelvic view of the uterus showing a hypoechoic leiomyoma distorting the posterior uterine contour. The endometrium is in the luteal phase.

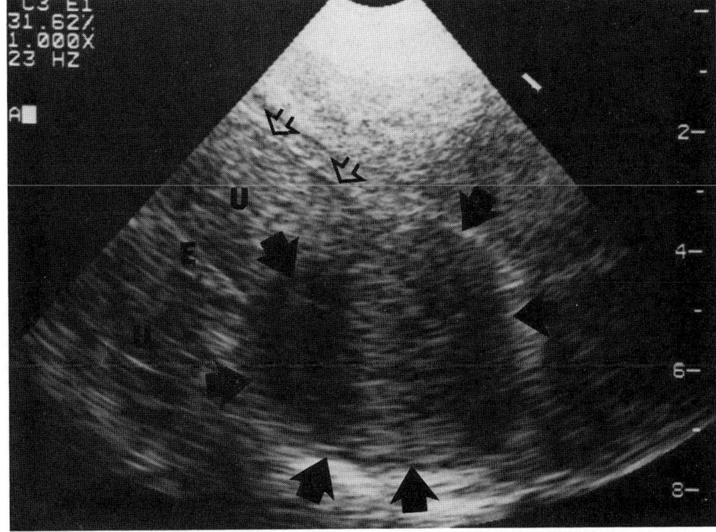

Fig. 5-8. Magnified AP-pelvic view of uterus (U) with large fundal fibroid (arrows) with distortion of the fundal contours and echo texture changes. The endometrium (E) is poorly developed. The cervix and lower uterine segment are not seen, but are to the left. The anterior wall of the uterus is at the top (open arrows). The posterior contour of the uterus is poorly defined.

gross or histologic pathology. In addition, adenomyosis is frequently associated with other common pelvic pathology, such as pelvic endometriosis (6 to 28 percent) or leiomyomata (19 to 56 percent).[18] Adenomyosis is suspected preoperatively, based on clinical evaluation, in only about 10 percent of cases.[19] Bohlman et al[19] noted uterine enlargement, especially with thickening of the posterior wall of the uterus, and an eccentric location of the endometrial cavity as potential ultrasonographic signs of adenomyosis. Calcification with acoustic shadowing or a decreased uterine echogenicity may also be associated with adenomyosis, especially if a leiomyoma can be excluded.

Adenomyosis may present either in a diffuse form or display a nodular pattern. Therefore, an ultrasound-defined roundish area in the uterine wall may not always be identified as leiomyoma. Fedele and colleagues[20] have evaluated the reliability of endovaginal ultrasound examination in the differential diagnosis of leiomyoma and adenomyoma. Their study was performed using 6.5-MHz probes in 405 women scheduled for myomectomy or hysterectomy because of symptomatic (menorrhagia, pelvic pain) uterine nodularities. Leiomyomas were defined as nodular heterogeneous structures with well-defined borders, whereas adenomyomas were recognized as heterogeneous circumscribed areas of the myometrium with indistinct margins, harboring anechoic lacunae. Special attention was paid to the pathologic analysis of the uterine nodularities of postoperative specimens. Data obtained from comparison of preoperative endovaginal ultrasound findings and postoperative pathologic observations are shown in Table 5-6.

Walsh et al[21] reported irregular cystic spaces 5 to 7 mm in size that disrupted the normal echo pattern of the uterus in patients with adenomyosis. This honeycomb pattern was thought to consist of blood-containing cavities. A honeycomb or polycystic myometrial pattern was noted in 36 percent of patients with adenomyosis. However, Seidler et al[18] did not find this honeycomb pattern in any of their eight patients with adenomyosis. Their most common finding was a diffuse uterine enlargement, with a few patients demonstrating a contour irregularity of the uterus.

Table 5-6. Reliability of Transvaginal Ultrasound Examination of the Uterus for the Diagnosis of Leiomyoma and Adenomyoma

	Adenomyoma (%)	*Leiomyoma (%)*
Sensitivity	87	96
Specificity	98	83
Positive predictive value	74	98
Negative predictive value	99	36

(Adapted from Fedele et al,[20] with permission.)

Table 5-7. Suggestive Ultrasound Findings of Adenomyosis

Diffuse uterine enlargement
Thickened posterior wall
Eccentric endometrial cavity
Hyperechoic density with acoustic shadow
Irregular cystic spaces, 5–7 mm
Disruption of homogeneous echo pattern

Although clinical diagnosis and ultrasound findings of adenomyosis may be found to be only suggestive (Table 5-7), Fedele and colleagues have attempted to clarify the use of endovaginal ultrasound in the diagnosis of diffuse adenomyosis, i.e., in the presence of endometrial glands and stroma in the myometrium.[22] Forty-three women presenting with menorrhagia, an enlarged uterus with no evidence of leiomyoma at clinical and transabdominal ultrasound examination, and normal endometrial biopsy findings were scanned to search for diffuse adenomysosis. Ultrasound criteria of the disease were as follows: visualization of one or more heterogeneous myometrial areas with indistinct margins that contained anechoic areas up to 3 mm in diameter. Sonographic findings were compared to anatomopathologic observations. The sensitivity and the specificity of 6.5-MHz endovaginal ultrasound examination of the uterus to diagnose diffuse adenomyosis were 80 percent and 74 percent, respectively. The positive predictive value (predictive value of a normal test) was 81 percent, whereas the negative predictive value (predictive value of an abnormal test) was 73 percent. In other words, transvaginal ultrasound may correctly identify diffuse adenomyosis in eight of ten women, when the disease is clinically suspected.

ULTRASOUND DIAGNOSIS OF CONGENITAL ANOMALIES OF THE UTERUS

The true prevalence of uterine malformations is not known. It has been suggested that only 25 percent of patients with uterine malformations experience reproductive problems (mainly uterine septa).[23,24] Many uterine malformations are clinically silent. Ultrasound can be helpful in diagnosing congenital anomalies of the uterus (also see Ch. 14). Nasri et al. studied 300 women using ultrasound and noted uterine malformations in 3 percent.[23]

Malini et al[25] have described the sonographic findings of congenital müllerian anomalies using the Buttram[24] classification (Fig. 5-9).

Class I: Segmental müllerian agenesis or hypoplasia
Cervical atresia: no cervix can be imaged, the uterus is round or oval with a short endometrial canal. The uterus is located high in the pelvis and may be displaced from the midline. Uterine agenesis: only a small remnant of fibrous tissue representing the uterus may be detected. There is no endometrial cavity or cervix. The differentiation between a small hypoplastic uterus and uterine agenesis may be difficult.

Class II: Unicornuate uterus
There is a distortion of the usual pear shape of the fundus and body of the uterus. The fundus appears asymmetric, with one cornual area appearing bulkier than the other. A rudimentary horn may be visualized. However, it must be differentiated from a bicornuate uterus. Marked uterine asymmetry and lateral displacement are suggestive of a unicornuate uterus (Fig. 5-10).

Class III: Uterus didelphys
Uterus didelphys appears as symmetric uterine halves or mirror images. Each half has an endometrial cavity and a cervix.

Class IV and V: Bicornuate uterus and septate uterus
Bicornuate uterus (class IV) and septate uterus (class V) are suggested by a broad uterine fundus or simultaneous visualization of two uterine horns or endometria. An anterior posterior/transverse diameter ratio of less than 0.6 is suggestive of a congenital anomaly, such as a bicornuate or septate uterus. Eccentric placement of a gestational sac in early pregnancy may also suggest a bicornuate or septate uterus. Mirror image artifacts should be ruled out, especially when using transabdominal sonography. A fibroid or an eccentric gestational sac in a cornual or ectopic pregnancy may be mistaken for a bicornuate or septate uterus (Fig. 5-11).

Nicolini et al[26] noted a 42.9 percent sensitivity and a 97.8 percent specificity in the diagnosis of congenital anomalies of the uterus using ultrasound. Most of the false-negative diagnoses involved minor malformations. There was one false-positive diagnosis among 89 patients. A ratio of the anterior posterior and maximal transverse diameter measured by transabdominal sonography was calculated. The mean for normal patients was 0.699 ± 0.102. This ratio was significantly decreased below the second standard

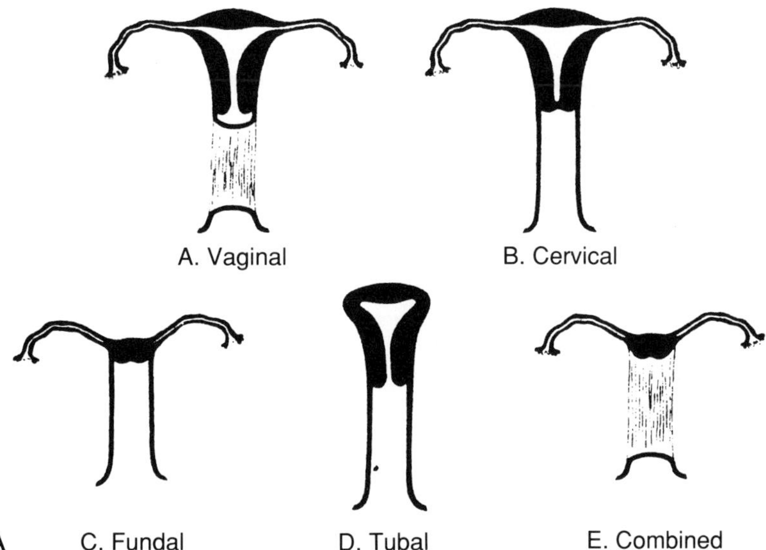

Fig. 5-9. **(A) Class I—Müllerian agenesis or hypoplasia.** *(Figure continues.)*

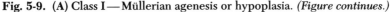

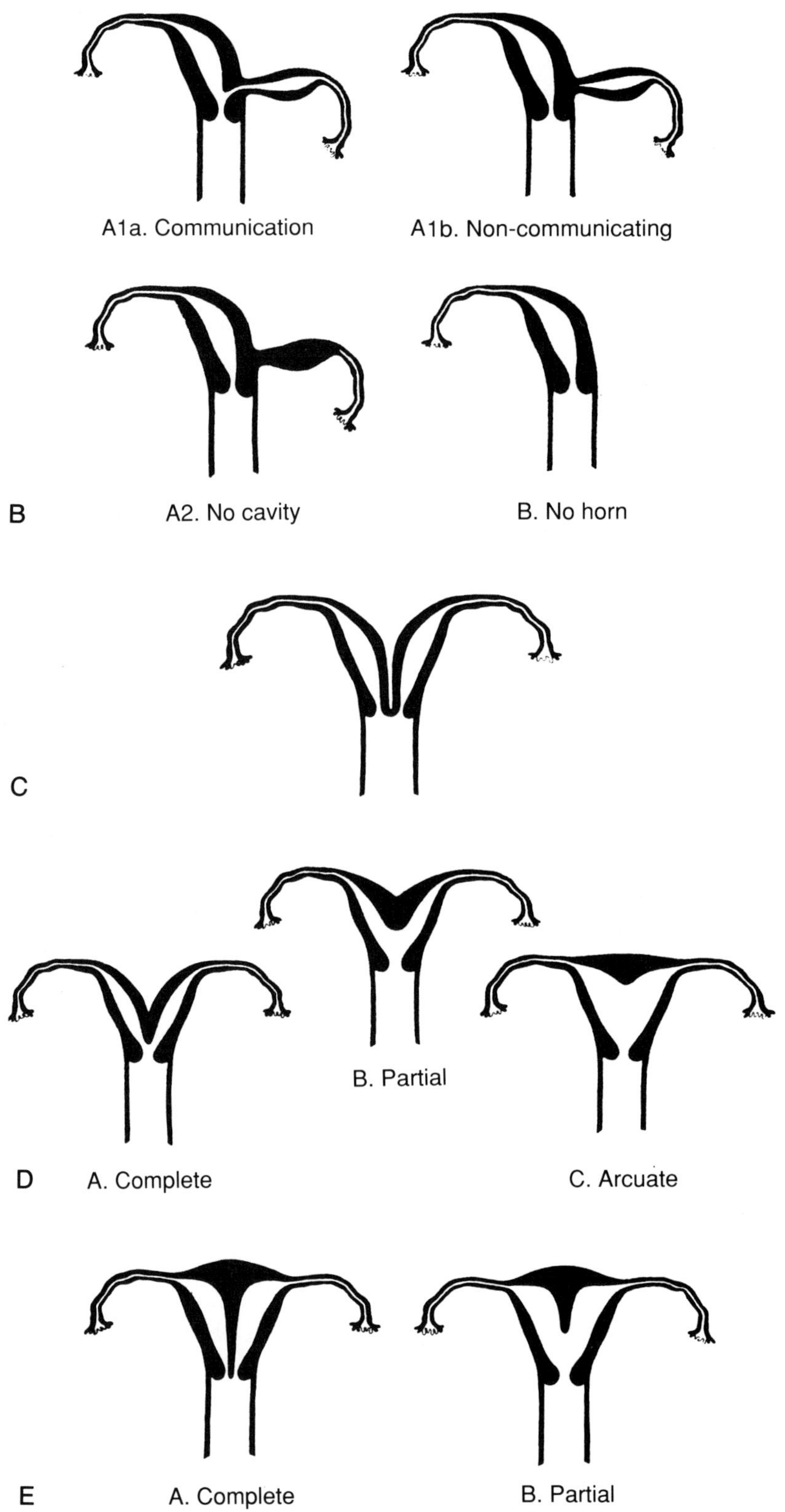

Fig. 5-9 *(Continued)*. (**B**) Class II—unicornuate uterus. (**C**) Class III—uterus didelphis. (**D**) Class IV—uterus bicornuate. (**E**) Class V—septate uterus. (From Buttram and Gibbons,[24] with permission.)

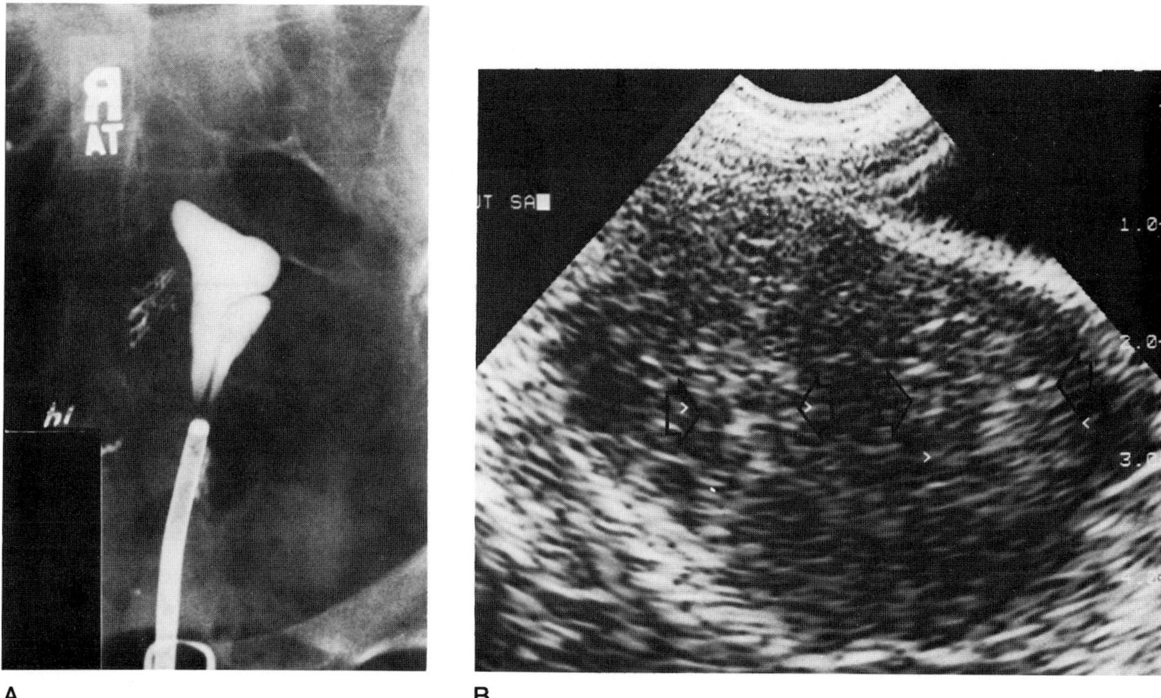

Fig. 5-10. (**A**) Hysterosalpingogram showing unicornuate uterus with rudimentary horn that is patent and communicates with the larger right uterine horn. There is no patency of the left tube from the rudimentary horn. (**B**) AP-pelvic transvaginal ultrasound of the same patient. Note the two endometrial cavities (open arrow and small arrowheads) and the irregular and distorted uterine shape. This image is of the lower segment of the uterus. The rudimentary horn appears almost as large as the main uterine bodies in this plane, which does not show the main body of the uterine fundus.

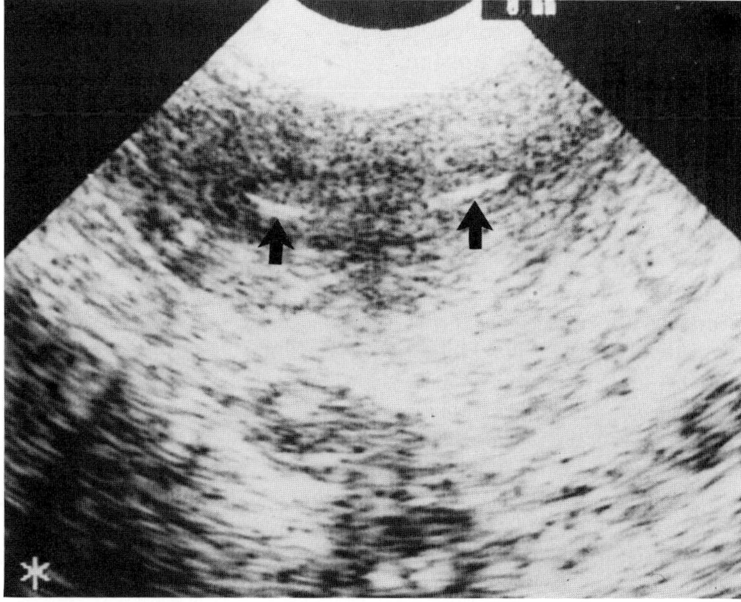

Fig. 5-11. T-pelvic view demonstrating a bicornuate uterus. Note two separate endometriums (arrows). The transverse diameter of uterus is widened.

deviation (SD) in one-third of the patients with uterus didelphys or complete septate uterus and below the first SD in 42 percent of the patients. The mean ratio in patients with class I anomalies was also significantly decreased (0.546 ± 0.132). Patients with minor müllerian malformations had a ratio similar to normal patients. These investigators thought that the unicornuate uterus was the most difficult to recognize by ultrasound.

Fedele et al[27] studied 14 patients with a hysterosalpingographic diagnosis of unicornuate uterus and noted a sensitivity of 85.7 percent and a specificity of 100 percent using ultrasound in diagnosing the presence of a rudimentary horn. Sonography was better than laparoscopy in diagnosing a cavity in a rudimentary uterine horn. However, the sonographer was already aware that the patient had a unicornuate uterus.

In a series of 50 patients, sonography was noted to be diagnostic for a congenital anomaly in 28 percent, confirmatory in 60 percent, and incorrect in 12 percent.[25] A sonogram was considered diagnostic when an anomaly had not been suspected before scanning or no studies adequate for diagnosis could be done (for example, when there was an imperforate hymen and a hysterosalpingogram could not be performed), and the anomaly was later confirmed by surgery. A confirmatory examination was one in which the diagnosis had already been made by other means and was confirmed sonographically. Incorrect examinations included those in which a congenital anomaly was known to exist but could not be demonstrated by sonogram, or the sonographic diagnosis was proved inaccurate by follow-up studies.

The prevalence of uterine malformations in the general population has not been established clearly. However, the frequency of uterine abnormalities in a group of 300 women referred for endovaginal ultrasound examination for different indications was assessed by Nasri and colleagues.[23] Using 5-MHz transducers, they assessed the external shape of the uterus, presence and aspect of the endometrium, presence of endouterine septum (40 percent of all the uterine abnormalities), and the presence and aspect of adnexal organs. Six women (2 percent) had a partial uterine septum, and 2 women (1 percent) had a complete uterus didelphys. Only 21 of the 300 (7 percent) had been referred for infertility evaluation. Ultrasound seems to be the least invasive method of distinguishing among all types of uterine abnormalities.

Subclasses or variations in the unicornuate uterus are important, since the prognosis for achieving a pregnancy or the potential for complications will vary depending on the anatomic variations. Variations in the unicornuate uterus include the presence or absence of a rudimentary horn, whether the rudimentary horn is functional and lined by endometrium or no cavity is present, and whether the rudimentary cavity communicates with the developed unicornuate horn. The presence of an endometrial cavity in a rudimentary horn and the lack of communication of the rudimentary horn with the unicornuate uterus dramatically increase the risk of endometriosis and the potential for pelvic adhesions.

Obstruction of the lower genital tract with a normal upper tract results in a hematocolpos or hydrocolpos after menarche. A cystic mass in the region of the vagina with elevation and anterior displacement of the uterus is noted. Obstructive lower genital tract lesions are generally better imaged by transabdominal sonography. However, the better image quality of the uterus and endometrium makes the transvaginal sonographic approach potentially very useful for other anomalies.

The association of renal and genital tract anomalies must be kept in mind. About one-fourth of patients with genital tract anomalies will also be noted to have urinary tract anomalies, and one-half to three-fourths of patients with urinary tract anomalies will also have genital tract anomalies.[28–31] In those essential cases where ultrasound allows the diagnosis of unicornuate uterus, laparoscopy may be performed to assess whether there is true or incomplete aplasia of the second horn. If communication between a normal and a rudimentary horn can be identified, it should be clipped to prevent development of a pregnancy obtained by transperitoneal migration of spermatozoa.

UTERINE VESSELS

It is common to visualize large veins running longitudinally and transversely within the myometrium (Fig. 5-12). A large fundal vein may occasionally be seen when imaging the uterus in the trans-pelvic plane. Frequently a large vein is running longitudinally in the posterior myometrium in the midline; it is best imaged in the midline AP-pelvic plane. In addition, several large veins can be noted in the broad ligament adjacent to the uterus in the coronal area at the level of the fallopian tube and ovary. There is also a com-

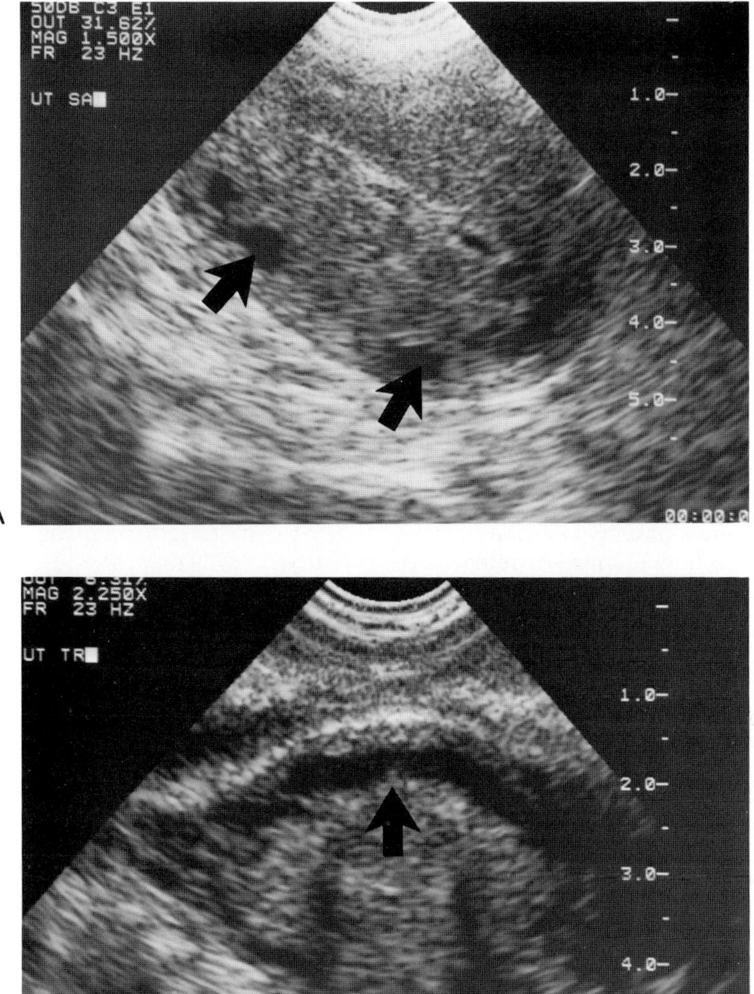

Fig. 5-12. (**A**) AP-pelvic view of the uterus showing a dilated vein in the posterior myometrial wall (arrows). This vein is tortuous, and only a few slices of the vein are noted in any one plane. (**B**) T-pelvic view showing large dilated vein in the anterior and fundal myometrium (arrow).

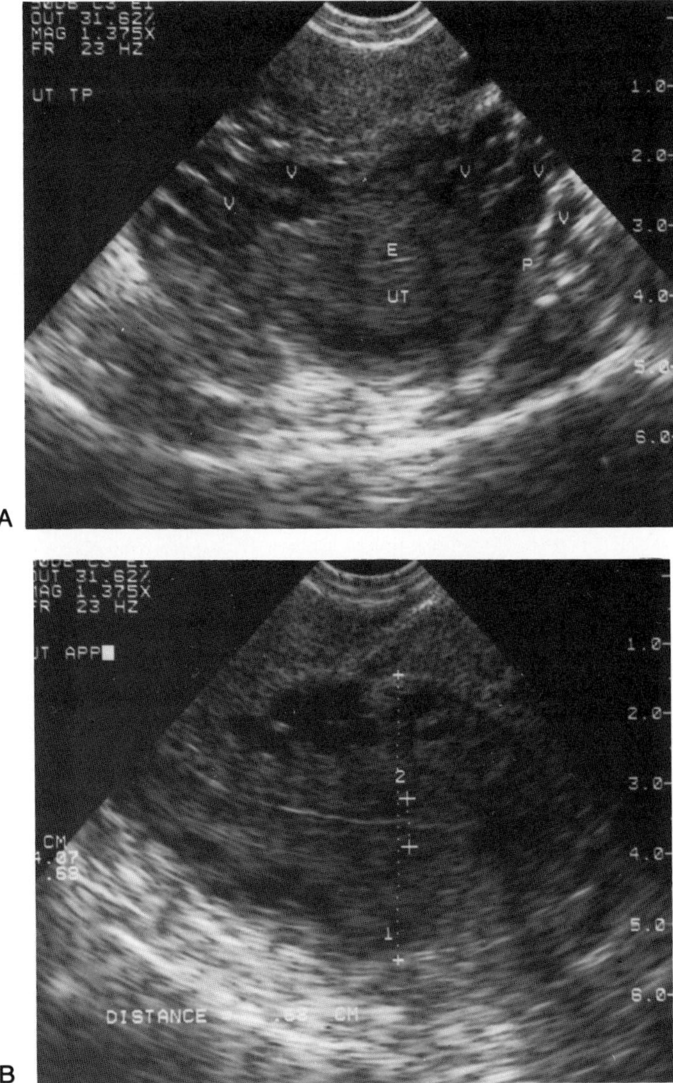

Fig. 5-13. Patient with pelvic pain. (**A**) T-pelvic view showing multiple dilated veins in the broad ligament at about the level of the internal cervical os (V). The lower uterine segment (UT) is central, with the endocervical canal or lower endometrial cavity (E) on the right. The peritoneum is noted (P) with a retroperitoneal vein (V). The levator muscle is below the vein in the lower right. (**B**) AP-pelvic view showing dilated veins in the myometrium. Cursor line 1 defines the anterior posterior dimension of the uterine fundus. Cursor line 2 defines the endometrium. The cervix is toward the left. The hyperechoic echoes in the lower portion of the photograph are small bowel in the cul-de-sac and posterior pelvis.

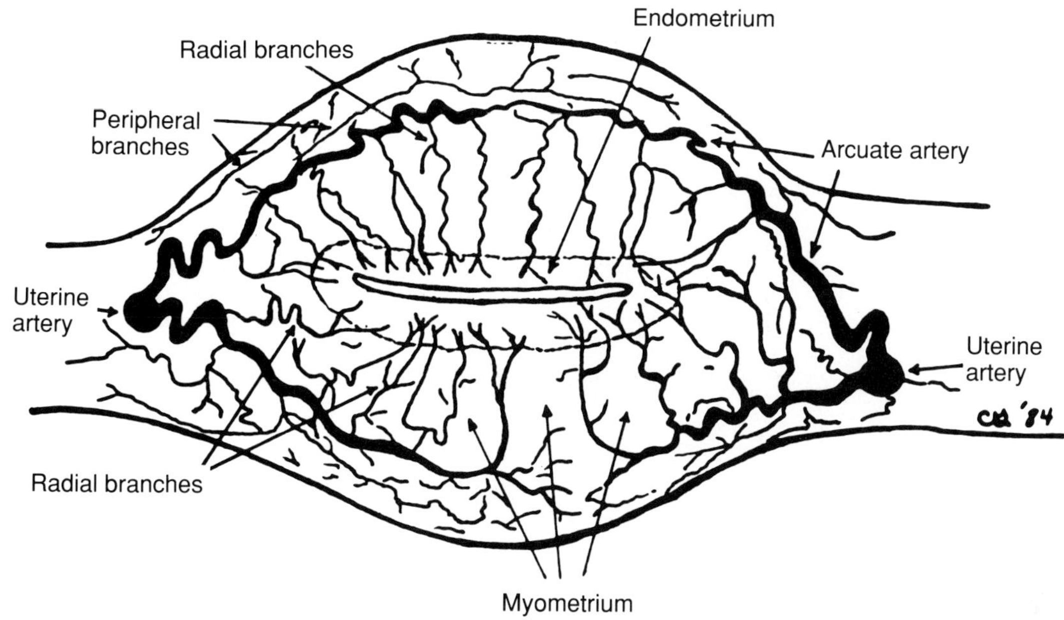

Fig. 5-14. Rendering of a miduterine cross-section of a uterus showing arterial system. There is a venous system that approximately parallels this arterial system. (From DuBose et al,[32] as adapted from Sampson,[33] with permission.)

plex of large veins at the level of the internal cervical os laterally on both sides of the uterus. Such venous complexes should not be mistaken for pelvic pathology. DuBose et al[32] have suggested that the uterine vessels are easiest to visualize 1 to 2 weeks after the onset of the last menstrual period and are most difficult to image just before or during the menstrual period.[33] This difficulty is thought to result from the vasoconstricting hormonal influence during the late luteal phase and the vasodilating action of estrogen on the uterus with an increased blood supply during midcycle. Varicosities involving both the vessels within the myometrium or the broad ligament vein may occur (Figs. 5-13 and 5-14).

ARCUATE ARTERY CALCIFICATION

Uterine artery calcification was first reported using x-ray by Camiel et al[34] in 1967 and was suggested to be associated with atherosclerotic disease. Occhipinti et al[35] reported calcification involving the arcuate branches of the uterine artery in eight patients in 1991. All eight patients were either hypertensive, diabetic, or both. In addition, three patients were receiving hemodialysis. Such calcifications are not rare. We have noted at least a half dozen such cases over the past 5 years.

Calcification generally consists of multiple hyperechoic densities, often with posterior shadowing within the myometrium. It usually involves multiple vessels at about the same level in the myometrium. As a consequence, the calcifications tend to form a linear configuration on a longitudinal image plain (AP-pelvic plain) or a circular configuration in the trans-pelvic plain. This type of pattern is quite distinct from calcification associated with a leiomyoma in which the calcifications tend to be randomly distributed in the leiomyoma or occur at the periphery and outline the leiomyoma. The association of arcuate artery calcification with atherosclerotic disease and diabetes warrants clinical evaluation for such underlying problems.

UTERINE TUMORS AND CYSTS

Sarcomas of the uterus comprise less than 5 percent of all uterine cancers. Malignant degeneration of a leiomyoma is rare and occurs in only 0.2 percent of pa-

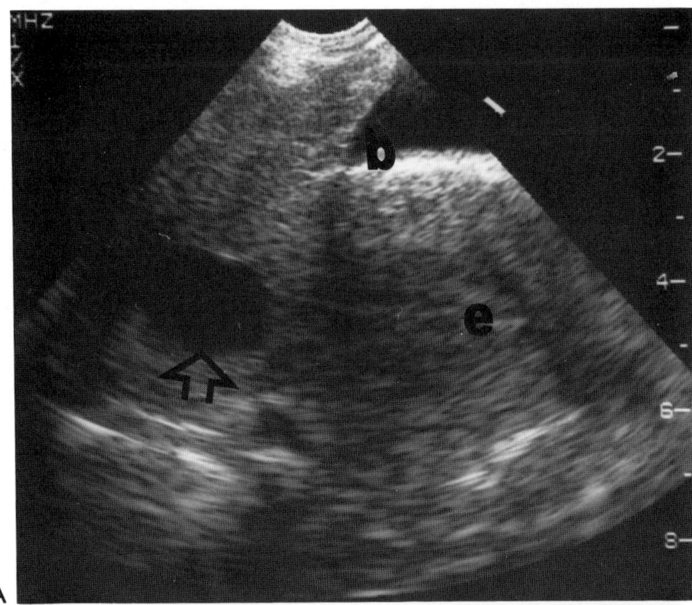

A

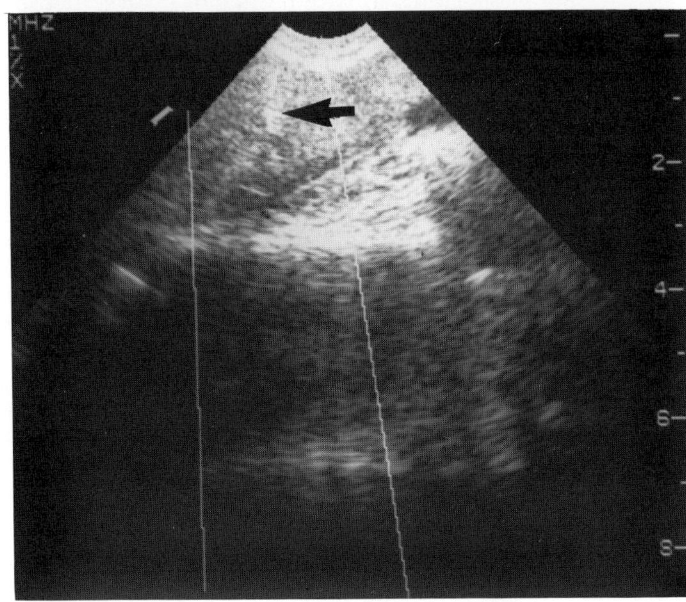

B

Fig. 5-15. (**A**) AP-pelvic view of the uterus. A 2-cm cyst is present in the posterior wall of the lower uterine segment and cervix (open arrow). The cyst was first noted 2 years previously, but was not seen during laparoscopy. (**B**) Transvaginal needle aspiration was done. Note the needle in the myometrium (arrow). The lines are electronically generated needle biopsy guides. *(Figure continues.)*

Fig. 5-15 *(Continued)*. (C) After removal of the needle, a small area of fluid remains following aspiration (open arrow). Cytology of the cyst aspirate was benign. e, endometrium; b, bladder.

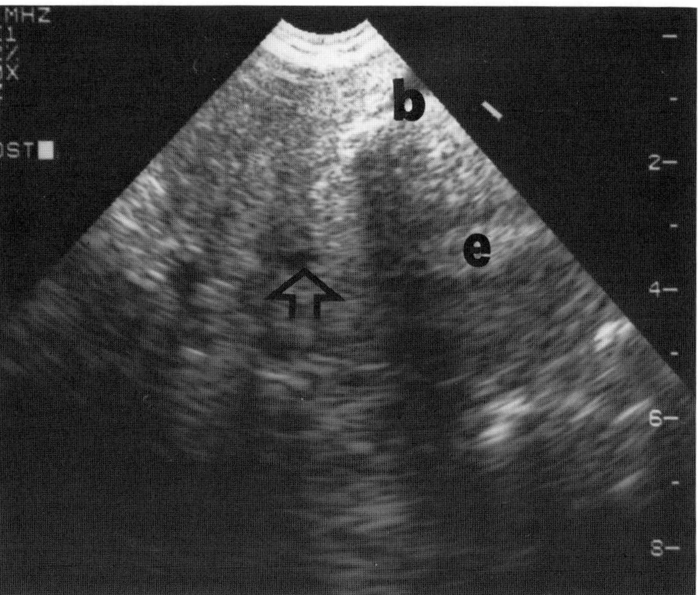

tients. Cystic lesions in the uterus usually occur in degenerating leiomyomas, but may rarely occur independent of a myoma (Fig. 5-15).

ULTRASOUND IN THE DIAGNOSIS AND PREVENTION OF UTERINE PERFORATION OR RUPTURE

Chen et al[36] evaluated 40 patients with previous cesarean sections using transvaginal ultrasound in the third trimester of pregnancy. A normal cesarean section scar imaged by ultrasound was considered to be a homogeneous acoustic reflection consisting of three layers: the chorioamniotic membrane and decidualized endometrium, a middle myometrial layer, and the outer visceral-parietal layer. About half of the patients had a normal scar. Thinning was defined as a scar less than 5 mm thick and was noted in about 13 percent of patients. Thickening of the scar was noted in 20 percent of patients. Ballooning of the scar was defined as an outward bulging of the scar and was noted in 10 percent of patients. A wedge defect in the scar consisted of a sonolucent wedge-shaped defect in the scar and was noted in 5 percent of patients. Although this study demonstrates the capability of ultrasound to evaluate the lower uterine segment and cesarean section scar area, the clinical significance of the findings are not known since most of the patients were delivered by repeat cesarean section. The suggested implications are that about three-fourths of patients had a scar with normal or greater thickness with no loss of integrity, whereas about one-fourth had scars that were either thin or showed some structural abnormalities that would raise concern for vaginal birth after cesarean section. However, despite the logic of the conclusion, the data do not confirm that ultrasound imaging of a previous scar can be utilized in the decision-making process whether a patient should have a repeat cesarean section or may be allowed to have a vaginal birth.

In fact, there is some controversy over the normal thickness for a cesarean section scar or the normal lower uterine segment at term. Fukuda et al[37] studied the anterior lower uterine segment in patients without a previous cesarean section and in 216 patients with a previous cesarean section. The mean thickness of the lower uterine segment in patients without a previous cesarean section at 40 weeks' gestation was 3.36 mm, with the thinnest lower uterine segment (mean -2SD) of 1.98 mm. Fukuda and colleagues suggested that a lower uterine segment of greater than 2 mm was normal; however, up to 6.3 percent of normal patients (no previous cesarean) had lower uterine segments that were 2 mm or less in thickness. Fukuda's group also found a good correlation between ultrasound measurements of the cesarean section scar thickness and measurements made using ophthalmic calipers at the time of the cesarean section and found ultrasound to have a 91.3 percent sensitivity and a 98.7 percent specificity compared to operative findings in predicting a normal scar area (no thinning) or thinning or loss of continuity. Ultrasound thus seems to be a relatively accurate technique for evaluating a previous cesarean section scar.

Unfortunately, the current clinical approach to the patient with a previous cesarean section is to confirm that the patient has a low transverse uterine incision, review the operative report if possible, and counsel her on the relative risks of repeat cesarean section versus vaginal delivery. If the patient elects vaginal delivery, she is given a trial of labor. The current clinical approach does not evaluate the cesarean section scar either before or during labor. This is clearly an area that sonographic evaluation might be of considerable benefit. However, it is also an area that needs much more study before reasonable and reliable recommendations can be made regarding the use of ultrasound in evaluating previous cesarean section scars or even the lower uterine segment in normal pregnant patients.

Sonography has also been utilized to diagnose uterine rupture in the second and third trimester of pregnancy and uterine perforation after suction curettage. Sonography may demonstrate a hematoma or loss of the uterine wall integrity.[38] Foster et al[39] noted an echo-poor area with echogenic material (fetal material) in the uterovesical space following uterine perforation from a suction curettage.

Real-time transabdominal ultrasound may also be utilized during a dilatation and curettage or suction curettage to help determine the location of the curett or suction cannula and to locate tissue in the uterine cavity, to help prevent perforation, and to ensure that the uterine cavity has been evaluated or evacuated adequately. Although the use of ultrasound is frequently not necessary for most cases, it can offer considerable information and help guide the procedure in patients with a large uterus or those with a large amount of tissue that must be removed, especially when there is a thin uterine wall. Ultrasound may also be of value in patients with a small uterus, but with a stenotic or deformed endocervical canal. We have frequently utilized ultrasound in the office to help guide endometrial biopsies in patients with stenotic endocervical canals. The catheter tip is easily visualized during real time, and ultrasound imaging can help maneuver the catheter tip into the endometrial cavity. For example, in a recent case, repeated attempts to insert an endometrial biopsy catheter in a patient with a markedly retroverted uterus were unsuccessful despite the use of a tenaculum and traction to help straighten the uterus. The catheter could be felt to be hitting a solid structure. Transabdominal ultrasound revealed that despite traction the uterus was still partially retroverted and that the catheter was hitting the anterior wall of the upper endocervical canal. It was also obvious that further pressure or attempts to insert the catheter in the direction it was following would result in a uterine perforation. Further traction was placed on the uterus, the catheter was partially withdrawn to separate it from its position against the anterior wall, and utilizing a twisting motion the catheter was maneuvered under direct visualization into the uterine cavity. Knowledge of the location of the catheter tip in relationship to the uterine wall and the direction that the catheter was taking allowed us to be much more aggressive in maneuvering the catheter and successfully completing the procedure while minimizing concern for uterine perforation.

REFERENCES

1. Callen PW: Ultrasonographic evaluation of pelvic disease. p. 209. In Goldberg HI (ed): International Radiology and Diagnostic Imaging Modalities. Department of Radiology, University of California, San Francisco, 1982
2. Fleischer AC, James AE, Jr, Millis JB, Julian C: Differential diagnosis of pelvic masses by gray scale sonography. AJR 131:469, 1978
3. Gray H: Anatomy of the Human Body. 30th Ed. Lea & Febiger, Philadelphia, 1985
4. Weiner JJ, Newcombe RG: Measurement of uterine volume: a comparison between measurements by ultrasonography and by water displacement. J Clin Ultrasound 20:457, 1992
5. Goldstein SR, Horii SC, Snyder JR et al: Estimation of nongravid uterine volume based on a nomogram of gravid uterine volume: its value in gynaecologic uterine abnormalities. Obstet Gynecol 72:86, 1988
6. Haynor DR, Mack LA, Soules MR et al: Changing appearance of the normal uterus during the menstrual cycle: MR studies. Radiology 161:459, 1986
7. Zalud I, Conway C, Shulman H, Trinca D: Endometrial and myometrial thickness and uterine blood flow in postmenopausal women: the influence of hormonal replacement therapy and age. J Ultrasound Med 12:737, 1993
8. Nussbaum AR, Sanders RC, Jones MD: Neonatal uter-

ine morphology as seen on real-time US. Radiology 160:641, 1986
9. Krantz KE, Atkinson JP: Gross anatomy. Ann NY Acad Sci 142:551, 1967
10. Sample WF, Lippe BM, Gyepes MT: Gray-scale ultrasonography of the normal female pelvis. Radiology 125:477, 1977
11. Orsini LF, Salardi S, Pilu G et al: Pelvic organs in premenarcheal girls: real-time ultrasonography. Radiology 153:113, 1984
12. Ivarsson SA, Nilsson KO, Persson PH: Ultrasonography of the pelvic organs in prepubertal and postpubertal girls. Arch Dis Child 58:352, 1983
13. Gompel C, Silverberg SG: Pathology, Gynecology and Obstetrics. 2nd Ed. JB Lippincott, Philadelphia, 1977
14. Bowie JD: Ultrasound of gynecologic pelvic masses: the indefinite uterus and other patterns associated with diagnostic error. J Clin Ultrasound 5:323, 1977
15. Walzer A, Flynn E, Koenigsberg M: Sonographic appearance of a prolapsing submucous leiomyoma. J Clin Ultrasound 11:101, 1983
16. Dudiak CM, Turner DA, Patel SK et al: Uterine leiomyomas in the infertile patient: preoperative localization with MR imaging versus US and hysterosalpingography. Radiology 167:627, 1988
17. Gross BH, Silver TM, Jaffe MH: Sonographic features of uterine leiomyomas: analysis of 41 proven cases. J Ultrasound Med 2:401, 1983
18. Seidler D, Laing FC, Jeffrey RB, Jr, Wing VW: Uterine adenomyosis—a difficult sonographic diagnosis. J Ultrasound Med 6:345, 1987
19. Bohlman ME, Ensor RE, Sanders RC: Sonographic findings in adenomyosis of the uterus. AJR 148:765, 1987
20. Fedele I, Bianchi S, Dorta M et al: Transvaginal ultrasonography in the differential diagnosis of adenomyoma verus leiomyoma. Am J Obstet Gynecol 167:603, 1992
21. Walsh JW, Taylor KJW, Rosenfield AT: Gray scale ultrasonography in the diagnosis of endometriosis and adenomyosis. AJR 132:87, 1979
22. Fedele I, Bianchi S, Dorta M et al: Transvaginal ultrasonography in the diagnosis of diffuse adenomyosis. Fertil Steril 58:94, 1992
23. Nasri MN, Setchell ME, Chard T: Transvaginal ultrasound for diagnosis of uterine malformations. Br J Obstet Gynecol 97:1043, 1990
24. Buttram VC, Jr, Gibbons WE: Müllerian anomalies: a proposed classification (an analysis of 144 cases). Fertil Steril 32:40, 1979
25. Malini S, Valdes C, Malinak R: Sonographic diagnosis and classification of anomalies of the female genital tract. J Ultrasound Med 3:397, 1984
26. Nicolini U, Bellotti M, Bonazzi B et al: Can ultrasound be used to screen uterine malformations? Fertil Steril 47:89, 1987
27. Fedele L, Dorta M, Vercellini P et al: Ultrasound in the diagnosis of subclasses of unicornuate uterus. Obstet Gynecol 71:274, 1988
28. Banner EA: The ectopic kidney in obstetrics and gynecology. Surg Gynecol Obstet 121:32, 1965
29. Doroshow LW, Abeshouse BS: Congenital unilateral solitary kidney: report of 37 cases and a review of the literature. Urol Surv 11:219, 1961
30. Collins DC: Congenital unilateral renal agenesis. Ann Surg 95:715, 1932
31. Fortune CH: The pathological and clinical significance of congenital one-sided kidney defect, with the presentation of three new cases of agenesia and one of aplasia. Ann Intern Med 1:377, 1927
32. DuBose TJ, Hill LW, Hennigan HW, Jr et al: Sonography of arcuate uterine blood vessels. J Ultrasound Med 4:229, 1985
33. Sampson JA: The escape of foreign material from the uterine cavity into the uterine veins. Am J Obstet Gynecol 13:265, 1918
34. Camiel MR, Berkan HS, Alexander LL: Roentgen visualization of uterine artery calcification. Radiology 88:138, 1967
35. Occhipinti K, Kutcher R, Rosenblatt R: Sonographic apperance and significance of arcuate artery calcification. J Ultrasound Med 10:97, 1991
36. Chen H, Chen S, Hsieh F: Observation of cesarean section scar by transvaginal ultrasonography. Ultrasound Med Biol 16:443, 1990
37. Fukuda M, Shimizu T, Ihara Y et al: Ultrasound examination of caesarean section scars during pregnancy.
38. Kushnir O, Izquierdo LA, Sigman RK et al: Vaginal sonography in the diagnosis of uterine rupture. J Ultrasound Med 9:169, 1990
39. Foster BB, Siu CM, Murray JB, Chung MH: Transabdominal and transvaginal ultrasonography of uterine perforation following suction curettage. J Can Assoc Radiol 40:318, 1989

6

The Endometrium

Melvin G. Dodson

The endometrial cavity should be visualizable as a separate entity within the uterus in virtually all menstruating patients. The endometrial cavity is generally centrally located in the uterus. The cyclic histologic changes and changes in thickening of the endometrium with hormonal stimulation that occur during the normal menstrual cycle result in characteristic sonographic images that can generally be used to distinguish the different phases of the menstrual cycle. Menses, the follicular phase, and the luteal phase each produce a characteristic ultrasound endometrial pattern. The sonographic transition between the follicular phase and the luteal phase after ovulation takes several days and also generally produces a characterized image pattern that can be distinguished. In addition, several abnormal endometrial patterns can be recognized that suggest abnormal anatomic changes in the endometrium, such as cancer, polyps, or submucosal leiomyoma, or abnormal physiologic changes, i.e., chronic anovulation with very low serum estrogen or anovulation with normal serum estradiol.

The hormonal and ovulatory status of the patient can be assessed by evaluating sonographic endometrial patterns. An evaluation of the endometrium and of follicular development in the ovary should be included. Ovulation is reflected in the endometrium by luteinizing changes secondary to progesterone, which result in a change in the endometrial ultrasound pattern from a three-line endometrium characteristic of estrogen stimulation and the proliferative phase, to a transitional pattern, and finally to a hyperechoic pattern characteristic of the luteal phase.

The ultrasound endometrial pattern can also be utilized during ovulation induction and IVF or other assisted reproductive technologies as a prognostic indicator for the potential of a pregnancy. A thin and/or poorly developed endometrium is associated with a poor pregnancy rate. Another physiologic aberration that can be recognized readily is a lack of synchrony between follicular development in the ovary and/or endometrial development and/or the last menstrual period (LMP).

An intrauterine device (IUD) used for contraception can be easily imaged within the endometrial cavity, as well as perforation of the myometrium. The use of birth control pills results in a characteristic unstimulated endometrial sonographic pattern consisting of a single hyperechoic line representing the endometrial cavity and endometrium. This central endometrial echo in a patient taking birth control pills is generally thicker than the single-line endometrium seen during late menstruation. Endometrial motion can also be observed and may correlate with menstrual cycle physiology and/or sexual function.

This chapter reviews each of these patterns and how the recognition of abnormal endometrial patterns may be utilized in diagnosis and/or therapy. However, it is just as important to be able to recognize the normal cyclic endometrial pattern throughout the normal menstrual cycle. Doing so enables the physician to recognize the difference between an abnormal pattern and normal pattern but where there is a lack of synchrony with the follicular development in the ovary (Table 6-1).

MENSES

During early menses, the endometrium still resembles the hyperechoic (white) endometrium characteristic of the luteal phase. However, sometimes small anechoic (black) areas can be noted within the white hyperechoic endometrium, indicating blood and the breakdown of the endometrium (see discussion of the premenstrual endometrium). Some posterior en-

Table 6-1. Correlation of Normal Menstrual Cycle Anatomy and Physiology with Ultrasound Endometrial Patterns

Anatomy/Physiology	*Ultrasound Pattern*
Menses	
Early	*Hyperechoic:* Resembles a luteal phase endometrium with anechoic areas indicating endometrial breakdown
Mid-menses	Mixed pattern with hyperechoic and anechoic areas indicating blood and tissue. Endometrium per se noted as two thin hyperechoic lines outlining the endometrial cavity
Late	Single line: Thin single line representing the endometrial cavity
Follicular phase	
Early	*Three-line:* The two outer hyperechoic lines represent the endometrial-myometrial junction. The center line is the endometrial cavity.
Late	*Three-line:* Thickening of the anechoic endometrial layer between the hyperechoic three lines.
Luteal phase	
Early	*Transitional:* Thickening of the hyperechoic three lines and irregular hyperechoic filling of the previously anechoic endometrial layers
Late	*Hyperechoic:* Uniform hyperechoic (white) endometrium
Premenstrual	*Hyperechoic:* With small anechoic collections.
Postmenopausal	*Single line:* Similar to late menstrual endometrium. Normally less than 5 mm thick

hancement characteristic of a luteal phase endometrium may still be present, although the degree of posterior enhancement and endometrial thickening is generally less than noted when the endometrium is fully developed during the luteal phase. The small anechoic areas begin to coalesce and are often mixed with hyperechoic reflections of menstrual debris. As menses progresses, the hypoechoic central echo representing blood and tissue and the thickened hyperechoic endometrium disappears. After most of the endometrial tissue has been passed, the endometrial cavity may be imaged as an anechoic area (usually representing blood) surrounded by a thin hyperechoic line—thought to represent the endometrial-myometrial junction and what remains of the endometrium (basalis layer) (Fig. 6-1). During heavy menstrual flow, the anechoic central echo may fill and distend the entire endometrial cavity. By day 3 to 7 of menstruation, the endometrial complex is visualized as only a very thin hyperechoic single-line reflection representing the endometrial cavity (Figs. 6-2 and 6-3). This single-line endometrium is usually only 1 to 3 mm thick (Fig. 6-4). A hypoechoic halo 2 to 3 mm thick surrounding the endometrium is also generally visualized.[1] This halo has been attributed to a vascular network at the interface of the endometrium and myometrium. It probably also represents the basalis layer of the endometrium. The halo is prominent several days after the onset of menstruation and remains throughout the follicular phase, but it is not present during the luteal phase.

After sloughing of the endometrium and before significant estrogen stimulation, the entire endometrial echo complex is visualized as only a thin hyperechoic straight line surrounded by the endometrial halo.

ULTRASOUND CHANGES DURING THE FOLLICULAR AND LUTEAL PHASE

Sakamoto[2] described in 1985 some of the characteristic sonographic images noted during the normal menstrual cycle. Several different ultrasound signs have been described to help differentiate a proliferative phase from a secretory phase endometrium (Fig. 6-5).[3] The proliferative endometrium is characterized by (1) the presence of a well-defined three-line sign, (2) a hypoechogenic functional layer, and (3) minimal or absent posterior acoustic enhancement. The three-line sign is formed by the central hyperechoic reflection representing the endometrial cavity and the additional hyperechoic reflections (one on each side of the central reflection) representing the endometrial-myometrial junction (Fig. 6-6A). There is also a surrounding hypoechoic halo, as noted above. During the luteal phases, the endometrium is hyperechoic, with posterior enhancement and absence of the three-line sign and halo (Fig. 6-6B).

Early Proliferative Phase

Very early in the follicular phase, the endometrium may still be imaged as a single hyperechoic line similar to the late menstrual endometrium. However, a surrounding anechoic area is generally noted that may be several millimeters thick and seems to represent the early proliferative endometrium. Very early

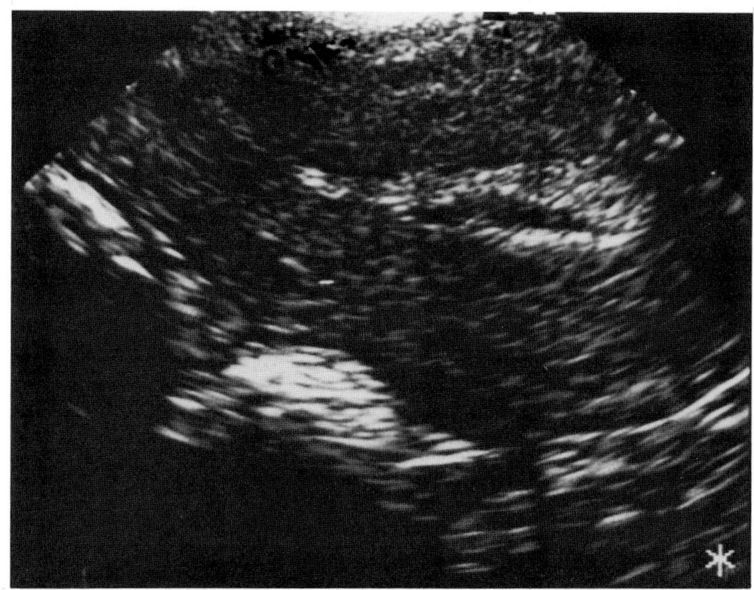

Fig. 6-1. AP-pelvic view of the uterus during heavy menses (day 1 of the cycle) showing an anechoic area within the endometrium representing blood. There is still a large amount of endometrium that has not been sloughed. The endometrium still has the hyperechogenic characteristics of a luteal phase endometrium. The estradiol was 95 pg/ml, and the serum progesterone was 10.6 ng/ml.

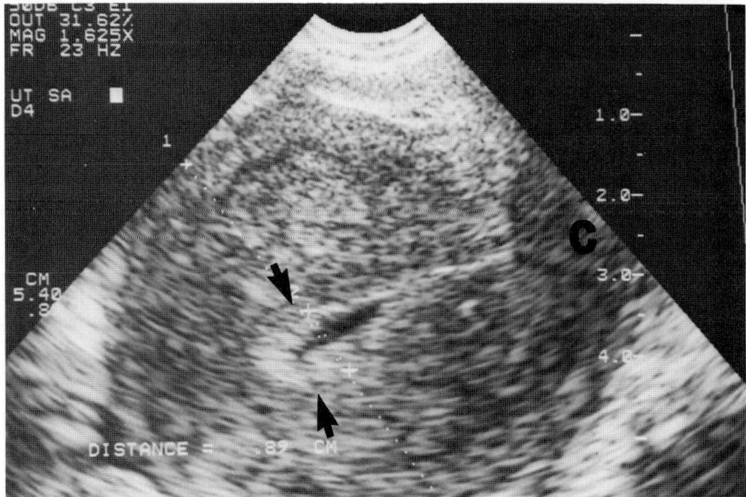

Fig. 6-2. AP-pelvic view of retroverted uterus with a menstrual endometrium on day 4. The cervix (C) is to the right and anterior. Note blood in the endometrial cavity with a small amount of luteal phase endometrium still present surrounding the blood (arrows).

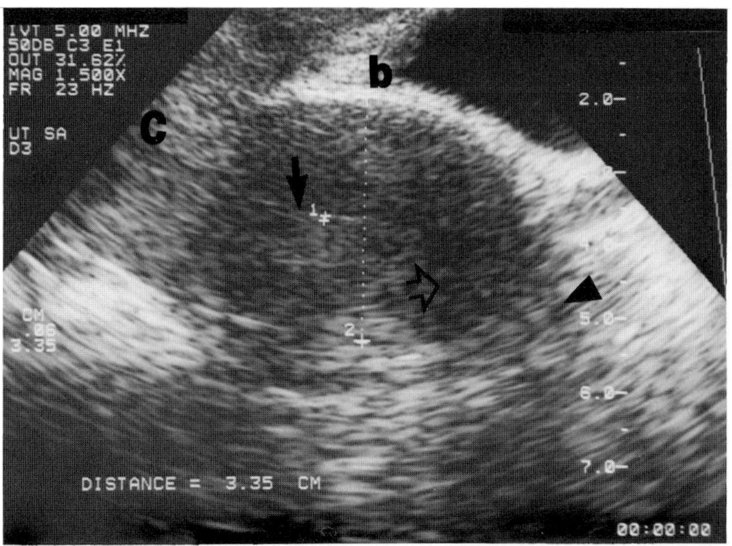

Fig. 6-3. AP-pelvic view of the uterus showing a thin single-line endometrium (arrow) 0.6 mm thick on menstrual day 3. The anterior posterior diameter of the uterus is 3.35 cm. Note the bladder angle (b), which is collapsed, and a small amount of urine in the bladder at top right of photograph. There is a weak critical angle artifact (arrowhead) shadow. There is some fundal shadowing artifact from the bladder angle (open arrow).

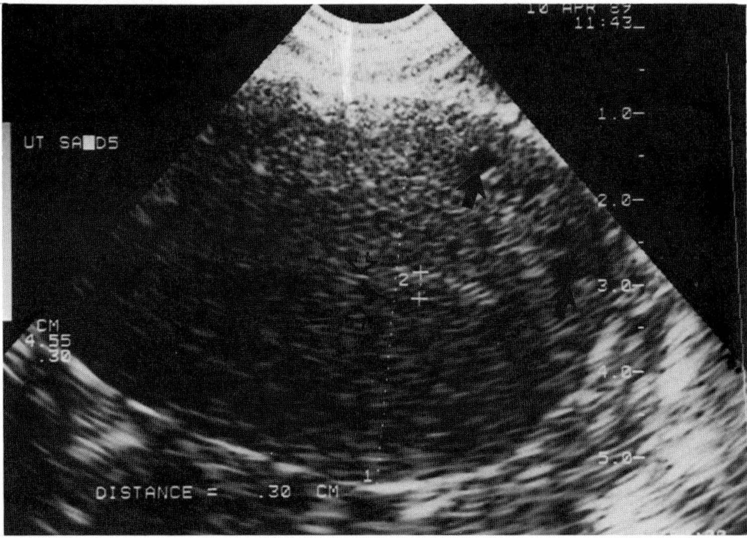

Fig. 6-4. AP-pelvic view of the uterus showing a day 5 single-line endometrium that is 0.3 mm thick. This endometrium is beginning to thicken, and there is some early suggestion of the three-line sign seen during the follicular phase (open arrows). The anechoic areas in the fundus are veins (arrow).

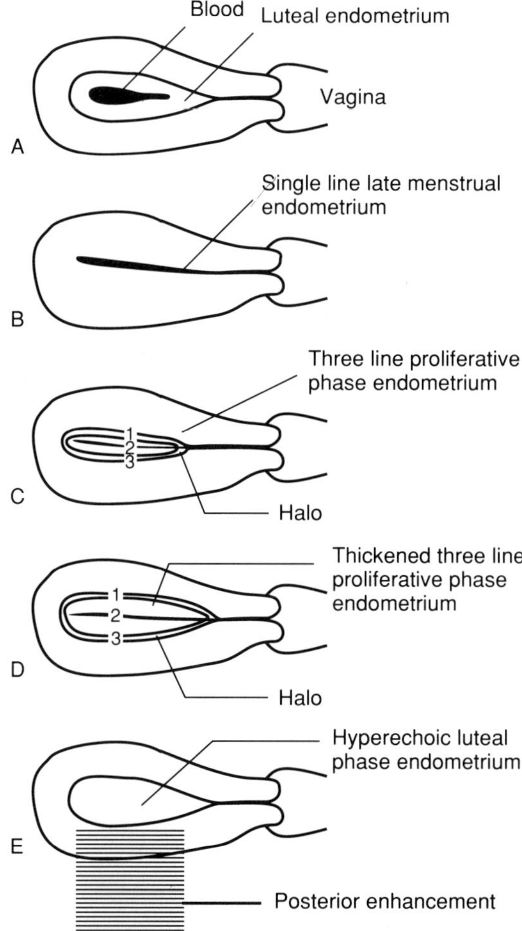

Fig. 6-5. Diagram of endometrial changes through a normal menstrual cycle. **(A)** Early menstrual endometrium. An anechoic collection of blood is present in the endometrial cavity. The endometrium still shows some of the sonographic characteristics of a hyperechoic luteal phase endometrium. **(B)** After sloughing of the endometrium later in menses (usually by day 3–5), the endometrium is imaged as a single hyperechoic line representing the endometrial cavity. **(C)** Estrogen stimulation results in an early follicular endometrium that is imaged as three separate lines. The central line (2) represents the endometrial cavity. There is an anechoic halo 1- to 2-mm thick around the endometrium. **(D)** The late proliferative endometrium is thickened and fully developed. **(E)** The secretory endometrium is hyperechoic with loss of the three-line sign and surrounding anechoic halo. There is generally posterior enhancement.

in the follicular phase the hyperechoic outer lines at the endometrial-myometrial junction may not be present. However, within a short time, the endometrial-myometrial junction becomes hyperechoic, and the endometrium is imaged as a three-line endometrium characteristic of the follicular phase of the menstrual cycle.

The development of the hyperechoic echo at the endometrial-myometrial junction generally does not occur all at the same time. Initially a thin hyperechoic (white) echo is noted in several areas surrounding the hypoechoic (dark) endometrium per se. However, within a short time the hyperechoic echo becomes more prominent eventually surrounding the entire endometrium and forming the outer two echoes of the sonographic three-line image pattern characteristic of the proliferative endometrium in the follicular phase of the normal menstrual cycle. Some authors refer to this pattern as a layered endometrium. I prefer the term three-line since it is descriptive of the sonographic pattern noted.

The three-line sign consists of three hyperechoic, relatively parallel lines. The general hypoechogenic character of the functional layer of the proliferative endometrium is thought to be related to the simple configuration of the glands and blood vessels. The central echogenic line of the three-line sign represents the endometrial cavity. The outer lines represent the endometrium and the interface between the endometrium and myometrium (Fig. 6-6A). These outer lines may thicken as the estrogen stimulation increases and the follicular phase progresses.

In the follicular phase, the halo, which is about 2 mm thick and surrounds the endometrium, is present. It can generally be imaged as a thin anechoic line just outside the outer hyperechoic echo at the endometrial-myometrial junction.

Generally no posterior enhancement (a white area behind or distal to the structure being imaged, see discussion below) is associated with a three-line endometrium in the follicular phase. A follicular phase endometrium greater than 6 mm thick has been associated with a serum estradiol level over 200 pg/ml and a developing follicular diameter in the ovary generally of 14 mm or greater.[4] However, these correlations are, at best, rough estimates.

Late Proliferative Phase

There is continued thickening of the endometrial echo complex in the late proliferative phase. The halo is still present. The endometrial complex is still

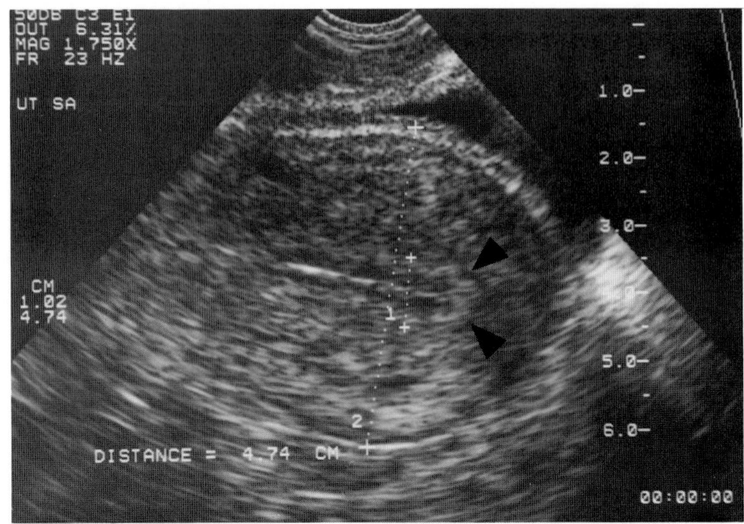

B

Fig. 6-6. (**A**) AP-pelvic image of uterus on day 15 of a natural cycle showing a follicular endometrium 1.02 cm thick with a three-line sign. A small amount of halo can be seen (arrowheads). (**B**) The same patient 3 days later with an early luteal phase endometrium (between cursor line and arrowheads). Note the loss of the three-line sign and development of a hyperechoic endometrium with some early posterior enhancement (arrow).

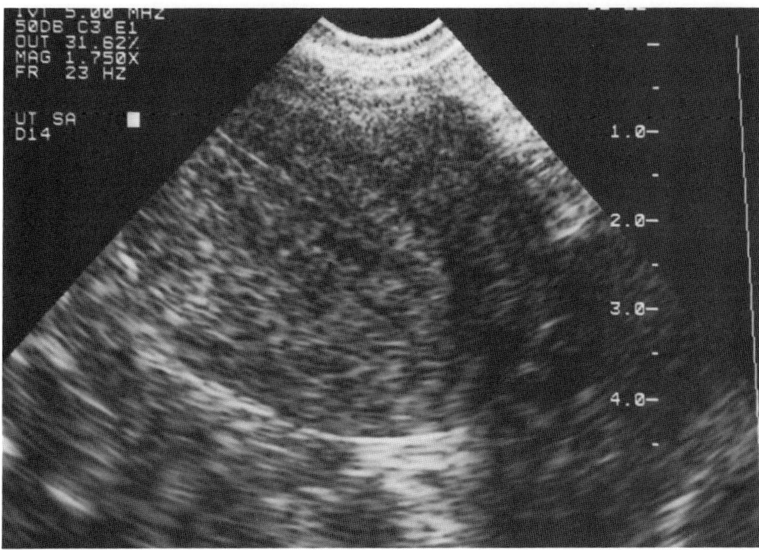

Fig. 6-7. AP-pelvic view of uterus on day 14 of a normal cycle showing a 1.16-cm-thick follicular endometrium with thickening of the outer lines at the endometrium-myometrium interface. There was a 21- by 18-mm follicle in the left ovary.

imaged as three parallel lines (the three-line sign), but the outer lines may begin to thicken. The total endometrial thickness increases and may reach 10 mm or greater in total thickness. There is no posterior enhancement (Fig. 6-7). Cervical mucus may occasionally be imaged as a hypoechoic density in the endocervix near the time of ovulation.

Luteal Phase

In the early luteal phase after ovulation, the outer lines of the three-line endometrium thicken, and the anechoic functional layer representing the endometrium per se begins to fill in with irregular hyperechoic areas. This sonographic transitional phase last several days. It is sometimes difficult to distinguish the sonographic transitional phase from a late follicular phase three-line endometrium. Since the histologic changes from a proliferative to a secretory endometrium constitute a continuum of microscopic changes, it is reasonable that the sonographic pattern reflects a slow continuum of changes before the fully developed sonographic image of the luteal phase endometrium is noted. The hyperechoic "fill-in" of the transitional endometrium continues until the endometrium is imaged as a homogeneous hyperechoic density with posterior enhancement characteristic of the sonographic luteal phase (Fig. 6-8). The three-line sign is no longer present. The three hyperechoic lines that are characteristic of the follicular phase have blended into the uniform hyperechoic (white) sonographic luteal phase endometrium. The rate of increase of thickness slows, and the endometrial echo complex soon achieves its greater anterior posterior dimension. The echogenicity of the endometrium becomes hyperechoic after coiling and lengthening of the endometrial glands, the production of mucus, and increased tortuosity of the glands and blood vessels (Fig. 6-9).

Acoustic enhancement is a hyperechoic or white echo distal to an object being imaged. It might be viewed as an acoustic artifact imaged as a "white shadow" that is associated with some physical characteristics of the tissue being imaged. Interestingly, acoustic enhancement is usually associated with cystic or fluid-filled structures that are hypoechoic such as an ovarian cyst. Yet, it is characteristically seen posterior to the hyperechoic sonographic luteal phase endometrium. Acoustic enhancement occurring posterior to a hyperechoic "solid" structure is unusual and is thought possibly to be related to the increased vascularity of the endometrium. However, probably other physical properties of the endometrial tissue are involved. Posterior acoustic enhancement is best assessed in the anterior posterior-pelvic (AP-pelvic) image plane, since some posterior enhancement may be noted in a trans-pelvic (T-pelvic) plane (when the sound beam is directed across the pelvis

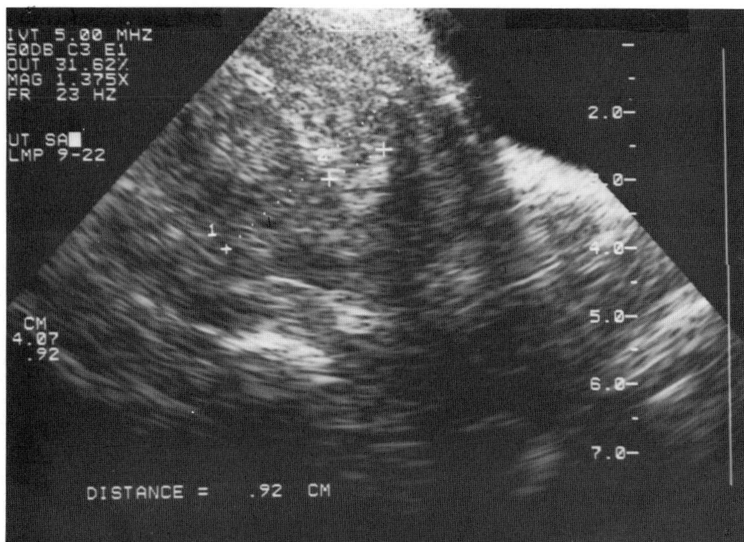

Fig. 6-8. A 31-year-old woman G3 on day 14 of a cycle. AP-pelvic view of uterus shows very early luteal phase endometrium. The endometrium is becoming hyperechoic. However, the central endometrial echo is still present. The endometrium has not progressed into a fully developed luteal phase endometrium. Serum estradiol was 97 pg/ml, and progesterone was 5.2 ng/nl.

from one side to the other) even during mid- to late follicular phases. It is not known why acoustic enhancement is sometimes noted below the follicular phase endometrium in the T-pelvic plane.

Several reports have noted no correlation between endometrial thickening and the serum progesterone value. Therefore, endometrial thickness cannot be utilized as a "sonographic assay" for progesterone levels. However, the change from a proliferative endometrium to the normal sonographic hyperechoic secretory endometrium is progesterone dependent and usually only occurs when the serum progesterone level is 1.5 ng/ml or higher.[4] Serum progesterone levels before ovulation are generally less than 1 ng/ml and rise to 5 to 20 ng/ml after ovulation.[5] The sonographic image of the endometrium evaluates the end organ response and acoustic properties of the tissue, and not the serum progesterone per se. Moreover, it must also be appreciated that the sonographic measurement of endometrial thickness and the sonographic pattern are providing data on parameters that have not been available in the past. Although serum progesterone is a valuable biochemical marker of normal menstrual physiology, it does not necessarily reflect luteal phase endometrial thickness and is only one parameter of menstrual physiology. In fact, in one study a poor correlation was even noted between serum progesterone levels and endometrial maturation, regardless of whether the chronological dating of the menstrual cycle was assigned from the day of the LH surge or from the onset of the next menses. Recently, studies have been published that correlate endometrial thickness and sonographic patterns with outcome in ovulation induction and assisted reproductive cycles. A thin endometrium (generally less than 6 mm in thickness) or an abnormal pattern for the follicular phase, such as a hyperechoic endometrium or a single-line endometrium, is associated with a decreased pregnancy rate. However, despite the fact that the significance of the biochemical markers and histologic evaluation of the endometrium is reasonably understood, the significance of the sonographic patterns and measurements in relation to reproductive physiology is still being studied. When all the sonographic signs are present suggesting a follicular or luteal phase (as noted above), there is a 93 percent agreement between the sonographic pattern and the endometrial histologic finding of a proliferative or secretory endometrium (Table 6-2).[3]

THE PREMENSTRUAL ENDOMETRIUM

Before menstruation, small anechoic areas may be noted in the endometrium (Figs. 6-10 and 6-11). These small premenstrual anechoic collections probably represent areas of hemorrhage into the endome-

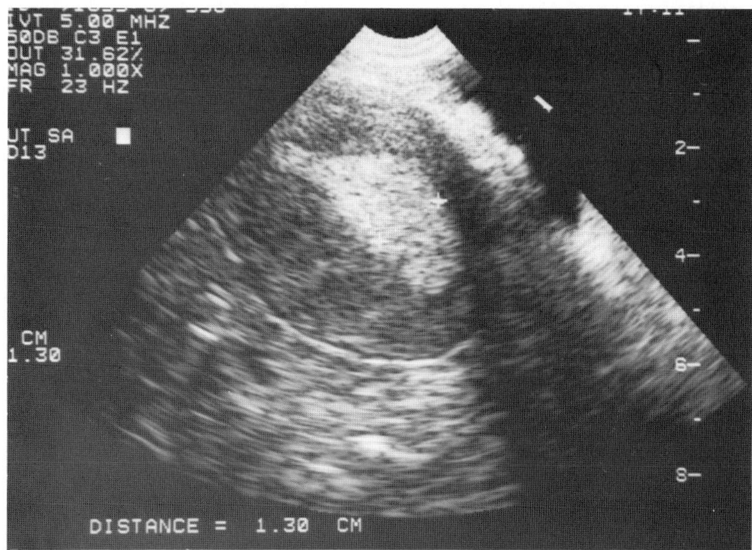

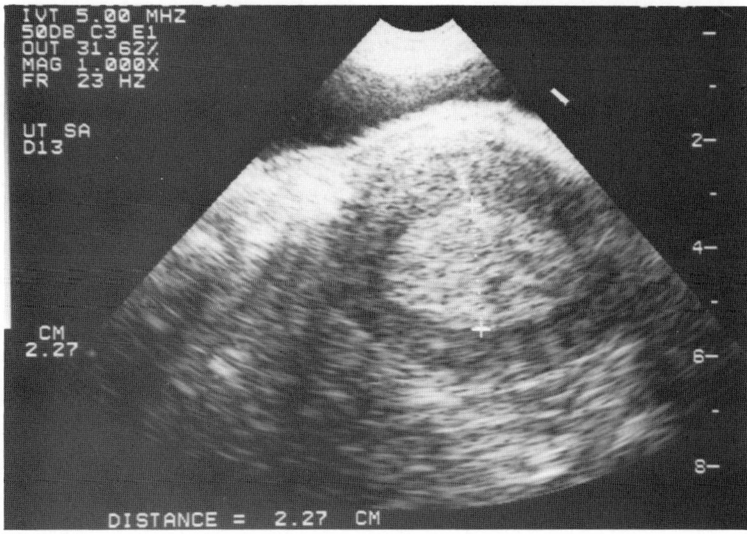

Fig. 6-9. (**A**) AP-pelvic view showing luteal phase endometrium 1.30 cm thick. There is a shadow from the bladder angle. (**B**) On T-pelvic view the endometrium is 2.27 cm thick. The difference in measurement from the AP-pelvic view probably results from variation in the image slice. Note that the posterior uterine wall is relatively thin compared with the anterior wall on the T-pelvic view, whereas the posterior wall is thicker than the anterior wall in the AP-pelvic view (see discussion in Ch. 5).

Table 6-2. Summary of Ultrasound Changes of the Endometrium During the Normal Menstrual Cycle†

Early menses (days 1–4)	Hypoechoic central echo (blood and menstrual debris) with a thick hyperechoic endometrial echo and posterior enhancement similar to the luteal phase
Late menses (days 3–7)	Single hyperechoic thin lines (central endometrial echo) Hypoechoic halo Hypoechoic central echo representing blood is gone Anterior posterior thickness of the entire endometrial echo complex is only 1–3 mm
Early follicular phase (days 5–9)	Halo present Relatively thin anterior posterior endometrial thickness (<6 mm) No posterior enhancement Three-line sign
Late follicular phase (days 10–14)	As above with thicker endometrial echo complex (>6 mm)
Luteal phase	Maximum endometrial thickness Hyperechoic endometrium Loss of halo Loss of three-line sign Prominent posterior enhancement

† Also see Fig. 6-5.

trium with endometrial degeneration and herald the onset of vaginal bleeding. However, the author has noted such collections as long as 7 days before evident vaginal bleeding.

SONOGRAPHIC ENDOMETRIAL PATTERNS IN USERS OF BIRTH CONTROL PILLS

Patients taking birth control pills usually have a somewhat thickened single-line endometrium (Figs. 6-12 and Fig. 6-13). Generally the endometrium is 3 to 5 mm thick and can be distinguished from the single-line endometrium noted during menses, which is thinner (generally 1 to 3 mm thick). This sonographic pattern reflects the endometrial response to simultaneous stimulation with both estrogen and progesterone as noted in patients taking birth control pills or in postmenopausal patients on estrogen replacement therapy when combined with progesterone.

A thickened single line is the term used in this text to describe the sonographic image characteristically noted in patients taking birth control pills. It can be thought of as a thickened menstrual or single-line endometrium, which it resembles, or as a very thin hyperechoic luteal phase type endometrium resulting from estrogen stimulation followed by progesterone or simultaneous estrogen progesterone (which is, in fact, how it is formed). Therefore, the birth control endometrial ultrasound pattern can be described as either a thick single-line endometrium or as a very thin luteal phase endometrium. It is a hyperechoic (white) image.

During menses, the patient taking birth control

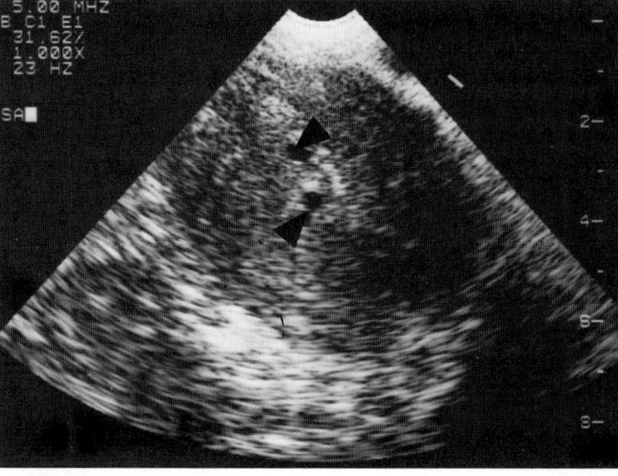

Fig. 6-10. A 46-year-old woman with vaginal spotting for 6 months after jogging. Transvaginal ultrasound on day 26 of cycle shows a luteal endometrium with two small anechoic areas. Patient began to menstruate the next day. The small anechoic areas probably represent mass collections of blood clots and the beginning of menstruation. Endometrial biopsy 2 weeks later showed proliferative glands and a follicular phase endometrium.

Fig. 6-11. AP-pelvic view of a uterus. The endometrium shows several small anechoic areas or premenstrual degeneration consistent with early breakdown of the endometrium before menstruation (arrows).

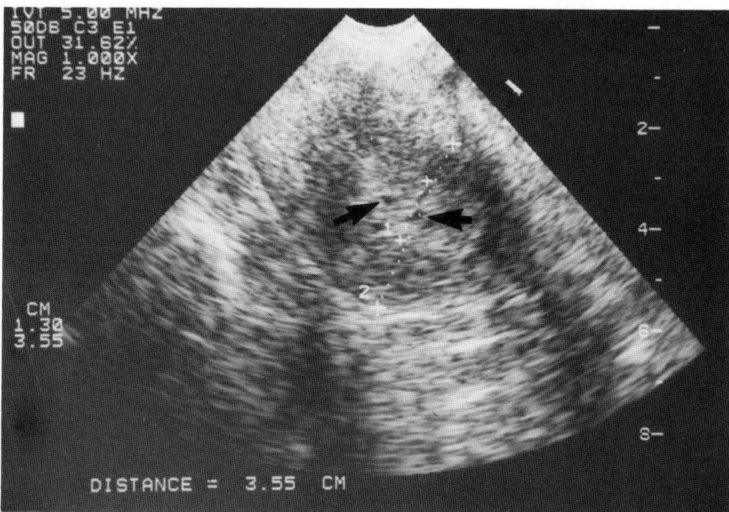

pills has the usual single-line endometrium characteristic of menses. However, occasionally a patient on birth control pills with breakthrough bleeding is noted to have a thin single-line (menstrual) endometrium, rather than the thickened single-line endometrium, because the bleeding has sloughed most of the endometrial tissue. Sometimes the patient taking birth control pills has a true single-line endometrium that cannot be distinguished from a menstrual endometrium. The few patients whom I have seen with these findings were experiencing only minimal spotting or no withdrawal bleeding after the end of a pill packet. Unfortunately, studies have not yet been done to evaluate the sonographic endometrial patterns and to correlate the sonographic findings with clinical findings, such as a missed period at the end of a birth control pill packet.

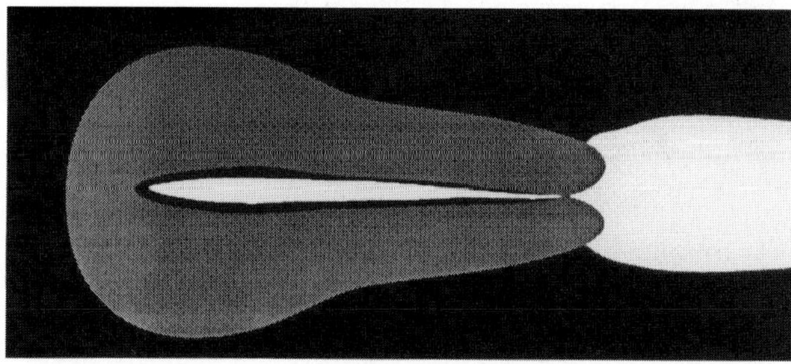

Fig. 6-12. The endometrium of a woman taking birth control pills is imaged as a thickened single line and is similar to a single-line menstrual endometrium, but is thicker. The ultrasound imaged endometrium generally noted in association with birth control pills might also be characterized as a very thin hyperechoic luteal phase endometrium. In fact, the thickened single-line endometrium imaged in patients taking birth control pills reflects the combined effect of concomitant estrogen and progesterone administration on the endometrium.

Despite the use of birth control pills, follicular development and ovulation occasionally occur. A patient taking birth control pills with a fully developed sonographic follicular (three-line) or luteal (hyperechoic) endometrium should be evaluated for an ovarian follicle, estrogen-producing cyst or tumor, or corpus luteal cyst. The presence of an endometrial pattern other than a thickened single-line endometrium in a patient taking birth control pills should be investigated. The patient reported in Figure 6-14 had a three line endometrium (characteristic of the proliferative phase of a natural cycle) despite the fact that she was on birth control pills. She was experiencing bleeding and had a small cyst or follicle in the ovary that was probably hormonally active, resulting in a sonographic endometrial pattern suggesting the follicular phase (three-Line) endometrium, rather than the expected thickened single-line endometrium generally noted when using birth control pills.

Transvaginal sonography can be of value in evaluating the patient on birth control pills experiencing breakthrough bleeding. In a study of patients with menometrorrhagia by Dodson, June 1994, one-third of patients taking birth control pills were noted to have an anatomic finding associated with the bleeding, such as an ovarian cyst or developing follicle. In

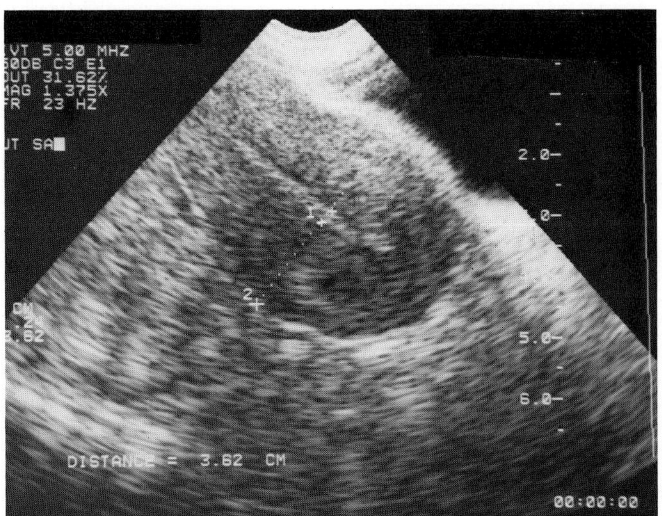

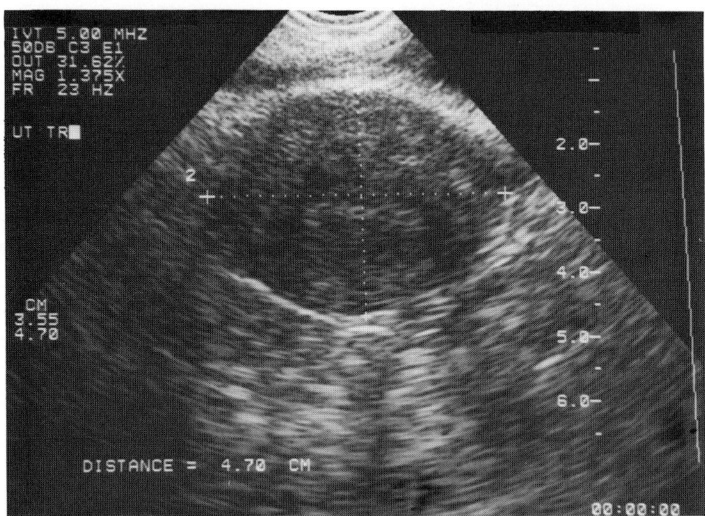

Fig. 6-13. (A) AP-pelvic view of uterus with an anterior posterior diameter of 3.6 cm. The bladder is to the right. The endometrium is 2.4 mm thick. This thickened single-line endometrium, is generally seen in patients taking oral contraceptives. The patient was taking Triphasil (levonorgestrel and ethinyl estrodiol). **(B)** T-pelvic view of the same patient. Uterine dimensions are normal.

one patient on birth control pills, no endometrial image was noted, suggesting an atrophic endometrium. The estrogen content of the birth control pills was increased for this patient to control the bleeding.

ABNORMAL ENDOMETRIAL PATTERNS

A number of other abnormal sonographic endometrial patterns can be recognized, providing valuable diagnostic information or suggesting the need for further evaluation (Table 6-3, Fig. 6-15).

Abnormal endometrial patterns may be associated with either anatomic pelvic pathology or physiologic aberrations in the normal menstrual cycle. Recognizable pathology includes endometrial carcinoma, hyperplasia, endometrial polyps, or pedunculated or submucosal leiomyomas protruding into the endometrium. Pathology involving the endometrium is frequently imaged as an abnormally thickened endometrium or a mixed hyper- and hypoechoic pattern that clearly does not fit into one of the normal sonographic endometrial patterns described above. Occasionally

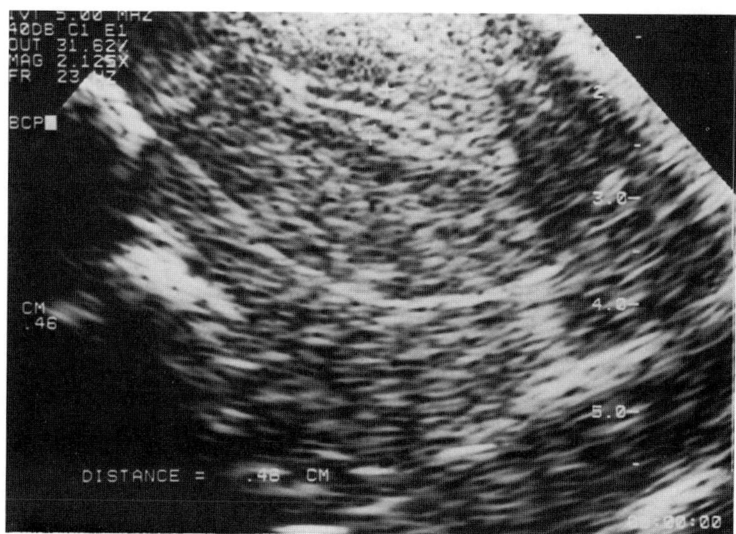

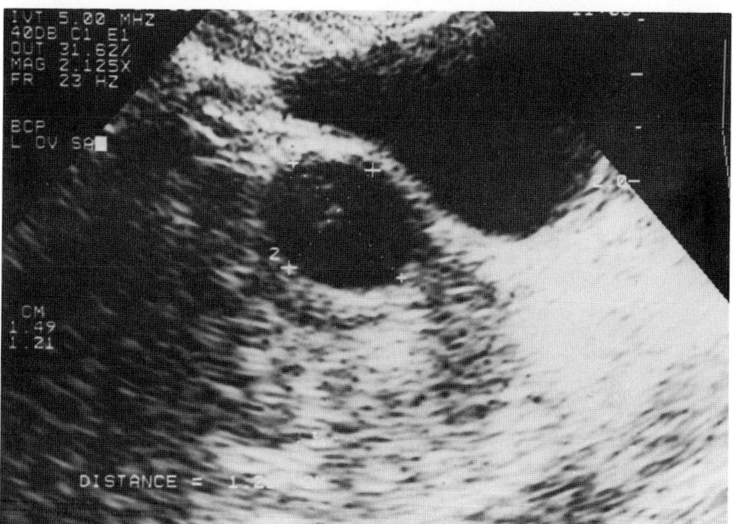

Fig. 6-14. Patient taking birth control pills with breakthrough bleeding for 10 weeks. **(A)** AP-pelvic image of the uterus. Note the thickened follicular endometrium rather than a thickened single line endometrium normally seen in patients taking birth control pills. The endometrium shows the three-line sign characteristic of a proliferative endometrium rather than the expected thickened single-line endometrium. **(B)** AP-pelvic image of the left ovary. A follicle (1.4 by 1.2 cm) is present in the left ovary. Additional estrogen from the developing follicle was probably responsible for development of the follicular endometrium. This follicle or small cyst developed despite the fact that the patient was taking birth control pills.

an endometrial polyp or leiomyoma is distinctly outlined by surrounding blood and can be imaged clearly. Usually the sonographic pattern is nonspecific, but can often be recognized as abnormal and can indicate the need for additional evaluation techniques, such as an endometrial biopsy, hysteroscopy, hysterosalpingography, or D&C. Patients with endometrial adhesion, such as Asherman's syndrome, may have a distorted endometrial pattern with areas where no endometrium can be imaged mixed with areas that appear more normal. Hematometra secondary to cervical stenosis or cervical carcinoma can be recognized as an anechoic area (fluid-filled) indicating a distended endometrial cavity. Occasionally, when the endometrium is atrophic and/or very thin, no endometrium is visualized by sonography. This is occasionally seen in postmenopausal women.

ATYPICAL ENDOMETRIAL PATTERNS

Hyperechoic Thickened Endometrium

This pattern is generally uniformly hyperechoic (white) and cannot be distinguished from the normal hyperechoic luteal phase sonographic endometrial

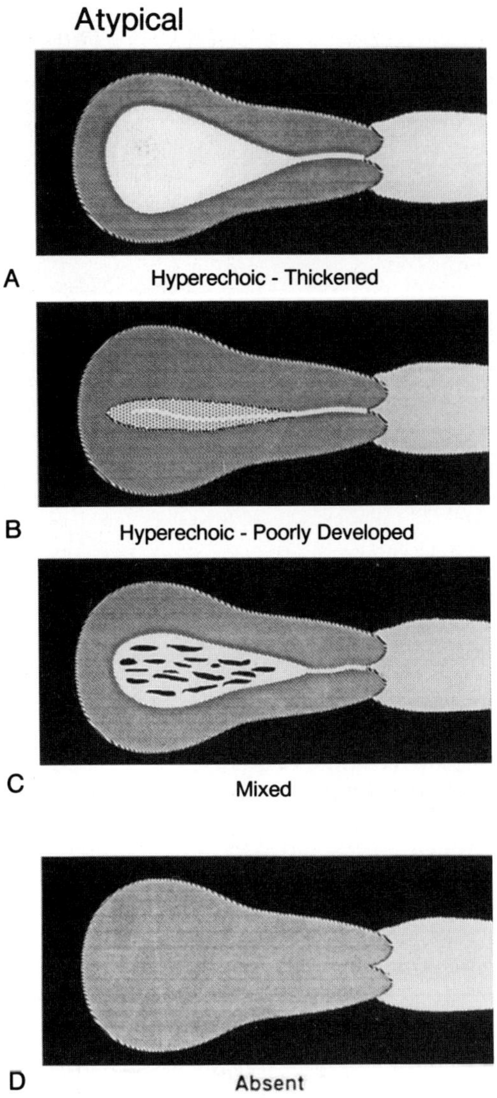

Atypical

A Hyperechoic - Thickened

B Hyperechoic - Poorly Developed

C Mixed

D Absent

Fig. 6-15. Ultrasound endometrium atypical does not fit into any of the normal endometrial patterns. (**A**) *Hyperechoic* and *thickened:* The hyperechoic thickened endometrium may be associated with endometrial carcinoma, adenomatous hyperplasia, or endometrial polyps, on leiomyomas projecting into the endometrial cavity. (**B**) *Hyperechoic* but *poorly developed* endometrium is characterized by a "washed out" appearance. It is generally thinner than a normal hyperechoic luteal phase endometrium, and there is often persistence of the central hyperechoic echo representing the endometrial cavity. This type of endometrium is seen with chronic low level estrogen stimulation often in association with anovulation. (**C**) *Mixed* endometrium is often associated with endometrial polyps or leiomyomas and is characterized by anechoic and hyperechoic areas. (**D**) *Absent* endometrial echo may be seen in postmenopausal patients or occasionally in patients on BCP contraceptive therapy.

Table 6-3. Atypical Ultrasound Imaged Endometrial Patterns

Hyperechoic
- Thickened: ≥ 17 mm in thickness[a]
- Poorly developed: Less hyperechoic and/or thinner than the usual luteal phase endometrium. The central hyperechoic echo of the endometrial cavity is generally still present.

Mixed
- A combination of endometrial ultrasound imaged findings often with multiple anechoic and/or hyperechoic areas. Does not fit any of the normal ultrasound imaged patterns or other atypical endometrial categories.

Absent or partially absent endometrial echo
- No echo representing the endometrial cavity present.

[a] Thickened endometrium may also normally be seen in early pregnancy.

pattern. However it is much thicker (equal to or thicker than 17 mm, (Fig. 6-16). This atypical variant can be associated with endometrial carcinoma, endometrial hyperplasia, or polypoid leiomyomas projecting into the endometrial cavity. In a patient with abnormal bleeding, a biopsy would be of value in ruling out hyperplasia or carcinoma; the pregnancy test should be negative before doing a biopsy. A proliferative endometrium would suggest chronic anovulation with normal or elevated estrogen—polycystic ovarian disease (PCOD), exogenous estrogens, or an estogen secreting ovarian tumors. A patient with a proliferative endometrium may be treated with progesterone to induce menses (chemical curettage). Persistence of a thickened endometrium after progesterone withdrawal would warrant hysteroscopy and/or D&C.

Hyperechoic Poorly Developed Endometrium

This pattern resembles the normal ultrasound pattern of the hyperechoic luteal phase endometrium, but is much less hyperechoic and often much thinner. However, the major characteristic of this pattern is not the thinness of the endometrium but rather the decreased echogenicity. In fact, occasionally the poorly developed endometrium is as thick as a normal luteal phase endometrium; however, with a little experience it is easy to recognize that it does not represent a normal luteal phase pattern (Fig. 6-17).

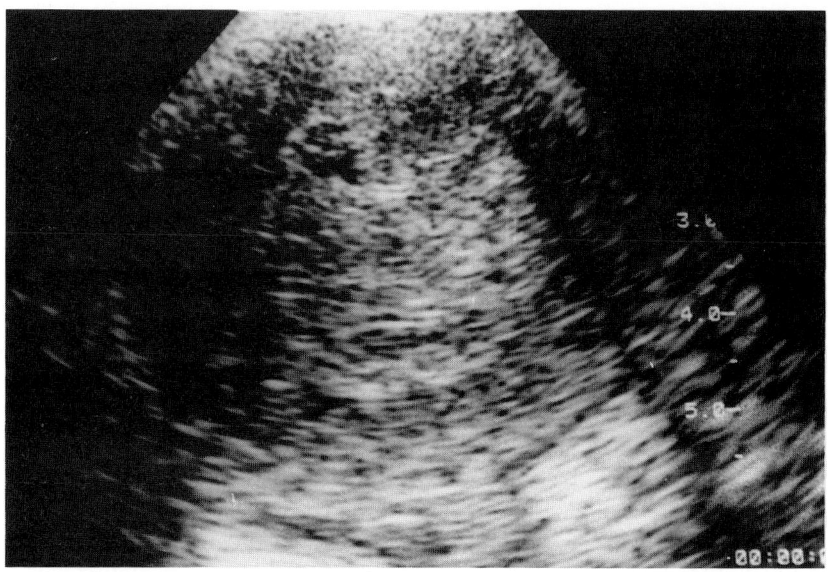

Fig. 6-16. Atypical, hyperechoic, thickened endometrium. The patient had an endometrial adenocarcinoma.

The poorly developed hyperechoic endometrium is uniformly white, but much less so than the normal luteal phase endometrium. In addition to the "washed out" or less hyperechoic (less white) appearance, the central hyperechoic echo representing the endometrial cavity is generally still evident within the surrounding hyperechoic endometrium. This type of atypical ultrasound endometrial pattern is, in my experience, one of the most frequently encountered abnormal patterns. It is commonly associated with chorionic anovulation, but there is a significant amount of circulating estrogen. This pattern may be seen in some patients with PCOD; however, a few PCOD patients develop a hyperechoic thickened pattern.

This atypical, poorly developed hyperechoic pattern can be quite confusing, particularly when a sonographer first begins to recognize the various en-

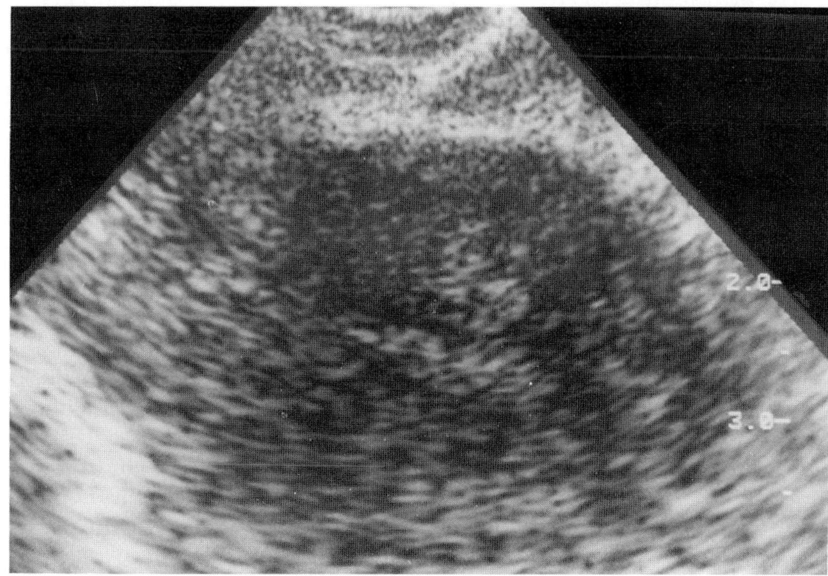

Fig. 6-17. Atypical, hyperechoic, poorly developed endometrium. The endometrium is thinner than a normal luteal phase endometrium, with persistence of the central hyperechoic echo representing the endometrial cavity. Although the endometrium is hyperechoic, it is much less reflective than the normal hyperechoic luteal phase endometrium. This type of endometrium is frequently associated with PCOD or chronic anovulation with chronic low level estrogen stimulation.

dometrial patterns and to correlate these patterns with normal or abnormal menstrual physiology. Since the normal luteal phase secretory endometrium is imaged sonographically as a hyperechoic area (white area of increased reflection), there is a natural tendency to equate the hyperechoic endometrium with a progesterone effect and ovulation. Unfortunately, this is not always true. I have noted many patients with hyperechoic sonographic endometrial patterns (but generally poorly developed as described here) with very low serum progesterone (below 1 ng/ml) and anovulation.

The hyperechoic poorly developed pattern seems to be associated with chronic anovulation with at least a moderate amount of estrogen present. This is in contrast to the persistence of a three-line endometrium pattern that continues to be imaged late into the luteal phase of a cycle and suggests estrogen stimulation, but a lack of ovulation in that particular cycle. Another explanation for a three-line endometrium in the late luteal phase of the menstrual cycle is a lack of follicular development until late in the cycle. The absence of a developing follicle would require a search for another mechanism. However, if the patient is imaged shortly after ovulation and follicle collapse but before luteal changes have occurred in the endometrium, a three-line endometrium (and no follicle) will be noted. It will not be possible in a single ultrasound examination to distinguish between an anovulatory cycle (with enough E_2 to stimulate the endometrium) and late ovulation. However, if a repeat ultrasound is done in 7 to 10 days, late ovulation can be diagnosed by the development of a hyperechoic luteal phase endometrium.

The use of ultrasound imaging and pattern recognition of the different endometrial patterns, although based on reasonable patient experience, still need more study to sort out the vagaries and subtleties. In a recent study by the author of 45 patients with menometrorrhagia in which the sonographic endometrial pattern and pelvic sonographic findings were compared to clinical findings, endometrial biopsy, and serum progesterone levels, there was an excellent correlation (89 percent). However, in two patients the sonographic pattern did not correlate with the ovulatory status and was wrong!

Although the sonographic pattern of the endometrium can be of considerable value in many clinical situations, it is important to recognize the limitation of the tool and to re-emphasize the obvious sonographic axiom that the images produced are the results of the reflection, absorption, transmission, scatter, etc. of sound waves by biologic tissues. Although the sound wave/tissue interaction can give a considerable amount of valuable information regarding the size, location, and character of the target tissue, the images are not pictures of the tissue per se, but are literally only a reflection. We see, in essence, a platonic view of the anatomy.

It is not clear why the secretory endometrium is generally hyperechoic. Although there seems to be a good correlation between a histologic secretory endometrium and a sonographic hyperechoic pattern, there is a poor correlation between serum progesterone levels and endometrial thickness. This may be due to the fact that endometrial thickness is primarily a function of estrogen stimulation with only a minimal additional thickening occurring in the luteal phase. From this viewpoint, endometrial thickness would be more of a reflection of the level and duration of estrogen stimulation with only a minimal effect produced by progesterone. Although as a generality this is probably true, the physiology is clearly more complex since I have seen patients undergoing clomiphene citrate ovulation induction with a relatively thin three-line endometrium (5 mm) but high serum estradiol levels (800 ng/ml). Therefore, the endometrial response to estrogen stimulation is also an important factor.

One possible explanation for the hyperechoic ultrasound luteal phase pattern is the presence of mucus within endometrial glands. However, mucus produced by endocervical glands that is abundant at midcycle in the endocervical canal is usually imaged as an anechoic echo, rather than being hyperechoic. Perhaps, some other particular physiochemical characteristic of the mucus or tissue, such as its water or salt content causes this pattern, or perhaps the hyperechoic pattern results from some entirely different character of the sound wave/tissue interaction. More research is needed in this area.

Mixed Pattern

In an atypical mixed pattern, hyperechoic and anechoic or hypoechoic areas occur together. This pattern is seen in patients with endometrial polyps, submucosal leiomyomas protruding into the endometrial cavity, incomplete abortions, and sometimes in patients without organic pelvic or endometrial disease (Fig. 6-18). This pattern often results from a mixture of blood and tissue within the endometrial cavity. When the pattern is persistent (in several menstrual cycles), it is often associated with anatomic changes

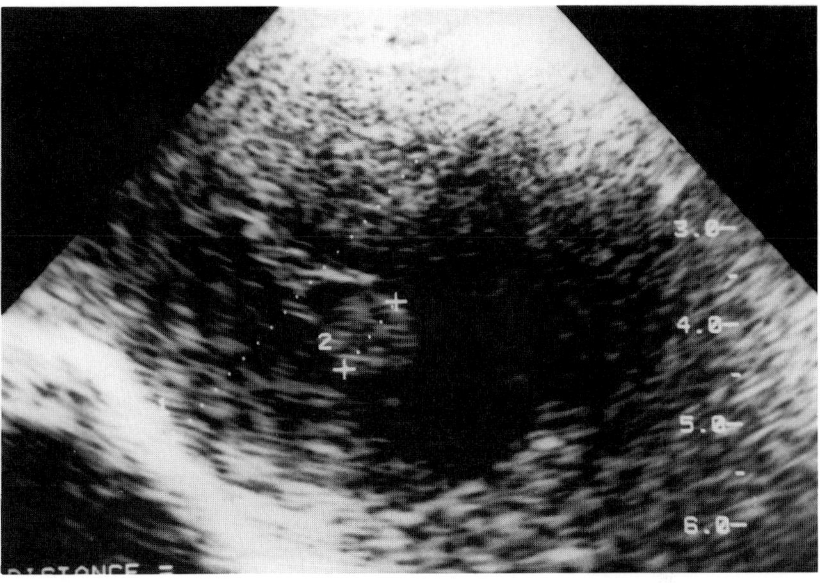

Fig. 6-18. The atypical mixed ultrasound-imaged endometrium has hyperechoic and hypoechoic areas and may be seen with endometrial polyps, leiomyomas, incomplete abortions, and other conditions. NOTE: Hyperechoic endometrial polyp is outlined by anechoic fluid.

rather than hormonal or physiologic aberrations, such as anovulation.

Anechoic Pattern

An anechoic pattern consists of a central anechoic echo surrounded by a (usually thin) hyperechoic rim. The anechoic area generally represents blood or fluid distending the endometrial cavity and may be seen in association with cervical stenosis or cervical carcinoma, particularly in the postmenopausal patient. This type of pattern can sometimes be seen during normal menses, but is transient and usually not as large (Figs. 6-19 A&B). The importane in the postmenopausal patient is obvious since they should not be menstruating. Hematometra is generally imaged by ultrasound as an anechoic endometrial pattern.

Absence of an Endometrial Echo

Another atypical endometrial variant consists of an absent or partial absence of any endometrial echo imaged by ultrasound (Fig. 6-15). This type of atypical endometrial pattern is most commonly associated with menopause, especially in patients 15 to 20 years after menopause who are not on hormone replacement therapy. It may also be seen in patients with very low estrogen levels and occasionally in patients on birth control pills (Table 6-4).

NORMAL ENDOMETRIAL PATTERNS ASSOCIATED WITH CLINICAL ABNORMALITIES

Menstrual Cycle Dys-synchrony

Abnormal endometrial patterns not characteristic of either menstruation or the follicular or luteal phase or a normal pattern that does not correlate with the menstrual cycle as dated from the LMP or the follicular development in the ovary suggests a hormonal irregularity and/or ovulatory dysfunction. These patterns can give the clinician considerable information that can be invaluable in the diagnosis and treatment of amenorrhea, missed or late menses, abnormal vaginal bleeding, and/or infertility. In a normal cycle, the endometrial pattern, follicular development, and menstrual cycle day should all be consistent. When these findings are inconsistent, dys-synchrony may be present.

A normal endometrial pattern, such as the single-line, three-line, and hyperechoic pattern, which is a normal finding during menses, the follicular phase, and the luteal phase of a menstrual cycle, respec-

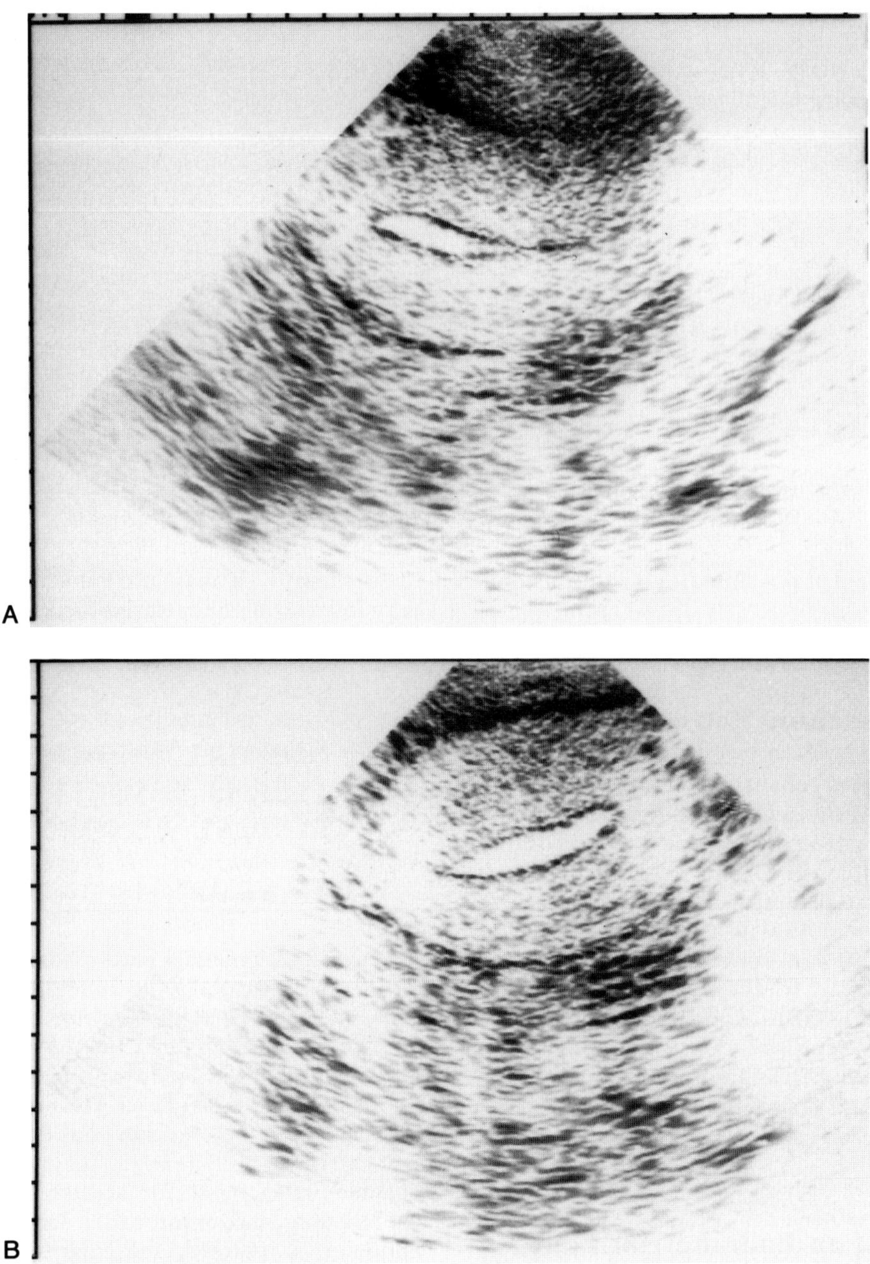

Fig. 6-19. **(A)** AP-pelvic image. **(B)** Trans-pelvic plane image of an anechoic endometrium filled with fluid with a very thin hyperechoic endometrium.

Table 6-4. Abnormal Endometrial Patterns

Pattern	*Characteristics*	*Clinical Association*
Hyperechoic thickened	Usually thicker than 17 mm	Hyperplasia, carcinoma, polyps, leiomyomas
Hyperechoic, poorly developed	Uniformly hyperechoic (white), but less than a normal sonographic luteal phase endometrium with persistence of the central line representing the endometrial cavity	PCOD, chronic anovulation
Mixed pattern	Presence of both hyperechoic and hypoechoic areas	Polyps, submucosal leiomyomas protruding into the endometrial cavity, incomplete abortions, mixed blood and tissue
Hypoechoic	Distended endometrial cavity with anechoic material, usually blood or fluid surrounded by thin hyperechoic endometrium	Hematometria, pyometria (usually filled with a fine grained echotexture) associated with cervical stenosis or cervical cancer
Absent	No endometrium imaged	Atrophic and/or very thin endometrium: low serum E

tively, may represent an abnormal pattern under some clinical circumstances. The sonographic endometrial pattern should be consistent with the LMP and with ovarian function, such as follicular development. Dys-synchrony may indicate an abnormality in menstrual cycle physiology, such as anovulation, and/or may be associated with clinical problems, such as menometrorrhagia, missed or late periods etc.

As an example, a thin single-line endometrium is a normal and expected pattern in a menstruating patient and in the postmenopausal patient, but indicates a minimally stimulated endometrium (low serum estradiol levels and anovulation) or a lack of an endometrial response when present during the luteal phase of the cycle (day 14 to 28). A single-line endometrium also indicates a lack of endometrial stimulation or an atrophic unresponsive endometrium in an amenorrheic patient. Recognition of the endometrial pattern is not only helpful in diagnosis but can also be used in the clinical management. The patient with amenorrhea and a single-line endometrium (less than 5 mm thick) will generally not menstruate when treated using the common approach of a progesterone challenge. This type of patient with a very thin endometrium needs estrogen followed by progesterone to induce menses (after an appropriate endocrine evaluation depending on the clinical circumstances).

As another example, a three-line endometrial pattern that correlates with estrogen stimulation and an endometrial proliferative response is a completely normal and expected finding in the first half of the menstrual cycle. However, the presence of the same finding in a patient with a history of a LMP 25 days before the sonographic examination suggests the possibility of a physiologic aberration, such as an anovulatory cycle or inadequate progesterone to luteinize the endometrium appropriately. In fact, I have noted the same pattern in some patients who have missed their period, have a positive pregnancy test, and have an ectopic pregnancy. However, this sonographic pattern is not noted in all ectopic pregnancies and although the three-line pattern is clearly recognizable in some patients with an ectopic pregnancy, there is often increased echogenicity of the endometrial layers with the three-line pattern blending into the atypical poorly developed pattern described above. However, a thick hyperechoic sonographic endometrial pattern is expected in a normal pregnancy, and the imaging of an unexpected pattern, such as a three-line endometrium or a variation, should alert the clinician to a potential problem.

Likewise, a hyperechoic endometrial pattern 12 mm thick would be a normal and expected finding in a patient late in her menstrual cycle, but would be an abnormal pattern for a postmenopausal patient where the endometrial thickness would be expected to be 5 mm or less. It would also be an unexpected finding in the early follicular phase and would possibly suggest the need for further evaluation depending on the clinical circumstances. A hyperechoic endometrial pattern in the early follicular phase may result from anatomic abnormalities as discussed above, but may also occur in a patient with a corpus luteal cyst from the previous cycle, with the "menses" representing abnormal bleeding.

These examples indicate that the same endometrial pattern can be normal or abnormal depending on the circumstances and emphasize the need to interpret

Table 6-5. Normal Endometrial Patterns That Are Not in Synchrony with the Menstrual Cycle, Suggesting an Abnormal Menstrual Physiology

Pattern	*Normal Association*	*Abnormal Association*
Single line	Menses, postmenopausal	When present during the follicular or luteal phase, indicates a lack of E_2 stimulation or endometrial response. May be associated with amenorrhea or irregular bleeding.
Three line	Follicular phase	When present during the luteal phase, suggests anovulation. May be associated with bleeding, infertility, or ectopic pregnancy (with a positive pregnancy test).
Hyperechoic	Luteal phase	When present during the follicular phase, suggests persistence from a previous cycle. May be associated with a corpus luteal cyst and abnormal bleeding or an anatomic abnormality (also see description of abnormal patterns that this pattern can resemble, such as atypical hyperechoic poorly developed pattern).

the pattern in the context of the total clinical findings (Table 6-5).

Consistency of Endometrial Pattern

The endometrial pattern should also be consistent with the findings in the ovary. It has long been recognized that the follicular phase of the menstrual cycle is associated with a developing follicle in the ovary and correlates with endometrial histologic (proliferative) changes. Likewise, the histologic term "proliferative phase" is used to describe this part of the menstrual cycle; it emphasizes endometrial histology. Sonographically, we can image both the ovarian and endometrial changes, and both should be consistent and in synchrony. For example, a well developed three-line endometrium on day 10 to 12 of a normal menstrual cycle should be associated with a developing follicle in the ovary. If a follicle is not present, the patient has either ovulated very early in her cycle, or a follicle has not yet developed. If a follicle develops later in the particular cycle, the patient will not ovulate until very late in the cycle and the cycle will be longer than expected, or the cycle is an anovulatory cycle. If knowledge of the ovulatory status is important, as for example in an infertility patient, serial ultrasound evaluations will reveal the patient's ovulatory dynamics—early cycle ovulation, late cycle ovulation, anovulation, etc. (see Ch. 18). The knowledge of the ovulatory status can also be important in many other clinical situations, such as abnormal bleeding or spotting, amenorrhea, and a late or missed period; these are very common problems seen by gynecologists.

As another example, the presence of an anechoic area 25 to 35 mm in diameter in the ovary on day 25 of a menstrual cycle associated with a sonographic luteal phase (hyperechoic) endometrium suggests that the patient has ovulated, and is producing enough progesterone to luteinize the endometrium. The most likely diagnosis of the ovarian cyst is a corpus luteal cyst; a neoplasm would also have to be considered, but is much less common and can often be differentiated based on other anatomic findings (see Ch. 7). Tumors would generally not produce progesterone and luteinize the endometrium. However, the patient may produce progesterone despite the presence of a tumor.

MENOMETRORRHAGIA

The status of the endometrium and the ovaries can be very helpful in determining the etiology of menometrorrhagia and the best approach to therapy. The endometrium may be imaged as a single-line endometrium indicating anovulation with only low level estrogen stimulation. A single-line endometrium can also be seen at the end of a normal menstrual period after sloughing of the endometrium. An anechoic area within the endometrium characteristic of a fluid collection suggests active bleeding or that bleeding will occur in the near future (Fig. 6-20).

A well developed follicular (3-line) endometrium suggests adequate estrogen stimulation and follicular development. Bleeding may also occur as a result of systemic disease, coagulation problems, estrogen stimulation followed by estrogen withdrawal, or chronic estrogen stimulation from a follicular cyst, estrogen-producing neoplasm, or exogenous estrogen administration. Chronic unopposed estrogen stimulation may result in an endometrium that is neither clearly follicular nor luteal but is atypical (Fig.

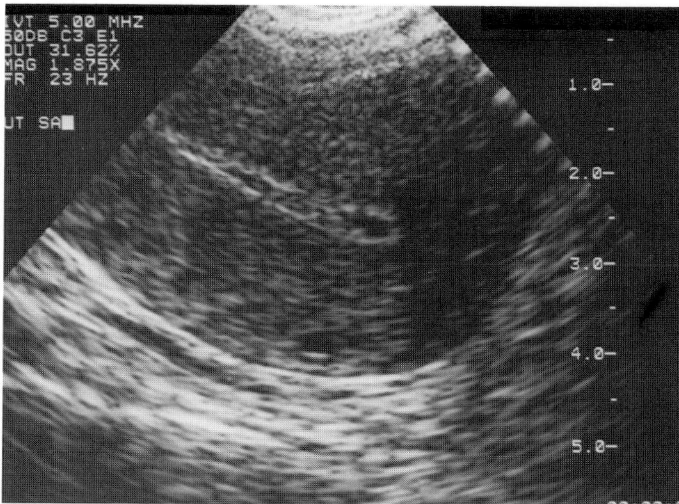

Fig. 6-20. AP-pelvic view of uterus showing menstrual-type endometrium with blood still in the endometrial cavity in a patient with menometrorrhagia. The three-line sign is not present. The serum estradiol was 52 pg/ml. The serum progesterone was less than 1 ng/ml. Note the two thin hyperechoic lines. Endometrial biopsy showed an early proliferative endometrium consistent with low level estrogen stimulation.

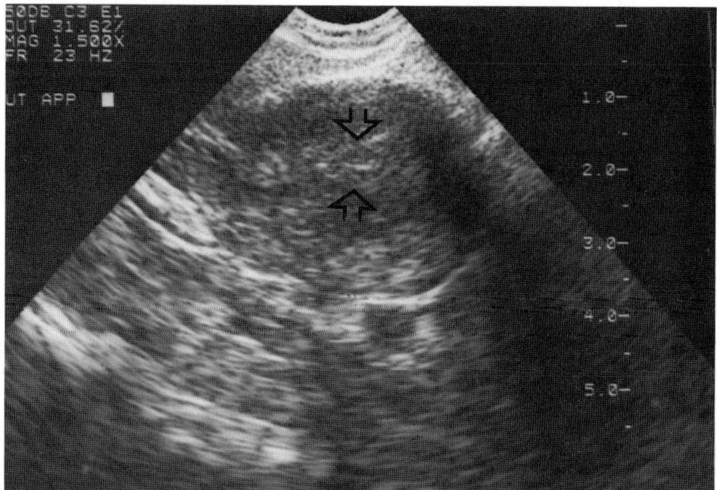

Fig. 6-21. A 25-year-old woman G0 with bleeding for 36 days. She was not using contraceptives. Transvaginal ultrasound examination showed no follicle or ovarian cyst. The endometrium (AP-pelvic) showed a nonspecific or atypical pattern that can be seen after prolonged low level estrogen stimulation or with low level progesterone stimulation during the luteal phase. The serum estradiol was 54.0 pg/ml with a progesterone of 0.2 ng/ml. Human chorionic gonadotropin was negative. The follicle stimulating hormone (7.6 mIU/ml) and luteinizing hormone (10.7 mIU/ml) were normal. Note that the central endometrial cavity is imaged but that the pattern is not characteristic of a follicular or luteal phase endometrium. There is a central echo probably representing the endometrial cavity and a diffuse hyperechoic area. However, the endometrium is less intense than generally seen in a well-developed luteal phase endometrium with adequate progesterone stimulation. An outer halo is absent. This atypical endometrium is consistent with anovulation and chronic low level estrogen stimulation.

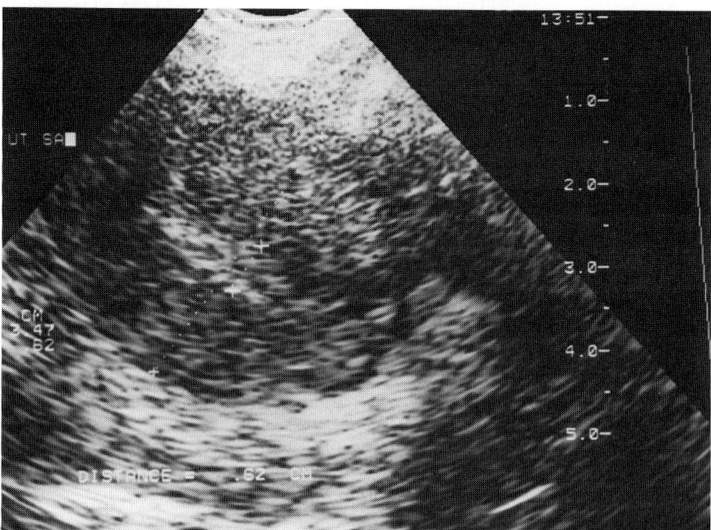

Fig. 6-22. AP-pelvic view of the uterus showing a poorly developed luteal endometrium 0.62 cm thick in a patient with menometrorrhagia. The serum estradiol was 134 pg/ml, and the progesterone was 5.3 ng/ml.

6-21). A luteal phase endometrium may be associated with bleeding when there is inadequate progesterone to support the endometrium (Fig. 6-22). Bleeding may occur with a luteal phase endometrium when a corpus luteal cyst is present that does not produce adequate progesterone for continued support of the endometrium. Bleeding may occur secondary to leiomyomas, polyps, or carcinomas (see below), from early pregnancy or complications of pregnancy (see Ch. 12), or with an ectopic pregnancy (see Ch. 15). It may also occur secondary to retained secundinae after delivery (Fig. 6-23).

ENDOMETRIAL THICKNESS

Since linear measurement of endometrial thickness really measures two layers of endometrium (the anterior and posterior wall, Fleischer et al[6] have suggested that such measurements should be divided by two. Care must be taken when interpreting or reporting such measurements to specify whether the full thickness of both layers of endometrium or only one layer is being measured. Since it is generally simpler just to measure the full endometrial thickness, this is usually the measurement reported. Unless otherwise stated, full thickness measurements of the endometrium are used in this text.

Endometrial thickness can generally be measured quite accurately. Varner et al[7] noted no more than a 1-mm variation between different examiners. However, it is important to evaluate the whole endometrium and to measure the thickest portion. Care must be taken not to measure the endometrium in an oblique plane, which will result in an increase in thickness. Because the uterus is generally anteverted or retroverted, measurements in the trans-pelvic plane (see Ch. 1) with the sound beam directed across the pelvis from side to side are more likely to result in an oblique cut and an inaccurate measurement. One clue suggesting that an image is in an oblique plane is when one uterine wall is much thicker than the other. Probably the best plane for evaluating and measuring the endometrium is the AP-pelvic plane, with the sound beam directed between the anterior abdominal wall and the back or buttocks. This gives a long axis image of the uterus. However, rotation of the transducer can still produce a distorted measurement plane, and care in technique must be taken regardless of the imaging plane.

Forrest et al[3] noted the average thickness of the proliferative endometrium to be 8.4 ± 2.2 mm, whereas the secretory endometrium is 9.6 ± 3.4 mm. The range of endometrium thickness reported varies between 6.2 and 13 mm (full thickness). Fleischer et al[8] noted that sonographic measurements of endometrial thickness were within 10 to 15 percent of actual

Fig. 6-23. A 21-year-old woman seen in the emergency room with heavy vaginal bleeding of 1 day duration. She had a normal spontaneous vaginal delivery 7 weeks earlier. The pregnancy test was weakly positive. On physical examination, there were 200 ml of blood in the vagina and on her perineal pad. The cervical os was open and the uterus was clinically 8 weeks size. AP-pelvic (**A**) and T-pelvic (**B**) views. Transvaginal ultrasound revealed a mixed echo density of 3.8 by 2.1 cm filling the endometrial cavity, suggesting retained placental tissue. Although markedly hyperechoic, there are also small anechoic and hypoechoic areas, and the margins are irregular, giving a moth-eaten appearance. A suction curettage was done, and 5 ml^3 of tissue was obtained that showed degenerating and infarcted chorionic villi with calcification. (**C**) One day after the curettage, the endometrium is now only 9 mm thick. However, the uterus shows a mixed echo pattern in the area of the endometrium with poorly defined borders.

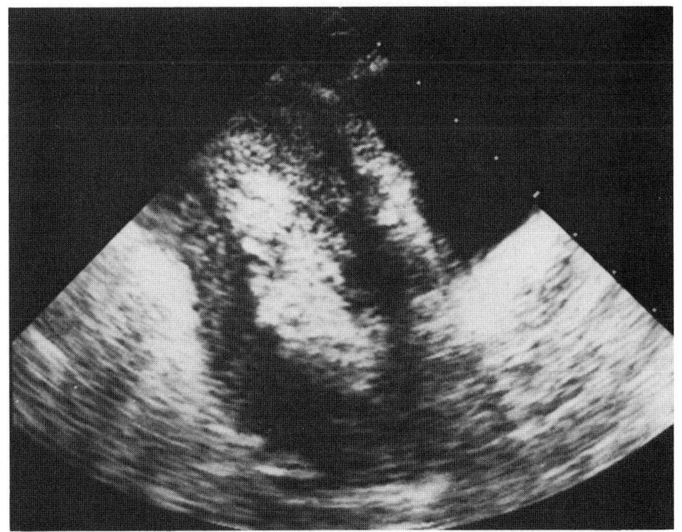
A

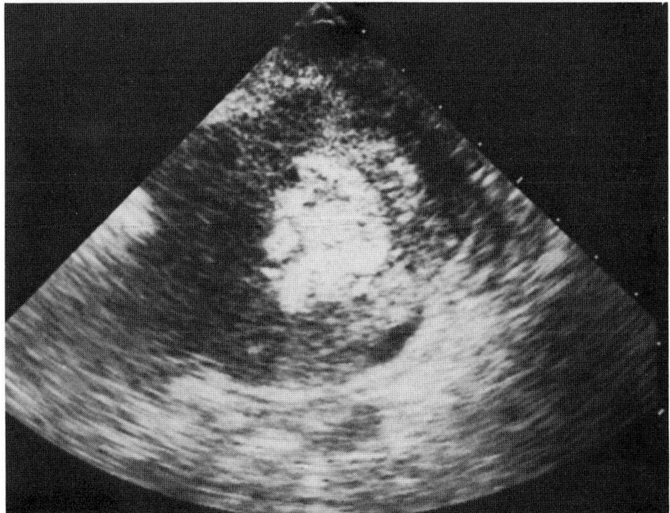
B

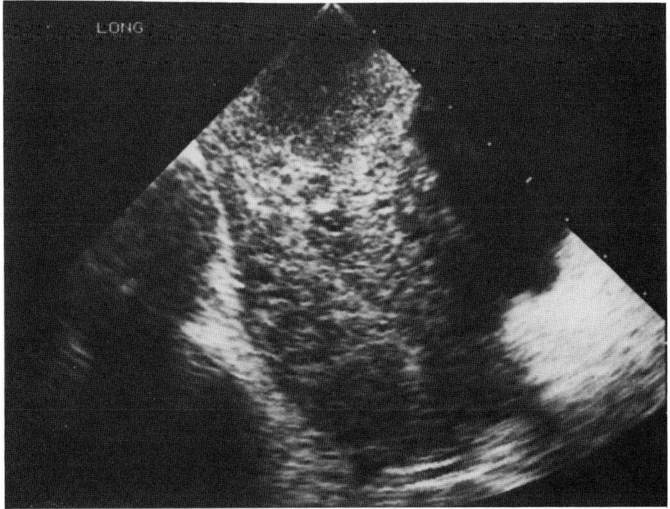

C

Table 6-6. Endometrial Thickness

Menstrual Phase	*Full Thickness (mm)*
Menstrual (late)	0.5–1
Proliferative (follicular)	4–8
Periovulatory	6–10
Secretory (luteal)	10–12

(Modified from Fleischer et al,[8] with permission.)

measurements from hysterectomy specimens. Total double layer thickness ranged from 4 to 12 mm with an average of 7.5 mm (Table 6-6).[8]

Although there is generally a small increase in endometrial thickness in the luteal phase after ovulation, the difference in thickness of the follicular and luteal phase endometriums is not statistically significant. The greatest increase in thickness occurs between the early and late proliferative phases, with only minimal additional thickening occurring during the secretory phase.

In a study using nuclear magnetic resonance (NMR) imaging, the cross-sectional area of the endometrium (calculated as the product of the long axis of the endometrial cavity and the maximal perpendicular dimension) increased by 50 to 150 percent during the follicular phase, with an average daily increase of 4.4 percent per day.[9] Wiczyk et al[10] noted a mean endometrial thickness of 5.1 ± 0.1 mm on day 4, which increased to 11.5 ± 0.5 mm on day 24. However, NMR measurements may be measuring a different myometrium-endometrium interface than ultrasound. Variation between sonographic measurements may also occur when the halo in the follicular phase is included in the measurement.

Endometrial thickness per se has not been found to be an accurate indicator of potential conception. In a group of IVF patients being stimulated with human menopausal gonadotropin followed by human chorionic gonadotropin, there was no statistical difference in endometrial thickness in conceptional versus nonconceptional cycles.[6]

Calculating the endometrial volume, Giorlandino et al[11] found no correlation with hormone levels (estradiol or progesterone) in either natural or stimulated cycles. There was some correlation ($R = 0.29$) between endometrial thickness measured in the anterior posterior diameter and serum estradiol levels. No correlation was noted between the endometrial thickness and serum progesterone levels. However, progesterone at concentrations of at least 1.5 ng/ml has been reported to produce the characteristic sonographic luteal phase endometrium.

ENDOMETRIAL MOTION

The endometrium can be seen to move during real-time ultrasonographic imaging. This movement can be quite impressive when first seen by a novice sonographer during real-time scanning. Birnholz[12] reported endometrial movement in 19 of 26 women (73 percent). Endometrial movement has been reported to be most pronounced 2 to 3 days after sexual intercourse. de Varies et al[13] noted that the uterus in the sexually mature individual is "never motionless."

Contractions of the inner one-third of the myometrium are found in 76 percent of examinations, with a frequency of 3.3 contractions (range, 0.5 to 9.0) per minute and an average length of the contraction of 7 mm (range, 4.0 to 10.0 mm). The contractions were usually retrograde, with the contraction wave moving from the cervix toward the fundus, except during menstruation when contractions were antegrade and moved from the fundus toward the cervix. Contractions were also noted in about half of early pregnancies and were also retrograde, except in one patient with an inevitable abortion who had antegrade contractions.

Lyons et al[14] noted that 80 percent of contractions were retrograde and that the frequency and amplitude of the contractions increased through the follicular phase to the periovulatory period and then decreased until menstruation. Abramowicz and Archer[15] also reported endometrial contractions that took the form of back-and-forth movements with progression toward the fundus that reminded them of intestinal peristalsis. More endometrial movements were noted in IVF patients with stimulated cycles than in patients with natural cycles. However, natural cycle patients had more contractions than patients on oral contraceptives. Peristalsis increased from the early follicular phase to midcycle and decreased in the luteal phase (Fig. 6-24).

POSTMENOPAUSAL ENDOMETRIUM

The endometrial echo in the postmenopausal woman is generally no more than a thin linear echo generally 1 to 3 mm in thickness. Postmenopausal bleeding in

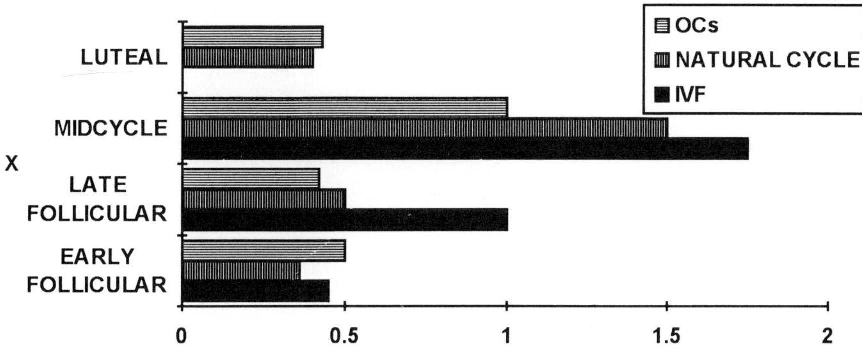

Fig. 6-24. Endometrial peristalsis* (Data from Abramowicz and Archer.[15])

such patients is usually from an atrophic endometrium (Fig. 6-25). Occasionally, in some postmenopausal patients, the endometrium may not be imaged or may be imaged as an incomplete thin line. This generally reflects an atrophic endometrium.

Varner et al[7] studied 80 postmenopausal women. Most were asymptomatic; however, 15 were evaluated for postmenopausal bleeding. All 60 patients (75 percent) with ultrasound endometrial thickness of 4 mm or less had endometrial biopsies showing minimal estrogen stimulation, an atrophic endometrium, or no tissue. Two women with endometrial thickness of 5 mm also had histologic evidence of minimal estrogen stimulation. Varner et al[7] noted that an endometrial thickness of 4 mm had a 96.7 percent sensitivity, 100 percent specificity, and a 100 percent positive predictive value for histologic findings of a minimally estrogen stimulated endometrium. Patients with endometrial thickness of greater than 4 mm had a variety of different histologic findings. No obvious morphologic features were noted that could clearly distinguish between a proliferative or hyperplastic endometrium, or endometrial carcinoma. Among patients with an endometrial thickness of greater than 4 mm, 40 percent had endometrial pathology (17 percent of the asymptomatic patients and 75 percent of the patients with postmenopausal bleeding).

A fluid collection within the endometrial cavity imaged as an anechoic area or an increase in endometrial thickening greater than 5 mm in a postmenopausal patient not on hormonal replacement therapy warrants investigation (Fig. 6-26). McCarthy et al[16] considered distension of the endometrial cavity by a volume of greater than 2 ml to be abnormal in post-

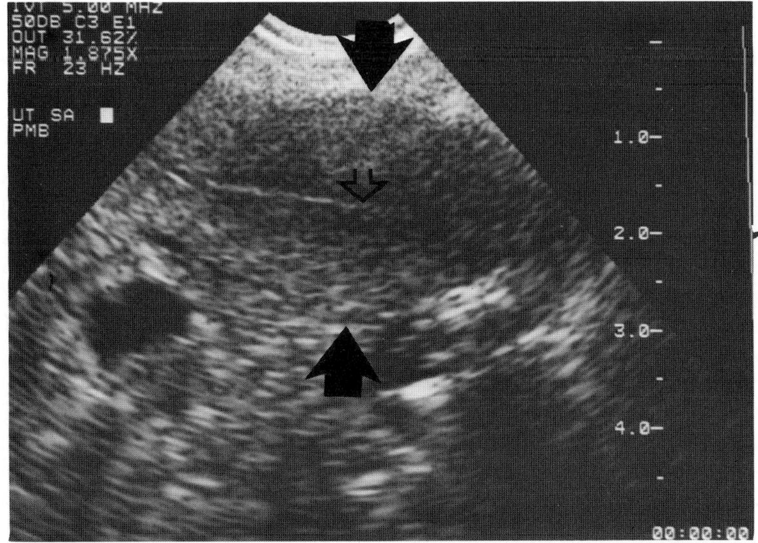

Fig. 6-25. A 59-year-old woman with postmenopausal bleeding with a prominent but thin single-line endometrium (open arrow) with a prominent halo. Biopsy showed an atrophic endometrium. Large arrows delineate the anterior posterior limits of the uterus.

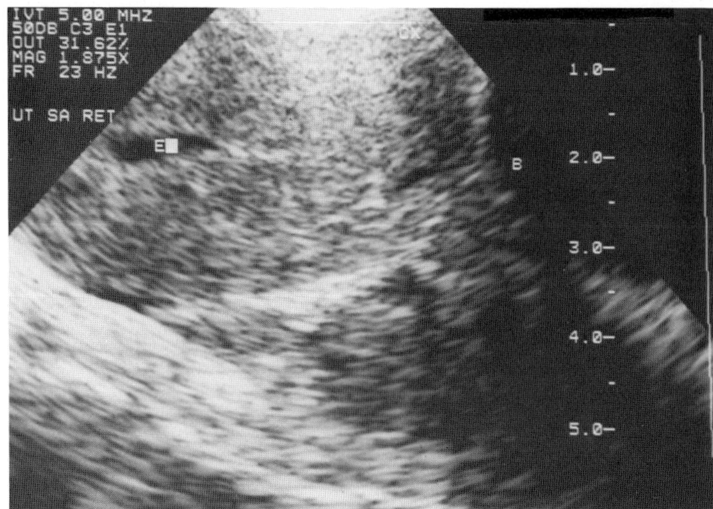

Fig. 6-26. A 53-year-old woman 2 years postmenopausal taking Premarin (1.25 mg/day) from days 1 to 25 and Provera (10 mg/day) from days 10 to 25 each month. The patient noted occasional spotting while taking her hormones. AP-pelvic plane image shows a small retroverted uterus with an early menstrual endometrium. Endometrial biopsy showed a secretory endometrium probably secondary to her estrogen and progesterone therapy.

menopausal women. Distension was estimated using the formula for a prolate ellipsoid (.5 × length × width × height). Distension of the endometrial cavity in the postmenopausal period is frequently due to obstruction of the outflow tract. However, benign processes were responsible for the obstruction in 75 percent of cases.

Johnson et al[17] noted that prominent endometrial echoes in postmenopausal women were associated with endometrial pathology in 83 percent of cases. Unfortunately, this report did not define exactly what constituted a prominent endometrial pattern.

Postmenopausal Bleeding

Postmenopausal bleeding PMB is a common clinical problem. About 5 percent of outpatient gynecologic visits in Great Britain are for postmenopausal bleeding. This condition is very significant because it is frequently associated with underlying pelvic pathology and must be thoroughly investigated. Abnormalities will be noted in one-fifth to one-third of postmenopausal patients, with 5 to 10 percent having endometrial carcinoma.[18]

In the past, the traditional approach for evaluating the patient with PMB has been a D&C. However, with the development of newer and better techniques for sampling the endometrium and with the increasing demand to cut costs, most patients with PMB are now managed on an outpatient basis utilizing endometrial sampling. In addition to the cost, inconvenience factors, and the frequent use of general anesthesia for a D&C, it is becoming better appreciated that a D&C is neither as benign nor as accurate as once thought. Studies show about 10 percent of endometrial lesions are missed during a D&C. Adequate endometrial specimens (almost as accurate as a D&C specimen) can generally be obtained from a variety of outpatient sampling techniques. Adequate histologic samples were obtained in 85 to 99 percent of specimens using the Vabra aspirator (Berkley Medevices, Inc.) and from 91 percent using the Pipelle (Unimar, Inc.) compared to 79 to 94 percent of D&C's.[19]

In a study of 45 patients with PMB, Smith et al[20] found ultrasonographic evaluation to be 100 percent sensitive with a 100 percent negative predictive value in detecting endometrial pathology. However, there were 14 false-positive ultrasound findings. Therefore, the specificity was only 61 percent, and the positive predictive value was only 39 percent.

Nasri et al[18] studied 103 patients with postmenopausal bleeding. Endometrial carcinoma was diagnosed in 6 percent of these PMB patients, hyperplasia was noted in 10 percent, and polyps in another 10 percent. In 63 percent of these patients the endometrium was atrophic, and the ultrasound endometrial thickness was 5 mm or less. In 31 percent, the endometrial histology was abnormal and was more than 5 mm thick. In 6 percent of patients the endometrium was atrophic but thicker than 5 mm due to intracavity fluid. However, the actual thickness of the endometrial walls was only 1 to 2 mm in these patients. Thickening due to fluid distension of the uterine cavity must be distinguished from true thickening of the endometrium. This can generally be done easily since the fluid within the cavity outlines the hyperechoic endometrium, which can be distinguished and measured as a separate entity. However, Nasri et al[18] also reported on three patients with distension of the endometrial cavity due to a pyometrium. Two of these patients had invasive squamous cell carcinoma of the cervix.

Pyometrium may be suggested by the presence of a mixed echotexture or increased echodensity of the pus compared to the completely anechoic appearance of fluid. Similar echodensities are seen in endometriomas and often indicate a dense (more reflective) fluid than serum. In a small study, Goldstein et al[21] noted minimal endometrial tissue from 11 patients with ultrasound endometrial thickness of 5 mm or less, whereas 65 percent of patients with a thicker endometrium had pathologic findings.

These studies confirm that ultrasonographic evaluation of the endometrium is a very sensitive technique for detecting endometrial pathology in the postmenopausal patient. An endometrium less than 5 mm in thickness measured utilizing the transvaginal sonographic technique is uncommonly associated with significant endometrial pathology. The patient with an endometrium thicker than 5 mm or with an abnormal echotexture pattern needs histologic sampling. Moreover, the sonographic evaluation should never be limited only to the endometrial thickness since additional significant pathology, such as ovarian neoplasms or cancers, and benign findings, such as endometrial polyps, leiomyomas, hematometra, or pyometria, may also be noted.

It is important that the histologic and sonographic findings are consistent. For example, a patient with a sonographic thick endometrium with an endometrial biopsy showing inadequate tissue for histologic evaluation needs further assessment, such as a repeat biopsy or hysteroscopy and/or D&C.

Some clinicians have began to utilize sonographic evaluation to decide which patients should undergo biopsy and which patients can simply be followed. This can be a particularly useful approach in the elderly patient in poor medical condition and the PMB patient with a very stenotic cervical os in which an endometrial sampling cannot be done in the office. However, the number of reports utilizing this approach and the numbers of patients involve are still quite limited.

ENDOMETRIAL CARCINOMA

Endometrial cancer is now the most common gynecologic malignant disease. About 2.2 percent of women eventually develop endometrial cancer. In 1980 there were 37,000 new cases with 3,300 deaths.[22] More than 70 percent of cases occur in women over the age of 50, and only 5 percent of cases occur in women under the age of 40.

The most common presenting symptoms of endometrial carcinoma is intramenstrual or postmenopausal bleeding, which is noted in 90 percent of cases. Because most endometrial cancers present with early bleeding, ultrasound has not played a major or even important role in early diagnosis in the past.[23]

Chambers and Unis[24] found sonographic signs suggestive of adenocarcinoma in 66.7 percent of patients with endometrial cancer. Suggestive signs of cancer included a distended uterine cavity, an enlarged uterus, a fluid-filled obstructed uterus, prominent or variable echogenicity of the endometrial cavity, or a lobular uterus (Table 6-7).

Hematometra, hydrometra, and pyometra in endometrial carcinoma may result from obstruction of the normal drainage of the uterus. The ultrasound finding of obstruction is asymmetric enlargement of the uterus with an enlarged, generally anechoic uterine cavity. Scott et al[25] reported on 11 cases of obstruction, all of which were secondary to uterine cancer or radiation therapy generally for cervical carcinoma. Hydrometra from obstruction may occur during, immediately after, or even many years after radiation therapy. It may or may not be associated with recurrent neoplasm.

Using as a normal uterine size 3 by 8 cm (anterior posterior and longitudinal) as suggested by Fleischer, Requard et al[23] found uterine enlargement in 71 percent of 21 patients with adenocarcinoma of the endometrium (Fig. 6-27).[26] Uterine size in these cancer

Table 6-7. Ultrasound Signs Suggestive of Endometrial Carcinoma

Enlarged uterus
Distended uterine cavity
Lobular uterus
Hypo- or hyperechogenic of uterine body
Loss of incomplete central hyperechoic line

(Data from Requard et al[23] and Chambers and Unis.[24])

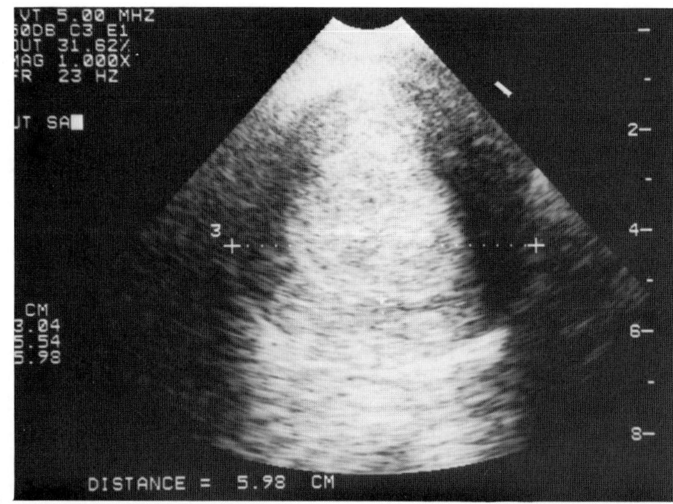

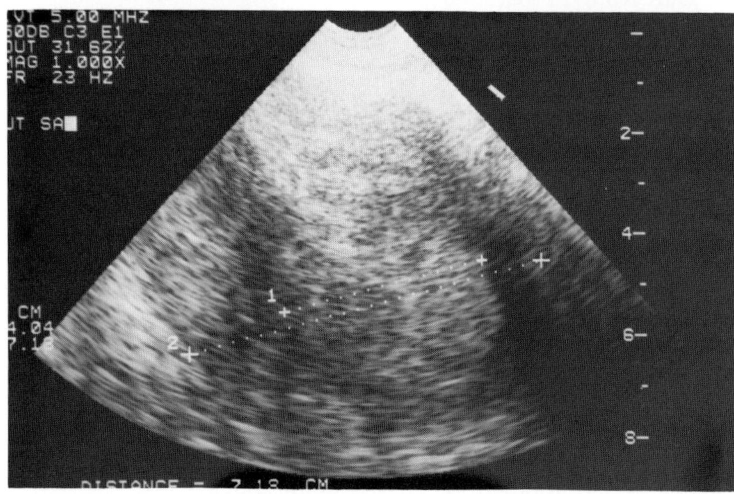

Fig. 6-27. A 34-year-old woman with heavy periods and a hemoglobin of 4.1. **(A)** T-pelvic image showing a large hyperechoic endometrium 3 cm thick and comprising about one-half of the anterior posterior thickness of the uterus. There is prominent posterior enhancement. The uterus is enlarged (anterior posterior diameter is 5.5 cm, transverse diameter is 6 cm). **(B)** AP-pelvic view again showing a marked thickening of the endometrium (4.0 cm). The anterior posterior diameter of the uterus is 7.2 mm in the fundal region. **(C)** AP-pelvic view of the lower uterine segment and cervix. Tumor involves the cervix, which is markedly thickened (see cursor line 1; 5.2 cm). A small area of bladder can be seen in the upper right. The endometrium in the lower uterine segment is irregular and measures 3 cm in thickness (see cursor line 2).

patients ranged from 2 to 5 cm (anterior posterior uterine diameter) to 9 to 14 cm (cervical-fundal uterine diameter) with an average of 5.5 by 8.7 cm (Fig. 6-28).

Requard et al[23] have emphasized the importance of the central uterine echo in the diagnosis of endometrial carcinoma. In an AP-pelvic image plane, the uterine cavity in the postmenopausal patient is generally seen as a single-line resting endometrium. However, the single-line endometrium was absent in 48 percent of patients with endometrial cancer and was incomplete (consisting of a dash-blank image of the endometrium) in another 48 percent in Requard et al's series.[23] However, this finding has been uncommon in my experience. The most common finding of endometrial carcinoma in the authors experience is

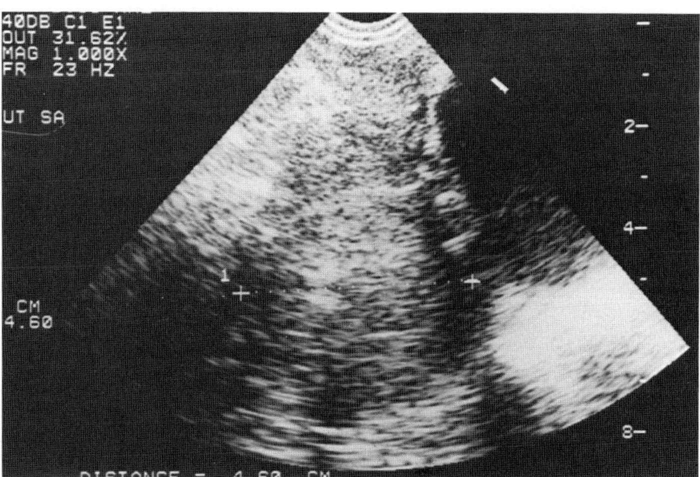

Fig. 6-28. AP-pelvic view of the uterus in a 79-year-old woman with vaginal spotting for 3 months. The uterus is in midposition and enlarged, with an anterior posterior dimension of 4.3 cm. Although only minimally enlarged for a menstruating woman, it is very large for a 79-year-old postmenopausal patient. The endometrium is seen as an irregular and poorly defined hyperechoic area. Dilatation and curettage revealed an endometrial carcinoma. D&C was done because of a stenotic cervical os requiring dilitation.

an atypical thickened hyperechoic endometrium (see above). If the sonolucent ring surrounding the resting endometrium is intact, the carcinoma, if present, is generally limited to the endometrium. Although preliminary, these data suggest that an intact endometrial halo is a good prognostic sign. A uterus of normal size and shape or a uterus with only minimal enlargement or dilatation is generally (94 percent of cases) associated with earlier stages of endometrial carcinoma (stage I and II disease). A lobular or an enlarged uterus with a mixed echo pattern or very thickened endometrium is more commonly noted in patients with advanced disease (stage III and IV disease).

In a more recent study using transabdominal real-time ultrasound, Fleischer et al[27] were able to estimate correctly the depth of myometrial invasion within 10 percent of actual measurement of the gross specimen in 70 percent of cases (Fig. 6-29). The distance from the luminal echo to the most distal interface thought to represent the tumor-myometrium junction was measured and divided by the total thickness of the myometrium. If the lumen could not be defined, then the total anterior posterior diameter of the myometrium was divided by the total endometrial width. When superficial invasion (less than one-half of the myometrium invaded) and deep invasion (greater than one-half of the myometrial thickness involved) were compared, the sensitivity of ultrasound was 100 percent and the specificity was 80 percent, with an overall accuracy of 80 percent in diagnosing the depth of myometrial invasion.[27] As noted above, preservation of the endometrial halo generally indicates superficial invasion. Absence of a halo is frequently associated with deep invasion. Poorly differentiated tumors (grades II and III) tend to be hypoechoic, whereas polypoid tumors are hyperechoic.

Unfortunately, in the early stages of endometrial carcinoma, no distortion or anatomic changes may be noted in the endometrial cavity, and therefore there may be no sonographic signs of early malignant disease. In addition, false-positive sonographic signs of cancer may result from cervical stenosis and obstruction or endometrial polyps. Since some cases of endometrial cancer may be missed with an ultrasound ex-

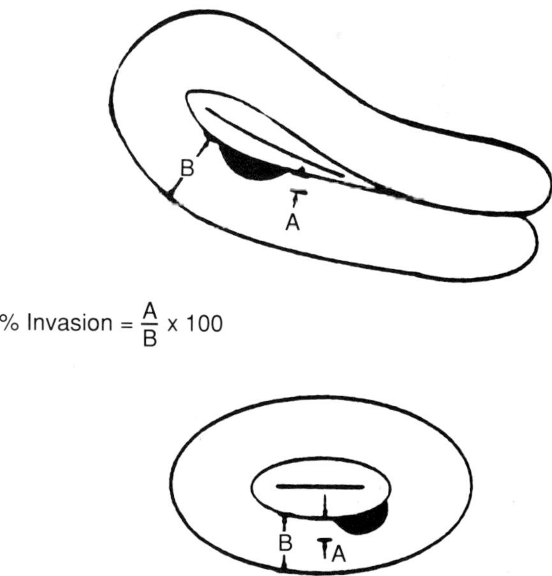

Fig. 6-29. Calculation of percent myometrial invasion. Tumor invasion is represented by the black areas. (From Fleischer et al.,[27] with permission).

amination, sonography must be combined with other methods for diagnosing endometrial cancer. However, recently Ross[28] reported on 60 postmenopausal bleeding patients, and all 6 patients with endometrial cancer were diagnosed correctly using ultrasound. No tumors were missed. In addition, two bladder tumors and one ovarian cancer were diagnosed that were not clinically suspected.

Schurz et al[29] diagnosed two endometrial carcinomas among 60 postmenopausal patients with bleeding. The endometrium was thickened and inhomogeneous and had an irregular border with the myometrium. In postmenopausal patients receiving hormonal replacement, two-thirds showed sonographic changes of a proliferative endometrium during estrogen therapy and secretory changes during progesterone therapy (Fig. 6-30). No sonographic changes were noted in one-third of the patients receiving hormonal therapy. Endometrial hyperplasia presenting as a thickened endometrium may also be

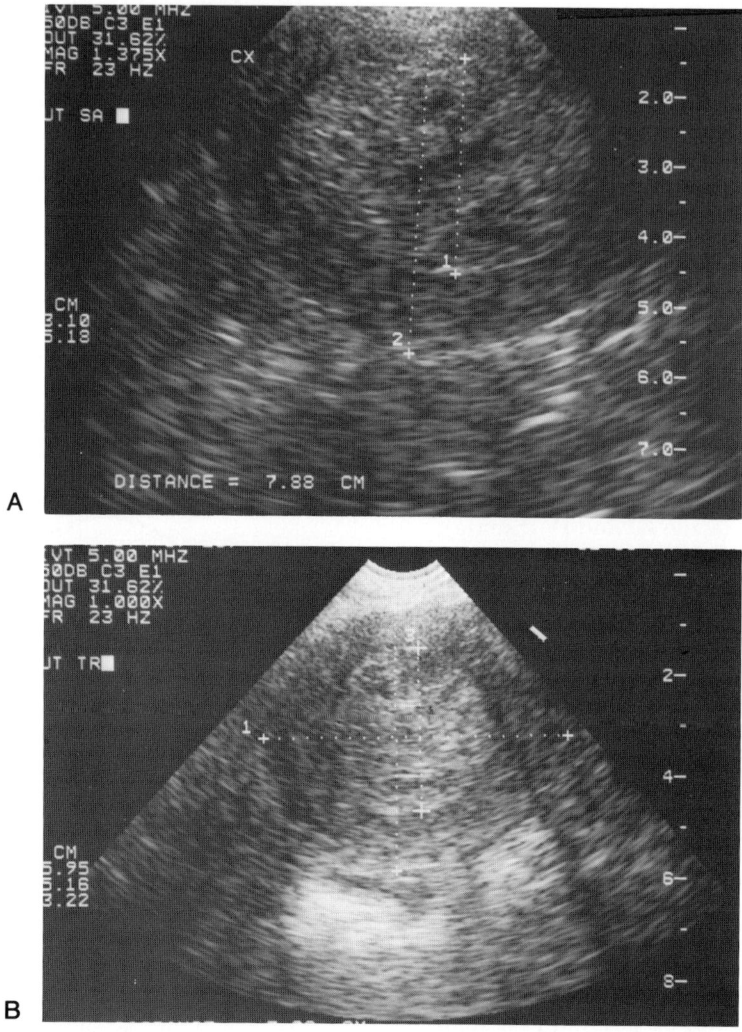

Fig. 6-30. (**A**) AP-pelvic and (**B**) T-pelvic views of the endometrium in a postmenopausal patient with bleeding. There is a hyperechoic endometrial mass 3.1 to 3.22 cm thick with an enlarged uterus (T-pelvic plain measurement of width, 5.95 cm; anterior posterior diameter(s) (thickness), 5.16 cm). Biopsy revealed an adenocarcinoma of the endometrium. The tumor involves 60 percent of the myometrial thickness.

noted in the postmenopausal patient and suggests the need for an endometrial biopsy before initiating hormonal replacement therapy. Ultrasonographic findings of a thickened endometrium or fluid collection with uterine enlargement should prompt endometrial biopsy and further evaluation as indicated.

Transvaginal ultrasound is rapidly becoming an important tool for evaluating postmenopausal bleeding and also for screening the postmenopausal patient for both ovarian and endometrial cancer and other pelvic pathology. It is also of value for gauging the depth of myometrial invasion of endometrial cancer.

REFERENCES

1. Callen PW, DeMartini WJ, Filly RA: The central uterine cavity echo: a useful anatomic sign in the ultrasonographic evaluation of the female pelvis. Radiology 131:187, 1979
2. Sakamoto C: Sonographic criteria of phasic changes in human endometrial tissue. Int J Gynaecol Obstet 23:7, 1985
3. Forrest TS, Elyaderani MK, Muilenburg MI et al: Cyclic endometrial changes: US assessment with histologic correlation. Radiology 167:233, 1988
4. Ayers JWT, Knight L, Grady E, Peterson EP: Transvaginal sonographic endometrial morphology—the bioassay of ovarian steroidogenesis in spontaneous and induced cycles. Abstract P-123. Presented at the 44th Annual Meeting of The American Fertility Society, Atlanta, GA, October 10-13, 1988
5. Speroff L, Glass RH, Kase NG: Clinical Gynecologic Endocrinology and Infertility. 3rd Ed. Williams & Wilkins, Baltimore, 1983
6. Fleischer AC, Herbert CM, Sacks GA et al: Sonography of the endometrium during conception and nonconception cycles of in vitro fertilization and embryo transfer. Fertil Steril 46:442, 1986
7. Varner RE, Sparks JM, Cameron CD et al: Transvaginal sonography of the endometrium in postmenopausal women. Obstet Gynecol 78:195, 1991
8. Fleischer AC, Kalemeris GC, Entman SS: Sonographic depiction of the endometrium during normal cycles. Ultrasound Med Biol 12:271, 1986
9. Haynor DR, Mack LA, Soules MR et al: Changing appearance of the normal uterus during the menstrual cycle: MR studies. Radiology 161:459, 1986
10. Wiczyk HP, Janus CL, Richards CJ et al: Comparison of magnetic resonance imaging and ultrasound in evaluating follicular and endometrial development throughout the normal cycle. Fertil Steril 49:969, 1988
11. Giorlandino C, Gleicher N, Nanni C et al: The sonographic picture of endometrium in spontaneous and induced cycles. Fertil Steril 47:508, 1987
12. Birnholz JC: Ultrasonic visualization of endometrial movements. Fertil Steril 41:157, 1984
13. de Varies K, Lyons EA, Ballard G et al: Contractions of the inner third of the myometrium. Am J Obstet Gynecol 162:679, 1990
14. Lyons EA, Taylor PJ, Zheng XH et al: Characterization of subendometrial myometrial contractions throughout the menstrual cycle in normal fertile women. Fertil Steril 55:771, 1991
15. Abramowicz JS, Archer DF: Uterine endometrial peristalsis—a transvaginal ultrasound study. Fertil Steril 54:451, 1990
16. McCarthy KA, Hall DA, Kopans DB, Swann CA: Postmenopausal endometrial fluid collections: always an indicator of malignancy? J Ultrasound Med 5:647, 1986
17. Johnson MA, Graham MF, Cooperberg PL: Abnormal endometrial echoes: sonographic spectrum of endometrial pathology. J Ultrasound Med 1:161, 1982
18. Nasri MN, Shepherd JH, Setchell ME et al: The role of vaginal scan in measurement of endometrial thickness in postmenopausal women. Br J Obstet Gynecol 98:470, 1991
19. Chambers JT, Chambers SK: Endometrial sampling: when? where? why? with what? Clin Obstet Gynecol 35:28, 1992
20. Smith P, Bakos O, Heimer G, Ulmsten U: Transvaginal ultrasound for identifying endometrial abnormality. Acta Obstet Gynecol Scand 70:591, 1991
21. Goldstein SR, Nachtigall M, Snyder JR, Nachtigall L: Endometrial assessment by vaginal ultrasonography before endometrial sampling in patients with postmenopausal bleeding. Am J Obstet Gynecol 163:119, 1990
22. Barber HRK: Manual of Gynecologic Oncology. JB Lippincott, Philadelphia, 1980
23. Requard CK, Wicks JD, Mettler FA, Jr: Ultrasonography in the staging of endometrial adenocarcinoma. Radiology 140:781, 1981
24. Chambers CB, Unis JS: Ultrasonographic evidence of uterine malignancy in the postmenopausal uterus. Am J Obstet Gynecol 154:1194, 1986
25. Scott WW, Jr, Rosenshein NB, Siegelman SS, Sanders RC: The obstructed uterus. Radiology 141:767, 1981
26. Fleischer AC, James AE, Jr, Millis JB, Julian C: Differential diagnosis of pelvic masses by gray scale sonography. AJR 131:469, 1978
27. Fleischer AC, Dudley BS, Entman SS et al: Myometrial invasion by endometrial carcinoma: sonographic assessment. Radiology 162:307, 1987
28. Ross LD: Pelvic ultrasound—should it be used routinely in the diagnosis and screening of postmenopausal bleeding? J R Soc Med 81:723, 1988
29. Schurz B, Metka M, Heytmanek G et al: Sonographic changes in the endometrium of climacteric women during hormonal treatment. Maturitas 9:367, 1988

7

The Ovary

Melvin G. Dodson

The rapid development of ultrasonography in detecting and evaluating ovarian size, follicular developments, or ovarian pathology and the use of ultrasound for aspiration of follicles for in vitro fertilization can be readily appreciated by the fact that the ovary and follicles were first visualized using sonography in 1972.[1]

IMAGING THE OVARY

Transvaginal ultrasound localization of the ovary has previously been discussed (see Ch. 3). The ovaries are generally imaged between the uterus and pelvic side wall at the level of the internal iliac vessels.

However, the ovaries may be in the cul-de-sac, higher in the pelvis, or adjacent and/or affixed to the uterus. Abnormal positioning and/or fixation of the ovary may suggest adhesions (Fig. 7-1). After a vaginal hysterectomy, the ovaries may be in the midline and adherent to the apex of the vagina (Fig. 7-2). The ovaries should be scanned in both the anterior posterior-pelvic (AP-pelvic) and trans-pelvic (T-pelvic) planes. The largest ovarian diameters in the T-pelvic and AP-pelvic planes should be recorded (Fig. 7-3). The ovarian volume can then be calculated (see below). The presence, number, and size of follicles should be noted. Enlargement of the ovary or the presence of an ovarian cyst should be characterized as to the echogenicity relative to the uterus: anechoic, hyperechoic, hypoechoic, or isoechoic. Cystic areas should be evaluated for septations, nodularity, or papillar projections. Characteristics of the cyst as multilocular or unilocular should be noted.

Ultrasonography may be used to confirm and evaluate follicular development and ovulation and conversely can be used to diagnose anovulation or dysfunctional ovulation. It is also used for monitoring patients during ovulation induction with clomiphene citrate and is an indispensable monitoring technique when inducing ovulation with gonadotropins (Pergonal, Metrodin) or pulsatile gonadotropin releasing hormone by pump administration.

OVARIAN DIAMETER AND VOLUME

The adult ovary is 2.5 to 5 cm long, 1.5 to 3.0 cm wide, 0.6 to 1.5 cm thick (average, 4 by 2 by 0.8 cm), and weighs 2 to 3.5 g.[2,3]

Ultrasonographic estimates of ovarian volume correlate with anatomic in situ measurements. Campbell et al[4] compared the ultrasonographic measurement of ovarian size with direct surgical measurement the following day. The correlation coefficient was 0.97.

Several techniques for determining the volume of the ovary have been used. A commonly used technique for estimating the volume of an ovary is to apply the formula for an ellipsoid: $(d_1) \times (d_2) \times (d_3) \times 0.523$.[5] This formula for calculating ovarian volume is particularly useful when there is greater than 0.5-cm difference in any of the three planes measured: length, width, and height. If all three planes are within 0.5 cm, the formula $4/3\pi r^3$ (the formula for a sphere) may be accurately utilized for calculating ovarian or follicular volume.[6] Wiczyk et al,[7] using the volume of an ellipsoid, reported a maximum normal ovarian volume of 6 cm^3 with a mean of 3.7 ± 0.8 cm^3 on day 12 of a natural cycle. Sample et al[8] reported the volume of the average adult ovary to be 4 cm^3 with a range from 1.8 to 5.7 cm^3. Munn et al[9] reported a mean ovarian volume of 6.48 ± 2.90 cm^3 with a normal range from 2.15 to 13.84 cm^3. The 99 percent confidence limit for normal ovarian volume is

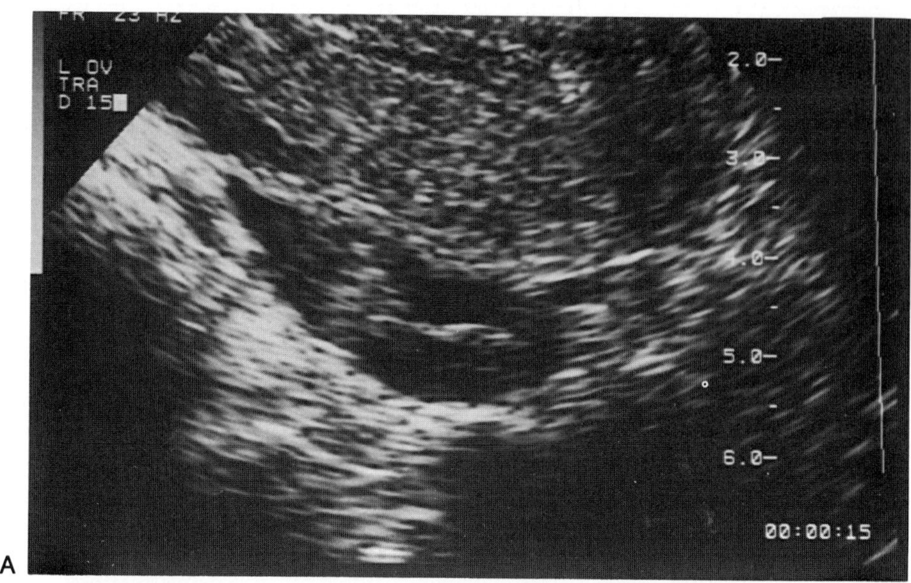

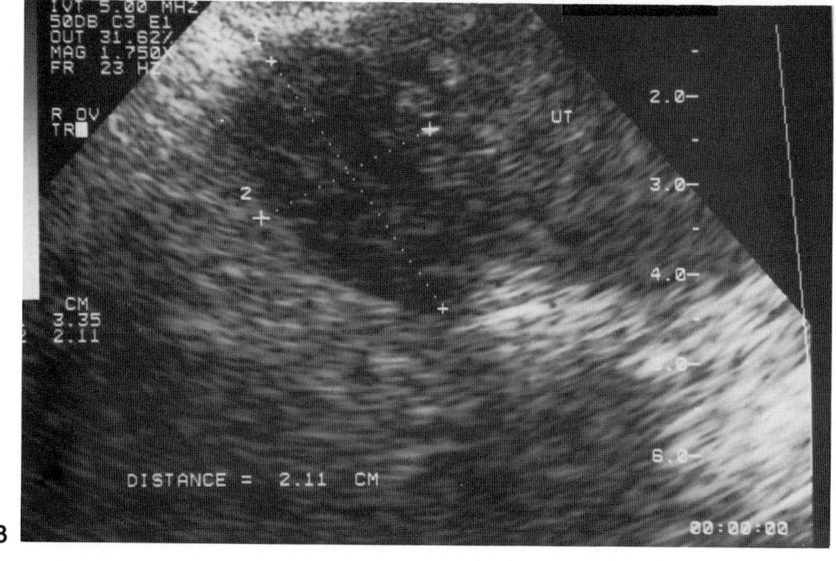

Fig. 7-1. (**A**) Anterior posterior-pelvic (AP-pelvic) view of an ovary in the cul-de-sac and posterior to the uterus. The endometrium is follicular. (**B**) Ovary adjacent to the uterus. There is no free space between the ovary and uterus, suggesting adhesions. The ovary and uterus could not be separated by manipulation of the uterus and/or ovary.

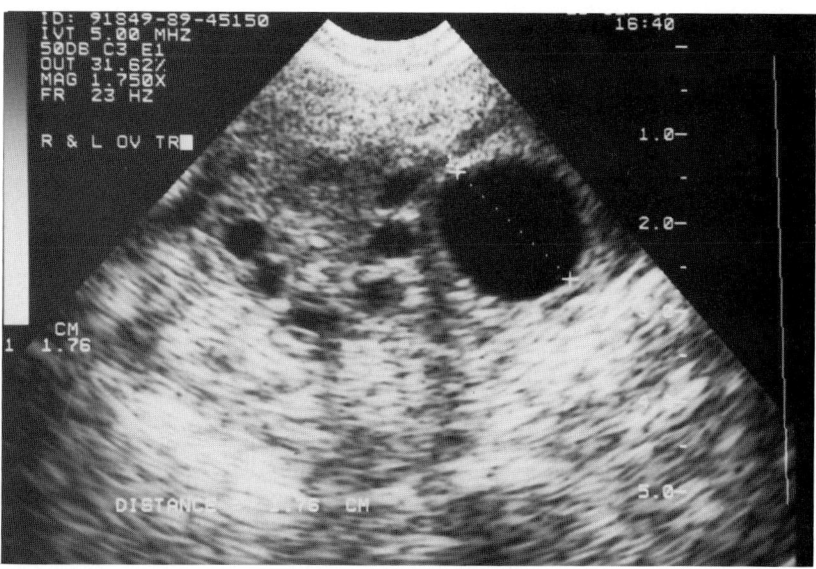

Fig. 7-2. A 34-year-old woman G3 who had had postvaginal hysterectomy with a complaint of pelvic pain. The uterus is surgically absent, and both ovaries are approximated in the midline. There is a 1.76-cm follicle or cyst in the left ovary. There are multiple preovulatory follicles in the right ovary.

4.96 to 8.00 cm^3. Therefore, the upper limit of the normal adult ovarian volumes is about 8 cm^3.[2,9–12] Abdominal and transvaginal measurements of ovarian volumes have been noted to be comparable.[13,14]

Ovarian volume has been demonstrated to vary during the menstrual cycle. The ovarian volume and largest diameter are greatest in the follicular phase before ovulation. Granberg and Wikland[15] reported an ovarian volume of 5.8 ± 2.9 cm^3 in the preovulatory phase (days 11 to 16) compared with 3.1 ± 2.2 cm^3 in the early follicular or luteal phase. However, they noted that an error of 2 mm in each diameter measurement would result in a 25 percent increase or decrease in ovarian volume in a normal ovary and as much as a 50 percent change in the volume of the smaller postmenopausal ovary. Therefore, they recommend using the largest ovarian diameter as the better biometric measurement of ovarian size. The average ovarian length in their study was 3.0 ± 0.5 cm.

Ovarian size varies with the age of the patient, and hormonal status. Contraceptive methods, such as birth control pills, may also affect ovarian volume. The ovarian volume and longest diameter are largest in the 30 to 49 age group and decrease in menopause (Fig. 7-4).

As noted in our discussion of uterine size (see Ch. 5), the ultrasound diagnosis of ovarian enlargement is only meaningful if it is associated with a pathologic process or gives additional information about the physiologic or hormonal status of the patient. Ovarian measurements outside the normal limits should stimulate a thorough evaluation for an explanation, such as a cyst, benign neoplasm, carcinoma, endometrioma, infection, or polycystic ovarian disease.

I use a volume of 8 cm^3 as the upper limit of normal in a menstruating woman. Ovaries larger than 8 cm^3 are frequently noted in patients with polycystic ovarian disease (PCOD) (average ovarian volume of 16 cm^3 with an upper limit of 30 cm^3), when there are multiple developing follicles after clomiphene citrate (Clomid) or menotrophic stimulations in patients with functional cysts (such as a corpus luteal cyst), or in patients who develop ovarian hyperstimulation after the use of Clomid or gonadotropins.[16] Also, the remaining ovary may enlarge when its sister ovary has been surgically removed. One ovary twice the volume of the opposite ovary is generally considered abnormal. An ovary may appear larger if there are adhesions to adjacent structures that may then appear sonographically to be part of the ovary. A pedunculated fibroid may be mistaken for an ovary.

Significant ovarian enlargement that is not readily explainable warrants further investigation. If the ovary is significantly enlarged, but there is a probable explanation (PCOD, functional cyst, etc.), a minimum evaluation may be a repeat transvaginal ultrasound in 6 to 8 weeks during the early follicular phase of the menstrual cycle. In PCOD, the diagnosis may be confirmed by clinical criteria or endocrine parameters (see Ch. 18).

If an enlarged ovary persists or increases in size or a definitive diagnosis cannot be made, laparoscopy or laparotomy may be indicated, depending on the clini-

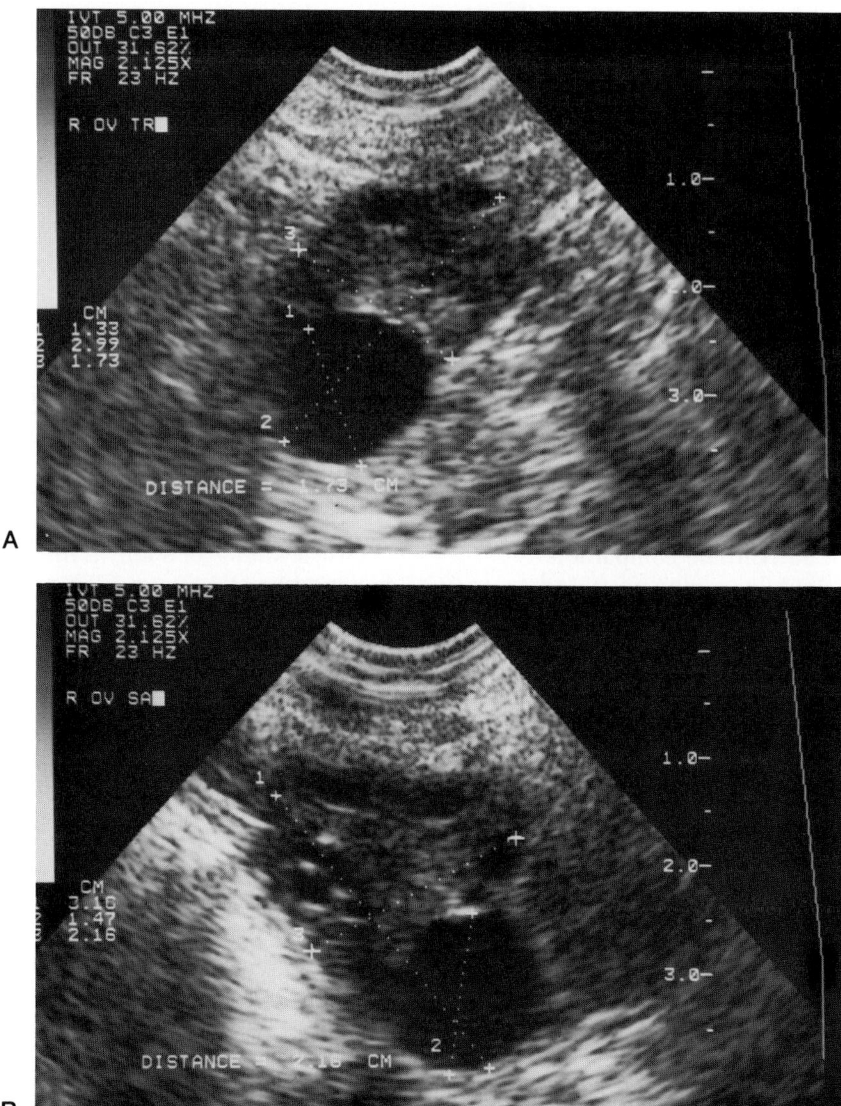

Fig. 7-3. (**A**) Trans-pelvic (T-pelvic) image of the right ovary measuring 2.99 by 1.73 cm (cursor lines 2 and 3). There is a follicle with a 1.33-cm diameter (cursor line 1). (**B**) AP-pelvic image of the same ovary measuring 3.16 by 1.47 cm (cursor lines 1 and 3). Follicle measures 1.47 cm in this plane (cursor line 2).

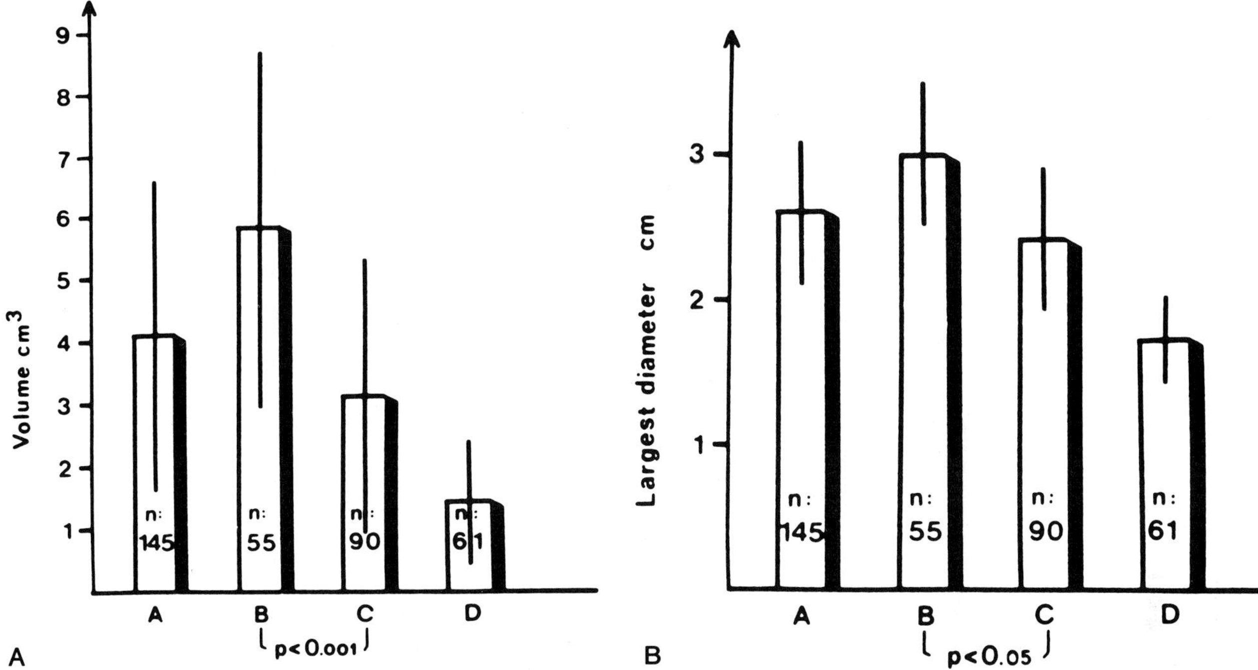

Fig. 7-4. (A) Ovarian volume as measured by ultrasound in relation to ovarian function. A, ovulating ovaries; B, preovulatory ovaries; C, luteal phase ovaries; D, menopausal ovaries. (B) The largest ovarian diameter as measured using ultrasound in relation to ovarian function. A, ovulating ovaries; B, preovulatory ovaries; C, luteal phase ovaries; D, menopausal ovaries. *(Figure continues.)*

cal circumstances and sonographic findings. A significantly enlarged ovary without an explanation should be viewed with suspicion, particularly in the older or postmenopausal patient.

OVARIAN VOLUME IN CHILDREN

Neonatal ovaries in anatomic studies vary from 0.5 to 1.5 cm in length and from 0.3 to 0.4 cm in thickness.[17] As might be expected, the ovary in a child increases in size with age, with the greatest increase around menarche. Transvaginal ultrasound is contraindicated in the neonate and young child because of the small vaginal size and hymen. In addition, it is particularly difficult to visualize the ovaries of a newborn using transabdominal ultrasound, since the neonate rarely has sufficient urine in the bladder.

By the age of 4 years, small cysts may be present in the ovary. Salardi et al[18] noted four or more small cystic areas less than 9 mm in size in very young children. By the age of 12 years, larger follicles (greater than 9 mm) may be noted but with some microcysts still present.

In younger patients (ages 13 to 20), the mean ovarian volume is 4.0 cm^3 with a range from 1.8 to 5.7 cm^3 (Table 7-1).[8]

IMMATURE FOLLICLES

Small follicles may be noted to appear and disappear throughout the entire menstrual cycle and may even be present during menstruation.[7,22,23] Most of these follicles remain nonovulatory and measure 0.3 to 1.0 cm in diameter. Bomsel-Helmreich et al[24] have documented and evaluated these small nonovulatory follicles histologically. These small nonovulatory follicles can be seen routinely when imaging the ovary using a 5- or 7.5-MHz transvaginal transducer.[7]

Although a small cohort of these small ovarian follicles will increase in size during the follicular phase, most will not increase in size beyond 10 mm and they

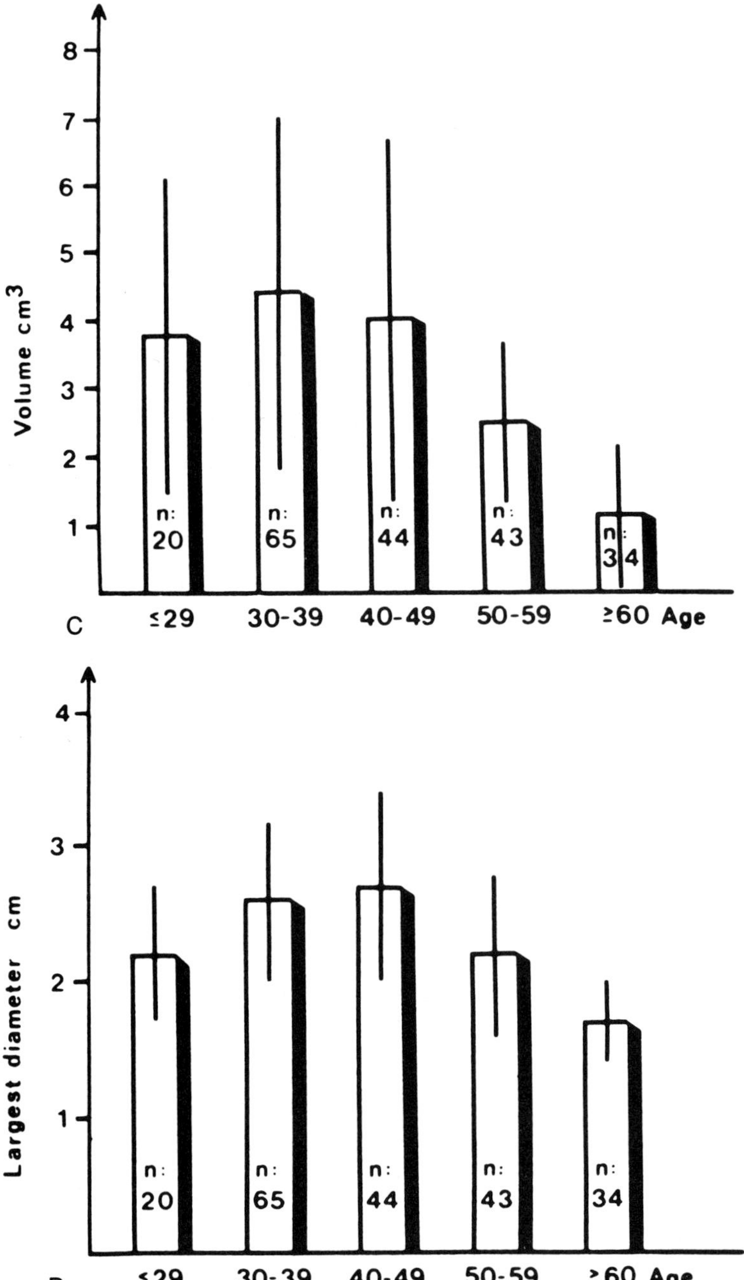

Fig. 7-4 *(Continued)*. **(C)** Ovarian volume as related to 10-year age cohorts. **(D)** The largest ovarian diameter as related to 10-year age cohorts. (From Granberg and Wikland,[15] with permission.)

Table 7-1. Ovarian Volume and Age

Age	*Volume (cm³)*
Neonatal[8,19]	0.16
6 mon – 2 yrs[8,19]	0.4
4 yrs[20]	0.8
7 – 9 yrs[8,19]	0.74
10 yrs[20,21]	0.7 – 2.2
13 – 14 yrs[8,19,20,21]	1.43 – 4.2
17 yrs[21]	5 – 6
13 – 20 yrs (postpubertal)[8]	4.0 (range, 1.8 – 5.7)
Adults[9]	6.48 ± 2.9 (range, 2.15 – 13.84)
Postmenopausal	<2.5

(Data from Sample et al,[8] Munn et al,[9] Simkins,[19] Orsini et al,[20] and Ivarsson et al.[21])

will not ovulate. The consistent absence of these small nonovulatory follicles and normal follicular development on serial pelvic ultrasonographic examinations suggest chronic anovulation or a perimenopausal or postmenopausal status. However, multiple small subcapsular follicles are often seen in patients with PCOD and therefore do not necessarily indicate an ovulatory status. In order to diagnose PCOD, there should be more than 11 such follicles in each ovary.

FOLLICULAR DEVELOPMENT

Follicles destined to ovulate increase linearly in diameter from menstrual day 5 to ovulation at a rate of 2 mm/day.[25] Before ovulation, the dominant follicle will obtain a mean diameter of 20.2 mm with a range of 18 to 24 mm. There is a good correlation between plasma estradiol concentrations and follicular diameter in a normal menstrual cycle. However, early in the cycle, it is not possible to determine which follicle will eventually become the dominant follicle and ovulate. Taylor et al,[26] using real-time pulsed image-directed Doppler ultrasound of the ovarian artery, noted a decrease in vascular impedance indicating increased blood flow in the ovarian artery on the side that eventually developed the dominant follicle. This change in vascular resistance and blood flow was noted even before the dominant follicle could be determined by direct imaging.[26] Only one dominant follicle generally develops (93 percent of cycles). However, two or more follicles have been reported in up to 7 percent of unstimulated cycles.[27]

Imaging of the cumulus oophorous was first reported in 1979.[25] Sonographically, the cumulus oophorous has been reported to consist of a crescent-shaped hyperechoic rim with an internal sonolucent area.[27] Hilgers et al[27] imaged the cumulus mass 1 to 5 days before follicular rupture. The cumulus complex measured 5.1 to 5.7 mm in diameter. However, there remains considerable controversy whether the structures imaged are artifacts or truly represent the cumulus.

OVULATION

Confirmation of ovulation is an important component of any infertility evaluation. The timing of ovulation is also critical in performing intrauterine insemination and donor semen insemination and in timing sexual intercourse to maximize the potential for pregnancy when using Clomid or Pergonal. Although basal body temperature (BBT) measurements have been the most commonly used techniques for timing ovulation in the past, recent studies have noted a BBT nadir preceding the day of ovulation in only 10 percent of cycles.[28] Even though the BBT is an inexpensive method of evaluating a patient for ovulation, the amount of diagnostic information gleaned from the BBT is minimal compared with serial ultrasound scanning.

Vermesh et al[28] correlated ovulation with the luteinizing hormone (LH) surge and sonography using the transvaginal probe. Disappearance of the dominant follicle occurred on the day after the LH surge in all cases. The mean cross-sectional area of the dominant follicle was 432 ± 39.2 mm² in stimulated (Clomid) cycles and 287 ± 13.8 mm² in spontaneous cycles. The mean largest follicular diameter in Clomid cycles was 25.4 ± 1.3 mm compared with 20.8 ± 0.6 mm in natural cycles. Interestingly, the largest follicle is not always the one ultimately destined to ovulate. The correlations among serum LH, estradiol, and transvaginal follicular growth in stimulated and natural cycles are shown in Figures 7-5 and 7-6.

Endocrine parameters can be very useful in predicting ovulation. The estradiol peaks generally precede the LH peak by 24 hours (48 hours before ovulation), and the LH peaks (greater than 40 mIU/ml) generally precede ovulation by at least 24 hours and are associated with a declining serum estradiol level.[28]

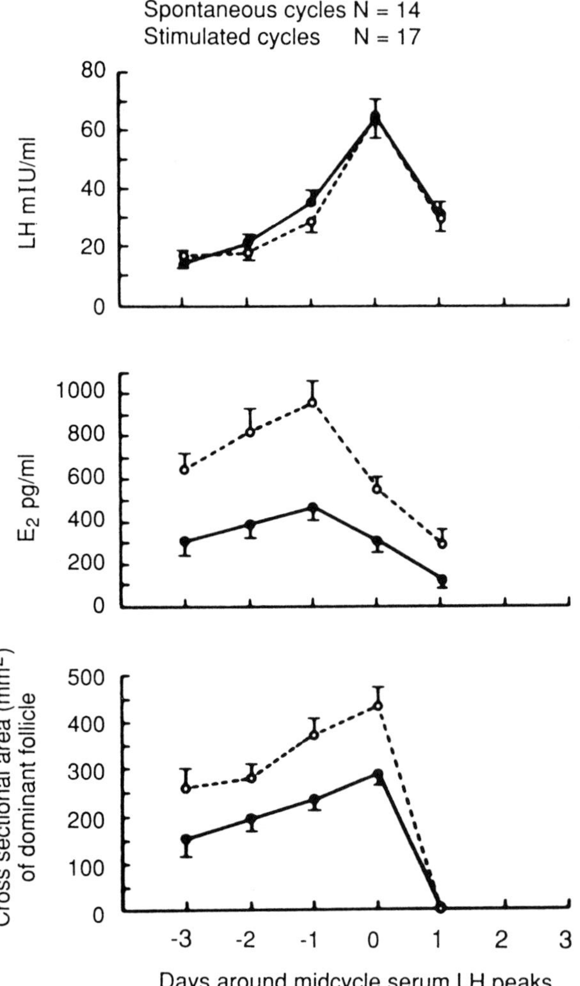

Fig. 7-5. Daily serum LH and estradiol levels and the cross-sectional area of the dominant follicle as seen by transvaginal ultrasound in spontaneous (O) and clomiphene citrate-stimulated (●) cycles. (From Vermesh et al,[28] with permission.)

The exact timing of ovulation after the LH surge may vary, and when multiple follicles are present, multiple ovulations may occur even over several days. Observations of ovulation by ultrasound or otherwise are quite rare in humans. de Crespigny et al[29] reported on four patients in whom actual follicular collapse was visualized using transabdominal ultrasound. Ovulation occurred at 28, 34, 34, and 35 hours after the onset of the LH surge, as determined by assaying urine LH levels every 3 hours. Follicular collapse occurred in less than 1 minute in two patients. In two other patients, there was a rapid initial release of fluid followed by a slower release of the remaining fluid over 7 and 35 minutes, respectively. A corpus hemorrhagicum developed within 1 hour of ovulation. Multiple ovulations were spread over an 8-hour period (28 to 35 hours) after the LH surge.[29] However, a urine LH assay done at 3-hour intervals was utilized. The ovulatory event seems to be relatively brief.

No consistent ultrasound marker of impending ovulation has been found. Although ultrasound does not enable the precise timing or prediction of when ovulation will occur, it does allow the visualization of the developing follicle and whether a dominant follicle is developing and progressing in size. The dominant follicle can be localized (right or left side), which is important when there is unilateral tubal obstruction or when one tube has been surgically removed as, for example, for an ectopic pregnancy. Ultrasound can give suggestive evidence that a follicle is approaching the time of ovulation based on its diameter. However, sonography is an excellent technique for confirming ovulation once it has occurred (Figs. 7-7 and 7-8). The disappearance of the follicle indicates ovulation.

Imaging of the endometrium can also be helpful in evaluating the hormonal status of a menstrual cycle. Thickening of the endometrium reflects estrogen production by the developing follicle, and luteinization of the endometrium indicates at least some progesterone production and suggests that ovulation has occurred. However, a luteinized but unruptured follicle still produces progesterone, despite the fact that ovulation does not occur. In this situation, the endometrium will be luteinized and serum progesterone will increase, but the follicle will persist on serial transvaginal ultrasound examinations. Unfortunately, endometrial thickness does not correlate in a linear fashion with serum estrogen levels nor directly with progesterone levels in the luteal phase. However, low levels of serum estrogen do not produce the characteristic sonographic follicular three-line endometrium (Fig. 7-9). Low level estrogen stimulation results in a resting or single-line endometrium, and in the absence of progesterone (less than 1.5 μg/ml), even an estrogen stimulated endometrium will not develop into a luteal (hyperechoic) endometrium.

By comparison with ultrasound, other commonly used methods of monitoring or predicting ovulation are also only relatively accurate. The LH surge suggests that ovulation should occur in about 24 hours if the peak of the LH surge is detected or in 36 hours if the beginning of the LH surge is noted. However, the

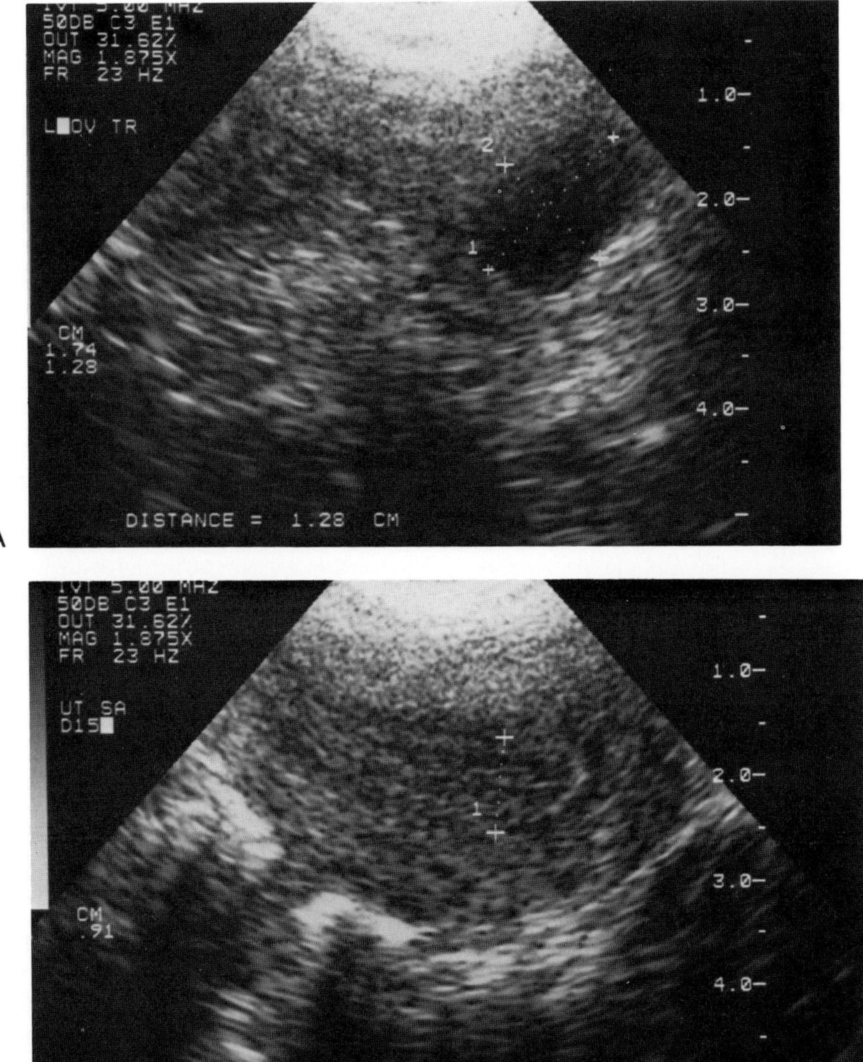

Fig. 7-6. On day 15 a follicle 1.74 by 1.28 cm in diameter is noted (**A**), and the endometrium is 0.91 cm thick (**B**). The serum estradiol was 180.0 pg/ml, and the LH was 22.2 mIU/ml. On day 16 the follicle was 1.71 by 1.55 cm, and the endometrium was 0.97 cm thick (not shown). The serum estradiol was 135.0 pg/ml, and the LH was 34 mIU/ml. *(Figure continues.)*

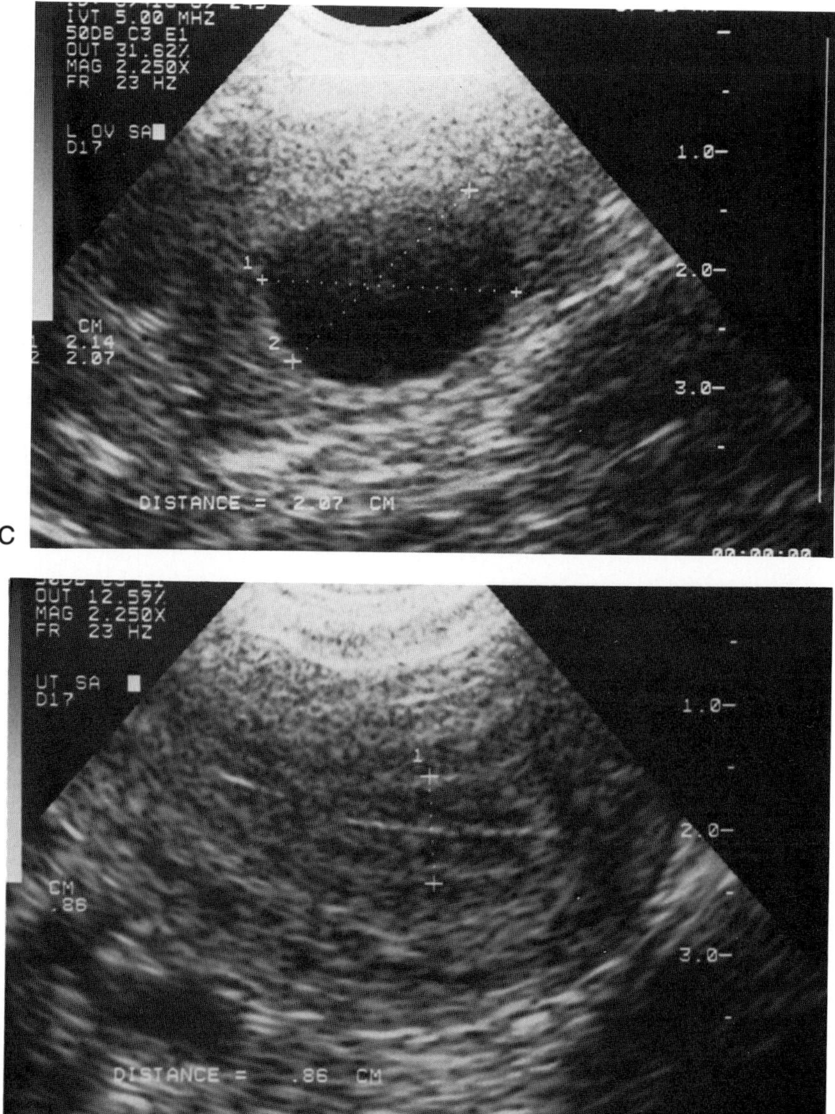

Fig. 7-6 *(Continued)*. On day 17 the follicle had increased to 2.14 by 2.07 cm (**C**), and the endometrium was 0.86 cm thick (**D**). The estradiol was 290 pg/ml. The morning LH level was 139 mIU/ml, and the evening LH level was 132 mIU/ml.

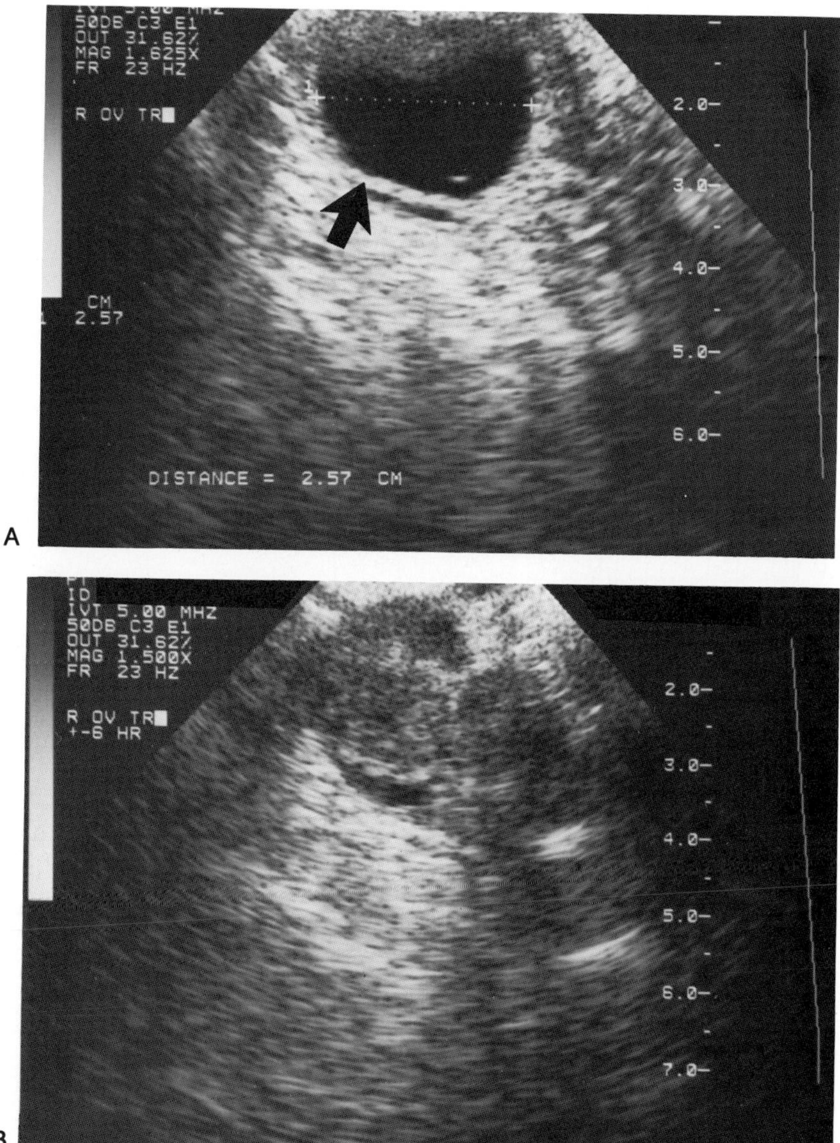

Fig. 7-7. **(A)** T-pelvic view of the right ovary on day 14 of a natural cycle shows a 2.57-cm follicle with double wall sign (arrow) and small internal echo, which has been suggested by some to represent a cumulus mass. **(B)** No follicle was noted about 6 hours later, indicating ovulation.

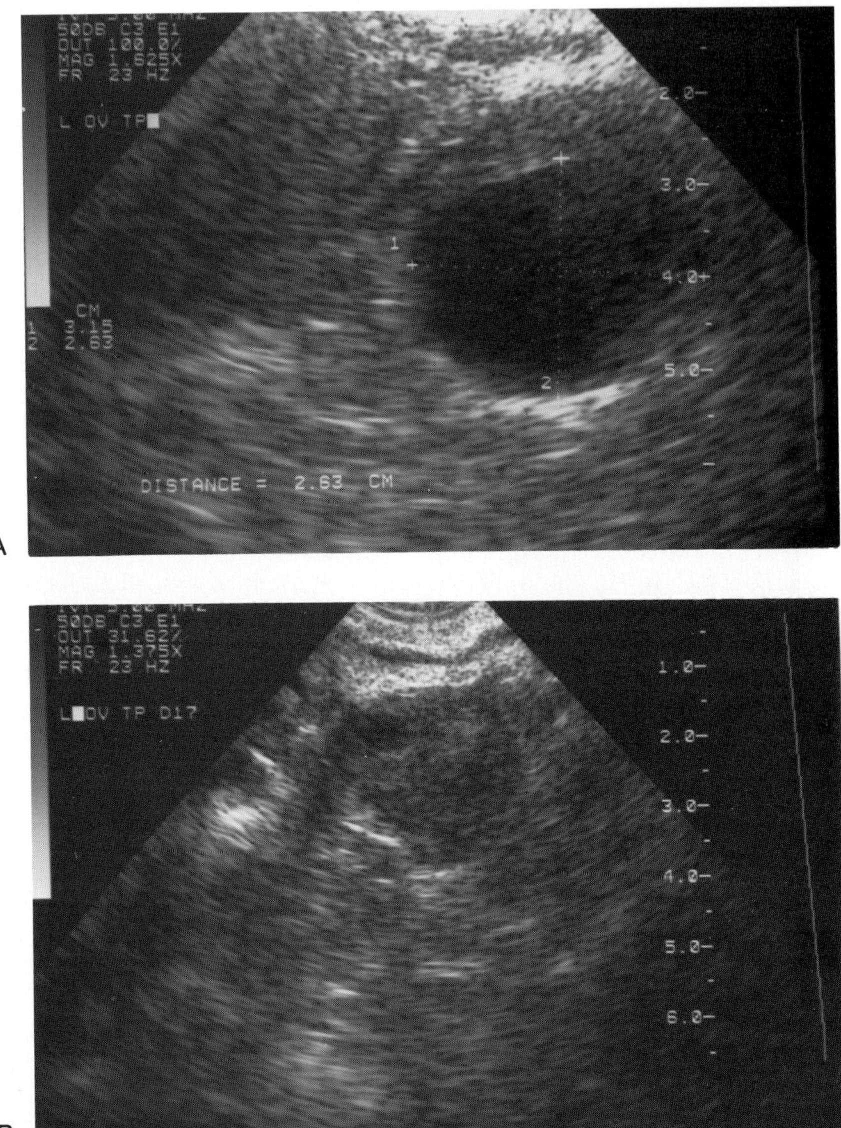

Fig. 7-8. (**A**) T-pelvic image of the left ovary showing a 3.2- by 2.6-cm follicle in the left ovary on day 16 of cycle after clomiphene citrate stimulation. (**B**) T-pelvic image of the left ovary on day 17 after ovulation.

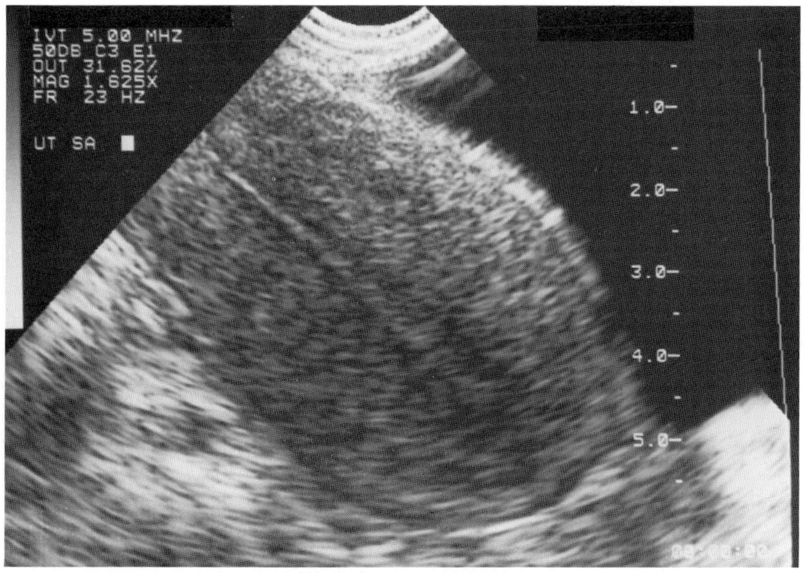

Fig. 7-9. AP-pelvic image of the uterus showing a single-line endometrium indicating low levels of estrogen stimulation.

interval from the LH surge to ovulation varies. An LH surge has been reported in luteinized but unruptured follicle syndrome without ovulation. However, serial LH determinations done every few hours probably allow the best prediction of the timing of ovulation currently available.

The BBT only vaguely suggests ovulation. Neither serial LH or BBT measurements confirm ovulation or give the additional information noted above with ultrasound monitoring. Although not practical or economic, serial sonography every few hours would also allow precise determination that ovulation has occurred.

In the human, ovulation and the initiation of corpus luteal formation is suggested by (1) the complete disappearance of the follicles, (2) a decrease in the size of the follicle, or (3) irregularity of the follicular contours with increased echogenicity within the follicle.[30] However, sometimes the follicular collapse may be missed, and a corpus luteal cyst or hemorrhagic

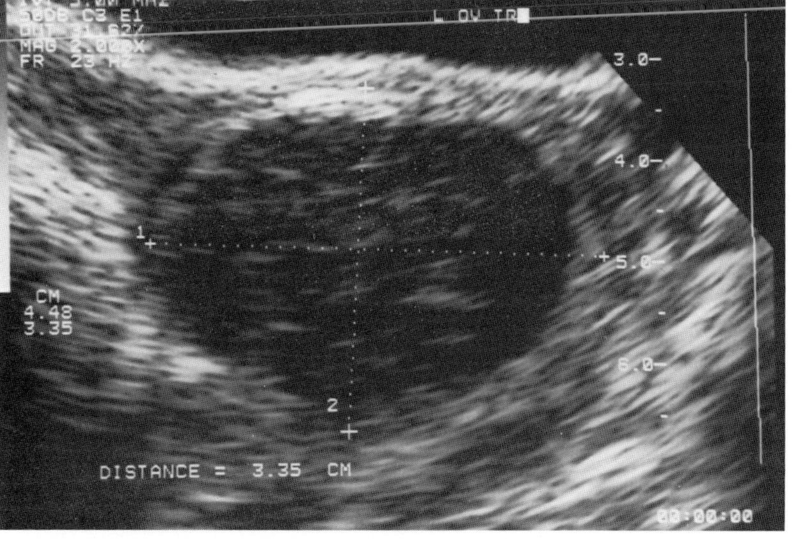

Fig. 7-10. T-pelvic view of the left ovary showing a 4.48- by 3.35-cm hemorrhagic corpus luteal cyst. Note the typical internal echo pattern of an organizing blood clot and the thick wall of the cyst. The cyst spontaneously resolved with the onset of menses.

A

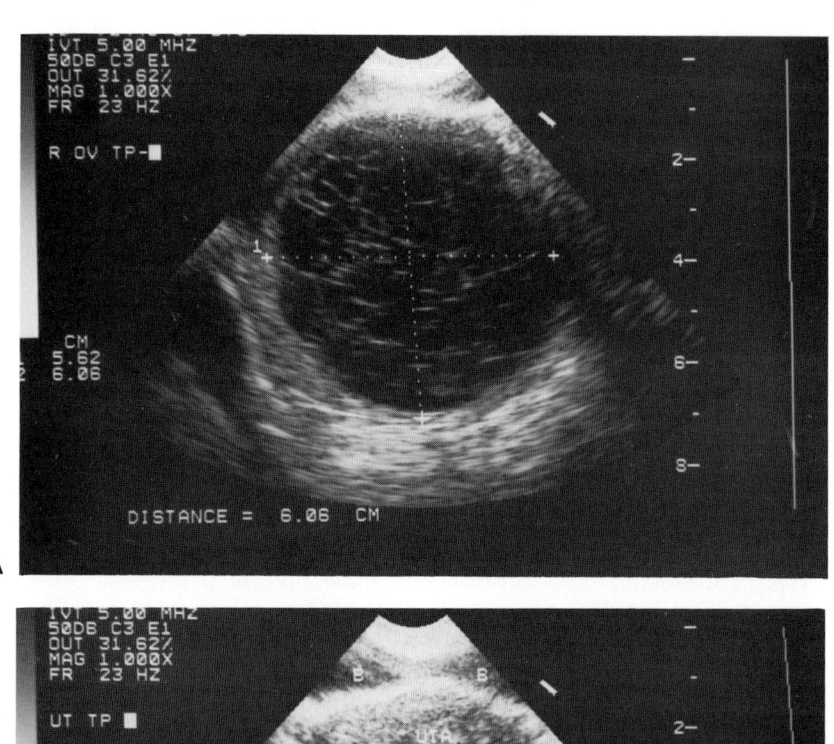

B

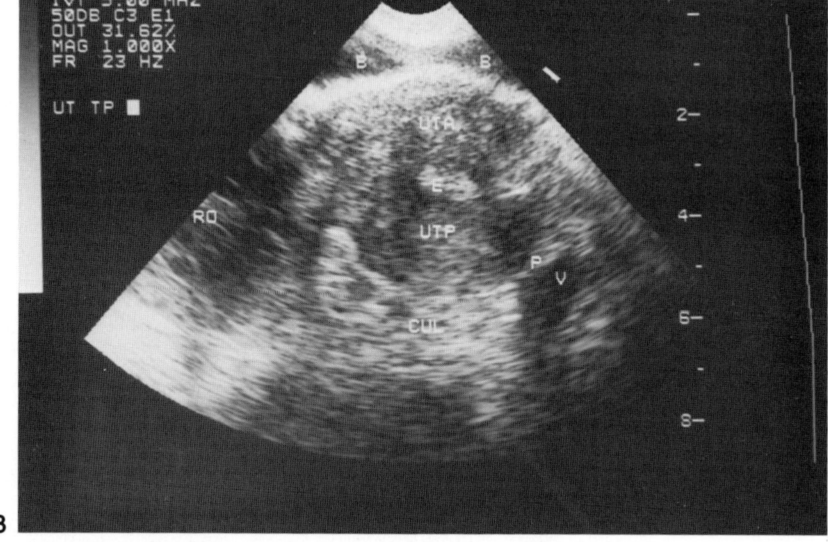

Fig. 7-11. (A) A 6- by 5.6-cm right corpus luteal cyst. Note the lacy pattern within the cyst. The internal iliac vein is to the left. **(B)** T-pelvic view. The large cyst has pushed the uterus against the left pelvic wall. UTA, anterior wall of the uterus; UTP, posterior wall of the uterus; E, endometrium; CUL, small bowel in the cul-de-sac; P, peritoneum; V, left internal iliac vein. The endometrium is luteinized. The serum estradiol was 30 pg/ml, and the serum progesterone was 10 ng/ml.

corpus luteum may form and appear as an anechoic area resembling a follicle. The presence of a hyperechoic area representing a blood clot or the speckled appearance of blood within the corpus luteum helps distinguish a preovulatory follicle from a corpus luteal cyst (Fig. 7-10). As noted above, the endometrium may also be helpful. The sudden appearance of increased cul-de-sac fluid is also suggestive evidence that ovulation may have occurred.

CORPUS LUTEUM

It is important that the sonographer be aware of normal follicular development and the appearance of corpus luteal cysts. Most hemorrhagic corpus luteal cysts present as heterogeneous echogenic ovarian masses that are predominantly anechoic, but that frequently contain hyperechoic material within the cyst (Fig. 7-11). The hyperechoic echoes represent a blood clot and may take many different and irregular forms. Sometimes the blood clot fills the cyst, but as the clot retracts, a separate anechoic area of serum is seen. Cul-de-sac fluid is present in 22 percent of women after ovulation (Fig. 7-12).[31] Sonographic imaging, particularly use of the transvaginal probe, allows visualization of small nonovulatory follicles of only 0.3 to 0.5 cm. A normal dominant follicle of 2.5 to 3.0 cm will appear quite large and may lead to the erroneous diagnosis of an ovarian cyst. Corpus luteal cysts are not pathologic but physiologic variants and may persist for 4 to 8 weeks. A corpus luteal cyst should not be surgically removed unless associated with significant and persistent intra-abdominal hemorrhage.

ORAL CONTRACEPTIVES

Most patients who have taken oral contraceptives on a long-term basis will not develop a dominant follicle and ovulate. The ovary will be imaged as a homogeneous structure without a dominant follicle. Frequently, even the small anechoic nonovulatory immature follicles may not be present. Occasionally, a dominant follicle will develop, and the patient may

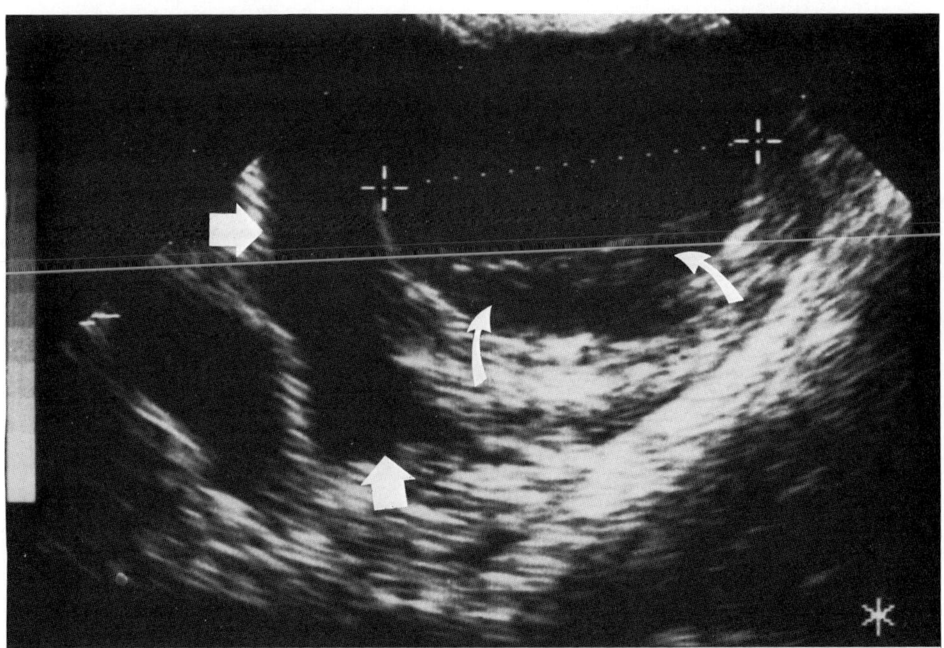

Fig. 7-12. Small corpus luteal cyst (3.4 cm) with layering of more solid material in the lower one-third of the cyst (curved arrows). The corpus luteal cyst had resolved when the patient was scanned 1 month later. Note the large amount of peritoneal fluid surrounding the cyst (arrows).

ovulate despite the use of oral contraceptives. Davis and Gosink[32] noted at least one ovarian follicle in 7 of 11 patients. The size of these follicles varied from 5 mm to 19 mm.

POSTMENOPAUSAL OVARY

Visualization and measurement of ovarian volume in the postmenopausal patient are sometimes difficult, but potentially afford early detection of ovarian cancer or neoplasm. Since there are usually no developing follicles or even preovulatory follicles in the postmenopausal ovary, the ovaries may blend with other pelvic structures and be difficult to recognize as a separate structure (Fig. 7-13), (for further discussion see Ch. 11). Ovarian volume and diameter decrease with age. The postmenopausal ovary measures only 1.5 by 1 by 0.5 cm and cannot be palpated during pelvic examination.

One percent of women over the age of 40 will develop ovarian cancer. The importance of early detection of ovarian cancer is evidenced by the fact that survival rates for stage I disease (limited to the ovary) are 80 to 85 percent, whereas survival rates for stage III and IV (advanced) disease are 14 and 5 percent, respectively.[4] Currently, there are no good screening methods to detect ovarian cancer at an early stage. Since ovarian cancer is generally asymptomatic until it has reached an advanced stage, most patients are not diagnosed until they have advanced disease. As a consequence, the overall survival rate for ovarian cancer is only 30 to 35 percent. Ultrasonography offers the capability of detecting even small increases in ovarian size and at least the potential for early diagnosis of ovarian cancer.

Postmenopausal ovaries are difficult to visualize because of their small size and lack of follicles, and the

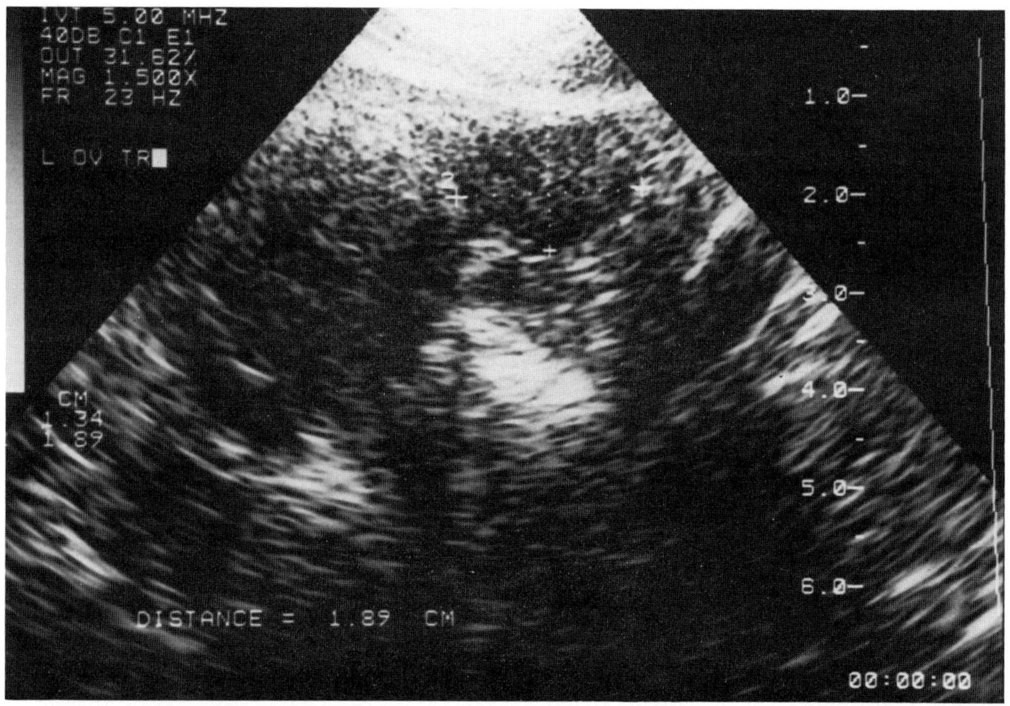

Fig. 7-13. A 42-year-old woman with a history of amenorrhea for 6 months who was being treated with Estraderm (estradiol) patches. The ovaries were both small (1.6 by 1.2 cm and 1.9 by 1.3 cm) and showed no follicular development of small immature follicles. The endometrium was a single line. The small ovaries with a lack of follicular development and a single-line endometrium are consistent with a postmenopausal status. The patient's follicle stimulating hormone was 44.7 mIU/ml, LH was 84.8 mIU/ml, and estradiol was 148 pg/ml.

normal postmenopausal ovaries may not be seen during the sonographic examination. Hall et al[33] visualized both ovaries in two-thirds of postmenopausal patients and at least one ovary in three-fourths of patients. Granberg and Wikland[13] found transvaginal sonographs to be slightly less accurate (23 percent) than abdominal ultrasound (34 percent) in visualizing the postmenopausal ovary. However, much clearer images were obtained using the transvaginal approach when the ovaries were localized. In seven patients in whom neither ovary could be visualized abdominally, both ovaries were identified in six of these seven patients transvaginally. When both the transvaginal and transabdominal techniques were used, the ovaries were visualized in all but one patient. Therefore, when there is difficulty in visualizing the postmenopausal ovary, the techniques of transabdominal and transvaginal ultrasound may be used to supplement each other.

In Hall et al's series,[33] the ovarian volumes in all postmenopausal patients were less than or equal to 2.5 cm^3. Granberg and Wikland[15] noted the mean ovarian volume in their series of postmenopausal women to be 1.4 ± 1.0 cm^3. Campbell et al[4] sonographically identified both ovaries in 84 percent of postmenopausal patients. The mean ovarian volume noted was 4.33 cm^3 with a range from 1.47 to 10.43 cm^3. One possible reason for the large difference in the size of the postmenopausal ovary between Hall et al's and Campbell et al's series may be the ages of the postmenopausal patients included in the respective studies.[4,33] Patients less than 3 to 5 years postmenopausal may still have appreciable ovarian volumes, as suggested by Barber and Graber.[34] Even follicular activity may occasionally be noted for the first 4 to 5 years after the menopause. The presence of a follicle or small anechoic area in the ovary during the first 5 years after menopause should not be mistaken for a pathologic process.[35] However, follicles that develop in a postmenopausal woman should rapidly disappear just as in any normal cycle. Persistence of even a small cyst must be viewed with concern.

Despite the difference in normal size reported for the postmenopausal ovary, there is a close correlation between the size of the right and left ovaries, with a mean difference of only 1.48 cm.^{3} Campbell et al[4] suggest that an ovary twice the size of its sister should be regarded as suspicious and warrant further evaluation. Postmenopausal ovaries with a volume larger than 5 cm^3, the presence of an anechoic cystic area, or a significant difference in size between the two ovaries probably warrant at least a repeat ultrasound examination in 1 to 2 months, and surgical intervention may be needed depending on the clinical circumstances. Difference in size between the ovaries is particularly important, since each ovary serves to some extent as a normal control for its sister. The inability to visualize an ovary after a thorough search is not significant, but a transabdominal scan should be done to insure that the ovary is not enlarged but out of the pelvis and out of the range of the transvaginal probe.

OVARIAN ENLARGEMENT

Abnormal enlargement of the ovary may result from (1) physiologic alterations, (2) non-neoplastic pathologic processes, and (3) benign or (4) malignant neoplasms (Table 7-2).

Physiologic alterations are, as the term implies, enlargements generally resulting from alteration of normal physiologic processes, such as follicular development or corpus luteum formation. These masses or cysts are very common, but are self-limiting, quite innocuous, and will spontaneously regress in 4 to 8 weeks (Figs. 7-14 and 7-15). Unfortunately, the factors leading to follicular or corpus luteal cyst formation are poorly understood. Functional cysts might simply be grown variants of normal follicles or corpus luteum and may represent the upper limits of variability of a bell-shaped curve of follicular or corpus luteal size. Hemorrhage into a developing corpus luteum may be an important factor in the formation of a corpus luteal cyst. Lack of ovulation with continued growth may contribute to the development of a follicular cyst that persists into what should be the luteal phase of a cycle (as judged from the last menstrual period) or even into the next cycle. Persistence of a functional cyst may cause a delay in menstruation or a missed menstrual period.

What size is necessary to justify a diagnosis of an

Table 7-2. Differential Diagnosis of Ovarian Cysts

Physiology
Developing follicles, follicular cyst, corpus luteal cyst
Non-neoplastic pathologic processes
Endometrioma
Infection, tubo-ovarian abscess
Ovarian ectopic pregnancy
Benign neoplasms
Malignant neoplasms

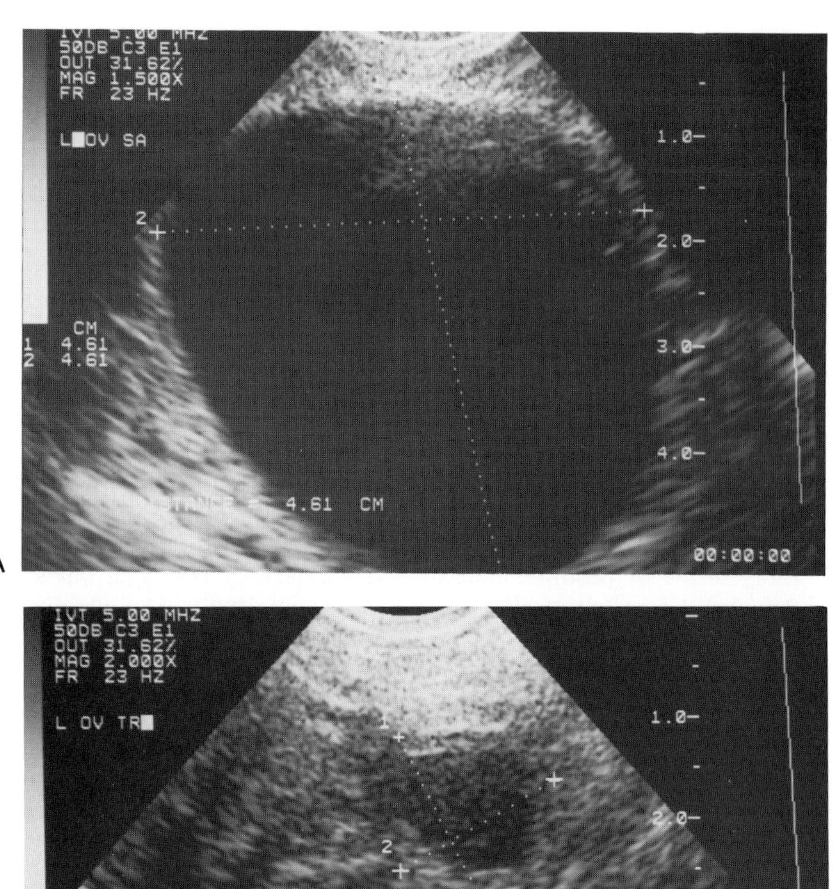

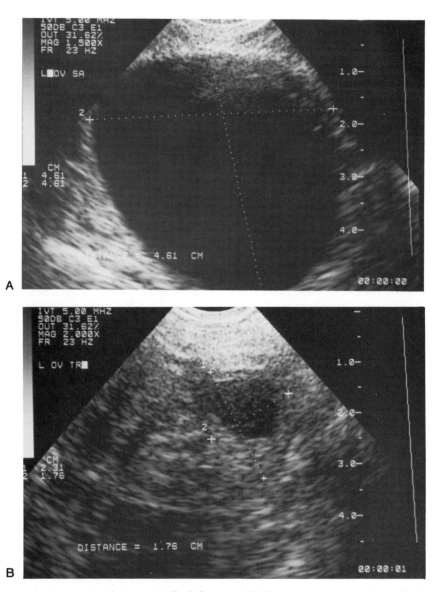

Fig. 7-14. **(A)** A 4.6- by 4.6-cm anechoic cyst in the left ovary. **(B)** The cyst spontaneously resolved 7 weeks later. The estradiol was 182 pg/ml, follicle stimulating hormone was 3.8 mIU/ml, LH was 13.9 mIU/ml, and progesterone was less than 1 ng/ml. Functional cysts are quite common and resolve spontaneously. About 5 percent of carcinomas can present as an anechoic cyst. However, an anechoic cyst without septations or nodularities of the cyst wall should not be operated on unless it is present for 6 to 12 weeks or there are other clinical considerations. The lack of internal echo, frequently seen with a corpus luteal cyst, estrogen production, and the lack of progesterone production suggest that this was a follicular cyst.

A

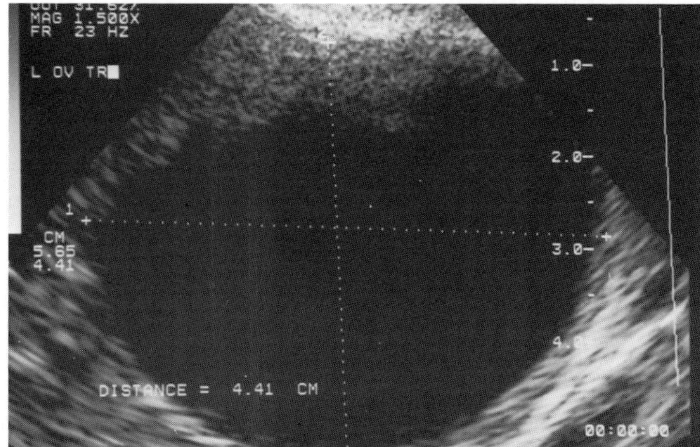

B

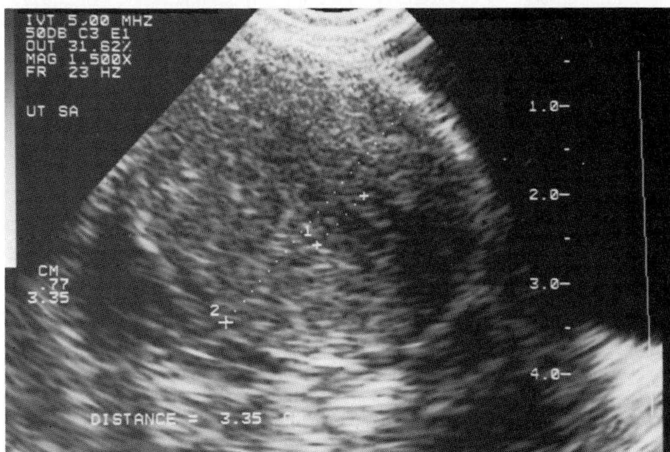

C

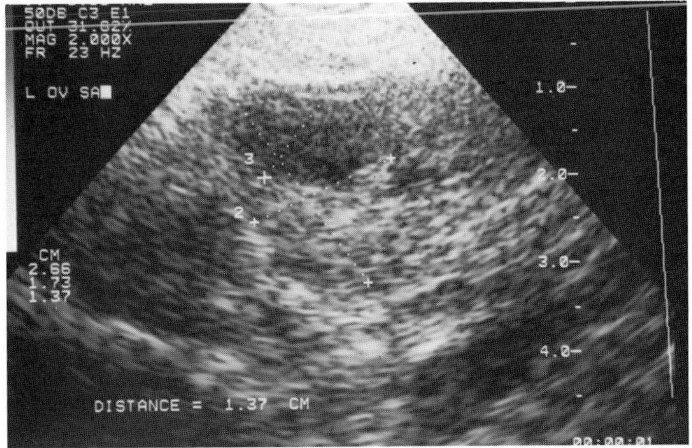

Fig. 7-15. A 45-year-old woman with a complaint of pelvic pain with an ultrasound examination on day 15 of her cycle. **(A)** A 5.7- by 4.4-cm anechoic cyst is noted in the left ovary. There are no internal echoes, and the cyst wall is smooth. **(B)** The uterus (AP-pelvic view) is normal with an anterior posterior diameter of 3.35 cm and a follicular endometrium measuring 0.77 cm. The serum estradiol was 182 pg/ml, with a progesterone level of less than 1 ng/ml, confirming the findings of a follicular endometrium and suggesting an estrogen-producing (probably follicular) cyst. The patient was treated with Provera (medroxyprogesterone acetate) (10 mg) for 10 days, with menses occurring after completion of therapy. The cyst resolved with the onset of menses. **(C)** Left ovary 7 days after the onset of menstruation.

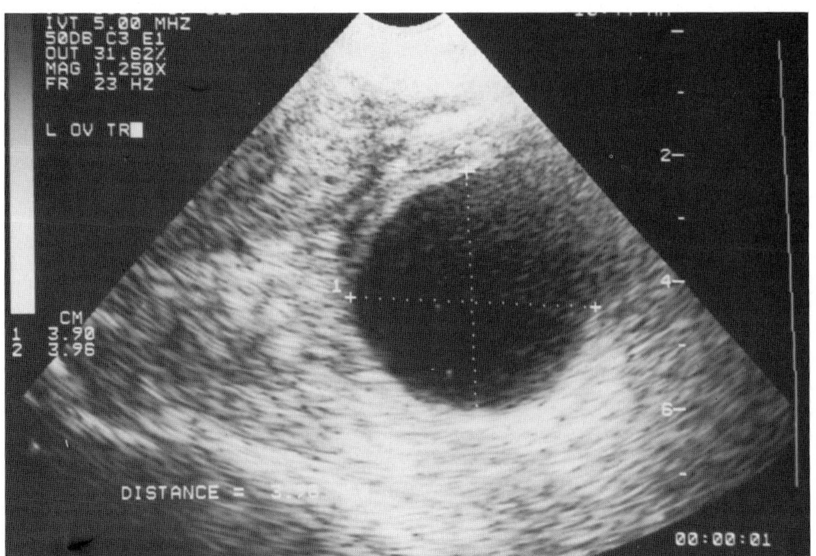

Fig. 7-16. A 4- by 4-cm follicle was noted on day 15 of a menstrual cycle. The follicle disappeared on day 16 of the cycle, suggesting ovulation. Distinguishing between a large follicle and a functional cyst may require serial scans to evaluate its biologic behavior. It may be impossible to differentiate a developing follicle from a functional cyst based on size alone, particularly for cysts or follicles 3 to 4 cm in diameter. This seems to have been a very large follicle that disappeared (ovulated) in midcycle.

ovarian cyst? Griffiths[36] suggested in 1979 that a follicle of 2.5 cm or greater constituted a follicular cyst. This was before the widespread use of ultrasound and particularly transvaginal ultrasound. This definition is clearly arbitrary, since the average diameter of a follicle at ovulation is 2.1 to 2.3 cm, and I have repeatedly noted follicles that enlarged to 3.0 cm and occasionally 3.5 cm to 4.5 cm that still ovulated at an appropriate time in the menstrual cycle and probably represented normal follicular variants (Fig. 7-16).[28]

In addition to the size criteria necessary to diagnosis an anechoic fluid-filled area as a cyst, its relation to the menstrual cycle, dynamic changes during the cycle, and life span are very important. For example, a 2.5-cm anechoic cystic structure imaged in the ovary on day 14 of a normal menstrual cycle is probably a dominant follicle nearing ovulation. However, the same 2.5-cm anechoic area in the ovary during menstruation is not normal and constitutes either a cyst or at least a temporal dyssynchrony between follicular development, the endometrium, and menstruation. However, it could be pathologic. Likewise, a 2.5-cm anechoic area present in the ovary on days 3 to 8 of a menstrual cycle that does not show a progression in size with resolution at midcycle may represent a functional cyst, a small endometrioma, or other non-neoplastic lesion or a neoplasm. A normal follicle should demonstrate a progressive increase in size of 2 to 3 mm per day and disappear after ovulation at midcycle.

Septations separating multiple anechoic areas within the ovary can represent either multiple developing follicles or a benign or malignant neoplasm (Fig. 7-17). Multiple follicles are uncommon in the ovary in a normal cycle, but may occasionally be noted. Nodularity or papillary excrescence along the cyst wall is definitely abnormal. A significant solid component or solid mass is also abnormal. However, blood clots in a corpus luteal cyst may appear as an irregular solid mass.

Although most follicles collapse and disappear after ovulation, the formation of a hemorrhagic cystic corpus luteum is quite common. These cysts tend to be somewhat larger than developing follicles or follicular cysts, but usually disappear with menses. Some corpus luteal cysts persist through an additional menstrual cycle. Probably one of the most important considerations in diagnosing a small anechoic mass in the ovary as a cyst is its persistence regardless of size and its failure to behave like a normal follicle.

A classic study on the importance of observing adnexal masses over time was published by Spanos.[37] Spanos observed for 6 weeks 286 patients with cystic adnexal masses diagnosed by pelvic examination. If the mass persisted, the patient was surgically explored. The mass persisted in 81 (28 percent) of patients. No patient with an adnexal mass that was observed and persisted for 6 weeks had a functional ovarian cyst. Seven patients (2.4 percent) of the total patients (8.6 percent of the 81 explored patients) had paraovarian cysts or hydrosalpinx. Malignant diseases were noted in 5 of the remaining 74 patients (6.8 percent of explored ovarian masses, 1.8 percent of diagnosed masses).

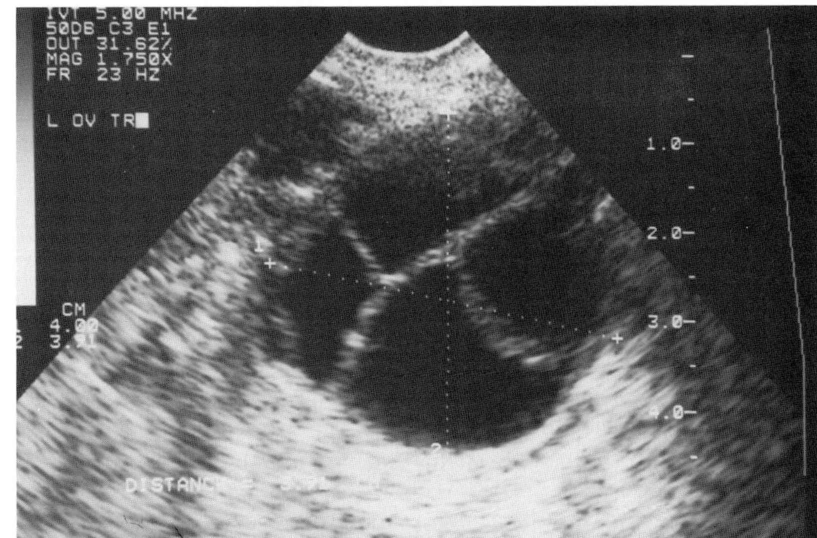

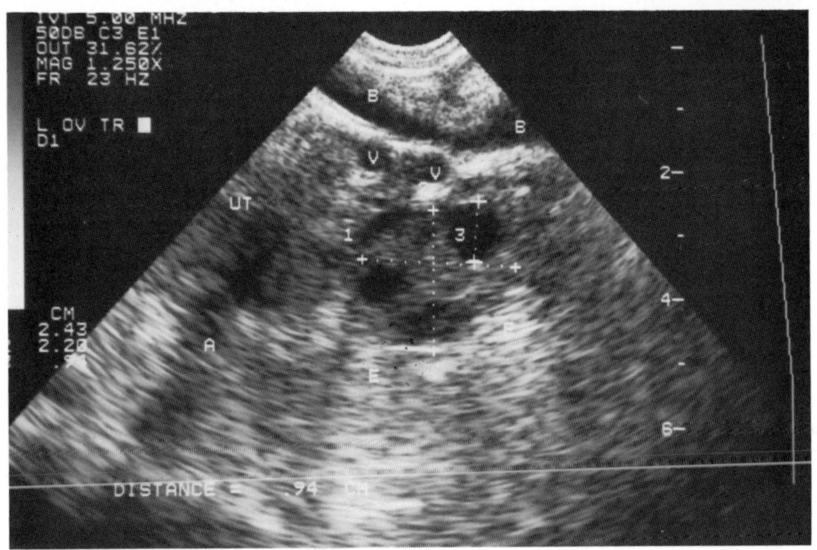

Fig. 7-17. A 24-year-old woman G2 with menometrorrhagia and abdominal pain. **(A)** T-pelvic view of the left ovary showing a 4- by 3.9-cm ovarian cyst with multiple septations. **(B)** The cyst resolved spontaneously 4 weeks later. The ovary is 2.4 by 2.2 cm with several small immature follicles. The uterus (UT) is to the left in the photograph. Some veins (V) in the infundibulopelvic ligament are present. There is some acoustic enhancement (E) posterior to the preovulatory follicles. B, bladder; A, an artifact shadow.

Andolf et al[38] evaluated the use of ultrasound for screening and detected ovarian enlargement in 805 women aged 40 to 70 years. Only 50 patients (6 percent) had a persistent abnormal repeat scan. Thirty-nine patients underwent surgical exploration, and 35 had significant pathology. The most common findings were cystadenomas in 12 of the 35 patients (34 percent). Ovarian carcinoma, borderline ovarian tumors, dermoids, endometriosis, and hydrosalpinx were some of the other findings.

Only 8 of the 35 patients (23 percent) had abnormal pelvic examinations, which again illustrates the potential value of ultrasound as an adjunct to the pelvic examination in gynecology. Andolf et al's data[38] would suggest that the ultrasonographic examination is four times as sensitive in detecting ovarian pathology as a pelvic examination during a routine screening examination in the asymptomatic patient. None of three borderline tumors or the one carcinoma of the ovary was detected during the pelvic examination. However, all were detected by sonogram. The difference in the rate of disappearance of the masses in Andolf et al's study compared with Spanos' study (6 percent versus 28 percent) probably reflects the fact that many smaller functional ovarian cysts were diagnosed using ultrasound. Most of the functional cysts disappeared spontaneously.[37,38]

The most important sign predicting pathology for

cystic pelvic masses is persistence of the lesion for more than 6 to 12 weeks. Even small persistent cystic structures of 3 to 4 cm are generally pathologic if they persist for 6 to 12 weeks. As noted by Spanos,[37] most small ovarian masses resolve spontaneously.

In three of the four patients who did not have any pathology in Andolf et al's study,[38] the last ultrasound examination had been done 5 to 6 weeks before surgery. The disappearance of four masses among 39 patients (10 percent) before surgery illustrates the importance of a repeat ultrasound examination at least a few days before surgery to confirm the persistence of the mass. This is particularly true if the mass is not clearly palpable during a pelvic examination on admission to the hospital or in the obese patient with a less than optimal pelvic examination. The fourth patient in Andolf et al's series[38] of patients who had a negative laparoscopy had been scanned before surgery and the sonogram was normal. However, a laparoscopy was still done for pelvic pain.

Generally, fluid-filled cystic masses without septations, papillary excrescence, or nodularity are benign. Hurwitz et al[39] reported on 52 women with clear pelvic cysts without septation(s) diagnosed by ultrasound that were 5 cm or larger and persisted for 4 to 8 weeks. There were no malignancies among the 52 patients. In patients surgically explored, benign ovarian neoplasms were present in 29 percent, simple cysts lined by cuboidal cells were found in 38 percent, and paraovarian cysts were present in 8 percent. One ectopic pregnancy and one endometrioma were found. In 15 patients the cysts were aspirated, and the cytology was benign. However, 1 of those 15 patients subsequently developed a serous cystadenoma. The aspiration of persistent ovarian cysts is still controversial at this time.

In pregnancy, corpus luteal cysts are quite common. However, cysts that persist into the second trimester have a higher risk of being neoplastic. Thorton and Wells[40] reported 14 sonographically diagnosed simple cysts larger than 5 cm in size in pregnancy; four were cystadenomas and three were borderline malignant neoplasms. All 15 cysts less than 5 cm in size resolved spontaneously.

MANAGEMENT OF ULTRASOUND-DETECTED OVARIAN MASSES

Sonographers should follow the same recommendation for conservative management of an ovarian cyst that has been used for years in gynecology. As a generalization, surgery should not be performed unless the cyst is larger than 6 cm and/or persists for 6 to 12 weeks.[41] As noted by DiSaia and Creasman, "Ninety-five percent of ovarian cysts less than 5 cm in diameter are non-neoplastic."[42] The exception to this rule is when there is a significant solid component, nodularity, or papillary projection noted on ultrasound.

The incidence of ovarian neoplasms has not suddenly changed with the development of ultrasound. However, what has changed is our ability to image and diagnose even very small cystic structures in the ovary. In the past, it was uncommon for a clinician to palpate a 3-cm follicle or cystic corpus luteum except in a very thin patient. Likewise, very small neoplasms or cancers were rarely diagnosed. Using transvaginal ultrasonography with magnification, a 3-cm cyst appears huge and fills the cathode ray screen. However, electronic caliper measurements quickly place the size of the cyst in perspective. With the exception of an occasional ruptured corpus luteal cyst with significant bleeding or a twisted cyst, both of which relatively uncommon, functional cysts do not require surgery. They will disappear spontaneously. The hallmark of management of small corpus luteal or functional cysts should simply be a follow-up ultrasound in 4 to 8 weeks to ensure resolution and to confirm the diagnosis that the cyst was, in fact, functional. Treatment with oral contraceptives may be used to accelerate involution.

OVARIAN CARCINOMA

There are approximately 18,000 new cases of ovarian cancer per year in the United States and 11,000 deaths.[42] Survival rates are particularly poor, with only a 5 to 20 percent 5-year survival rate for patients with advanced disease compared with an 80 to 85 percent 5-year survival rate for patients with stage I disease.[4,43] Unfortunately, 50 to 70 percent of ovarian cancers are not detected until they are at an advanced stage (stages III and IV). As discussed above, early detection is critical. However, except for a yearly pelvic examination, screening is uncommon. High risk groups for ovarian cancer include postmenopausal women, nulliparous women, and women with relatives with known ovarian or breast cancer.[15]

Requard et al[44] reported a 97 percent efficiency in detecting ovarian neoplasms using sonography. Only one case with diffuse peritoneal tumor implants but with normal-sized ovaries was not detected by ultrasonography. The ovarian neoplasms detected ranged from 3 to 21 cm in diameter. In a preoperative sonographic evaluation of 32 patients with malignant ovarian tumors, sonography accurately characterized the gross pathologic appearance in 84 percent of patients. Ascites confirmed at surgery was correctly diagnosed in 41 percent of patients. An additional 16 percent of patients had minimal ascites at surgery not detected by sonography. There were no sonographic false-positive diagnoses of ascites. Unfortunately, the efficiency of transabdominal ultrasonography in detecting omental or peritoneal tumors, which are common sites for the spread of ovarian carcinomas, is only 25 percent. Tumor involvement of retroperitoneal nodes was detected in only one of four cases. Sonography correctly staged only 48 percent of 25 patients.

In 1976 Kobayashi[45] reported sonography to be 70 percent accurate in distinguishing carcinoma of the ovary from other types of tumors in the pelvis. Achiron et al[46] noted that the presence of papillary projections, soft tissue nodules, and thick internal septae was suggestive of malignant disease. Poorly defined margins, ascites, or omental thickening suggest a poorly differentiated tumor.

Meire et al[47] evaluated the sonographic findings of 51 surgically evaluated adnexal masses. All lesions less than 5 cm that were unilocular and anechoic were benign. Of unilocular masses larger than 5 cm, only 2 of 19 were malignant (11 percent). Sixteen of 27 multilocular lesions (59 percent) were malignant. Masses with thin septa (less than 3 mm) were about equally benign and malignant (Fig. 7-18). However, seven of eight masses with thick septa (greater than 3 mm) were malignant. Most masses with thin septae and no nodules were benign. Tumors with nodules within the mass had an 83 percent chance of being malignant. Therefore, Meire et al[47] concluded that unilocular or multilocular masses with thin septa but no nodules were usually benign and that masses with multiloculations, thin septa, and nodules or with multiloculations and thick septa with or without nodules were usually malignant. Using their criteria, a correct diagnosis of benign or malignant ovarian neoplasm could have been made in 91 percent of cases. Although Meire et al's report[47] suggested that the thickness of septa is important, others have not found this criterion quite as useful in distinguishing malignant from benign neoplasms.[44]

DeLand et al[48] found sonography accurate in pre-

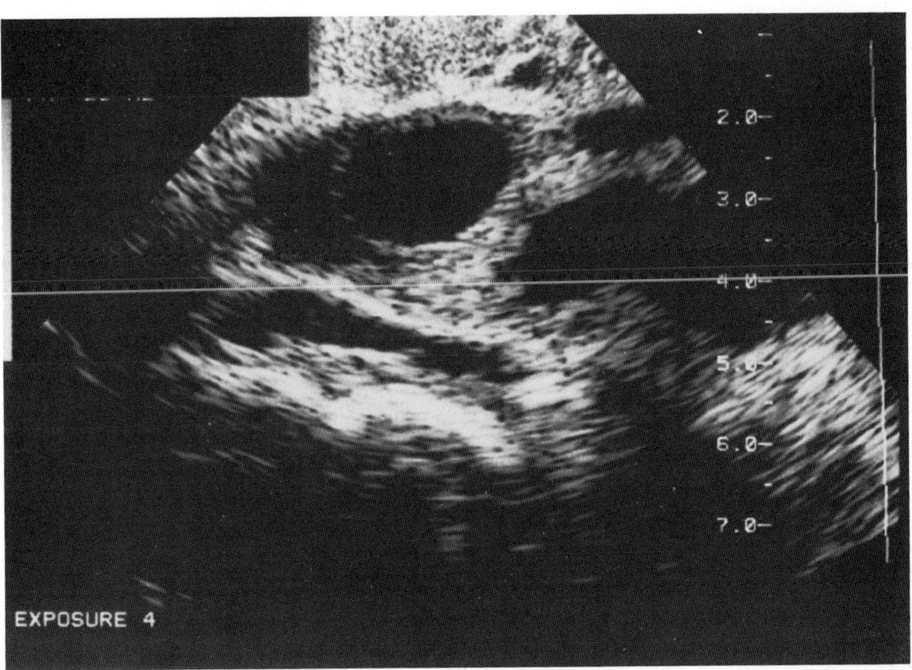

Fig. 7-18. AP-pelvic view of left ovarian cyst (10 by 7 by 7 cm) with thick septation. The tumor fills the cul-de-sac, with the uterus anterior. The septa in some areas are 7 mm thick. Multiple thick septations are uncommon in functional cysts. Ovarian hyperstimulation syndrome after Pergonal or Clomid (clomiphene citrate) therapy may produce multiple septa. However, they are generally thin. Some irregularity of the septal wall is noted, suggesting nodularity or papillar projections. The mass was a serous cystadenoma.

dicting the malignant nature of 13 of 14 carcinomas (93 percent) and the benign character of 43 of 46 ovarian cysts (94 percent). Seventy percent of tumors of the ovary had a complex or solid sonographic pattern, whereas only 1 of 38 (3 percent) was purely cystic. Completely anechoic ovarian masses have a high likelihood of being benign and are most commonly mucinous or serous cyst adenomas.[49] The possibility of malignancy increased as the amount of echogenic material in the mass increased. An exception to this rule were lesions with very echogenic foci consistent with a tooth, bone, or hair in a benign teratoma (Fig. 7-19). One-third of the totally solid tumors were malignant (Fig. 7-20). Only 4 of 72 (6 percent) completely anechoic ovarian masses were malignant in three studies.[47–49]

In summary, we can conclude that ultrasound is quite effective in detecting small ovarian cysts and masses (less than 5 cm) and is more effective than a routine pelvic examination for this purpose. However, screening for ovarian cancer by ultrasonography or pelvic examination has a relatively low yield

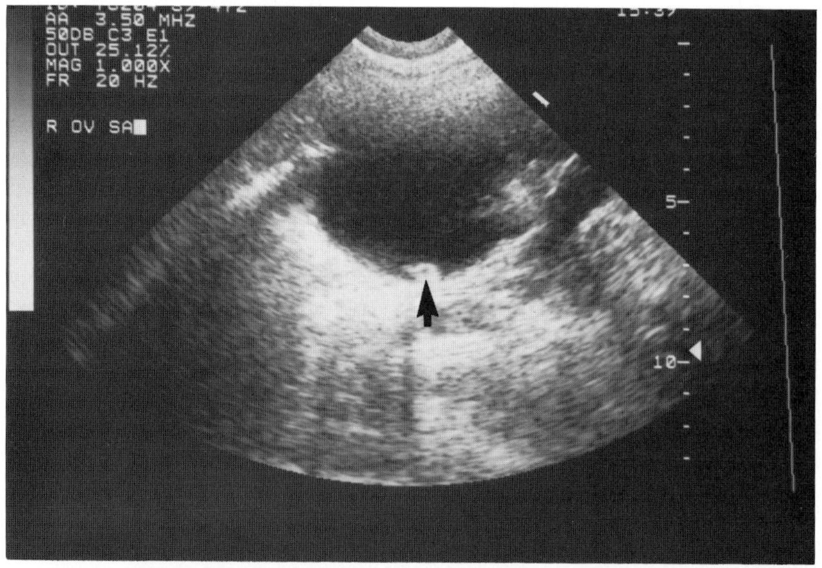

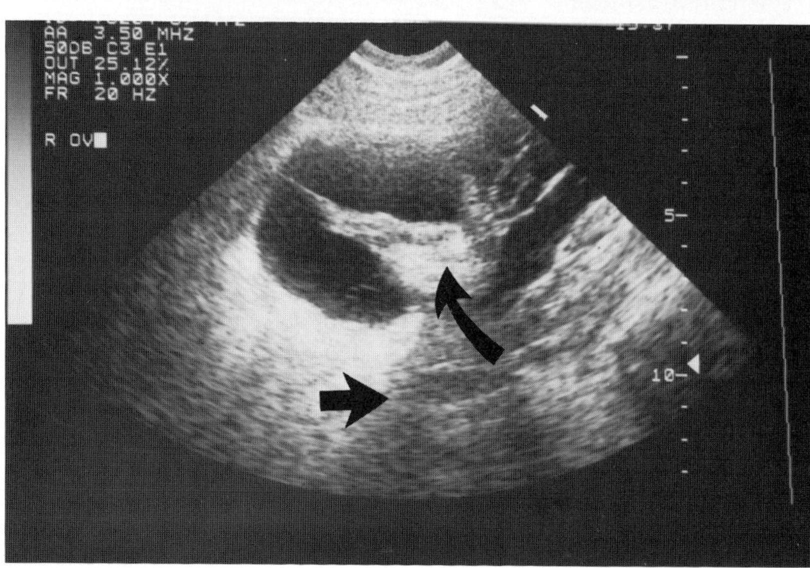

Fig. 7-19. (**A**) Note the nodularity of the cyst wall (arrow). (**B**) Thickened hyperechoic area (curved arrow) with posterior shadowing (arrow) representing hair within a dermoid.

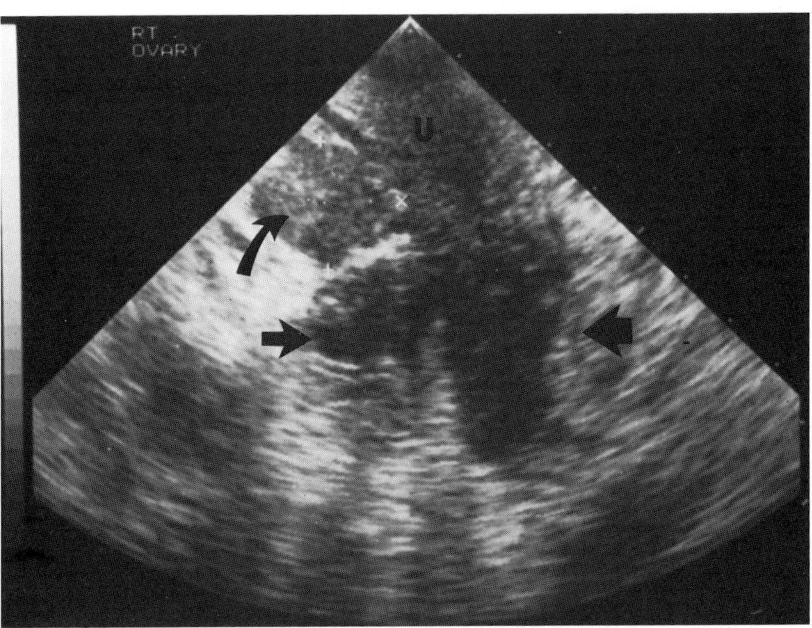

Fig. 7-20. T-pelvic image of a solid irregular mass in the cul-de-sac (large arrows). This mass is separated from but is adjacent to the ovary (curved arrow). The uterus (U) is at the top of the photo. This mass was a lymphoma.

(1.5/10,000) unless higher risk populations are screened (over 40 years old, family history of ovarian cancer, etc.). Most masses less than 5 cm in diameter are functional cysts and will disappear. A mass with thick septations, nodularity, papillations, or a significant solid component should be of concern and probably warrants surgical exploration (Fig. 7-21). Although ultrasound has an overall accuracy of over 90 percent in characterizing an ovarian mass, it is poor at staging ovarian cancer. Ovarian cancer is and should be staged surgically.

The three most common criteria for surgery for an ovarian cyst are its size, consistency, and persistence of the mass. Masses larger than 6 cm or with solid or semisolid components, significant nodularity, or papillary excrescence or masses that are present for longer than 6–12 weeks should be surgically explored. However, size per se is the least reliable factor in predicting neoplasm or malignancy, particularly in the 6 to 8 cm range with an anechoic cystic content and no nodularity of the cyst wall.

Some Families at High Risk for Cancer

Some families having a high risk for cancer have been reported.[50] Such families generally have site-specific cancers, such as ovarian cancer, breast and ovarian cancer, or a cancer family syndrome in which ovarian cancer may be associated with endometrial or colon cancer. The risk of ovarian cancer in some high risk members of ovarian cancer-prone families may approach 50 percent. Lynch et al[50] have suggested semiannual ultrasonographic surveillance for such individuals, with prophylactic surgery after childbearing. Those who refuse surgery should continue to have meticulous ultrasound and clinical surveillance.

Screening for Ovarian Cancer in Asymptomatic Patients

Unfortunately, ovarian cancer is rarely symptomatic in its early stages. As a consequence, detection of an early ovarian cancer is often serendipitous. The annual rate of 1.4 ovarian cancers per 10,000 women translates into only an occasional early case discovered during a routine pelvic examinations. Yet, early diagnosis and surgical removal are the most important factors known to improve prognosis.

There have only been a few studies using sonography as a tool for screening for early ovarian cancer.[5,38] In a sonographic study of 1,084 postmenopausal patients, only 3 percent were noted to have an abnormal ovarian morphology.[5] Histologic data were available for only 15 of these 34 patients. There was one clear cell carcinoma and five cystadenomas (Table 7-3).

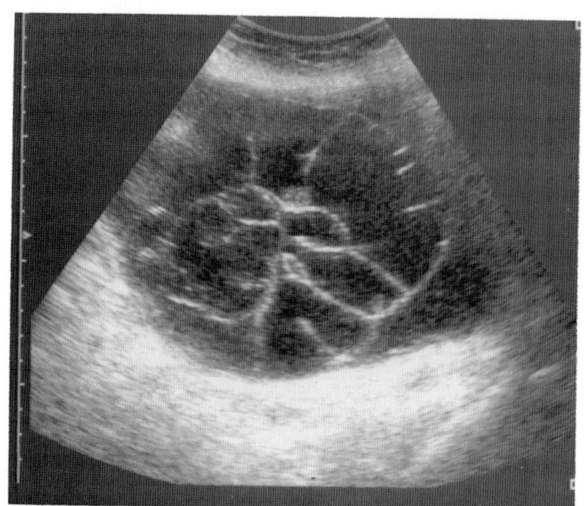

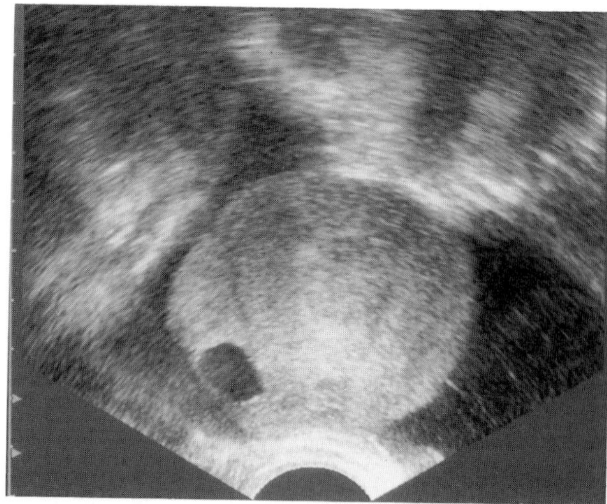

Fig. 7-21. (A) Ovarian serous cystadenoma, 130 mm × 90 mm. This was a fortuitous finding of an adnexal mass during a gynecological exam in a 92-year-old patient. Multiple septa are very suggestive of this type of tumor. (**B**) Krukenberg tumor of the left ovary in a 34-year-old woman. A gastric tumor had previously been diagnosed, and the patient presented with more than 6 L of ascitis. Note the highly echogenic, homogeneous aspect of the 50 mm × 60 mm mass englobing the whole ovary and the abnormally high amount of peri-ovarian fluid, corresponding to ascitis. (Both ovaries were involved) (Courtesy of I. Vial, M.D., Department of Obstetrics and Gynecology, CHUV, Lausanne, Switzerland).

It is not clear at this time whether ultrasound screening will be either efficient or cost-effective as a screening tool for ovarian cancer. However, perhaps at least some comparisons can be made with screening for breast cancer by mammograms. In women aged 40 and older, the lifetime risk for breast cancer (United States) is about 7 percent compared with 1.0 percent for ovarian cancer. Therefore, based only on incidence, ovarian cancer screening would be expected to be seven times less cost-effective. However, other considerations—for example, how long an ovarian cancer persists as sonographically detectable but remains asymptomatic and/or undetectable on pelvic examination, and localized to the ovary—will also affect cost-effectiveness. These data are simply not known at this time. The cost of a screening pelvic sonogram clearly will also be an important factor in estimates of cost-effectiveness.

Table 7-3. Postmenopausal Ultrasound Screening[a]

One	clear cell carcinoma
Three	serous cystadenomas
Two	mucinous cystadenomas
One	dermoid
One	fibroid
Two	endometriomas
Two	simple serous cysts
Three	follicular cysts

[a] Histology was available in only 15 of 34 patients.
(Modified from Goswamy et al,[5] with permission.)

OVARIAN VEIN THROMBOSIS

The diagnosis of ovarian vein thrombosis has generally been made on clinical findings, with only 20 percent of cases diagnosed preoperatively.[51] Puerperal ovarian vein thrombosis has an estimated frequency of 1 in 600 cases.[52] It is preceded by endometritis in 23 to 45 percent of cases.[52] Femoral venography, gallium scanning, ovarian vein phlebography, and intravenous pyelograms have been used to make the diagnosis in the past. More recently, computed tomography, nuclear magnetic resonance imaging, and ultrasound have become more reliable diagnostic techniques and are less invasive than venography. Savader et al,[51] using an abdominal 5-MHz sector transducer, reported the ultrasound appearance of the thrombosed ovarian vein as an anechoic to hypoechoic, round to oval mass, with an echogenic center representing the thrombosis. Baran and Frisch[53] used pulsed image-directed Doppler evaluation to demonstrate a lack of blood flow in the ovarian vein after thrombosis. Although the pelvic portion of the ovarian vein is easily visualized using transvaginal ultrasound, visualization of the abdominal portion and the inferior vena cava requires transabdominal scanning.

Computed tomography or nuclear magnetic resonance imaging may become the technique of choice for the diagnosis of pelvic thrombophlebitis. However, ultrasound is helpful in evaluating the patient with suspected pelvic thrombosis with fever and pain to rule out retained products of conception and/or tubo-ovarian abscess and may also help diagnose a thrombosis in pelvic vessels. Newer transvaginal probes with Doppler or color flow may be particularly useful in evaluating blood flow in pelvic vessels.[54]

REFERENCES

1. Kratochwil A, Urban G, Friedrich F: Ultrasonic tomography of the ovaries. Ann Chir Gynaecol Fenn 61:211, 1972
2. Hall DA: Sonographic appearance of the normal ovary, of polycystic ovary disease, and of functional ovarian cysts. Semin Ultrasound 4:149, 1983
3. Gray H: Anatomy of the Human Body. 30th Ed. Lea & Febiger, Philadelphia, 1985
4. Campbell S, Goswamy R, Goessens L, Whitehead M: Real-time ultrasonography for determination of ovarian morphology and volume: a possible early screening test for ovarian cancer? Lancet 1:425, 1982
5. Goswamy RK, Campbell S, Whitehead MI: Screening for ovarian cancer. Clin Obstet Gynaecol 10:621, 1983
6. Queenan JT, O'Brien GD, Bains LM et al: Ultrasound scanning of ovaries to detect ovulation in women. Fertil Steril 34:99, 1980
7. Wiczyk HP, Janus CL, Richards CJ et al: Comparison of magnetic resonance imaging and ultrasound in evaluating follicular and endometrial development throughout the normal cycle. Fertil Steril 49:969, 1988
8. Sample WF, Lippe BM, Gyepes MT: Gray-scale ultrasonography of the normal female pelvis. Radiology 125:477, 1977
9. Munn CS, Kiser LC, Wetzner SM, Baer JE: Ovary volume in young and premenopausal adults: US determination. Radiology 159:731, 1986
10. Deutsch AL, Gosink B: Normal female pelvic anatomy. Semin Roentgenol 17:241, 1982
11. Swanson M, Sauerbrei EE, Cooperberg PL: Medical implications of ultrasonically detected polycystic ovaries. J Clin Ultrasound 9:219, 1981
12. Hann LE, Hall DA, McArdle CR, Seibel M: Polycystic ovarian disease: sonographic spectrum. Radiology 150:531, 1984
13. Granberg S, Wikland M: Comparison between endovaginal and transabdominal transducers for measuring ovarian volume. J Ultrasound Med 6:649, 1987
14. Schwimer SR, Lebovic J: Transvaginal pelvic ultrasonography: accuracy in follicle and cyst size determination. J Ultrasound Med 4:61, 1985
15. Granberg S, Wikland M: A comparison between ultrasound and gynecologic examination for detection of enlarged ovaries in a group of women at risk for ovarian carcinoma. J Ultrasound Med 7:59, 1988
16. Jaffe R, Abramowicz J, Eckstein N et al: Sonographic monitoring of ovarian volume during LHRH analogue therapy in women with polycystic ovarian syndrome. J Ultrasound Med 7:203, 1988
17. Krantz KE, Atkinson JP: Gross anatomy. Ann NY Acad Sci 142:551, 1967
18. Salardi S, Orsini LF, Cacciari E et al: Pelvic ultrasonography in girls with precocious puberty, congenital adrenal hyperplasia, obesity, or hirsutism. J Pediatr 112:880, 1988
19. Simkins CS: Development of the human ovary from birth to sexual maturity. Am J Anat 51:465, 1932
20. Orsini LF, Salardi S, Pilu G et al: Pelvic organs in premenarcheal girls: real-time ultrasonography. Radiology 153:113, 1984
21. Ivarsson SA, Nilsson KO, Persson PH: Ultrasonography of the pelvic organs in prepubertal and postpubertal girls. Arch Dis Child 58:352, 1983
22. Hall DA, Hann LE, Ferrucci JT, Jr et al: Sonographic morphology of the normal menstrual cycle. Radiology 133:185, 1979
23. Smith DH, Picker RH, Sinosich M, Saunders DM: Assessment of ovulation by ultrasound and estradiol levels during spontaneous and induced cycles. Fertil Steril 33:387, 1980
24. Bomsel-Helmreich O, Gougeon A, Thebault A et al: Healthy and atretic human follicles in the preovulatory phase: differences in evolution of follicular morphology and steroid content of follicular fluid. J Clin Endocrinol Metab 48:686, 1979
25. Hackeloer BJ, Fleming R, Robinson HP et al: Correlation of ultrasonic and endocrinologic assessment of human follicular development. Am J Obstet Gynecol 135:122, 1979
26. Taylor KJW, Burns PN, Wells PNT et al: Ultrasound Doppler flow studies of the ovarian and uterine arteries. Br J Obstet Gynaecol 92:240, 1985
27. Hilgers TW, Dvorak AD, Tamisiea DF et al: Sonographic definition of the empty follicle syndrome. J Ultrasound Med 8:411, 1989
28. Vermesh M, Kletzky OA, Davajan V, Israel R: Monitoring techniques to predict and detect ovulation. Fertil Steril 47:259, 1987

29. de Crespigny LC, O'Herlihy C, Robinson HP: Ultrasonic observation of the mechanism of human ovulation. Am J Obstet Gynecol 139:636, 1981
30. Marinho AO, Sallam HN, Goessens LKV et al: Real-time pelvic ultrasonography during the periovulatory period of patients attending an artificial insemination clinic. Fertil Steril 37:633, 1982
31. Baltarowich OH, Kurtz AB, Pasto ME et al: The spectrum of sonographic findings in hemorrhagic ovarian cysts. AJR 148:901, 1987
32. Davis JA, Gosink BB: Fluid in the female pelvis: cyclic patterns. J Ultrasound Med 5:75, 1986
33. Hall DA, McCarthy KA, Kopans DB: Sonographic visualization of the normal postmenopausal ovary. J Ultrasound Med 5:9, 1986
34. Barber HRK, Graber EA: The PMPO syndrome, editorial. Obstet Gynecol 38:921, 1971
35. Ritchie WGM: Sonographic evaluation of normal and induced ovulation. Radiology 161:1, 1986
36. Griffiths CT: The ovary. p. 325. In Kistner RW (ed): Gynecology—Principles and Practice. 3rd Ed. Year Book Medical Publishers, Chicago, 1979
37. Spanos WJ: An operative hormonal therapy of cystic adnexal masses. Am J Obstet Gynecol 116:551, 1973
38. Andolf E, Svalenius E, Astedt B: Ultrasonography for early detection of ovarian carcinoma. Br J Obstet Gynaecol 93:1286, 1986
39. Hurwitz A, Yagel S, Zion I et al: The management of persistent clear pelvic cysts diagnosed by ultrasonography. Obstet Gynecol 72:320, 1988
40. Thornton JG, Wells M: Ovarian cysts in pregnancy: does ultrasound make traditional management inappropriate? Obstet Gynecol 69:717, 1987
41. Weingold AB: Pelvic masses. p. 559. In Kase NG, Weingold WB (eds): Principles and Practice of Clinical Gynecology. John Wiley & Sons, New York, 1983
42. DiSaia PJ, Creasman WT: Clinical Gynecologic Oncology. CV Mosby, St. Louis, 1981
43. Sigurdsson K, Alm P, Gullberg B: Prognostic factors in malignant epithelial ovarian tumours. Gynecol Oncol 15:370, 1983
44. Requard CK, Mettler FA, Jr, Wicks JD: Preoperative sonography of malignant ovarian neoplasms. AJR 137:79, 1981
45. Kobayashi M: Use of diagnostic ultrasound in trophoblastic neoplasms and ovarian tumors. Cancer 38:441, 1976
46. Achiron R, Schejter E, Malinger G, Zakut H: Observations on the ultrasound diagnosis of ovarian neoplasms. Arch Gynecol Obstet 241:183, 1987
47. Meire HB, Farrant P, Guha T: Distinction of benign from malignant ovarian cysts by ultrasound. Br J Obstet Gynaecol 85:893, 1978
48. DeLand M, Fried A, van Nagell JR, Donaldson ES: Ultrasonography in the diagnosis of tumors of the ovary. Surg Gynecol Obstet 148:346, 1979
49. Moyle JW, Rochester D, Sider L et al: Sonography of ovarian tumors: predictability of tumor type. AJR 141:985, 1983
50. Lynch HT, Albano WA, Lynch JF et al: Surveillance and management of patients at high genetic risk for ovarian carcinoma. Obstet Gynecol 59:589, 1982
51. Savader SJ, Otero RR, Savader BL: Puerperal ovarian vein thrombosis: evaluation with CT, UD, and MR imaging. Radiology 167:637, 1988
52. Brown TK, Munsick RA: Puerperal ovarian vein thrombophlebitis: a syndrome. Am J Obstet Gynecol 109:263, 1971
53. Baran GW, Frisch KM: Duplex Doppler evaluation of puerperal ovarian vein thrombosis. AJR 149:321, 1987
54. Rudoff JM, Astrauskas LJ, Rundoff JC et al: Ultrasonographic diagnosis of septic pelvic thrombophlebitis. J Ultrasound Med 7:287, 1988

8

Small Bowel, Sigmoid Colon, and Rectum

Melvin G. Dodson

SMALL BOWEL

The small bowel is almost invariably visualized in the normal pelvis posterior and superior to the uterus. Peristalsis is frequently noted. When the small bowel is full of fluid, the bowel wall is easily recognized and is normally less than 3 mm thick. Air in the small bowel appears as hyperechoic densities with shadowing and/or posterior reverberation artifacts. The small bowel content may consist of anechoic fluid, hyperechoic air, and bowel content with a mixed echo pattern (Figs. 8-1 and 8-2).

Generally, the small bowel found in the pelvis is from the terminal ileum. Valvulae conniventes are circular folds of mucosa 3 to 5 mm apart that may be seen as linear echo densities. The sonographic image of these mucosal folds is referred to as the keyboard sign and is characteristic of the jejunum. These folds generally are not seen in the ileum in the pelvis. Blood, ascites, or peritoneal fluid from a ruptured cyst after ovulation or sometimes normal peritoneal fluid will outline the small bowel. Large fibroids, pelvic adhesions, or ovarian masses may displace the small bowel from the cul-de-sac and posterior pelvis. Small bowel obstruction may result in dilatation of the small bowel. Crohn's disease may result in a thickened bowel wall or a "target" or "bull's-eye" pattern consisting of a thickened edematous bowel wall with a central bowel lumen (Fig. 8-3).[1] Appendicitis may also present as a target lesion. An appendicular abscess may be difficult to differentiate from a tubo-ovarian abscess.

Wang et al.[2] and others have sonographicically evaluated the normal and pathologic gut wall and have distinguished five distinct echo layers. The first, third, and fifth layers are echogenic, whereas the second and fourth layers are hypoechoic. Histologic correlation suggests that these sonographically recognizable layers represent distinct gut wall structures as noted in Table 8-1 and Fig. 8-4. These layers were distinguishable using a 8.5-MHz linear-array ultrasound transducer in an in vitro system. Although this in vitro study demonstrates the potential for ultrasound in distinguishing detailed histology, it is more common clinically to visualize the hyperechoic serosa and submucosa separated by the hypoechoic or anechoic muscularis propria. The mucosa and particularly the mucosal surface are often hard to distinguish depending on the bowel contents. The mucosa per se may be imaged as an anechoic to hypoechoic layer if the bowel is filled with echogenic material.

Because of the relatively low incidence of pathology (at least diagnosed sonographically), the small bowel is generally considered a rather boring structure. It is the ever present background that is not "seen." However, the skilled sonographer can often gain additional clinical information and "use" the small bowel to help outline other pelvic structures. For example, the peristalsis of the small bowel can often be used to outline the broad ligament to localize the ovary. The presence of increased fluid between bowel loops may indicate pelvic or abdominal inflammation, ascites, a recently ruptured ovarian cyst, intraabdominal bleeding, and neoplasm or malignancy (Table 8-2). Recognition of the bowel layers may help distinguish a loop of fluid-filled small bowel from a hydrosalpinx. An increase in bowel gas may be an explanation for a patient's abdominal pain.

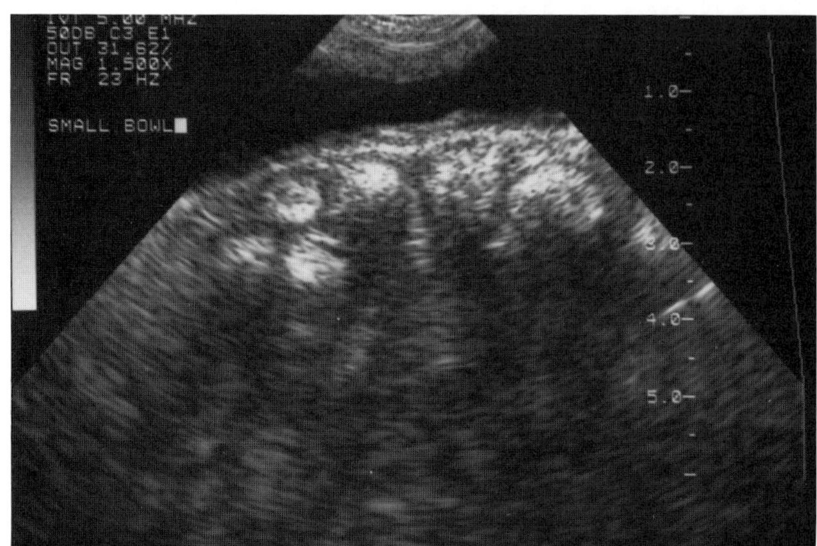

Fig. 8-1. Multiple loops of small bowel with air and bowel contents. The bladder is at the top of the photograph. Note the shadowing and reverberation artifact posterior to the bowel.

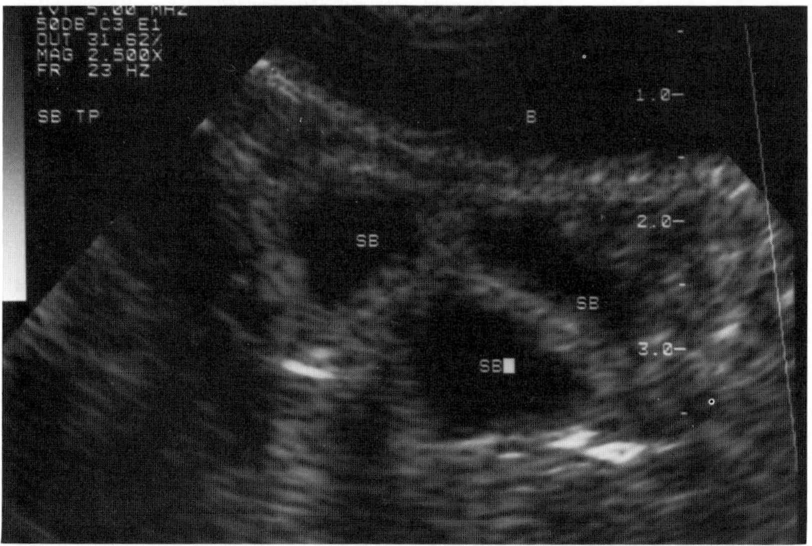

Fig. 8-2. T-pelvic view of several loops of small bowel. The bowel lumen is anechoic and probably contains fluid (SB). Note bladder above (B) and bladder wall. The bowel could be seen peristalting in real time.

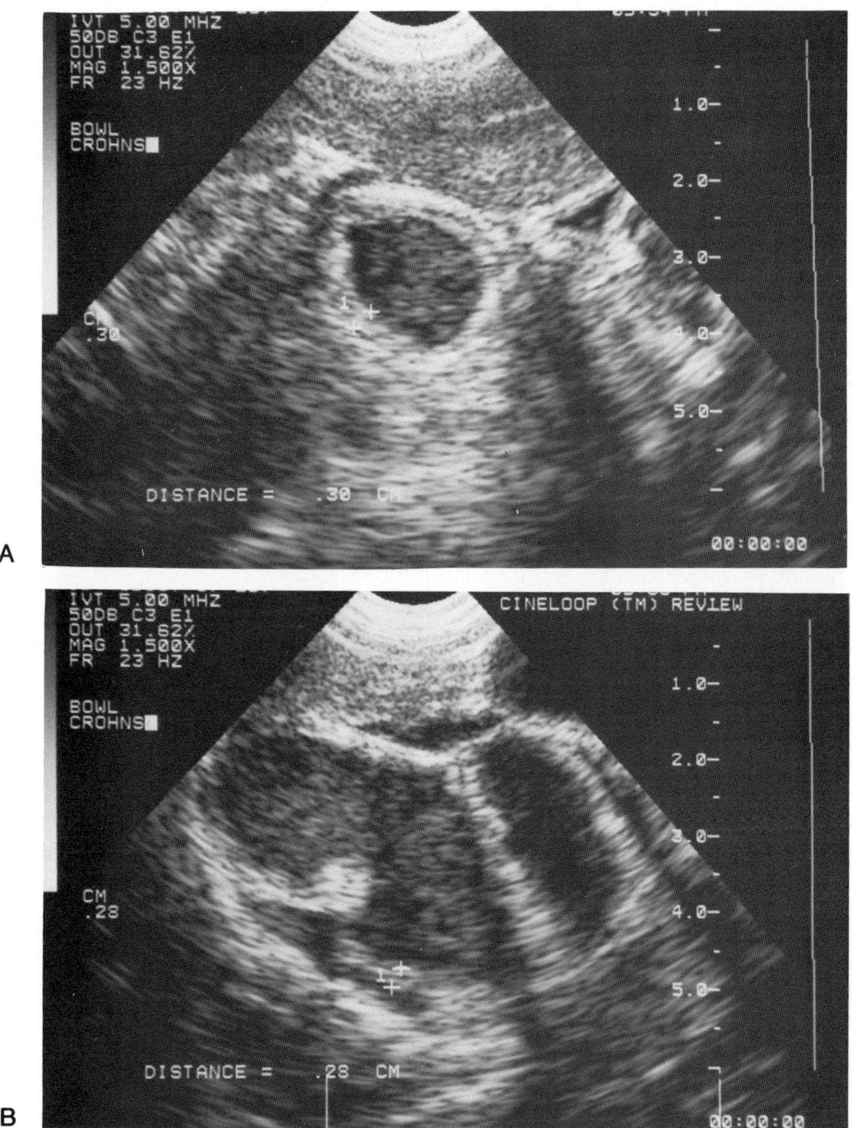

Fig. 8-3. **(A & B)** Bowel in the cul-de-sac with a thickened bowel wall (0.28 to 0.30 cm) in a patient with a long history of regional enteritis. In panel **A**, note uterus above imaged in the AP-pelvic plane with a single-line endometrium.

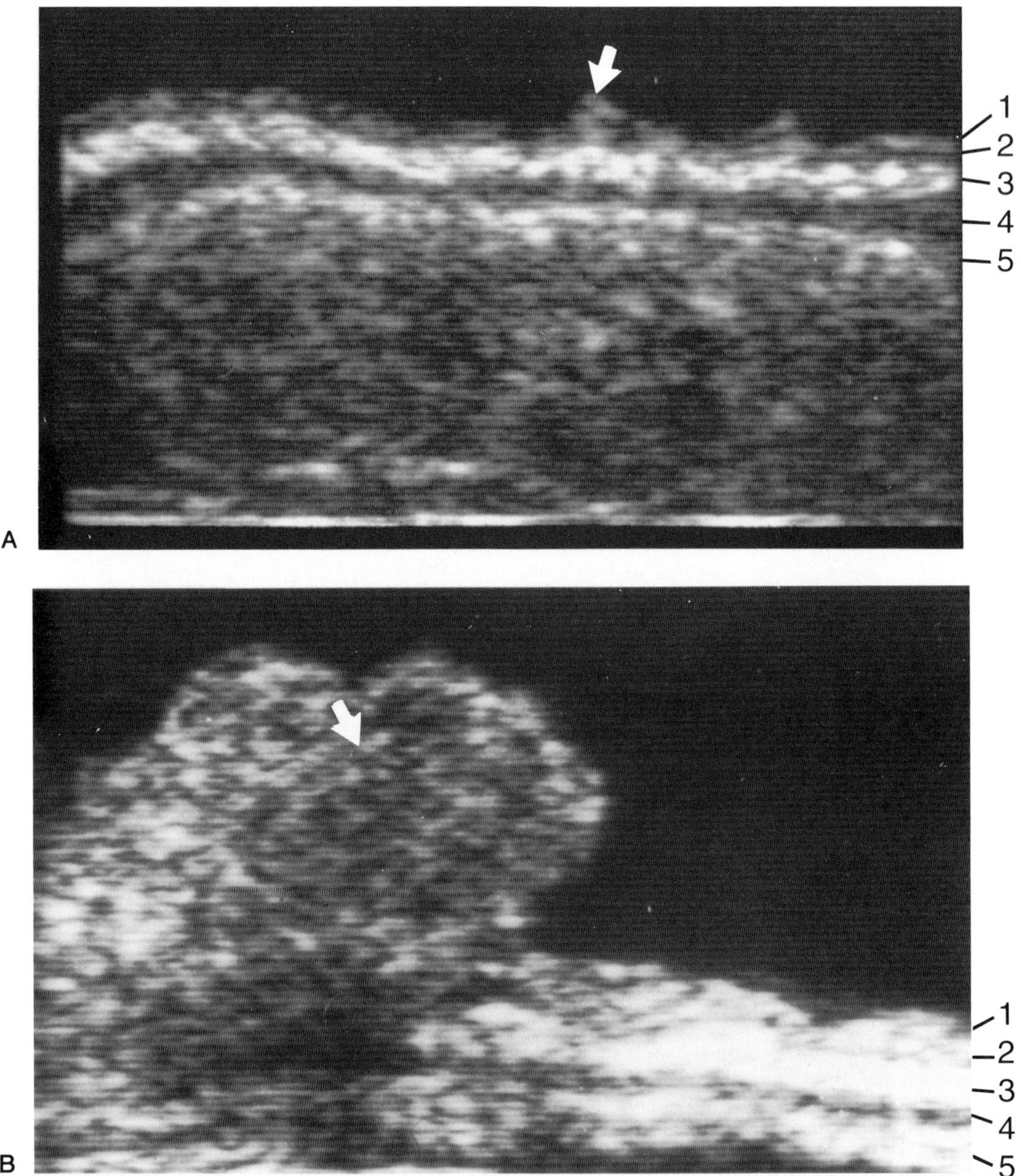

Fig. 8-4. (**A & B**) Ultrasound image of the intestinal wall and (**C & D**) corresponding histologic sections; **M**, mucosa; **SM**, submucosa; **MP**, muscularis propria (externa); **S**, serosa and subserosa. **A & C** represent a normal specimen except for a small tubular adenoma (open arrow). **B & D** show normal stratification on the right side of the specimen; a carcinoma on the left invades through the submucosa but not through the muscularis propia. See Table 8-1 for ultrasound echo character and histologic correlation. (From Wang et al,[2] with permission.) *(Figure continues.)*

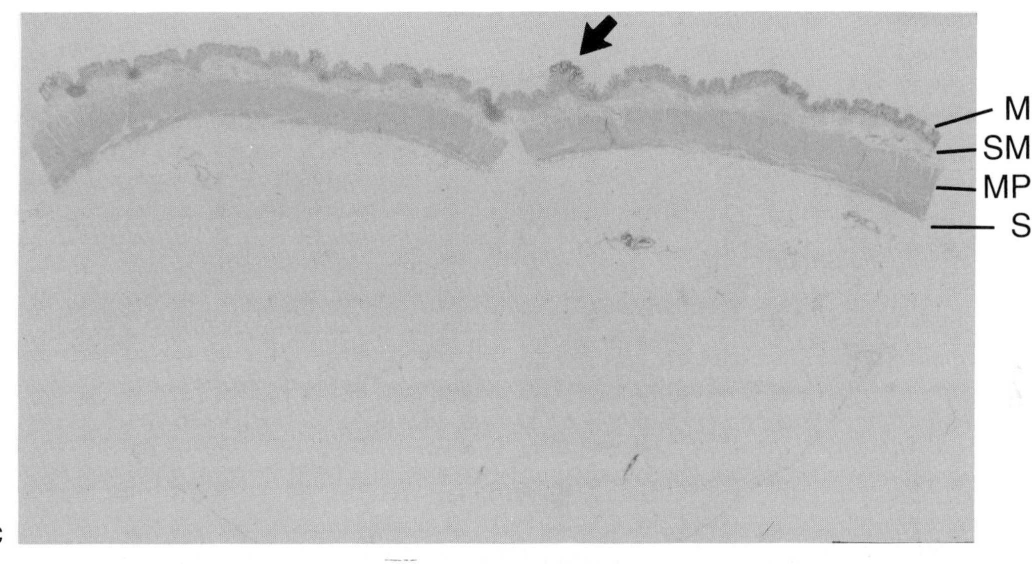

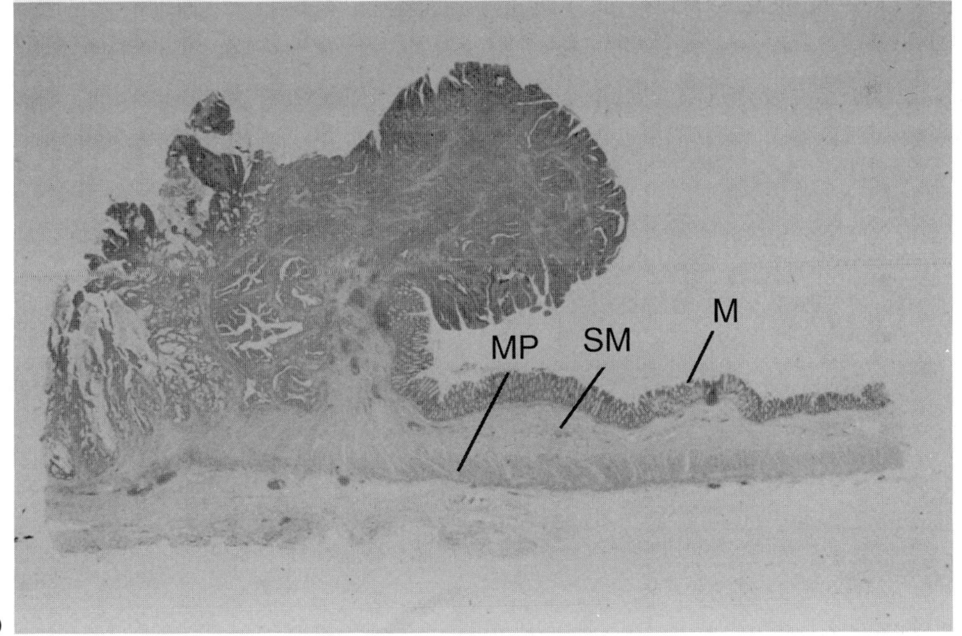

Fig. 8-4 *(Continued).*

Table 8-1. Sonographically Distinguishable Bowl Wall Layers

Layer (From the Mucosa)	*Echo Character*	*Histologic Correlation*
First	Hyperechoic	Mucosal surface
Second	Anechoic	Mucosa
Third	Hyperechoic	Submucosa
Fourth	Anechoic	Muscularis exterenia (propria)
Fifth	Hyperechoic	Serosa and subserosal fat

SIGMOID COLON

The sigmoid colon is a prominent pelvic structure noted posterior and to the left of the uterus and anterior to the sacrum. Stool may dilate the sigmoid and appear as a mixed echogenic structure. Gas may be noted in the sigmoid as a characteristic hyperechoic echo with posterior shadowing and/or reverberation artifacts. The hyperechoic gas and the posterior shadow below the gas sometimes make visualization of the left adnexa difficult. Unfortunately, there is no simple solution to the problem of visualizing the left adnexa when the sigmoid colon is full of gas. If necessary, the patient may be scanned at a later time in hopes that little or no gas will be present, or the patient may be given an enema to help expel the gas. It is important for the sonographer to recognize the stool-filled colon and not to mistake it for a mass during the transvaginal sonographic examination. A diverticular abscess also may present as a complex pelvic mass. Rubin et al[3] and Kurtz et al[4] recommended a water enema to differentiate pseudotumors composed of fluid- and feces-filled loops of bowel and to localize pelvic lesions when the diagnosis is not clear.

Table 8-2. Etiology of Increased Pelvic Fluid

Ruptured ovarian cyst
Ascites
Malignancy
Neoplasm
Infections
Intra-abdominal bleeding
Ruptured hemorrhagic corpus luteal cyst
Ectopic pregnancy
Ruptured viscous (liver, spleen)

In Wang and colleagues' in vitro study of the normal colon wall, the mucosa was about 0.6 mm thick, the submucosa was about 0.9 mm, and the muscularis propria was 1.8 mm thick.

Appendicitis

Because the appendix is generally not imaged by transvaginal ultrasound, this is one area where abdominal imaging is clearly superior. However, transvaginal ultrasound can play an important role in evaluating the female patient with suspected appendicitis by helping rule out other pelvic pathology as the etiology for pain, such as a tubo-ovarian abscess, hydrosalpinx, and ectopic pregnancy. Negative laparotomy or laparoscopy rates for suspected appendicitis of up to 45 percent are noted in women because of the many clinical gynecologic conditions that can mimic appendicitis. Transabdominal ultrasound may occasionally be of value in helping diagnose appendicitis.

Puylaert introduced graded compression ultrasound for the diagnosis of acute appendicitis.[5] Considerable skill and experience are needed to apply this technique. The linear array transducer (5.0 or 7.5 MHz) is used as a local compression device. The patient is asked to point with one finger to the most tender area. A normal appendix is rarely visualized and is generally less than 6 mm thick when it is visualized. An abnormal appendix is characterized by visualization of the appendix, a thickness of greater than 6 mm, a mural wall thickness of 3 mm or more, the

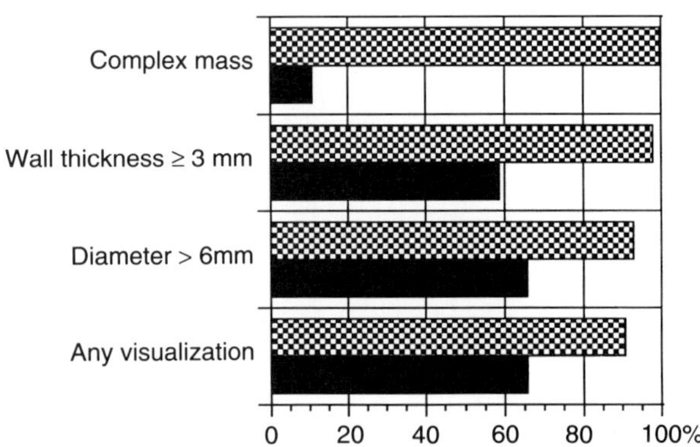

Fig. 8-5. Sensitivity and specificity of transvaginal ultrasound in the diagnosis of appendicitis. (Data from Worrell et al.[5])

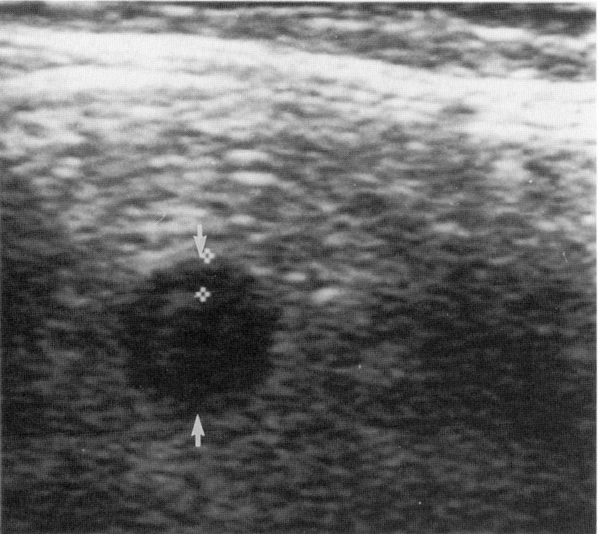

Fig. 8-6. Short-axis view of an inflamed appendix. White arrow indicates the appendiceal diameter, and the cursors demonstrate the thickened muscular wall. Appendicitis was surgically proven. (From Worrell et al,[5] with permission.)

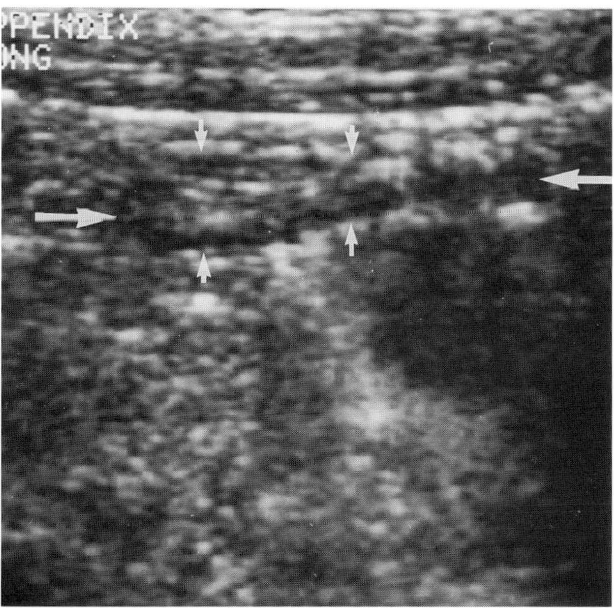

Fig. 8-7. Long-axis view of a normal appendix (outlined by white arrows). Note the thin muscular wall. A normal appendix was surgically proven. (From Worrell et al,[5] with permission.)

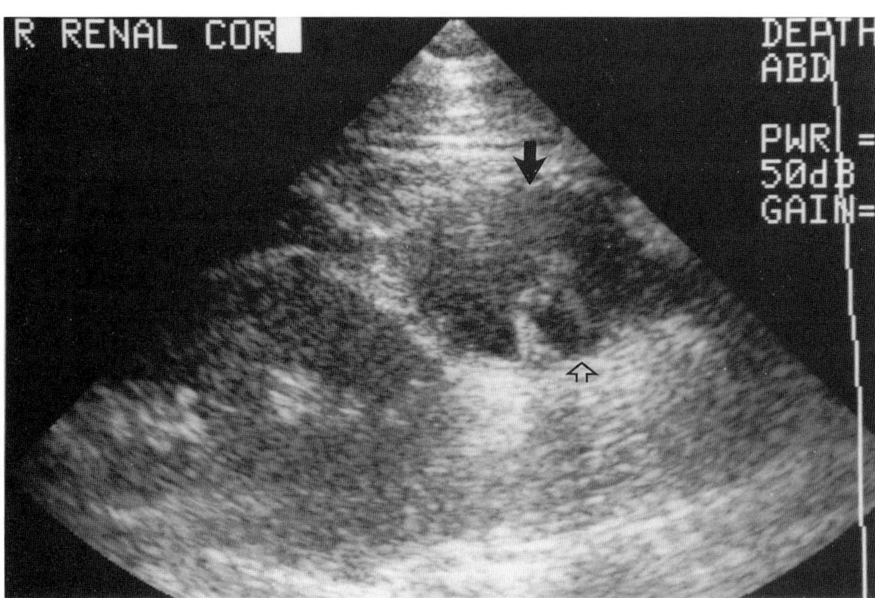

Fig. 8-8. Appendiceal abscess imaged as a complex mass. The appendiceal abscess was surgically proven. (From Worrell et al,[5] with permission.)

presence of periappendiceal fluid or appendicoliths, and/or reproducible pain with compression over the area of the appendix using the ultrasound transducer.[5,6]

Marn and Bree[6] studied 159 patients using this technique and noted a sensitivity of 90 percent, a specificity of 96 percent, and an overall accuracy of 94 percent. Worrell et al[5] reported on 200 consecutive cases of clinically suspicious appendicitis using the technique of graded compression ultrasound. The sonographic criteria utilized to diagnose appendicitis were (1) any visualization of the appendix, (2) appendiceal diameter greater than 6.0 mm, (3) muscular wall thickness greater than or equal to 3.0 mm, and (4) the presence of a complex mass. Only 54 percent of operated cases (82 operations) had appendicitis. Although the specificity for the ultrasound criteria was good, the best sensitivity of any single criterion was only 66 percent (Figs. 8-5 to 8-8).

Despite the potential value of ultrasound for diagnosis of appendicitis, the principal diagnostic approach is still the clinical findings.

RECTUM

Rectal Cancer

Transrectal ultrasound is recognized as one of the most sensitive techniques for the preoperative staging of rectal cancers, followed by computed tomography and nuclear magnetic resonance. Its accuracy in the diagnosis of rectal cancer in 12 patients was reported by Badea et al[7] to range between 81 to 94 percent. The tumor was visualized in all patients. The visualization was even better when the transvaginal examination was done after a cleansing enema. Transvaginal ultrasound was utilized to evaluate extension into the rectal wall, neighboring organs, and the rectovaginal space (Fig. 8-9).[7] It was also helpful in staging by demonstrating tumor extension (or lack of extension) into the posterior vaginal wall (Fig. 8-10) and by detecting perirectal lymph node enlargement (Fig. 8-11). Enlarged lymph nodes were noted in seven of nine patients with transvaginal ultrasound compared to six of nine using transrectal ultrasound. Lymph node extension was proven by surgery.

One advantage of transvaginal ultrasound was its ability to be used in all patients, whereas transrectal imaging could not be done in patients with rectal stenosis as the transducer could not be passed into the rectum. However, the transrectal technique had the advantage of better visualization of the rectal wall layers and better imaging of neoplastic infiltration, which could not be adequately imaged with transvaginal ultrasound. The authors felt that both ultrasound techniques were complementary to one another and improved preoperative staging when utilized together.

Transvaginal ultrasound may also be used to follow patients postoperatively and to detect early local recurrence of rectal cancer. The 5-year survival rate for

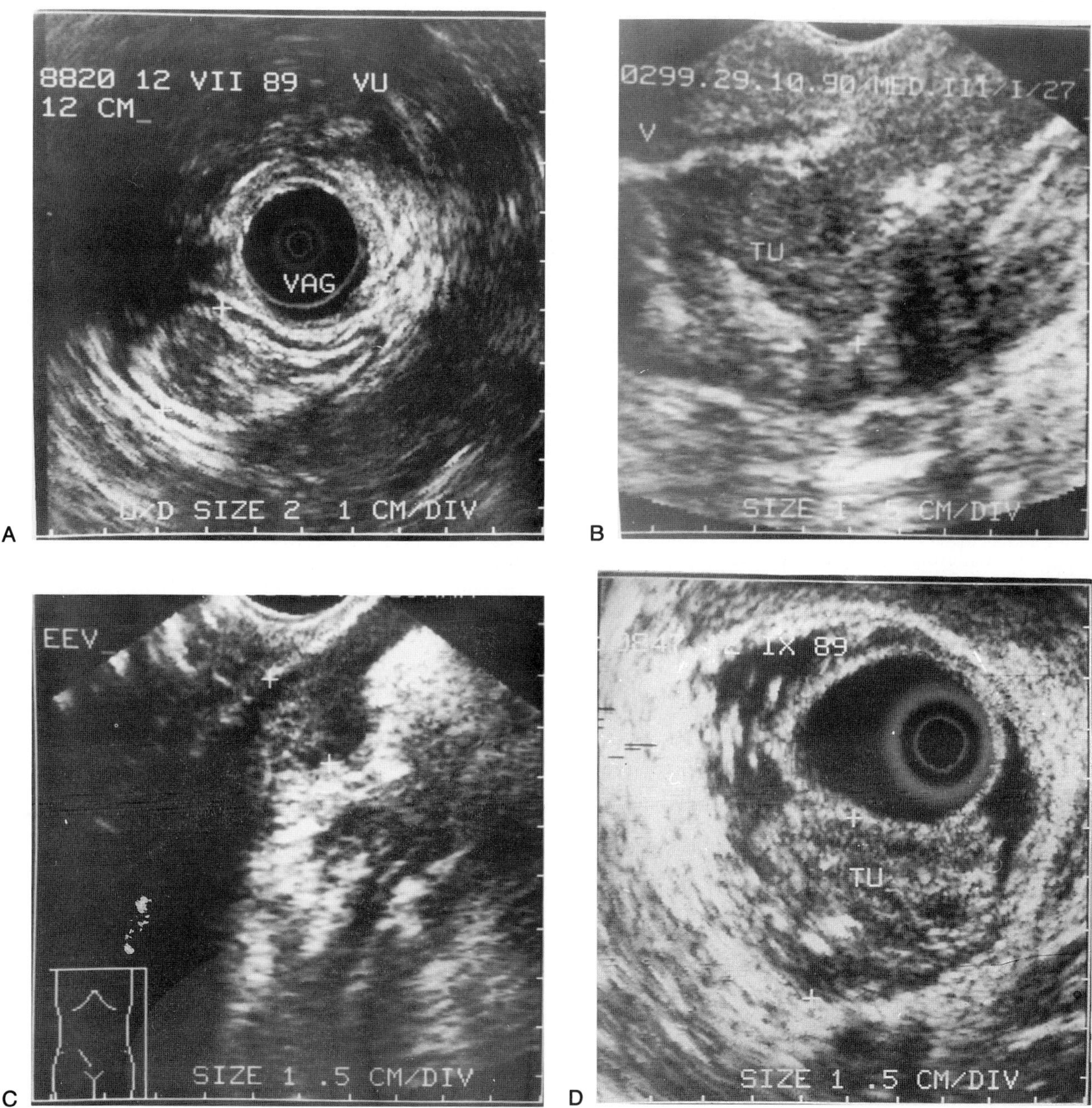

Fig. 8-9. (**A**) Transvaginal examination showing a polypoid rectal tumor between the cursors. VAG, vagina. (**B**) Longitudinal axis scan with a 7-MHz transducer demonstrating a rectal tumor. V, vagina; TU, tumor. (**C**) Transvaginal examination showing a stenosing rectal tumor. (**D**) Transrectal examination demonstrating a rectal tumor between the cursors. TU, tumor. (From Badea et al,[7] with permission.)

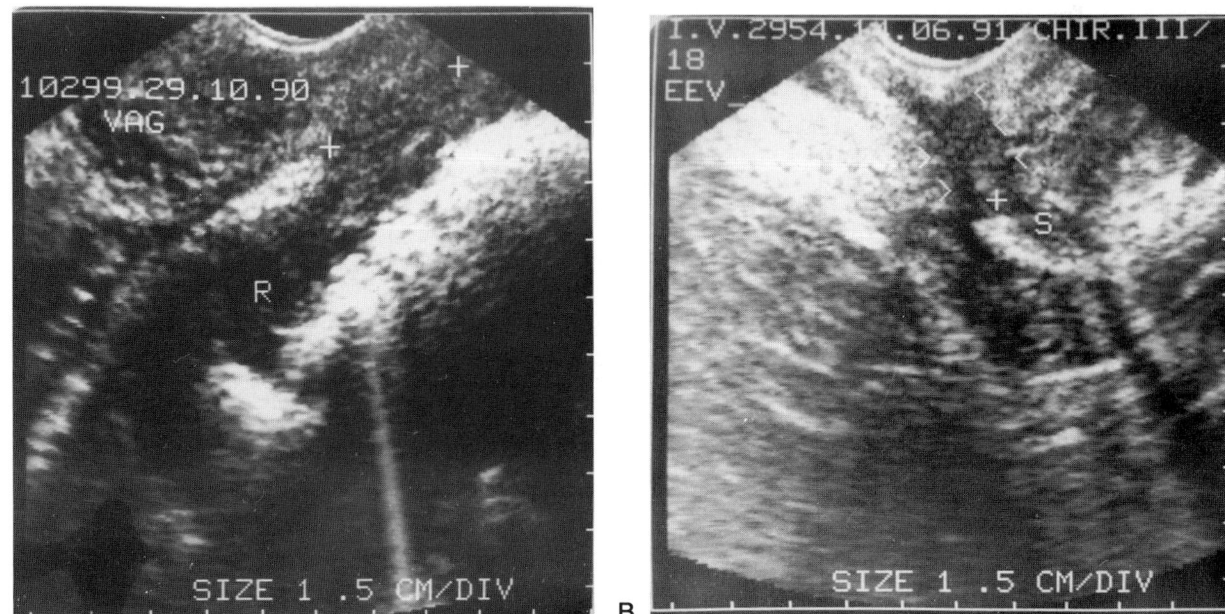

Fig. 8-10. **(A)** Rectal cancer invading into the vagina (markers) visualized from the vagina using a 7-MHz transducer. VAG, vagina; R, rectum. **(B)** Transvaginal examination demonstrating a rectovaginal fistula (between cursors) using a 7-MHz transducer. S, sigmoid. (From Badea et al,[7] with permission.)

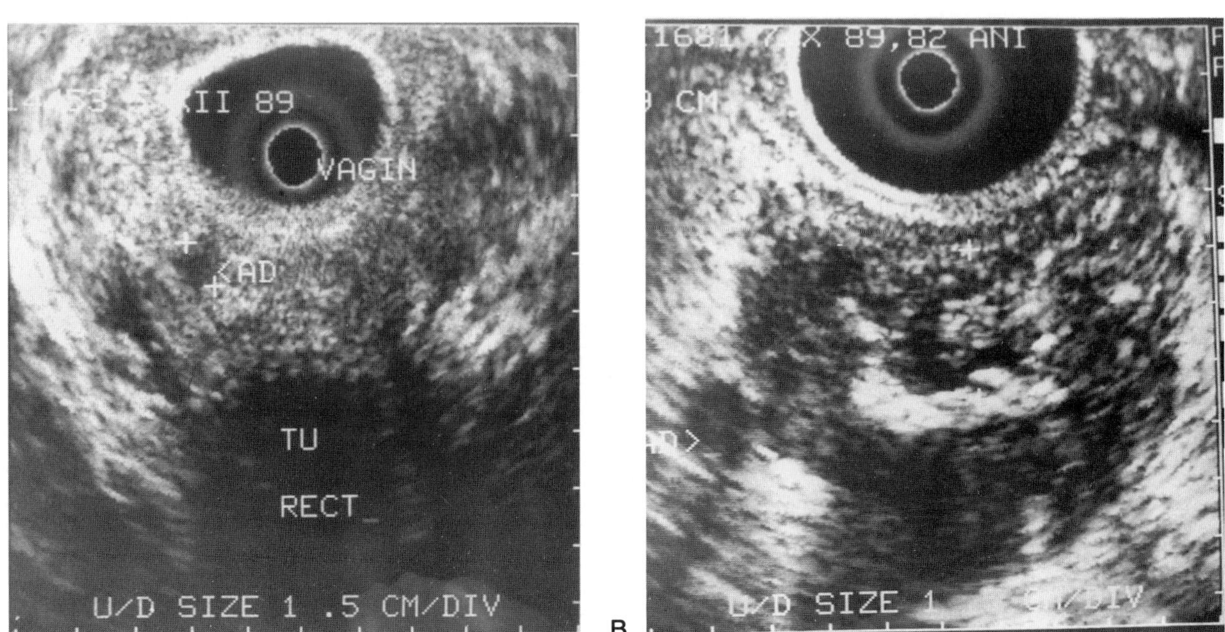

Fig. 8-11. **(A)** Transvaginal examination demonstrating a tumor and an enlarged adjacent lymph node (between cursors). **RECT**, rectum; **TU**, tumor; **AD**, lymph node. **(B)** Rectal cancer with a 13-mm enlarged lymph node. **AD**, lymph node. (From Badea et al,[7] with permission.)

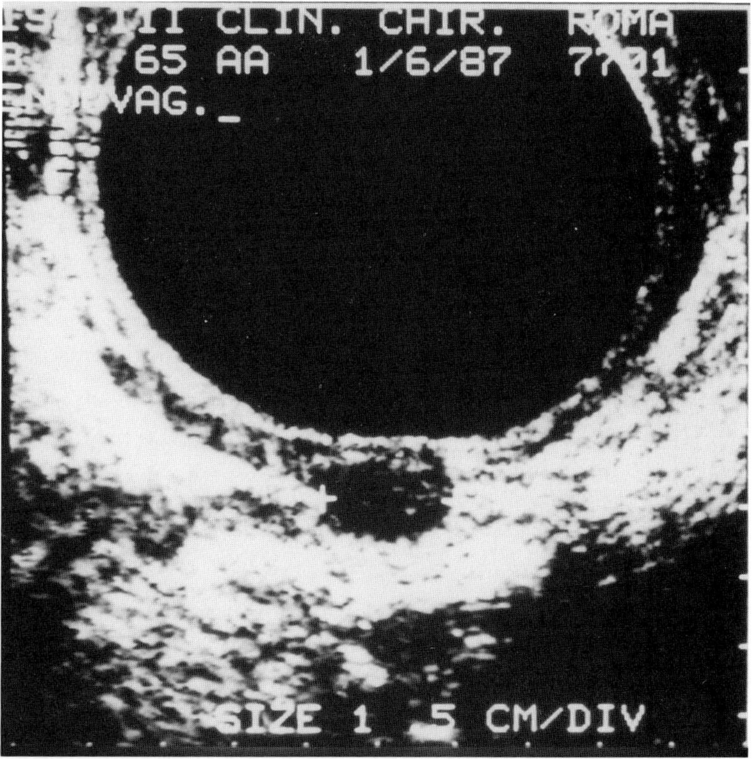

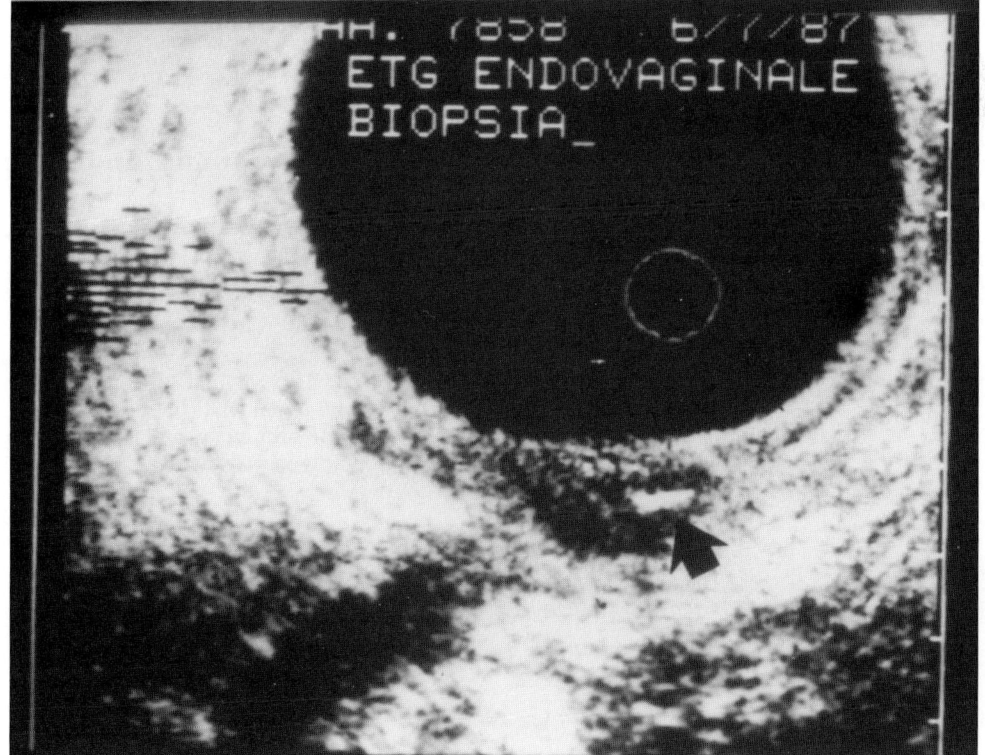

Fig. 8-12. (**A**) Transvaginal image of a small mass (<1 cm) exterior to the posterior wall of the vagina. (**B**) Transperineal biopsy confirming the diagnosis of recurrent tumor. Arrow indicates the biopsy needle. (From Masagni et al,[8] with permission.)

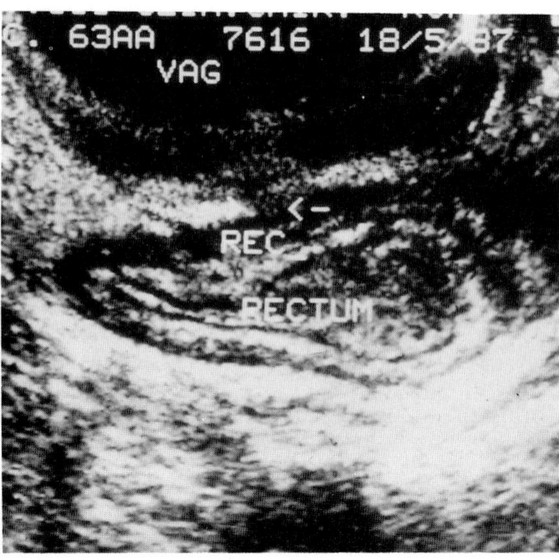

Fig. 8-13. Transvaginal ultrasound showing infiltration of tumor from the rectum into the vagina. VAG, vagina; REC, recurrent tumor. (From Masagni et al,[8] with permission.)

patients operated on for rectal cancer is approximately 50 to 60 percent. The poor prognosis results from local recurrence or the development of distant metastases. Local recurrence may occur in 6 to 32 percent of cases and is generally (70 to 80 percent) noted within 2 years after surgery. Early detection of local recurrence is critical and may allow reoperation and potential cure (Figs. 8-12 and 8-13). Mascagni et al[8] followed 120 patients (51 females) postoperatively for rectal carcinoma using endorectal and transvaginal ultrasound. Recurrence was noted in 14 percent (17) of patients. Ultrasound was 94 percent sensitive and 98 percent specific in detecting local recurrences. Recurrent neoplasms were generally imaged as a hypoechoic, nonhomogeneous mass with well defined margins.

In the Wang et al[2] in vitro study, all normal specimens with neoplasms were correctly identified sonographically (see Fig. 8-4). Of the neoplastic specimens, ultrasound was 92.5 percent accurate in demonstrating invasion of the submucosa and 77 percent accurate in detecting invasion of the muscularis externa. The use of transrectal and transvaginal ultrasound to diagnose, stage, and follow rectal tumors is a relatively new technique that shows considerable potential.

Rectosigmoid Endometriosis

Bowel involvement may occur in 3 to 18 percent of cases of endometriosis and may be submucosal, intramural, or involve the serosa. Lesions may be cystic,

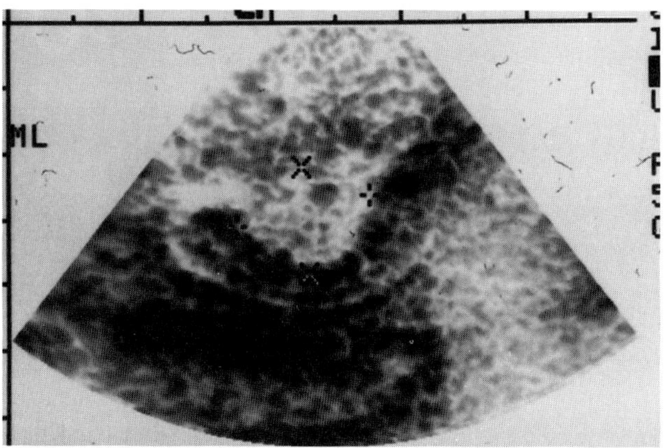

Fig. 8-14. Transvaginal ultrasound of endometriosis involving the rectal wall (between cursors). The mass is external to the submucosa and is primarily in the muscularis (Photograph courtesy of Dale Cyr.[9])

solid, or have a mixed appearance. Cystic areas result from repeated cyclic hemorrhage and are imaged sonographically as a hypoechoic mass generally with low level internal echoes with increased through transmission (posterior enhancement) (Fig. 8-14).[9] The walls may be irregular, and septations may be present. Small lesions of a few millimeters in size can not generally be detected.

Hauge et al[10] have reported a case of endometriosis involving the anal sphincter that was imaged using a 7-MHz rotating transducer in the anal canal (Bruel & Kjaer). Anosigmoidoscopy appeared normal. By ultrasound the endometriosis was imaged as a circumscribed hypoechoic area within the external anal sphincter and in close proximity to the internal sphincter. Using anal endosonography, the internal and external anal sphincter are generally easily recognized. The internal anal sphincter is imaged as a hypoechoic ring surrounded by the echogenic external anal sphincter.

REFERENCES

1. Hsu-Chong Y, Rabinowitz JG: Granolamatous enterocolitis: findings by ultrasonography and computed tomography. Radiology 149:253, 1983
2. Wang KY, Kimmey MB, Nyberg DA et al: Colorectal neoplasm: accuracy of US in demonstrating the depth of invasion. Radiology 165:827, 1987
3. Rubin C, Kurtz AB, Goldberg BB: Water enema: a new ultrasound technique in defining pelvic anatomy. J Clin Ultrasound 6:28, 1978
4. Kurtz AB, Rubin CS, Kramer FL, Goldberg BB: Ultrasound evaluation of the posterior pelvic compartment. Radiology 132:677, 1979
5. Worrell JA, Drolshagen LF, Kelly TC, Hunton DW et al: Graded compression ultrasound in the diagnosis of appendicitis: a comparison of diagnostic criteria. J Ultrasound Med 9:145, 1990
6. Marn CS, Bree RL: Advances in pelvic ultrasound: endovaginal scanning for ectopic gestation and graded compression sonography for appendicitis. Ann Emerg Med 18:1304, 1989
7. Badea R, Badea G, Dejica D, Henegar E: The role of transvaginal sonography as compared with endorectal sonography in the evaluation of rectal cancer: preliminary study. Surg Endosc 5:89, 1991
8. Mascagni D, Corbellini L, Urciuoli P, Di Matteo G: Endoluminal ultrasound for early detection of local recurrence of rectal cancer. Br J Surg 76:1176, 1989
9. Gorell HA, Cyr DR, Wang KY, Greer BE: Rectosigmoid endometriosis diagnosis using endovaginal sonography. J Ultrasound Med 8:459, 1989
10. Hauge C, Nielsen MB, Rasmussen OO, Christiansen J: Clinical findings and endosonographic appearance of endometriosis in the anal sphincter. J Clin Ultrasound 21:48–51, 1993

9

Acute Pelvic Inflammatory Disease

Melvin G. Dodson

The usual signs and symptoms of acute pelvic inflammatory disease (PID) are lower abdominal pain, lower abdominal tenderness, sometimes with rebound tenderness, adnexal and uterine tenderness, and tenderness to movement of the cervix. Fever, elevated leukocyte count, and elevated sedimentation rate may also be noted.[1] Unfortunately, the use of clinical criteria for the diagnosis of acute PID is relatively inaccurate. Jacobsen and Westrom, in what has become a classic study of acute PID, used laparoscopy to study 814 patients with clinical signs and symptoms of acute PID.[2] The clinical diagnosis was confirmed in only 65 percent of cases. In 12 percent of patients, other pelvic pathology was noted; however, in 23 percent of patients diagnosed as having acute PID, the pelvis was completely normal. This very large study suggests that about one-third of patients may have a false-positive diagnosis of acute PID when standard clinical criteria for diagnosis are utilized. In addition to false-positive diagnosis, false-negative diagnoses are also quite common. Jacobsen and Westrom also reported on 91 patients who underwent a laparoscopic evaluation for diagnosis other than acute PID who were noted to have pelvic inflammatory disease.[2]

ULTRASOUND IN THE DIAGNOSIS OF ACUTE PID

Transvaginal ultrasound may be utilized to evaluate carefully the pelvis in patients suspected of having acute PID and may be helpful in confirming the diagnosis and in evaluating the severity of the infection. Patients with mild disease generally have a normal ultrasound evaluation. In the early stages of uncomplicated acute pelvic inflammatory disease (PID), ultrasound findings are nonspecific. However, patients with acute PID often complain during the pelvic sonographic examination of pain and object to even the minimal pressure exerted by the transvaginal probe. Although care must be taken not to hurt the patient, the transvaginal probe may occasionally be utilized to determine the most tender pelvic structures that are inflamed or infected or which structures are associated with a patient's complaint of pain by combining the patient's responses to gentle pressure using the transvaginal probe and clinical interrogation of the patient during the examination while directly visualizing specific pelvic structures. The ultrasound findings in mild to moderate disease may include an indistinct central endometrial echo, increased endometrial fluid, an ill-defined uterine contour, enlarged ovaries with an indistinct contour, or periovarian fluid collection. Increased cul-de-sac fluid may be noted and may show increased echogenicity (Table 9-1). Again, all of the findings are nonspecific; however, they may be helpful when combined with the history and clinical findings. Ultrasound may also be very useful by eliminating other diseases as the etiology for the clinical findings.

In a series of 90 patients with acute PID evaluated by Bulas et al using ultrasound, 34 percent had normal findings.[3] Although some of these cases may have been false-positive clinical diagnoses, 84 percent had positive cervical cultures for *Neisseria gonorrhea* and/or *Chlamydiae trachomatis* and probably had mild disease. However, the relatively high incidence of

Table 9-1. Ultrasound Findings in Acute PID

- Mild
  - Ultrasound often normal
  - Pain from manipulation of the probe
  - Enlarged ovaries
  - Periovarian fluid
  - Indistinct ovarian borders
  - Indistinct uterine contour
  - Indistinct endometrium
  - Endometrial fluid
  - Increased cul-de-sac fluid
- Moderate/severe
  - Hydrosalpinx:
    - Sausage shaped
    - Fluid filled (anechoic)
    - Mucosal folds thickened
    - Thickened serosa
    - Separate from ovary
    - Double serosa (from tubal bending)
    - Concave wall adjacent to ovary
  - Tubo-ovarian abscess:
    - Complex mass with cystic and solid areas, borders often indistinct

normal ultrasound findings is consistent with clinical difficulty in diagnosing mild PID.

In a small series of 16 patients with laparoscopic confirmation of ultrasound findings, Patten et al[4] reported a 91 percent sensitivity and 93 percent accuracy in diagnosing ovarian/periovarian abnormalities. It is frequently possible to distinguish hydrosalpinx, pyosalpinx, and tubo-ovarian complex with recognizable but inflamed tubes and ovary from tubo-ovarian abscesses with a complex mass. Significant hydrosalpinx, pyosalpinx, or tubo-ovarian complex or abscesses that are associated with advanced disease are generally easily identified by transvaginal ultrasound. Hydrosalpinx, pyosalpinx or tubo-ovarian complex or abscess may be unilateral or bilateral.

In patients with advanced disease, a hypoechoic cystic structure with a thick wall, sometimes with gravitational layering of hyperechoic material within the ovary or tube, may be imaged. In addition, loculated fluid, representing pus, may be imaged outside and surrounding the ovary and/or tubes. The small bowel may be involved. A tubo-ovarian abscess consists of a complex mass involving the ovary, generally a hydrosalpinx or pyosalpinx, and loculated pus and small bowel. Hydrosalpinx can sometimes be delineated by the sausage shape of the mass. Lande et al[5] reported on five patients with tubo-ovarian abscesses, and all were noted to have a tube-shaped fluid collection during transvaginal ultrasound examination. The thickened wall of an ovarian abscess may vary from one area to another around the abscess cavity. The borders of the mass may be indistinct. Usually, at least some portion of the mass will involve the cul-de-sac. Uhrich and Sanders[6] have emphasized the irregularity of the mass wall in a tubo-ovarian abscess. As the disease progresses, multilocular masses are often noted. Commonly, it is difficult to outline the uterus. Although the ultrasound findings are nonspecific, the diagnosis of an abscess is usually quite evident in association with the clinical findings.

Serial ultrasound examinations can be utilized to follow patients with acute PID. In a patient with an initial normal ultrasound evaluation who is not responding to therapy, hydrosalpinx or other indications of disease progression may be noted sonographically that were not present on an earlier ultrasound examination. Serial examinations are particularly useful in following patients with advanced disease, such as a tubo-ovarian abscess, and in evaluating antibiotic response (Fig. 9-1).

Differential Diagnosis

Appendicitis or a diverticular abscess must be considered in the differential diagnosis. The appendix is generally not seen during a transvaginal ultrasound, since it lies outside of the pelvis. However, on transabdominal ultrasound a complex mass in the right lower quadrant surrounding the appendix may sometimes be visualized using the graded compression technique. Other signs of appendicitis include visualization of the appendix, appendiceal thickness of greater than 6 mm, or increased wall thickness 3 mm or greater (see Ch. 8). The linear array transducer may also be useful in diagnosing perihepatitis associated with acute PID (Curtis Fitz-Hugh syndrome). During the acute phase these patients generally have pain in the right upper abdomen in addition to the signs and symptoms of pelvic disease.

Acute perihepatic infection may be associated with thickening of the right anterior extrarenal tissue as described by Schoenfeld et al[7] (Fig. 9-2). The perirenal fascia cannot be identified separately by ultrasound and merges with the fat and adjacent renal and liver capsules and has been termed the right anterior extrarenal tissue. Its thickness in 72 normal women

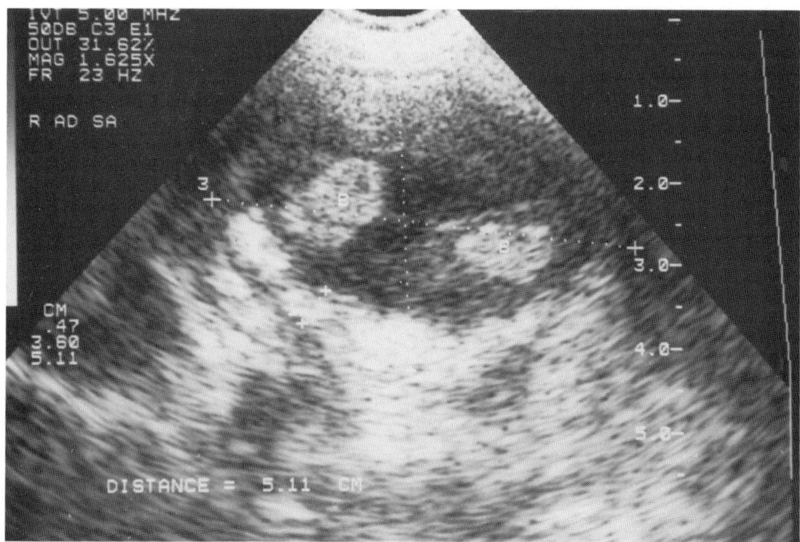

Fig. 9-1. A 30-year-old woman G1 P1 with a complaint of pelvic pain and low grade fever. Anterior posterior-pelvic (AP-pelvic) view of a 5.1 by 3.6 cm pelvic mass. Note the thick border inferiorly, possibly composed of small bowel. There are several hyperechoic loops of small bowel in the mass with surrounding fluid. The border of the mass is indistinct. The mass was fixed and tender to palpation on pelvic examination. The patient was treated with intravenous antibiotics for 7 days, and the mass decreased markedly in size and the patient became afebrile.

averaged 1.8 mm with a range from 1 to 5 mm. In patients with laparoscopically proven perihepatitis, this area measured 6 to 12 mm with an average of 7.7 mm. This tissue space measured 3 cm from the superior or inferior pole of the kidney.[7] Although thickening is suggestive of infection, the finding is nonspecific and may be noted in other inflammatory conditions, such as appendicitis, perforated ulcer, acute pancreatitis, acute cholecystitis, etc.

Other diagnoses to consider are a twisted ovary, ectopic pregnancy, endometrioma of the ovary, or an ovarian neoplasm. A twisted ovarian cyst may present with signs and symptoms similar to a tubo-ovarian abscess, including fever and pain, but is unilateral, and a twisted ovary is generally associated with an enlarged ovary that is easily imaged. With an ectopic pregnancy, a thick-walled complex mass may be noted in the adnexa. However, less than 1 percent of patients with an ectopic pregnancy have a fever, and almost all patients with an ectopic pregnancy have a positive serum beta-human chorionic gonadotropin (provided a assay sensitive to 5 to 10 mIU or greater is used).

Endometriosis may produce a complex mass that often contains a fine speckled pattern in cystic areas (see Ch. 6). However, a variety of sonographic patterns have been reported with endometriosis.[8] Endometriosis may be differentiated clinically by the absence of signs and symptoms of infection, such as fever, elevated leukocyte count, etc. (Table 9-2).

TRANSVAGINAL ULTRASOUND DRAINAGE OF PELVIC ABSCESSES

Pelvic sonography may play an important role in acute PID by proving or disproving the presence of a pelvic mass and by evaluating the mass for possible transvaginal drainage. There are an increasing number of reports about the use of transvaginal ultrasound for drainage of tubo-ovarian abscesses.[9-12] However, the primary treatment of acute PID is antibiotics. At this time, it is not clear whether aspiration of a tubo-ovarian abscess improves a patient's clinical response. Although the principle of drainage of an abscess is well known, there are no controlled studies using

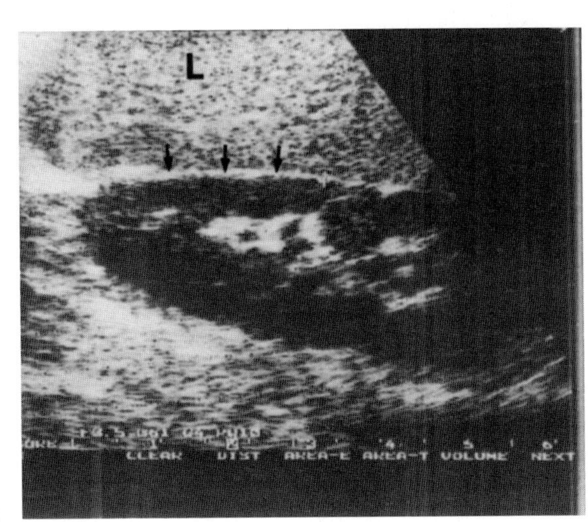

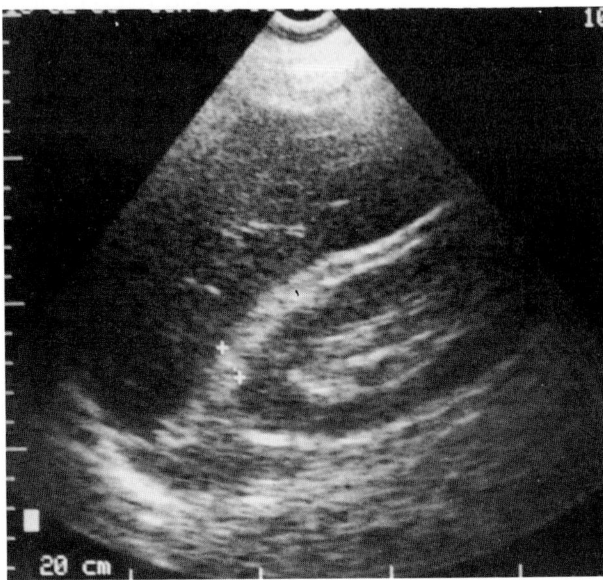

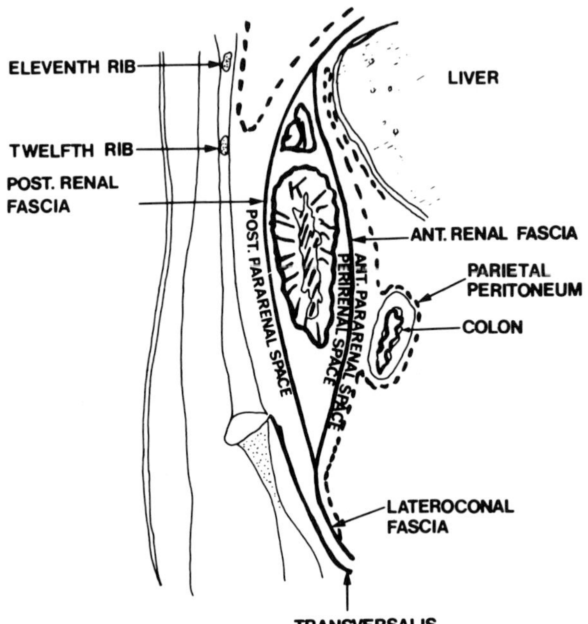

Fig. 9-2. **(A)** The normal right anterior extrarenal tissue as a thin echogenic line *(arrows)*. L, liver tissue. **(B)** A patient with perihepatitis demonstrating increased thickness (12 mm) combined with hyperechogenicity of the right anterior extrarenal tissue. **(C)** Sagittal section of the retroperitoneal fascia and spaces. K, kidney. (From Schoenfeld,[7] with permission)

Table 9-2. Differential Diagnosis of Acute PID

Appendicitis	Linear array transducer: visualization of normal appendix is uncommon, complex mass, appendix >6 mm, thick wall
Diverticular abscess	Complex mass, generally left side
Twisted ovary	Enlarged ovary on involved side only
Ectopic pregnancy	No intrauterine sac, positive hCG, fetus noted in tube, doughnut sign, complex mass, pelvic fluid and clots
Endometrioma	No fever, cyst filled with echoes
Ovarian neoplasm	Ovarian solid or cystic mass, wall nodularity, thick septum, ascites fluid
Functional ovarian cyst	No fever, simple unilocular cyst, hemorrhagic corpus luteal cyst, often has a complex structure with hyperechoic areas (clots), a lacy pattern, and anechoic fluid areas

transvaginal needle aspiration of pelvic abscesses that prove that such an approach gives a better or more rapid clinical response. The principle seems valid; however, good data are simply not available at this time.

The majority of patients treated with appropriate antimicrobials will respond rapidly without more aggressive or invasive therapy. Most patients will be afebrile and improved clinically within 48 hours of the initiation of treatment. This is particularly true for patients with mild to moderate disease. At this time, aspiration should probably be reserved for the patient with a demonstrable tubo-ovarian abscess who is not responding to antibiotic therapy within a reasonable period of time. However, additional research and experience with this technique are needed. Vaginal surgical drainage of tubo-ovarian abscesses that are pointing in the rectovaginal septum was a very common approach to treatment in the past. However, this type of therapy is relatively uncommon today and is almost invariably reserved for the patient who does not respond to antibiotic therapy and who has a fluctuant mass dissecting into the rectovaginal septum that is readily accessible to a vaginal surgical approach.

A multilocular tubo-ovarian abscess located higher in the pelvis would be difficult and perhaps dangerous to approach by vaginal drainage. This is particularly true if bowel is noted to lie between the abscess and the point of drainage. Although transvaginal ultrasound allows a better assessment of the extent of the abscess, much more accurate needle placement for

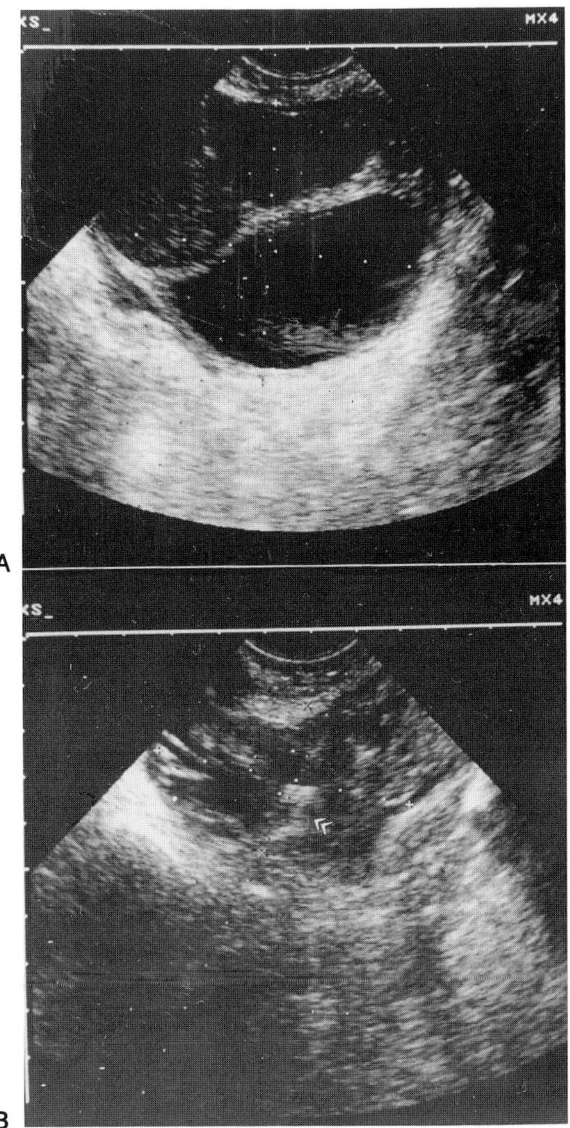

Fig. 9-3. (A) Tubo-ovarian abscess with cystic and solid areas. (B) The same abscess after ultrasound guided aspiration of 110 ml of pus. Arrowheads indicate the tip of the aspiration needle. (From Teisala,[9] with permission.)

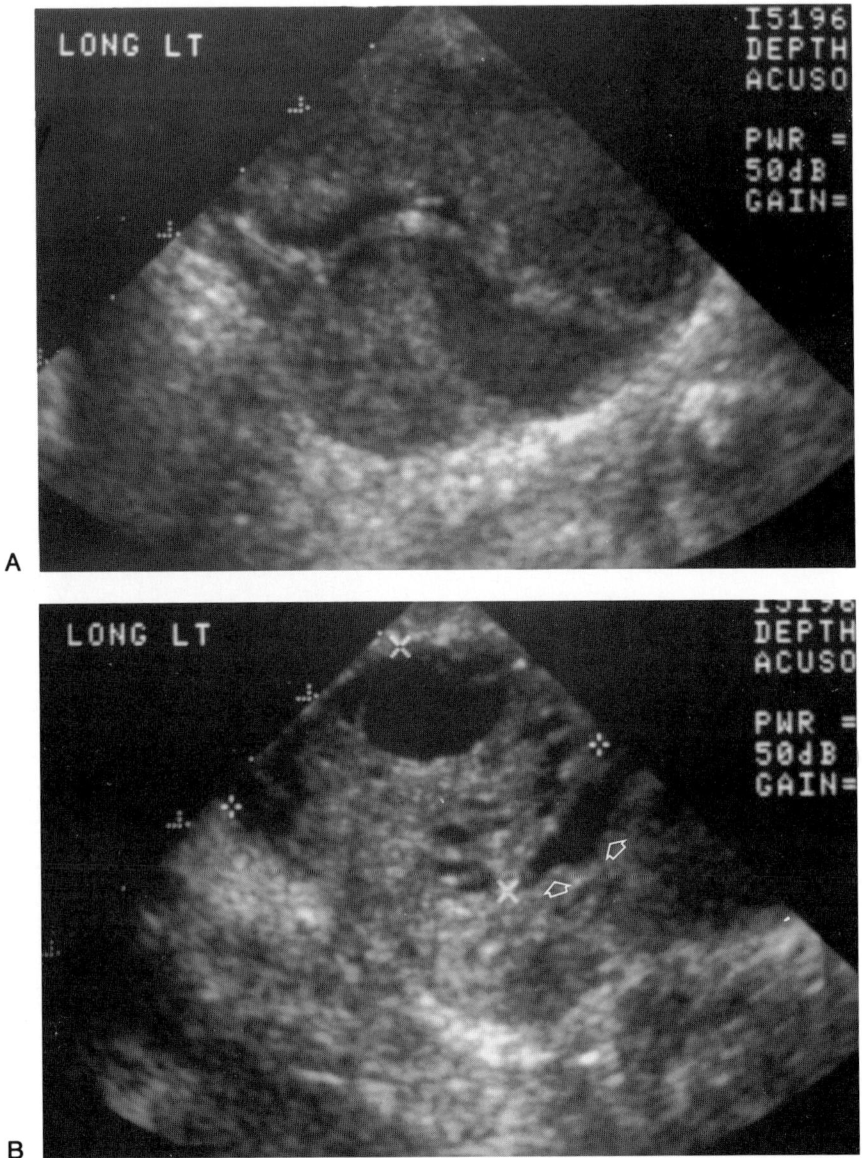

Fig. 9-4. **(A)** A patient with acute PID demonstrating a dilated, convoluted tube filled with echogenic material. **(B)** The ovary (between cursors) adjacent to the tube is shown. A small amount of periovarian fluid is present (arrows). *(Figure continues.)*

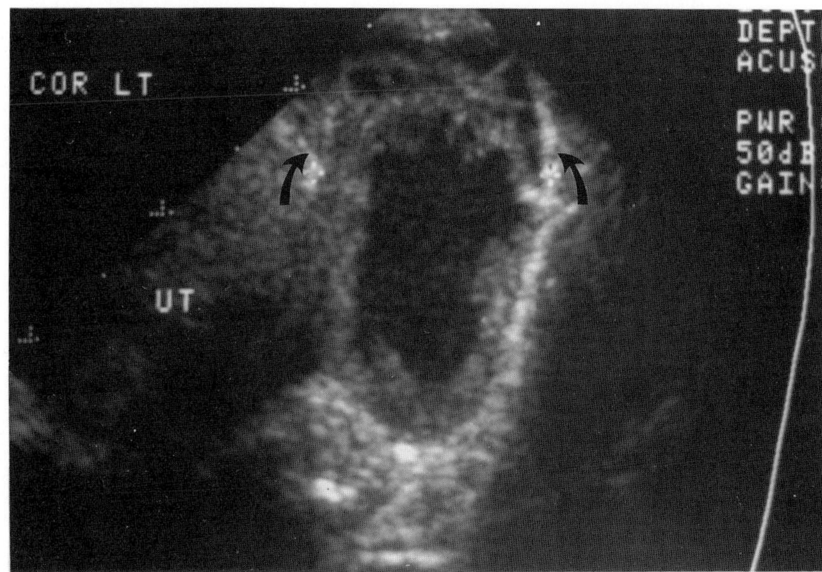

C

D

Fig. 9-4 *(Continued)*. **(C)** Scan done one week later shows low level echoes that remain within the dilated tube and the ill-defined margin between the ovary and tube (arrows). **(D)** Scan done 2 weeks later for persistent pelvic pain demonstrates a thin dilated fluid-filled tube (arrow). Laparoscopy confirmed a chronically inflamed hydrsalpinx. (From Bulas,[3] with permission)

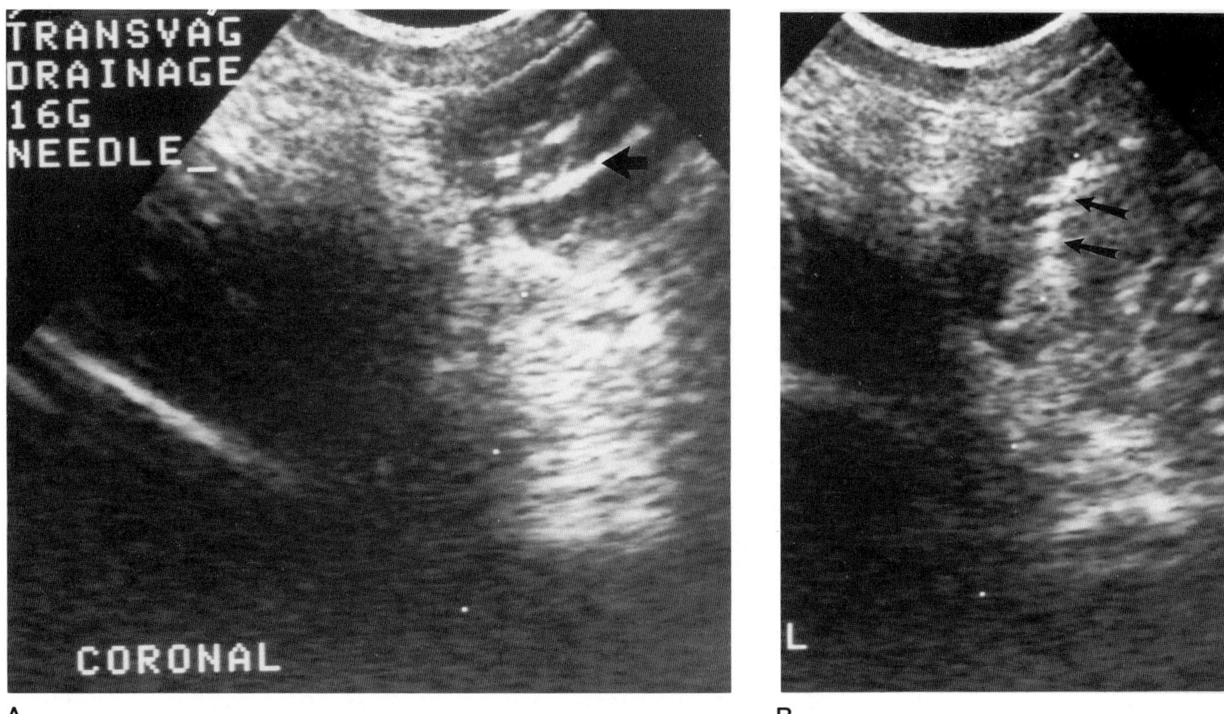

Fig. 9-5. **(A)** Twenty-six-year-old patient with Crohn's disease with a pelvic abscess after surgery. Transvaginal 7 French catheter (arrows) drainage using transvaginal ultrasound imaging; catheter was inserted by coaxial Seldinger technique though initial 18-gauge needle. **(B)** Postdrainage scan after evacuation of pus reveals the catheter (arrows) within the collapsed cavity. (From VanSonnenberg,[12] with permission)

needle aspiration, or more controlled and accurate access to the abscess cavity for catheter placement and drainage, proper patient selection is necessary.

Drainage may be done in an office or operating room depending on the clinical status of the patient, equipment available, etc. Local anesthesia may be used, but IV sedation and analgesia are probably adequate for most needle aspirations. However, catheter placement and more extensive manipulation may require spinal/epidural or general anesthesia depending on the clinical circumstances. The vagina is prepped with betadine. A needle guide attached to the transducer and an electronic tract guide on the monitor screen are very useful for determining the intended position of the needle. The intended needle path should take the shortest route that allows adequate access to the abscess cavity. Actual needle placement can generally be imaged in real time by using a needle tip that has been scored or etched. A variety of needle sizes have been used, including 22-, 20-, 18-, and 16-gauge (Figs. 9-3 and 9-4).[3,9] Thicker fluid collections or organized pus may require larger bore needles or catheters for adequate drainage (Figs. 9-5 and 9-6).[12] The cavity may be irrigated with normal saline. Aspirated material should be sent for culture. Teisala et al[9] reported positive cultures in 60 percent of patients after transvaginal ultrasound aspiration using a 16-gauge needle and IV diazepam analgesia (10 mg). The average volume of pus aspirated was 52 ml. *E. Coli* was the most common organism cultured. A variety of catheters have been used. VanDerKolk[11] used a 30 cm 20-gauge needle. A dilator was advanced over the needle, and then a Lunderquist wire was inserted through the needle, followed by an 8-French cope loop nephrostomy catheter (Cook, Bloomington, IN). Abscess diameters ranged from 4 to 6 cm. The distance from the inner aspect of the abscess wall to the transducer was never more than 2 cm. Catheters remained in place for 5 to 21 days.

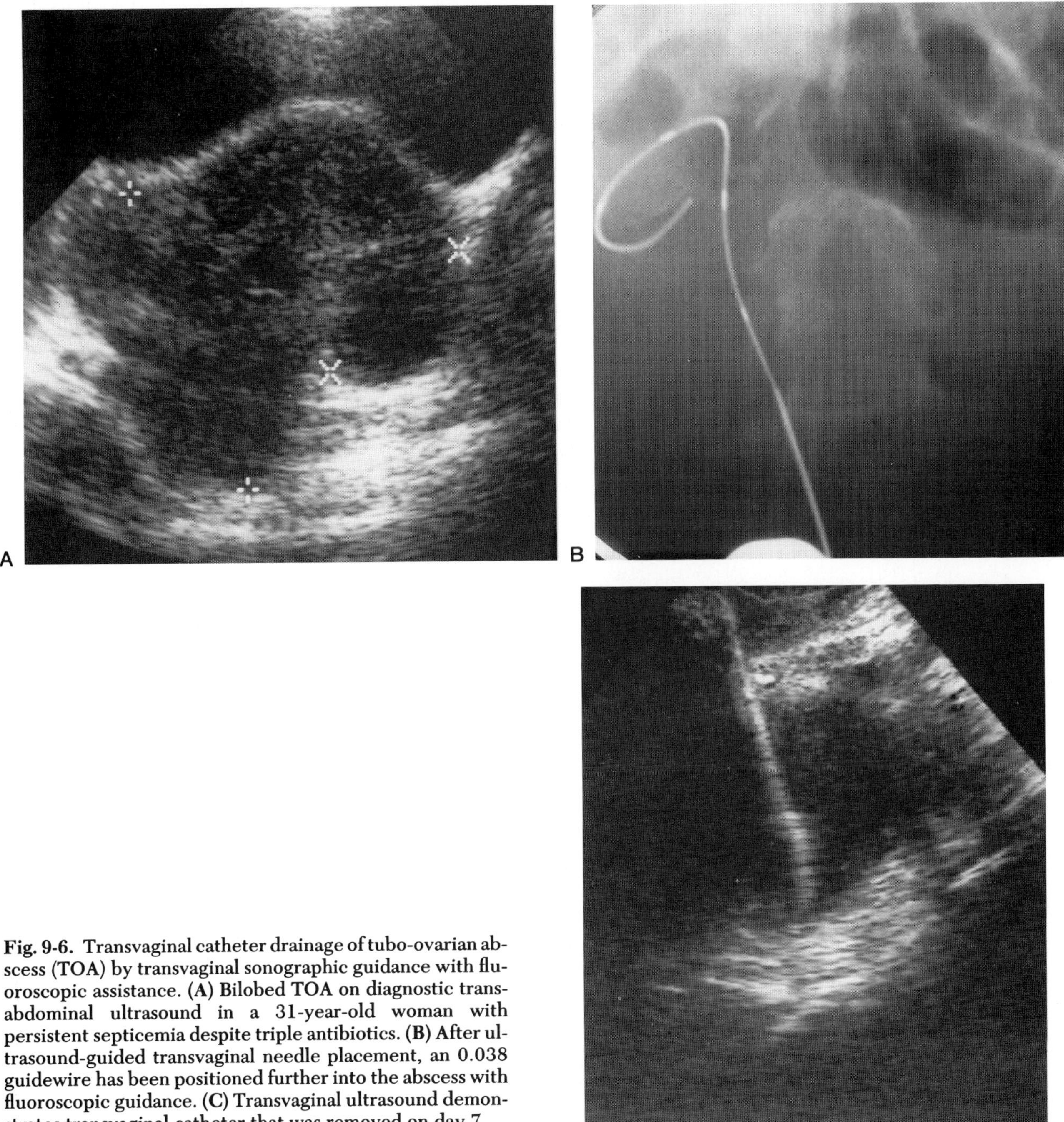

Fig. 9-6. Transvaginal catheter drainage of tubo-ovarian abscess (TOA) by transvaginal sonographic guidance with fluoroscopic assistance. (**A**) Bilobed TOA on diagnostic transabdominal ultrasound in a 31-year-old woman with persistent septicemia despite triple antibiotics. (**B**) After ultrasound-guided transvaginal needle placement, an 0.038 guidewire has been positioned further into the abscess with fluoroscopic guidance. (**C**) Transvaginal ultrasound demonstrates transvaginal catheter that was removed on day 7.

REFERENCES

1. Dodson MG: Optimum therapy for acute pelvic inflammatory disease. Drugs 39:511, 1990
2. Jacobson L, Westrom L: Objectivized diagnosis of acute pelvic inflammatory disease. Am J Obstet Gynecol 105:1088, 1969
3. Bulas DI, Ahlstrom PA, Sivit CJ et al: Pelvic inflammatory disease in the adolescent: comparison of tansabdominal and transvaginal sonographic evaluation. Radiology 183:435, 1992
4. Patten RM, Vincent LM, Wolner-Hanssen P, Thorpe Jr P: Pelvic inflammatory disease: endovaginal sonography with laparoscopic correlation. J Ultrasound Med 9:681, 1990
5. Lande IM, Hill MC, Cosco FE, Kator NN: Adnexal and cul-de-sac abnormalities: transvaginal sonography. Radiology 166:325, 1988
6. Uhrich PC, Sanders RC: Ultrasonic characteristics of pelvic inflammatory masses. J Clin Ultrasound 4:199, 1976
7. Schoenfeld A, Fisch B, Cohen M et al: Ultrasound findings in perihepatitis associated with pelvic inflammatory disease. J Clin Ultrasound 20:339, 1992
8. Lipsit ER: Inflammatory disease of the pelvis and postoperative fluid collections. p. 85. In Steel WB, Cochrane WJ (eds): Gynecologic Ultrasound. Churchill Livingstone, New York, 1984
9. Teisala K, Heinonen PK, Punnonen R: Transvaginal ultrasound in the diagnosis and treatment of tubo-ovarian abscess. Br J Obstet Gynaecol 97:178, 1990
10. Abbitt PL, Goldwag S, Urbanski S: Endovaginal sonography for guidance in draining pelvic fluid collections. AJR 154:849, 1990
11. VanDerKolk HL: Small, deep pelvic abscesses: definition and drainage guided with an endovaginal probe. Radiology 181:283, 1991
12. VanSonnenberg E, D'Agostino HB, Giovanna C et al: US-guided transvaginal drainage of pelvic abscesses and fluid collections. Radiology 181:53, 1991

10

Infertility

Melvin G. Dodson

About 15 percent of all couples experience difficulty achieving a pregnancy. A female factor is thought to be responsible for about 60 percent of infertility, and a male factor is responsible for about 40 percent. The major causes of female infertility include anovulation and ovulatory dysfunction, tubal damage and pelvic adhesions, endometriosis, endocrine abnormalities, and uterine factors, such as uterine leiomyomas, congenital anomalies, or endometrial adhesions. Less common causes of infertility include cervical factors and immunologic infertility. In about 10 to 15 percent of couples, the evaluation of both the male and the female is completely normal, and the etiology of the infertility cannot be determined. The use of ultrasound in the diagnosis and management of infertility has increased dramatically over the past 5 to 10 years and has become an integral part of the infertility diagnostic work-up and treatment.

INITIAL INFERTILITY EVALUATION

A systematic ultrasound evaluation of the uterus, cervix, endometrium, ovaries, adnexa, and cul-de-sac should be done with particular consideration of findings that might affect fertility. It is important to appreciate that ultrasound not only gives information regarding the status of the pelvic anatomy but also allows the assessment of functional problems that may be of particular importance in the infertility evaluation. (Table 10-1)

Uterus

Uterine size and position should be evaluated. The uterus should be evaluated for leiomyomas and congenital anomalies. Leiomyomas are quite common and are noted in up to 40 percent of women over the age of 35. However, they are not a common cause of infertility. Buttram and Reiter[1] in a review of nine published reports involving 1,698 myomectomies noted a history of infertility in 27 percent of these patients. In Buttram's personal series of 677 major operations, only 2.4 percent involved myomectomies in patients in which no other cause of infertility was found.[1] Leiomyomas as a cause of infertility was higher in blacks (9.1 percent) than in whites (1.8 percent).

About 40 percent of patients undergoing myomectomy for infertility will achieve a pregnancy. Buttram has noted that uterine size at the time of surgery is an important factor in determining whether a patient will be able to achieve a pregnancy after myomectomy.[1] All patients with an 8 weeks size uterus were able to achieve a pregnancy after myomectomy; however, no patient with a 10 to 16 week size uterus conceived. This study utilized the common practice in gynecology of estimating uterine size based on the pelvic examination with a comparison of size to the pregnant uterus. Ultrasound allows a more accurate assessment of uterine size.

Ultrasound also assesses accurately the specific size and location of leiomyomas. Surgery must be performed before leiomyomas reach a large size if fertility is to be preserved in a significant percentage of patients. However, pelvic surgery per se is associated with pelvic adhesions and infertility. This leaves the clinician with a therapeutic dilemma. If surgery is performed for small leiomyomas that are not a major contributing factor to the infertility, the patient's risk of infertility may actually be increased. Yet, if surgery is delayed and the leiomyoma is allowed to increase in size significantly, surgery may not be effective. Ultimately, the decision is a clinical one based on consid-

Table 10-1. Initial Ultrasound Evaluation

Organ	*Evaluate for*
Uterus	Size (as an indirect measure of hormonal and ovulatory status), leiomyoma, congenital anomalies
Cervix	Length, presence of cysts and cervical mucus
Endometrium	Thickness, cyclic changes (as a reflection of hormonal status and endometrial response), quality for implantation, polyps, adhesions
Adenexia	Hydrosalpinx, para-ovarian cysts
Ovary	Size, presence of immature follicles (< 10 mm), follicular development, ovulation, PCOD, dysfunctional ovulation

eration of the patient's age, length of infertility, size and location of the leiomyoma, and whether other factors that might be contributing to the infertility are present. Ultrasound can be utilized to monitor carefully the growth of small leiomyomas.

If preservation of fertility is a major concern, a leiomyoma that is rapidly increasing in size or is of significant size when initially evaluated should probably be removed without delay. The mechanism by which leiomyomas cause infertility is not known. Location of the leiomyoma may be an important factor. Leiomyomas located in the cornual or cervical region may compromise the tubal lumen or endocervical canal and cause infertility. A submucosal leiomyoma may cause atrophy or ulceration of the endometrium or result in vascular alterations that impair blood flow or cause improper nidation of the embryo. Transvaginal ultrasound is an excellent mechanism for localizing leiomyomas. The ultrasound diagnosis of leiomyomas is discussed in Chapter 5.

Leiomyomas may also result in an increased abortion rate. A summary of 1,063 pregnancies noted an abortion rate of 41 percent. Myomectomy reduced the abortion rate to only 19 percent, which approaches the spontaneous abortion rate noted in the general population (10 to 15 percent).[1]

Congenital anomalies of the müllerian system are noted in 2 to 3 percent of patients. Congenital uterine anomalies are the most common. About 25 percent of women with congenital uterine anomalies experience a problem with fertility.[2] Bicornuate uterus and uterus didelphys are generally readily diagnosed by ultrasound because of the presence of two endometrial cavities. The ultrasound diagnosis of unicornuate uterus is more difficult; however, a sensitivity of 85.7 percent and a specificity of 100 percent have been reported.[3] The diagnosis of septate uterus may also be difficult depending on how far the septum extends down into the uterine cavity. For a review of the use of ultrasound in the diagnosis of congenital uterine anomalies, see Chapter 5.

Fallopian Tubes and Adnexa

Pelvic adhesive disease is a significant cause of infertility. Pelvic adhesions requiring surgery have been reported in 44 percent of blacks and in 17.5 percent of white infertility patients.[1]

Ultrasound is not a sensitive or specific technique for the diagnosis of pelvic adhesions. However, the position of the ovary can suggest pelvic adhesions. Normally, the ovary is positioned along the lateral pelvic wall with several centimeters of space between it and lateral aspects of the uterus. This space is generally filled with small bowel. There is also often a small space between the ovary and the lateral pelvic wall, and the ovary can be moved by gentle pressure with the transducer tip away from the lateral pelvic wall. An ovary that is approximated against the uterus with minimal or no space between it and the uterus is suggestive of adhesions, provided that the uterus is not enlarged. Lack of motility of the ovary in relationship to the uterus and lateral pelvic side wall may also suggest adhesions. Generally, the transvaginal transducer can be used to separate the ovary from adjacent structures, such as the uterus, by using the transducer as a probe and gently pushing the ovary (or uterus) away from the adjacent structure. The space created is easily imaged. A "sliding organ sign" has been described.[4] If the ovary or uterus does not slide past each other when pressure is applied by the transducer, adhesions are suggested. Unfortunately, these "signs" are only suggestive of adhesions.

However, occasionally in patients with increased pelvic fluid, adhesions can be imaged directly as bands connecting different pelvic organs. The injection of normal saline may also be used to evaluate the patency of the fallopian tubes and allow direct imaging of peritubular and periovarian structures including adhesions. Deichert et al[5] have injected Ringer's solution to outline the uterus and evaluate the endometrial cavity followed by the intrauterine injection of a sonographic contrast media with transvaginal ultrasound imaging and pulsed wave Doppler to evaluate tubal patency. The contrast media (SH U 454, Echovist, Schering) consist of galactose microparticles with micrometer-sized air bubbles.[5] Complete agreement was noted between sonographic evaluation of tubal patency and laparoscopic chromotubation (see Ch. 17).

One of the most reliable ultrasound signs indicating tubal damage as an etiology of infertility is the presence of bilateral hydrosalpinx. The tube cannot generally be imaged as a separate structure in the absence of peritoneal fluid or of fluid in the tube (hydrosalpinx). However, when the tube is filled with fluid, it is easily imaged. Hydrosalpinx is imaged as a persistent anechoic "sausage-shaped" fluid collection generally adjacent to the ovary. Thickening of the tubal wall is often evident, and the tube is frequently bent back on itself, producing a "double wall" sign. Two separate walls are distinguishable, even though they are closely approximated. The double wall generally does not extend across the entire hydrosalpinx. A septum in an ovarian cyst generally extends from one wall to another or to another septum, and two separate walls cannot be distinguished. The mucosal folds of the fallopian tube, which are normally thin and delicate, become thickened and can be noted to project into the tubal lumen. Occasionally, the thickened mucosal folds extend from one tubal wall to the other, but more commonly they are imaged as projections into the lumen. When there is a space between the ovary and the hydrosalpinx, the diagnosis is easily made. However, the fluid-filled tube is frequently densely adherent to the ovary, and it is occasionally difficult to differentiate a hydrosalpinx from an ovarian cyst.

One ultrasound finding that may be helpful when the ovary and cystic areas are closely adherent is a "concave sign." The ovary and ovarian capsule are generally firmer than the hydrosalpinx. As a consequence, the hydrosalpinx bends over the ovary, and the hydrosalpinx outer wall is noted to be concave adjacent to the ovary and convex on its free wall away from the ovary. In contrast, ovarian cysts originate within the ovarian substance and below the ovarian capsule. Even when the cyst projects out from the ovary and the cyst wall is both adjacent to the ovarian stroma and along the surface, it's outer wall is still convex. In other words, an ovarian cyst is generally round like a balloon, whereas a hydrosalpinx adjacent to the ovary is "pushed in." A hydrosalpinx takes on the contour of the ovary in the area adjacent to the ovary, but is then "pushed out" like a cyst in areas not approximated against the ovary. A cyst wall will generally be convex on both the outer surface and inner surface unless the cyst is approximated against a harder surface.

The hydrosalpinx, although generally anechoic, may contain some internal echoes indicating debris. Para-ovarian cysts and hydatid of Morgagni will also be imaged as anechoic adnexal cysts. They can generally be differentiated from an ovarian cyst since they can be separated from the ovary. Generally, they have a smooth wall with no irregularity (as in a hydrosalpinx secondary to folding or in the presence of thickened mucosa folds). However, the most common problem is differentiating an atypical functional ovarian cyst from a hydrosalpinx. One of the most important differentiating findings is *persistence*. Hydrosalpoinx will persist, whereas functional cysts will resolve in 8 (rarely 10) weeks (Table 10-2).

Table 10-2. Ultrasound Findings in Hydrosalpinx and Ovarian Cysts

Hydrosalpinx	*Ovarian Cyst*
Tubular "sausage shaped"	Generally round
Separating space from the Ovary occasionally noted	No space between cyst and ovary (para-ovarian cysts are separable)
Double wall sign	Septum may appear similar but two separate adjacent walls are not imaged
Thickened mucosal folds generally project into lumen but do not extend from wall to wall	Nodularity of cyst wall may appear similar, but are uncommon except in malignancies
Concave cyst wall adjacent to ovary, convex away from the ovary	Convex wall *both* adjacent to the ovarian stroma on ovarian surface
Persists for >8–12 weeks	Functional cysts will resolve in 8–10 weeks, neoplasms will persist

Ovary: Ovulation, Anovulation, and Ovulatory Dysfunction

Ultrasound has become an important tool for confirming normal follicular development and ovulation or diagnosing anovulation and ovulatory dysfunction. Normal ovulatory function is characterized by follicular development with a progressive increase in follicular size by 1 to 2 mm per day until a dominant follicle of 18 to 25 mm develops. Ovulation is characterized by the disappearance of the follicle on ultrasound and formation of a corpus luteum or corpus luteal cyst. Normal cyclic endometrial changes should be noted in association with follicular development, with a single-line endometrium progressing to a three-line endometrium with progressive thickening (generally to 7 to 12 mm, full thickness measurement) and finally evolving into a hyperechoic ultrasound endometrium pattern characteristic of the luteal phase. Normal cyclic endometrial changes are associated with cyclic hormonal levels and are a good, although indirect, gauge of normal follicular function and endometrial response (see Ch. 6 for a discussion of the ultrasound findings and cyclic changes in a normal menstrual cycle and Ch. 7 for a discussion of the ultrasound findings associated with normal follicular development and ovulation).

No follicle will be noted to develop in the anovulatory patient. In addition, patients with chronic anovulation and low serum E_2 levels generally have a single-line endometrium that is only 1 to 2 mm thick, confirming the anovulation and the endocrine status. If the low serum E_2 levels are chronic, the uterus may be small and atrophic and resemble a postmenopausal uterus. However, a variety of other endometrial patterns can be seen in association with anovulation (see Ch. 6 and 11 for a detailed discussion).

Patients with polycystic ovarian disease (PCOD) generally are anovulatory and frequently (but not always) have enlarged ovaries with multiple immature (less than 10 mm in diameter) follicles. However, normal ovulatory patients should also have some immature follicles (generally, about five per ovary). In order to be reasonably sure of a diagnosis of PCOD, the ovaries should be enlarged (over 8 cm^3), and there should be 11 or more immature follicles (less than 10 mm in diameter) in each ovary. The endometrium may be a single line, but more commonly is hyperechoic, atypical, and thinner than the normal hyperechoic luteal phase endometrium, consistent with long term anovulation with normal but tonic serum E_2 levels (without the midcycle increase in E_2 associated with follicular development). The diagnosis of PCOD can be confirmed in the presence of clinical findings of infertility, obesity, hirsutism, and menstrual irregularities or amenorrhea and with laboratory findings, such as an elevated LH (or LH/FSH ratio over 3) and elevated androgens, e.g., testosterone and/or androstenedione (see Ch. 18).

The absence of any immature follicles (less than 10 mm in diameter) in an amenorrheic patient of 35 years or younger with very small ovaries (volume of 2.5 cm^3 or less), a very thin endometrium, and a small uterus suggest the diagnosis of premature ovarian failure. The diagnosis can be confirmed if the serum FSH is elevated (generally above 50 mIU/ml). Patients with resistant ovary syndrome have similar findings; however, small immature follicles are present in their ovaries. Likewise, the patient who is experiencing early menopause (between ages 35 to 50) has similar findings.

Luteinized but unruptured follicle (LUF) syndrome is characterized by follicular development, but without ovulation and disappearance of the follicle. Hormonal levels (including a mid cycle LH surge) are generally normal in patients with LUF syndrome.

Table 10-3. Ultrasound Evaluation of the Ovary in Infertility

Diagnosis	*Ovary*	*Endometrium*	*Comments*
Ovulation	Normal progressive (1–2 mm/day) follicular development (to 18–25 mm) with disappearance of the follicle	Three-line endometrium 7–12 mm thick becoming hyperechoic in the luteal phase	Serial ultrasound evaluations are generally necessary
Anovulation	No follicular development >10 mm	Single-line or three-line <6 mm thick; no change in the luteal phase	Generally low serum E_2, no LH surge, P <2.5 pg/ml
PCOD	Enlarged ovaries (>8 cm^3), multiple small immature follicles (<10 mm)	Generally atypical	Confirm by clinical findings and lab (LH, androgens)
LUF	Progressive follicular growth but with failure to ovulate	Normal cyclic changes and thickness	Normal hormonal findings
Premature ovarian failure	No follicular development, small ovaries, no immature follicles	Generally single line because of low E_2	Elevated FSH, low E_2
Resistant ovary	No follicular development, small ovaries, but immature follicles present	Generally single line because of low E_2	Elevated FSH, low E_2
Menopause	No follicular development, small ovaries, no immature follicles	Generally single line because of low E_2	Elevated FSH, low E_2

The presence of functional ovarian cysts (follicular or corpus luteal cyst) may be associated with short term (1 to 2 months) anovulation and/or menstrual irregularity, but is not a cause of infertility. In fact, the presence of a corpus luteal cyst is evidence that the patient is ovulatory. Ovarian neoplasms or cancer may (or may not) be associated with longer periods of anovulation and amenorrhea or menstrual irregularities. (Table 10-3)

Ultrasound is also an important technique for monitoring ovulation induction in anovulatory patients, in stimulation for IVF and other assisted reproductive technologies (particularly when using hMG), and for follicular aspiration in IVF (see Ch. 18 and 19).

ENDOMETRIUM: ENDOMETRIOSIS

Endometriosis is thought to be present in 5 to 20 percent of women of reproductive age and has been noted in 20 percent of laparoscopies for pelvic pain. Endometriosis may be the cause of 5 to 15 percent of all cases of infertility and of 30 percent of cases in which no other significant abnormalities are noted.[6] Symptoms suggestive of endometriosis include infertility, chronic pelvic pain, dysmenorrhea, and dyspareunia. Dysmenorrhea beginning after years of pain-free menses is particularly suggestive of endometriosis. However, many patients are asymptomatic or experience infertility as their only symptom. Common physical findings associated with endometriosis include an ovarian endometrioma or fixation of pelvic structures secondary to adhesions. The uterus may be retroverted. Nodularity and tenderness of the uterosacral ligaments are noted in one-third of patients with endometriosis.[7] Nodularity of the uterosacral ligaments is not generally imaged by ultrasound.

Small endometrial implants cannot be detected by ultrasound. The only reliable ultrasound finding of endometriosis is an endometrioma. Endometriomas consisting of blood-filled collections in the ovary lined by endometrial glands and stroma can generally be imaged and diagnosed by ultrasound (Fig. 10-1). Walsh et al[8] reported on 25 surgically confirmed cases of endometriomas and noted four patterns: cystic, polycystic, mixed, and solid. The cystic pattern was the most common. The inner cyst wall may be irregular and shaggy or smooth. However, in five patients with endometriomas reported by Sandler and Karo[9] none had a smooth, well-defined wall or a totally echo-free content characteristic of a simple cyst. The endometrioma cyst wall was generally shaggy and irregular, sometimes with septations. The polycystic pattern of endometriosis in the ovary consists of multiple small cystic cavities separated by septations. The mixed pattern consists of a predominantly cystic mass with focal clusters of echogenic tissue lining the cyst wall. A mixed pattern may be impossible to differentiate sonographically from pelvic inflammatory disease (PID).[9] A history of fever, clinical findings, and/or positive cultures for *Chlamydia trachomatis* and *Neisseria gonorrhea* may be helpful in making a diagnosis of PID.

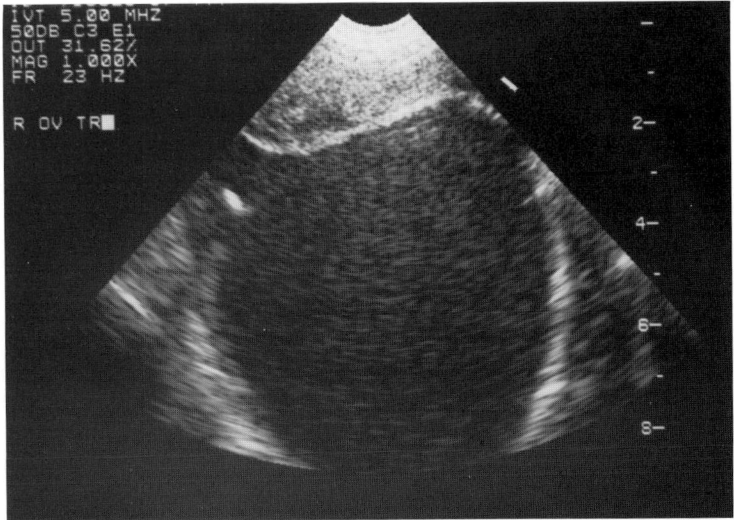

Fig. 10-1. Endometrium of the left ovary measuring 7.0 by 6.8 cm. Note smooth wall and echogenic pattern of the chocolate cyst consisting of old blood. This endometrioma was removed surgically.

Athey and Diment reported on the sonographic findings of 40 pathologically proven endometriomas.[10] Endometriomas are generally either round or ovoid (87 percent), but are occasionally bilobed or lobulated. Posterior acoustic enhancement is very common (87 percent). Some endometriomas are totally anechoic—with no internal echoes or septations (17 percent) or anechoic except for septations (10 percent), whereas others have scattered internal echoes with or without septations (30 percent) or diffuse low level echoes (17 percent). Solid endometriomas are uncommon (2 percent). Solid-appearing endometriomas may appear similar to solid ovarian neoplasms. Dependent echoes or "layering" may be noted (22 percent). The cyst walls are generally thin (80 percent), and septations are noted in 40 percent of patients.[10]

CA-125 may be of help in diagnosing endometriosis. Ca-125 has been reported to be elevated (above 16 U/ml) in 73 percent of women with infertility and endometriosis and in 80 percent of patients with pelvic pain. About 53 percent of women with endometriosis can be identified by elevation of CA-125, with a false-positive rate of only 7 percent when other clinical conditions, such as pregnancy and leiomyomas, are excluded.[7] In patients with a cyst 4 cm or larger, a CA-125 of 20 U/ml or greater was associated with an endometrioma in 96 percent of cases.

Endometriomas should be considered in the differential diagnosis of a cystic ovarian lesion, especially if the cyst persists or if there is a history of endometriosis, infertility, and dysmenorrhea. Hemorrhagic corpus luteal cysts (HCL) may be difficult to differentiate from an endometrioma. A helpful sonographic finding is the changing internal echo pattern of a HCL. This pattern is due to fibrinolysis of the hemorrhagic contents of the cyst with lysis of clots, changing proportions of cystic and solid components, and changes in the pattern of solid areas (clots).[2] Blumenfeld et al successfully diagnosed ten patients with endometriomas preoperatively by transvaginal ultrasound. Of 103 patients, the false-negative rate was less than 2 percent with no false-positive diagnoses.[2]

Endometriosis should also be considered if sonographic evidence is suggestive of adhesive disease. The adnexa may be adherent to the uterus or cul-de-sac secondary to adhesions. A hydrosalpinx may also be present. A honeycomb-appearing myometrium with irregular cystic spaces 5 to 7 mm in size representing adenomyosis has been reported to be present in 36 percent of patients with endometriosis.[2]

However, despite suggestive sonographic signs of endometriosis, laparoscopy remains the diagnostic technique of choice, particularly for small endometrial implants that cannot be imaged by ultrasound. Ultrasound is very sensitive for detecting small ovarian masses that might represent small endometriomas and is reasonably effective in evaluating such masses, particularly when combined with CA-125 as noted above. Sonography may be useful before laparoscopy or pelvic surgery to indicate when small endometriomas or suspicious ovarian masses are present in the ovary that should be evaluated at the time of surgery. Small endometriomas may not be apparent on the surface of the ovary at the time of laparoscopy, but can be easily localized before surgery using sonography. If the physician is not aware that there is a small cyst or area suspicious for endometriosis in the ovary, the endometrioma may be missed and appropriate treatment not done at the time of surgery.

REFERENCES

1. Buttram VC, Reiter RC: Uterine leiomyomata: etiology, symptomatology, and management. Fertil Steril 36:433, 1981
2. Blumenfeld Z, Nehemya Y, Bronshtein M: Transvaginal sonography in infertility and assisted reproduction. Obstet Gynecol Survey 46:36, 1990
3. Fedele L, Dorta M, Vercellini P et al: Ultrasound in the diagnosis of subclasses of unicornate uterus. Obstet Gynecol 71:274, 1988
4. Timor-Tritsch IE, Rottem S, Levron Y: The fallopian tubes. p. 45. In Timor-Tritsch IE, Rottem S (eds): Transvaginal Sonography. Elsevier Science Publishing Company, New York, 1988
5. Deichert U, Sclief R, van de Sandt M, Juhnke I: Transvaginal hysterosalpingo contrast sonography (HyCoSy) compared with conventional tubal diagnostics. Hum Reprod 4:418, 1989
6. Dawood MY: Endometriosis. p. 387. In Gold JF, Josimovich JB (eds): Gynecologic Endocrinology. 4th Ed. Plenum Publishing, New York, 1987
7. Speroff L, Glass RH, Kass NG: Endometriosis and infertility. In Clinical Gynecology, Endocrinology and Infertility. 4th Ed. Williams & Wilkins, Baltimore, 1989
8. Walsh JW, Tayloe KJW, Rosenfield AT: Gray scale ultrasonography in the diagnosis of endometriosis and adenomyosis. AJR 127:229, 1978
9. Sandler MA, Karo JJ: The spectrum of ultrasonic findings in endometriosis. Radiology 127:229, 1978
10. Atley PA, Diment DD: The spectrum of sonographic findings in endometriomas. J Ultrasound Med 8:487, 1989

11

Amenorrhea and Menometrorrhagia

Melvin G. Dodson

Ultrasound may help diagnose and plan treatment for patients with amenorrhea and menometrorrhagia. However, in order to utilize ultrasound imaging of the endometrium normal endometrial ultrasound patterns must be recognized. Table 11-1 and Figs. 11-1 through 11-5 review normal endometrial patterns,[1] and abnormal patterns are discussed in Chapter 6.

AMENORRHEA

Etiology

Amenorrhea is a common clinical problem. It is defined as an absence of periods for 3 months or longer (secondary) or the absence of menarche by the age of 16 years (primary). After excluding pregnancy, the etiologies of amenorrhea may be divided into three major categories: anatomic causes, ovarian failure, and endocrine abnormalities.[2] Endocrine abnormalities are by far the most common cause of amenorrhea.

Franks reported on the etiology of 100 consecutive cases of secondary amenorrhea.[3] Weight loss and PCOD were the most common causes cited (about two-thirds of cases). Ovarian failure, increased prolactins, and low gonadotropins accounted for about one-third of the cases of secondary amenorrhea (Fig. 11-6).

Anatomic Causes

Anatomic causes of amenorrhea include Asherman's syndrome and disorders of sexual differentiation, such as gonadal dysgenesis or müllerian agenesis or dysgenesis. Hysterosalpingography has been the most common technique utilized in the past for the diagnosis of Asherman's syndrome. Hysteroscopy is also a valuable technique for the diagnosis of Asherman's syndrome if the adhesions are not so extensive that they eliminate the endometrial cavity and prevent insertion of the hysteroscope. There has been much less experience utilizing ultrasound to diagnose this condition.

Transvaginal sonographic evaluation in patients with Asherman's syndrome may show a disordered endometrial echo pattern if the adhesions are extensive enough. In addition, ultrasound allows a detailed examination of the endometrium with measurement of endometrial thickness, as well as evaluation of the myometrium. Recently, sonosalpingography using contrast media or saline to better visualize the endometrial cavity and fallopian tubes has been described. Bonilla-Musoles et al studied 76 patients using saline solution or Dextran 60 as a distension media[4] (see discussion in Ch. 17). Two patients were noted to have endometrial synechiae. Sonosalpingography was more sensitive but less specific than HSG or hysteroscopy in the diagnosis of uterine cavity pathology. In addition to diagnosing Asherman's syndrome, ultrasound may provide information on the physiologic potential of the endometrium to menstruate. Patients with Asherman's syndrome may not withdraw to progesterone or even to estrogen stimulation followed by progesterone if the endometrial adhesions are extensive enough. Ultrasound may be utilized to evaluate the thickness of the endometrium and the potential for menstruation after progesterone challenge.[5] A very thin endometrium (1.5 mm or less) in a patient with amenorrhea often signifies an

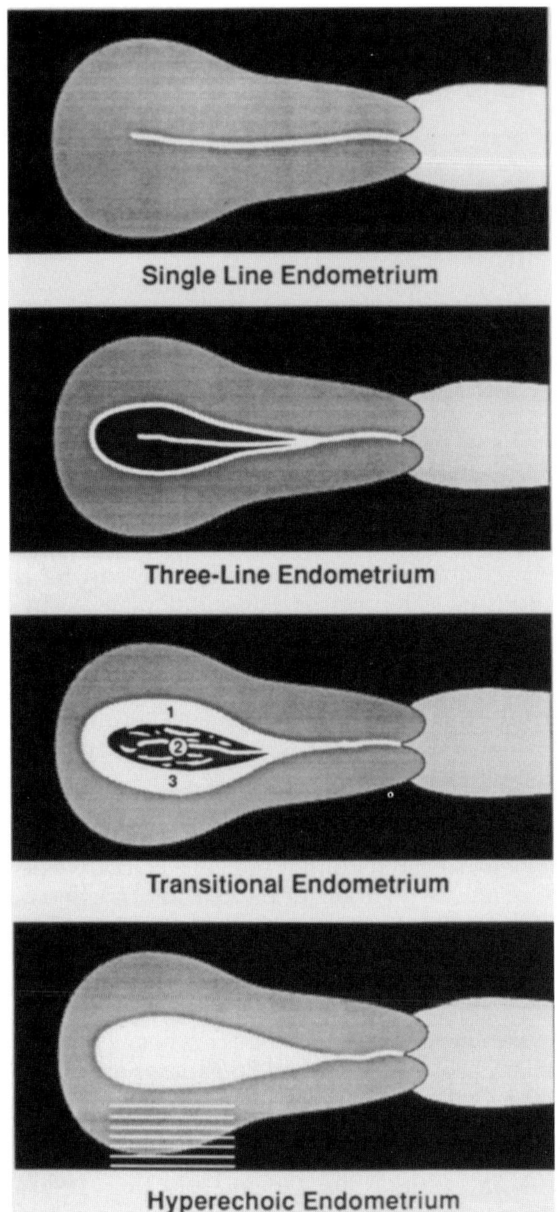

Fig. 11-1. Classification of the ultrasound-imaged endometrium through a normal menstrual cycle: menses *(single-line)* endometrium; proliferative (follicular) phase *(three-line)* endometrium; early luteal phase *(transitional)* endometrium; secretory (luteal) phase *(hyperechoic)* endometrium.

atrophic endometrium that will not withdraw to progesterone.

Gonadal dysgenesis may be inferred by the inability to visualize the ovaries and the effects of hypoestrogenism (small uterus and minimally stimulated single-line endometrium as discussed below). Ultrasound may also be used to diagnose müllerian anomalies as discussed in Chapter 5. However, transvaginal sonography may not be possible in patients with vaginal agenesis. This is one of the least common causes of amenorrhea.

Ovarian Failure

Ovarian failure may be suggested sonographically by anatomic findings associated with minimal estrogen stimulation. Patients with ovarian failure generally have a single-line endometrium and a small uterus and ovaries with low estrogen levels. Another important sonographic sign suggesting ovarian failure (which is also generally noted in the postmenopausal patient) is the lack of immature follicles—small follicles less than 10 mm in diameter. Unfortunately, small immature follicles continue to cause confusion. Even their name is quite confusing. I generally refer to these small follicles as immature follicles to distinguish them from the developing preovulatory follicles. Small immature ovarian follicles are a normal finding throughout the menstrual cycle in normal ovulating women. Yet, I continue to see patients diagnosed as having "ovarian cysts" by ultrasound based on the presence of these normal immature ovarian follicles.

Pache et al[6] have reported an average of five immature follicles per ovary with an average size of 5.1 mm in normal women. Patients with PCOD have an increased number of small immature follicles (average number 9.8, average size 3.8 mm); however, there is considerable overlap between normal patients and patients with PCOD (see the discussion in Ch. 7 and 18). More than 11 immature follicles in one ovary is very suggestive of PCOD.[3] Furthermore, their presence or absence can suggest the physiology and hormonal function of the ovary. The absence of any immature follicles suggests ovarian failure or menopause. The diagnosis of primary ovarian failure may be confirmed by an elevated follicle stimulating hormone (above 50 mIU/ml) in a patient under age 35.

Endocrine Abnormalities

By far endocrine aberrations are the most common cause of amenorrhea. Amenorrhea can result from a variety of systemic diseases that are endocrine in ori-

Table 11-1. Endometrial Classification[a]

Endometrium	*Description*	*Correlation*
Single-line endometrium	Single hyperechoic line representing the endometrial cavity (1–3 mm thick)	Noted at the end of menses, during the early follicular phase, in the postmenopausal period, and in patients with minimal estrogen stimulation, such as some anovulatory patients.
Three-line endometrium	Three hyperechoic relatively parallel lines. The central thin hyperechogenic line is the endometrium cavity. The outer lines occur at the acoustic interface of the endometrial-myometrial junction. The functional layer of the endometrium is hypoechoic or anechoic.	Correlates with estorgen stimulation, and is noted during the follicular phase.
Transitional endometrium	Thickening of the outer hyperechoic echo and increased echogenecity of the ultrasound imaged functional layer of the endometrium. The central hyperechoic echo of the endometrial cavity is still present.	Noted during the early luteal phase. Ultrasound image of the endometrial as it converts from a proliferative phase three-line endometrium following estrogen stimulation to a diffuse hyperechoic endometrium characteristic of progesterone effect.
Hyperechoic endometrium	Hyperechoic with loss of the three-line endometrium. Acoustic enhancement may be noted posterior to the hyperechoic endometrium.	Generally seen during the luteal phase and is associated with a progesterone response of an estrogen stimulated endometrium.
BCP endometrium	Thickened hyperechoic endometrium 3–5 mm thick.	Associated with simultaneous E_2 and P stimulation as with birth control pills.
Atypical endometrium	An ultrasound imaged endometrium that does not correlate with any of the above described normal patterns.	See Chapter 6 for detailed discussion and review.

[a] See diagrams in Figure 11-1 and in Figures 11-2 through 11-5.

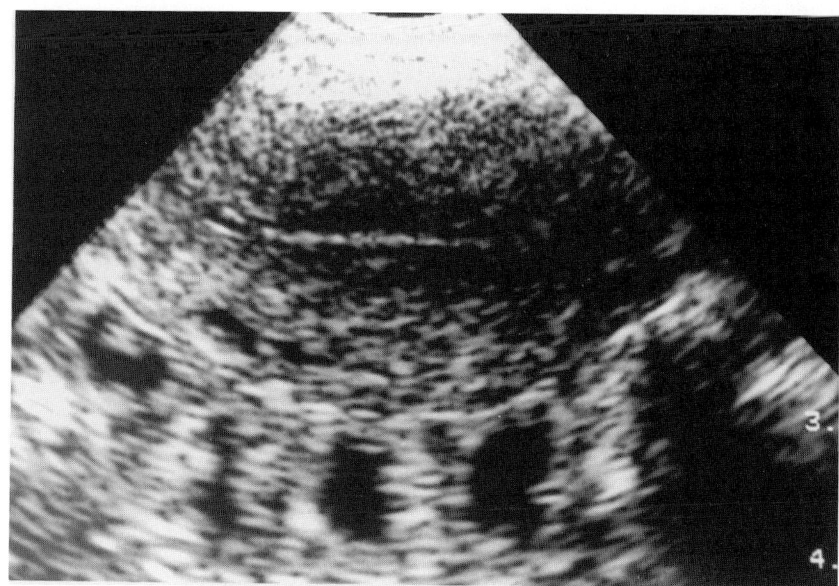

Fig. 11-2. Single-line (unstimulated or menstrual) endometrium. The endometrium is imaged as a single thin hyperechoic central line (echo) usually less than 3 mm thick that represents the endometrial cavity. The single-line endometrium is generally seen in association with menses, but is also noted in postmenopausal patients and in many chronically anovulatory patients with low serum estradiol levels.

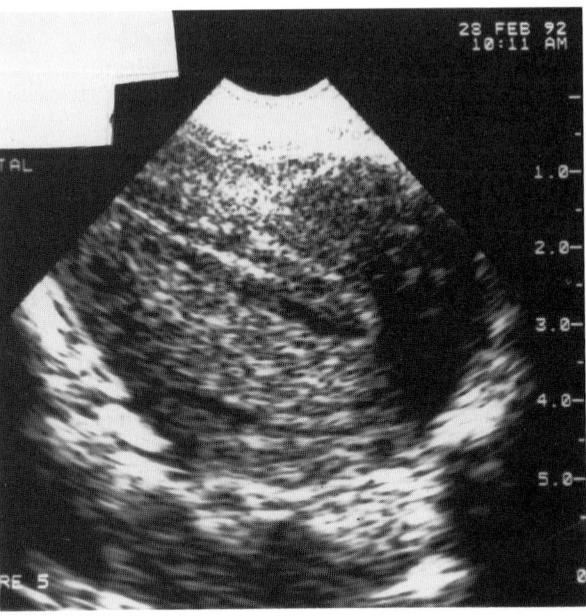

Fig. 11-3. A three-line endometrium consisting of a central hyperechoic echo representing the endometrial cavity and two outer lines (echoes) at the endometrial-myometrial junction. A three-line endometrium reflects estrogen stimulation and a proliferative endometrial response characteristic of the follicular phase of the menstrual cycle. The functional endometrial layer is hypoechoic and lies between the two outer hyperechoic echoes and the central hyperechoic echo.

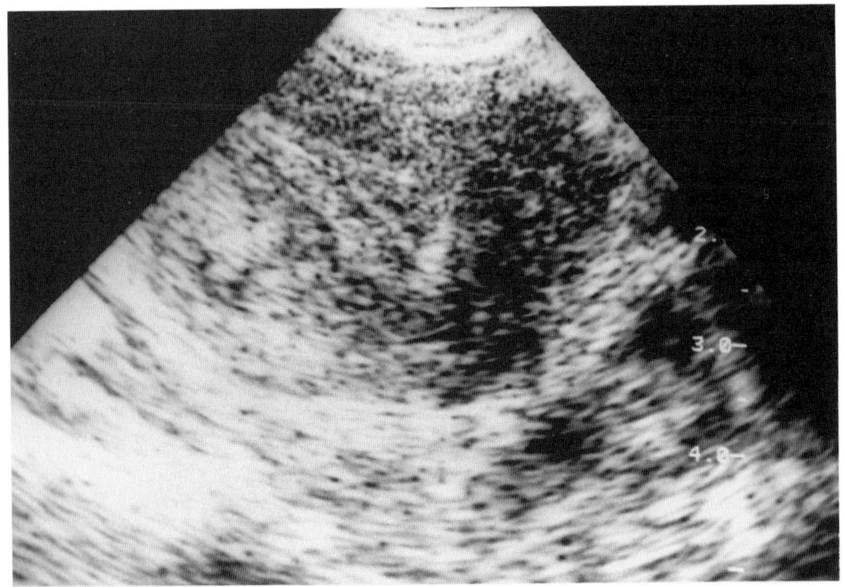

Fig. 11-4. A transitional endometrium is characterized by thickening of the two outer echoes of the three-line proliferative endometrium and increased echogenecity of the hypoechoic functional endometrial layers. A transitional endometrium is noted after progesterone stimulation of an estrogen-primed endometrium (three-line endometrium), but before a fully developed hyperechoic luteal phase endometrium has developed.

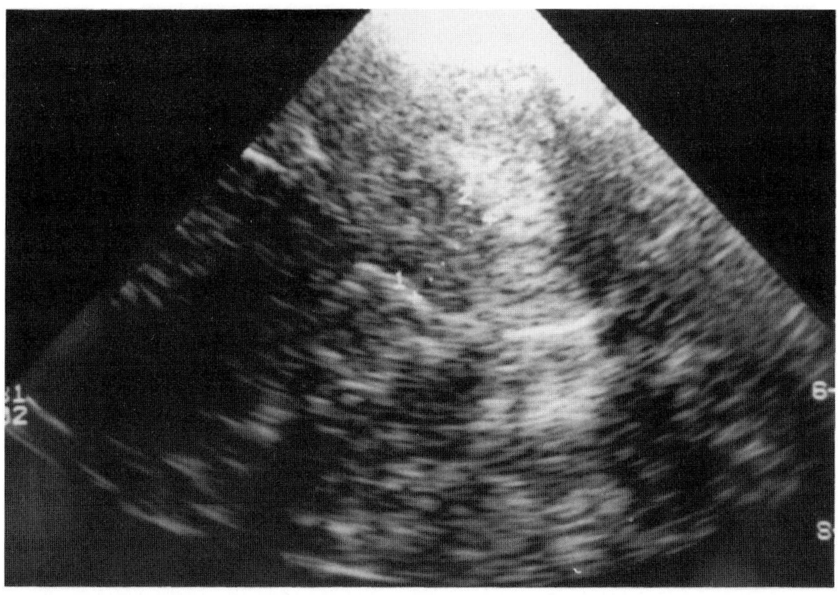

Fig. 11-5. A hyperechoic endometrium is imaged in the luteal phase (secretory endometrium) and generally reflects a progesterone effect on an estrogen-stimulated endometrium.

gin, such as hypothyroidism, or more commonly for chronic ovulation occurring secondary to a systemic division. Severe stress or psychological problems may also cause amenorrhea. Patients with amenorrhea associated with low levels of estrogen generally have a single-line endometrium similar to a late menstrual endometrium (Fig. 11-7). The minimally stimulated endometrium can be differentiated from the late menstrual endometrium based on the patient's history. The late menstrual endometrium is seen on days 2 to 7 during or after a menstrual period. The presence of a single-line endometrium not associated with menses suggests either a physiologic or anatomic abnormality manifested clinically as amenorrhea.

Normoestrogenic and hypoestrogenic amenorrhea patients can generally be distinguished by the response (menses or no bleeding) to a progesterone challenge. Morcos et al[5] reported on 70 patients with amenorrhea challenged with progesterone. An endometrial thickness of 1.5 mm or less by ultrasound imaging was associated with an absence of bleeding after a progesterone challenge. Ultrasound imaging had a 79 percent positive predictive value and a 98 percent negative predictive value (using a thickness of 1.5 mm) in predicting menses after a progesterone challenge.

However, not all patients with chronic amenorrhea have a single-line endometrium. Some patients, such as those with PCOD with long standing amenorrhea but with normal serum estradiol levels, have atypical and often thick sonographic endometrial patterns. These patients generally have withdrawal bleeding when challenged with progesterone. Not infrequently, a patient will miss one or two menstrual periods or even have amenorrhea associated with a luteinized (white ultrasound image) endometrium due to exogenous progesterone administration, or corpus luteal development after a single sporadic ovulation during a period of anovulation. One of the most common scenarios is the non-pregnant patient who has missed a menstrual period (occasionally even two periods) with a luteinized and thick endometrium and the presence of a corpus luteal cyst. Although missing only one or even two periods does not constitute amenorrhea per se, this is a very common clinical situation. Ultrasound can provide the diagnosis—a

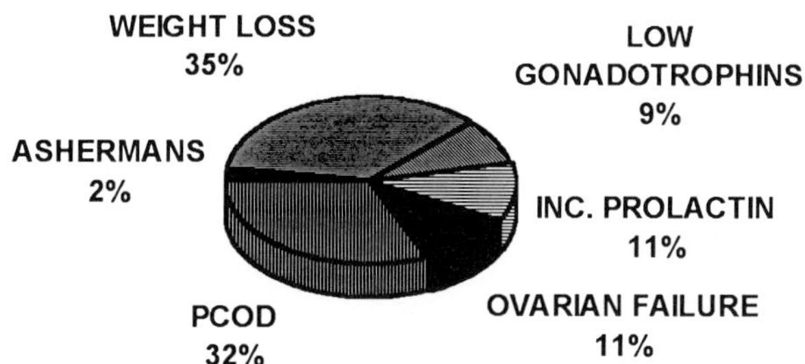

Fig. 11-6. Etiology of secondary amenorrhea. (Data from Franks[3] involving 100 consecutive patients with secondary amenorrhea.)

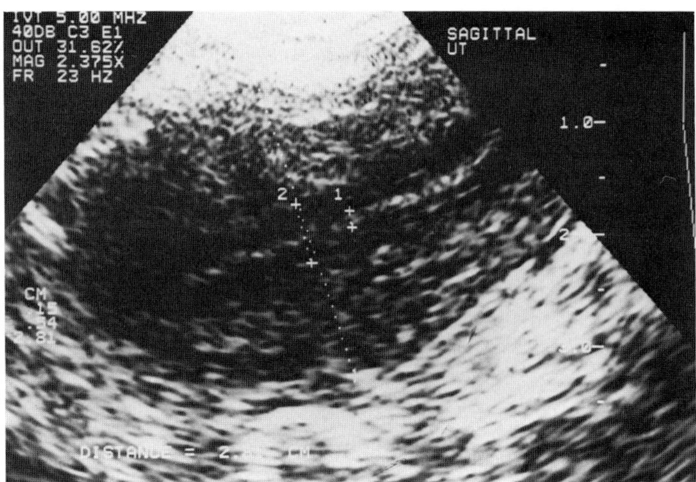

Fig. 11-7. A 26-year-old woman with amenorrhea for 1 year and galactorrhea. The AP-pelvic view of the uterus shows a single-line endometrium with a prominent halo. The endometrium is 1.5 mm thick. In the lower uterine segment there is some suggestion of the endometrium-myometrium junction forming the three-line sign. The prolactin was 70.4 ng/ml, follicle stimulating hormone was 3.0 mIU/ml, luteinizing hormone was 7.1 mIU/ml, and serum estradiol was 62.0 pg/ml. The patient withdrew on medroxyprogesterone acetate (10 mg/day) for 5 days. An NMR confirmed a microadenoma of the pituitary.

missed period due to a persistent corpus luteal cyst with a luteal phase endometrium. The patient can be reassured that spontaneous menses will ensue following collapse and disappearance of the cyst; sometimes irregular bleeding occurs even while the cyst is present. It must also be appreciated that ultrasound imaging and the patient's physiology are dynamic processes. A patient with one or two missed menses may not have a corpus luteal cyst because it collapsed the day before (or eve a few hours before) the ultrasound examination. Careful imaging of the ovary may reveal an echovariant area in the ovary (nonhomogeneous echo areas) where the cyst was located (Fig. 11-8; see also Fig. 1-3).

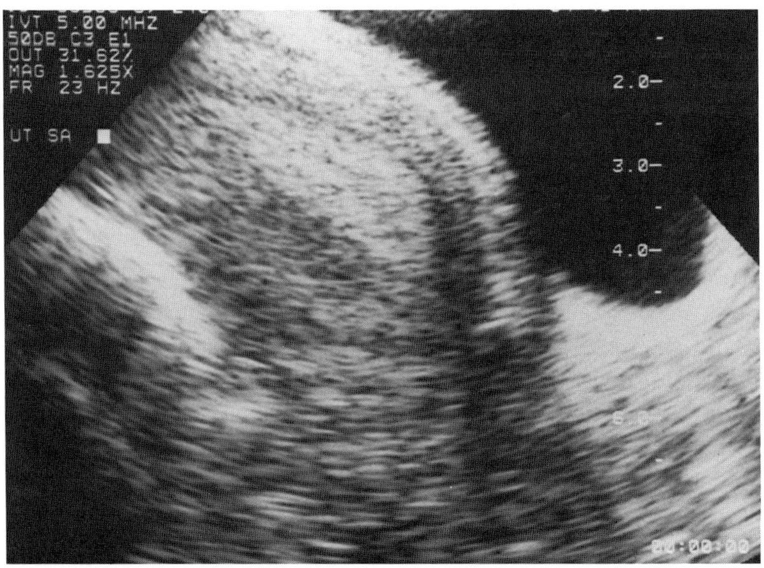

Fig. 11-8. An 18-year-old woman G1 P1 with no menses for 6 weeks. Patient experienced a period after discontinuing her birth control pills, but missed her expected next period. The AP-pelvic view of the uterus showed a well-developed endometrium consistent with the luteal phase. There were no cysts or follicles in the ovaries. She was told she would have a normal period within 2 weeks. The serum progesterone was 20.4 ng/ml. She had a spontaneous menses 11 days later. Without ultrasound examination this patient would have been diagnosed as having postpill amenorrhea with anovulation. The ultrasound examination revealed that the patient had ovulated and had a well-developed luteal endometrium and would have a spontaneous period. She had probably taken several weeks to develop a follicle after discontinuation of her birth control pills, and her cycle was simply reflecting several weeks of delayed follicular development before ovulation.

Table 11-2. Etiology of Menometrorrhagia

Classification of Menometrorrhagia	*Value of Ultrasound*
Pregnancy related	++++
Systemic disease	Minor
Drugs (nonhormonal) or anticoagulants	Minor
BCP (breakthrough bleeding)/hormone related	++
Postmenopausal bleeding	++++
Anatomic pelvic pathology	++++
Dysfunctional uterine bleeding	+++

MENOMETRORRHAGIA

Abnormal vaginal bleeding is a common clinical problem responsible for up to 20 percent of gynecologic office visits.[7] The etiology of abnormal vaginal bleeding is quite varied, but can be grouped into several large categories (Table 11-2). Such a classification system is a useful guide to a rational diagnostic and therapeutic approach to patients with menometrorrhagia. Despite the wide variety of potential causes of abnormal vaginal bleeding, the most common causes are a complication of pregnancy, anatomic lesions involving the pelvic organs, and aberrations of the normal menstrual cycle (generally associated with anovulation), which are generally grouped under the term "dysfunctional uterine bleeding."

Bleeding is also quite common in patients taking birth control pills and is generally considered a separate entity and is diagnosed as "breakthrough bleeding." Breakthrough bleeding from oral contraceptive therapy is usually viewed clinically as a nuisance complication of little medical significance and of no lasting consequences. However, in addition to the inconvenience of bleeding, patients are often concerned that there might be a more serious underlying problem. Ultrasound can be utilized to reassure the patient that her uterus, endometrium, and ovaries are normal and that the bleeding is truly only breakthrough bleeding.

Postmenopausal bleeding is also not uncommon and is approached clinically as a separate entity because of its significant association with endometrial carcinoma. The clinical approach centers around ruling out an endometrial cancer.

Sonography can frequently play an important role in determining the etiology of abnormal bleeding and in selecting appropriate therapy. This discussion is organized around the classification of menometrorrhagia in Table 11-2.

Pregnancy Related

Vaginal bleeding in association with an intrauterine pregnancy (IUP) is termed a threatened abortion and is noted in about one-fourth of pregnancies. About half of the patients experiencing a threatened abortion will eventually abort, whereas the pregnancy will progress successfully in the other half. Although very early pregnancy is best diagnosed utilizing a serum beta-hCG, ultrasound can image a gestational sac as early as the fifth gestational week and can often image a fetus in a normal pregnancy in a normally ovulating patient by the sixth gestational week (from the LMP). Ultrasound findings associated with bleeding in early pregnancy include a blighted ova; inevitable, incomplete, or missed abortion; twins; subchorionic hemorrhage; leiomyomas; pregnancy with an IUD; ectopic pregnancy; or gestational trophoblastic disease.

The presence of an intrauterine fetus with fetal cardiac activity imaged by transvaginal ultrasound is a very reassuring diagnostic finding that is associated with an abortion rate of only 1.3 to 2.6 percent.[8–10] Fetal cardiac activity can generally be noted as soon as the fetus is recognized as a distinct entity. The absence of discernible fetal cardiac activity by transvaginal ultrasound in a clearly recognizable fetus is generally associated with an inevitable abortion. Likewise, the presence of an intrauterine gestational sac 20 mm or larger without a yolk sac, or larger than 25 mm without a fetus, is generally associated with a blighted ova and an inevitable abortion. A distorted gestational sac or yolk sac may also be associated with an inevitable abortion (Table 11-3, see Ch. 13-15).

Ectopic Pregnancy

Bleeding is also noted in one-half to three-quarters of patients with ectopic pregnancies. Ectopic pregnancies represent about 1 percent of all pregnancies and are particularly important to recognize clinically since about 10 percent of all maternal deaths result from this complication. Transvaginal ultrasound has become an essential tool for the diagnosis of ectopic pregnancy. (see Ch. 15.)

Table 11-3. Ultrasound in Intrauterine Pregnancy (IUP)

Diagnosis	*Ultrasound Findings*
IUP	Confirm IUP, viability, gestational age, diagnose some congenital anomalies, twins
Threatened abortion	Confirm fetal presence, viability, ± subchorionic hemorrhage, ± normal uterus
Abortion	Confirm degenerating fetus or gestational sac, no FHT, ± abnormal yolk sac, ± subchorionic hemorrhage
Blighted ova	Confirm absence of fetus with sac ≥ 20-mm diameter
Gestational trophoblastic disease	Confirm absent fetus, multiple small cysts
Other	Confirm IUD, uterine leiomyoma, uterine congenital anomaly

Systemic Disease

Systemic disease is an uncommon cause of abnormal vaginal bleeding. The most common systemic diseases associated with bleeding are the endocrinopathies, such as hyper- or hypothyroidism, and the coagulation disorders, such as idiopathic thrombocytopenic purpura, i.e., Von Willebrand's disease.

Since these conditions are generally diagnosed by history and physical examination and appropriate laboratory or other tests, transvaginal ultrasound is of limited value except to confirm normal pelvic anatomy.

Drugs (Non-hormonal) or Anticoagulants

Nonhormonal drugs are an uncommon cause of abnormal bleeding, but must be considered. Patients receiving heparin or coumarin-like drugs may experience abnormal vaginal bleeding that is difficult to control. Psychopharmacologic agents and autonomic drugs that have an inhibitory effect on ovulation are common offenders, and morphine, reserpine, phenothiazines, monamine oxidase inhibitors, and anticholinergic drugs may also be associated with bleeding. The major role of transvaginal ultrasound is to rule out underlying anatomic pathology, such as leiomyomas, or to confirm normal pelvic anatomy.

Common Causes of Menometrorrhagia in Non-pregnant Patients

There are four common categories of abnormal vaginal bleeding in nonpregnant patients: bleeding from organic pelvic pathology (anatomic bleeding), dysfunctional bleeding (nonanatomic associated), bleeding associated with the use of hormones, and bleeding in the postmenopausal patient.

In a study of 45 patients with menometrorrhagia using transvaginal ultrasound, Dodson[1] noted a considerable difference in the etiology of bleeding when the history and physical examination were utilized as the primary evaluation procedure rather than sonography. Using the history and physical examination only, 7 percent of patients were postmenopausal, and in 22 percent of patients the bleeding occurred in patients taking hormones. A diagnosis of an anatomic abnormality by physical examination was noted in only 9 percent of patients. The remaining 62 percent of patients were diagnosed as experiencing dysfunctional uterine bleeding by exclusion with a normal physical and pelvic examination. These findings are in general agreement with the prevailing view that the majority of bleeding is dysfunctional in etiology, with only about 10 percent occurring secondary to organic pelvic pathology. However, when the transvaginal sonographic examination was utilized as a part of the evaluation process, the etiology of bleeding was quite different. Anatomic findings that could explain the bleeding were noted in 31 percent of patients. In addition, ovarian enlargement (ovarian volume greater than 8 cm^3 in the absence of a cyst or follicle) and the presence of multiple immature follicles suggesting PCOD were present in an additional 9 percent of patients.

Although bleeding in PCOD patients is anovulatory and is generally considered to result from the disturbed hormonal milieu noted in PCOD patients (and is usually considered a form of dysfunctional uterine bleeding), there is also an anatomic component relating to enlarged ovaries with the presence of multiple small cysts. Both the enlarged ovaries and multiple cysts can frequently be noted on the sonographic examination and can suggest the diagnosis of PCOD. In fact, the sonographic evaluation is probably the best current method—and certainly the least expensive and least invasive method—for accurately evaluating ovarian size and the size and number of small immature follicles within the ovary. Ovarian enlargement is one of the classic findings first utilized by Stein and Leventhal in their description of PCOD (Stein-Leventhal syndrome).[11] However, not all patients with PCOD have enlarged ovaries, and there is considerable overlap between the number of immature follicles noted in normal patients and PCOD patients.

In addition to anatomic findings by ultrasound, clinical and biochemical findings consistent with PCOD should be noted (see Ch. 18). If PCOD with ovarian enlargement is considered, 40 percent of patients experiencing menometrorrhagia had anatomic findings diagnosed by ultrasound. These findings are in marked contrast to the 5 to 10 percent incidence of anatomic findings generally thought to be associated with menometrorrhagia.

Anatomic Pelvic Pathology

Using transvaginal ultrasound, it is clear that the incidence of anatomic associated pelvic pathology and dysfunctional uterine bleeding is different than what has previously been reported based on evaluations utilizing only the history and physical examination or even compared to studies utilizing more extensive evaluation and invasive diagnostic procedures. Using transvaginal ultrasound evaluation, anatomic pelvic lesions are a more common and dysfunctional bleeding a less common cause of menometrorrhagia than generally considered. Several studies have reported that 14 to 19 percent of patients with a normal pelvic examination will be found to have organic pelvic pathology, rather than dysfunctional uterine bleeding, if more invasive diagnostic evaluations are done.[12–14] In a series of 500 cases, Benjamin[12] noted that 18.4 percent of patients with a normal pelvic examination were bleeding from systemic or endocrine disease or organic pelvic pathology.

Ovarian causes of abnormal uterine bleeding include functional ovarian cysts, neoplasms, or carcinomas. Ovarian cysts or neoplasms usually produce uterine bleeding by interfering with normal ovulation and therefore normal cyclic hormonal production; less commonly, they may interfere with the endogenous production of hormones per se. In my study noted above,[1] functional ovarian cysts were the most common anatomic finding associated with abnormal bleeding, accounting for 43 percent of the anatomic causes of bleeding, but they were usually small and not discernible on pelvic examination. If these small functional cysts were excluded, the higher incidence of anatomic lesions noted by sonographic evaluation (31 percent) was very consistent with previous reports using more invasive approaches (such as a D&C and other surgery) to diagnose the etiology of bleeding—18 percent anatomic lesions noted by ultrasound excluding functional ovarian cysts.

Functional ovarian cysts are very common and are self-limited. Bleeding can generally be controlled using oral contraceptives or hormonal therapy, such as estrogen or progesterone. A repeat sonographic evaluation should be done in 8 weeks to confirm resolution of the cyst. A follicular cyst is generally imaged as an anechoic cyst with a smooth internal wall with no septum, internal echoes, or wall nodularity.

Hemorrhagic corpus luteal cyst can present as an anechoic cyst similar to a follicular cyst or with a wide variety of bizarre internal echo patterns that can occasionally be difficult to differentiate from a neoplasm (see Ch. 7). The common internal echo patterns noted in a corpus luteum are (1) a "lacy pattern" representing a blood clot undergoing lysis (see Fig. 7-10 and 7-11) or (2) a complex anastomosing pattern resembling septum and solid areas separating anechoic areas and/or areas filled with low level echodensities, again representing clot retraction with areas of serum and/or blood between the clots.

Occasionally, "layering" at the bottom of a cyst is noted. This layering represents a completely lysed clot with red cells and debris at the bottom of the cyst and serum above (see Fig. 7-12). These patterns can sometimes be difficult to differentiate from a solid and cystic neoplasm. Color flow and Doppler evaluation of vessels can be of value in differentiating malignant from benign cysts. However, corpus luteal cysts can also be associated with neovascularization.

I have found three criteria to be of value in differentiating the occasional complex hemorrhagic corpus luteal cyst from a neoplasm. First, a rapidly changing (within several weeks) internal echo pattern is generally not seen with neoplasms. As the clots within a hemorrhagic cyst undergo lysis, the pattern changes. Although the echo architecture within a neoplastic cyst may evolve with time, these changes are generally slower—not as dramatic in a 2-week time span—and are usually associated with an increase in the size of the cyst, as well as consistency in the architectural pattern. Second, neovascularization of a corpus luteal cyst is generally limited to the cyst wall, and color flow is not usually noted within the substance of the cyst per se. In contrast, in a malignant neoplasm, color flow may be noted in septae and solid areas within the tumor. Doppler evaluation often reveals low impedance flow, which is a very valuable clue to the character of the cyst. The clots within a hemorrhagic corpus luteal cyst may present a very bizarre image pattern with septic and solid areas. However, they are not vascularized. Color flow is noted in the cyst wall, but not in the interior of the cyst. Third, persistence of the cyst indicates that it is not a functional cyst, such as a follicular or corpus luteal cyst. When the sonographic findings are questionable, persistence of a cyst is the sine qua non criterion for the diagnosis of pathology.

Although most texts note that a functional cyst will disappear within 6 to 8 weeks, I have seen functional cysts that have persisted for 10 to 12 weeks before resolving spontaneously.

A cyst with findings suggestive of a significant potential of malignancy or neoplasm with or without abnormal bleeding, or persistent ovarian cysts, should be evaluated and treated using the appropriate surgical approach (see Ch. 7).

By far, the most common uterine cause of bleeding is a leiomyoma. Other uterine etiologies, such as sarcomas, are quite rare. Ultrasound can be particularly valuable in diagnosing smaller leiomyomas that are not appreciated during the pelvic examination, although those smaller than 1 cm may not be seen during the sonographic evaluation. Ultrasound may also be utilized to document the size of smaller leiomyomas and to evaluate their growth by serial evaluations in patients with minimal or no symptomatology and/or those selecting conservative therapy. Very rapid growth should raise suspicion of a sarcoma. In addition, growing leiomyomas in a young patient who wishes to preserve fertility should be removed. Subserosal leiomyomas are less often associated with abnormal bleeding than are submucosal tumors.

Adenomyosis may be associated with hypermenorrhagia. Bird et al[15] reported adenomycosis in 39 percent of 200 consecutive hysterectomies.[15] Adenomyosis is associated with leiomyomas in about half the cases. However, it is difficult to diagnose using ultrasound (see Ch. 5). Diffuse uterine enlargement may be noted, and occasionally the isolated specific dilated endometrial gland may be imaged within the myometrium. Diffuse uterine enlargement with thickening of the posterior wall in the absence of a leiomyoma is suggestive of adenomyosis.[16] Walsh et al[17] have reported a honeycomb appearance consisting of small cystic spaces 5 to 7 mm in diameter in one-third of patients with adenomyosis; however, others have not confirmed these findings.[18]

Endometrial lesions, such as an endometrial polyp or carcinoma, may be associated with abnormal bleeding. Endometrial polyps have been reported to account for 6.8 percent of all cases of menometrorrhagia in women aged 20 to 40.[19] I noted endometrial polyps in 4 percent of all bleeding patients, which represented 14 percent of anatomic causes of menometorrhagia (excluding PCOD).[1] Endometrial carcinomas account for about 10 percent of bleeding in postmenopausal patients (not on hormonal replacement therapy), but is a much less common cause of bleeding in premenopausal patients.

Syrop and Sahakian[20] have noted that polyps are often imaged as hyperechoic or mixed-density lesions and are best imaged during the late proliferative phase of the cycle.[20] They have also reported on the use of fluid contrast injected under sonographic guidance to visualize endometrial polyps. The presence of endometrial polyps was confirmed in all patients by hysteroscopy and histologically using their technique (see Ch. 17). Fedele et al[21] noted that polyps are often hyperechoic and are difficult to diagnose during the luteal phase of the cycle or when they are small because they are often obscured by the hyperechoic endometrium.

Endometrial hyperplasia may also be responsible for menometrorrhagia. In one report of 1,000 patients with bleeding 27 percent had hyperplasia.[22] Ultrasound findings are not specific for hyperplasia, but this condition may be suspected when a particularly thick endometrium is noted in a patient with menometrorrhagia. In a report by Smith et al[23] involving 51 premenopausal patients with irregular bleeding, abnormal histopathologic lesions were noted in 6 percent. An endometrial thickness of equal to or more than 8 mm was considered abnormal. Using this criterion, sonography had a sensitivity of 67 percent and a specificity of 75 percent in diagnosing endometrial pathology, with a positive and negative predictive value of 14 percent and 97 percent, respectively. Although these findings are interesting, a false-positive diagnosis in almost one-fourth of patients limits the value of endometrial thickness as the sole criterion for ultrasound diagnosis of pathology. In fact, Forrest et al[24] noted that the average thickness of the proliferative endometrium is 8.4 $\pm$ 2.2 mm.

A better approach to evaluating the endometrium in the premenopausal patient with menometrorrhagia is to recognize abnormal endometrial patterns as noted above, as well as endometrial thickness, with consideration of the clinical history. Endometrial thickness seems to be very reliable as a single criterion for the diagnosis of pathology in the postmenopausal patient with bleeding, but is much less reliable in the premenopausal patient. An endometrium thicker than 5 mm in the postmenopausal patient should undergo biopsy.

When used as the sole parameter for evaluation in the premenopausal bleeding patient, it is less clear what endometrial thickness would yield the best sensitivity and specificity for endometrial pathology. An endometrial thickness of 17 mm is almost always abnormal (with a negative pregnancy test) and generally warrants biopsy, and a thickness greater than 14 mm should begin to raise concerns for the potential of an abnormality. However, a prudent approach is to repeat the sonographic evaluation on days 3 to 6 after menses. If the patient is experiencing irregular bleeding to the extent that menses cannot be distinguished from the irregular bleeding, a repeat ultrasound can be done in 3 weeks. Again, persistence of a very thick endometrium warrants further investigation and generally biopsy (negative pregnancy test).

Treatment with a progestational agent, such as medroxyprogesterone acetate 10 mg for 10 days, generally controls bleeding in a patient with a thick endometrium and allows a repeat evaluation of the endometrium after completion of the progestin and withdrawal bleeding (chemical curettage). The patient with an estrogen primed and thicker endometrium is a particularly good candidate for progesterone therapy. However, biopsy is indicated in the older patient or any patient in whom a carcinoma is suspected or with an abnormally thick endometrium. Persistence of a thick endometrium after progestin withdrawal (a chemical curettage) warrants further evaluation, including an endometrial biopsy and/or hysteroscopy. Unfortunately there are still very limited data from control studies available on the nuances and vagaries in the application of transvaginal ultrasound to the patient experiencing menometrorrhagia (Table 11-4).

Table 11-4. Common Anatomic Causes of Menometrorrhagia

Ovarian functional cysts
Ovarian neoplasms
Ovarian malignancies
Uterine leiomyomas
Adenomyosis
Endometrial polyps
Endometrial hyperplasia
Endometrial carcinoma

Dysfunctional Uterine Bleeding

Dysfunctional uterine bleeding (DUB) has been defined as nonmenstrual bleeding from the uterine endometrium that is unrelated to anatomic lesions. DUB is the most common cause of menometrorrhagia. After excluding pregnancy, systemic disease, and drugs or exogenous hormones, most premenopausal patients with a normal pelvic examination are classified as having DUB. The diagnosis of DUB is not made in a definite or direct manner, but indirectly by excluding all other diagnoses. Therefore, DUB is a diagnosis of exclusion and is only as accurate as our ability to eliminate other etiologies of bleeding. Moreover, utilizing the current clinical approach without ultrasound, the diagnosis of DUB is inaccurate about one-third of the time. The reason that clinicians have not been aware of the inaccuracy of the diagnosis of DUB probably is that half of the undiagnosed anatomic lesions are small functional cysts that are self-limiting, resolve spontaneously, and often respond (at least in terms of control of the abnormal bleeding) to some of the same hormonal therapies that are used to treat DUB. In other words, we have frequently had the wrong diagnosis, but the right treatment. Those patients diagnosed as experiencing DUB who are bleeding from other anatomic etiologies will often continue to bleed, will eventually be evaluated by more invasive techniques, such as a D&C, laparoscopy, hysteroscopy or hysterectomy; and the correct diagnosis will finally be made.

Transvaginal ultrasound can be used to increase the accuracy of the diagnosis of DUB. The presence of a normal sonographic examination gives more assurance that the diagnosis of DUB is, in fact, correct. Yet, a clinician who is a diagnostic nihilist might legitimately say "Who cares," since the treatment works part of the time and the correct diagnosis is eventually made most of the time. In fact, a clinician may utilize a "blind" diagnostic approach to abnormal uterine bleeding and eventually "feel" (literally and figuratively) his or her way to a correct diagnosis of anatomic bleeding versus DUB most of the time. In retrospect, by necessity, this is exactly what we have been doing clinically in the past before the availability of transvaginal ultrasound. However, the sonographic evaluation allows a rapid, more accurate, and relatively noninvasive approach to differentiating anatomic bleeding from DUB.

In addition, sonographic evaluation of the endometrium can also provide data indirectly on the hormonal status of the patient and, of even more pragmatic value, can indicate to which hormonal treatment the patient is most likely to respond. In fact, since the bleeding is from the endometrium, knowledge of the status of the endometrium in terms of its thickness and character is probably at least as valuable as information regarding the hormonal status of the patient.

Although dysfunctional uterine bleeding has often been considered to be synonymous with anovulatory bleeding, Kempers[25] notes that 10 percent of menometrorrhagia in DUB patients is associated with ovulation. However, the clinical diagnosis of dysfunctional ovulatory bleeding is rarely made. Often, the ovulatory status of the patient and generally whether the DUB is associated with an anovulatory cycle or an ovulatory cycle can be determined by sonographically evaluating the endometrium and ovary.

In my study[1] utilizing ultrasound to evaluate patients with menometrorrhagia, 40 percent of the patients were experiencing DUB as compared to the 62 percent of patients who would have been diagnosed as experiencing DUB based on the usual clinical approach that uses the history and physical examination only. Anovulation was noted in 56 percent of DUB patients (22 percent of all bleeding patients), whereas ovulatory DUB was noted in 44 percent of patients (18 percent of all menometrorrhagia patients). The ovulatory status of patients was generally confirmed using serum progesterone and/or endometrial biopsies.[1]

Although a relatively small study (45 patients), its sample reflects an unselected population of nonpregnant patients in a general obstetrics and gynecology practice experiencing abnormal bleeding. Utilizing sonographic characterization of the endometrium as described above and discussed in detail in Chapter 6, five endometrial patterns were noted in patients with DUB. Each pattern is associated with a somewhat different hormonal stimulation/endometrial response and/or ovulatory status (Table 11-5).

Table 11-5. Sonographic Endometrial Patterns and Their Usual Hormonal Status and Treatment

Endometrial Pattern	*Hormonal Status*	*Treatment*
Single-line	Low E_2	Estrogen followed by progesterone
Three-line	Low, normal E_2	Progesterone
Atypical, poorly developed	Low, normal E_2	Progesterone
Hyperechoic	Normal E_2 and P	No treatment, ? biopsy
Hyperechoic thickened	May be associated with polyps, leiomyomas, or carcinoma	Biopsy indicated depending on the clinical situation
Absent endometrium	No endometrium imaged	Indicates an atrophic endometrium

DUB With a Single-Line Ultrasound Endometrial Pattern A single-line endometrium was associated with DUB in 39 percent of patients (Fig. 11-9). This pattern reflects either low serum estrogen levels or a lack of response by the endometrium to normal levels of estrogen and is generally associated with chronic anovulation. It can also be noted when all of the endometrium has been sloughed (as during normal menses) and is similar to the minimally stimulated endometrium noted in some patients with amenorrhea and in the postmenopausal patient.

The common denominator in all of these clinical conditions is the low estrogen level. This pattern was noted in about half of patients with anovulatory DUB. These patients generally do not respond to progesterone or progestational agent therapy, which is frequently utilized in the treatment of DUB. There is minimal endometrium present, and progesterone requires an estrogen-primed proliferative endometrium to be effective in controlling bleeding. Likewise, a D&C in this type of patient will be of little value since there is very little endometrium that can be removed. In fact, a D&C would subject the patient to high costs, anesthesia, and surgical risks, such as uterine perforation, with little diagnostic or therapeutic benefit. A D&C may even increase the possibility of the development of Asherman's syndrome since the thin endometrium will rapidly be removed and curettage of the remaining raw myometrial surface may lead to scar formation.

Office endometrial biopsy is less costly and less objectionable, but again is of minimal benefit in the presence of a thin single-line sonographic-imaged endometrium. It should probably be reserved for the case where documentation of the endometrial status is important or when there is some question regarding the sonographic diagnosis. These patients are best treated with estrogen followed by progesterone or an

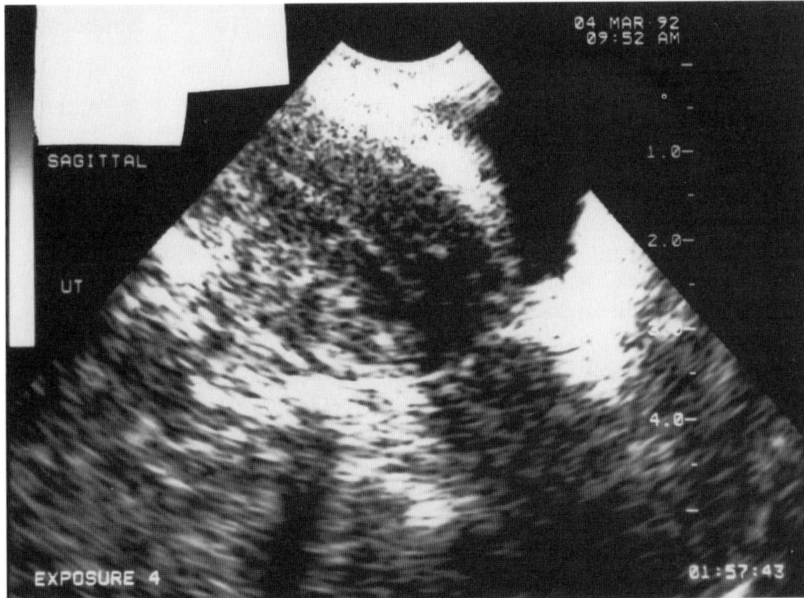

Fig. 11-9. Single-line endometrial pattern.

estrogen/progesterone combination (birth control pills).

DUB With a Three-Line Ultrasound Endometrial Pattern
A three-line endometrium was noted in 11 percent of bleeding patients (Fig. 11-10). This pattern indicates estrogen stimulation and an endometrial response. A normally developing follicle is generally not present in the ovary in a patient with DUB. (Multiple small immature follicles less than 10 mm should not be confused with the presence of a developing preovulatory follicle.) Bleeding with this type of endometrial pat-

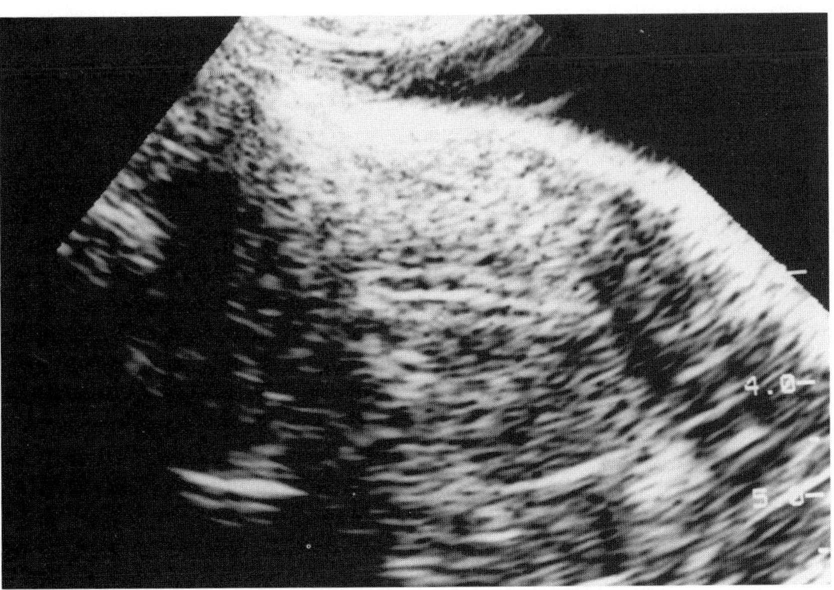

Fig. 11-10. Three-line endometrial pattern.

tern generally responds to progesterone therapy (with sonographic development of a hyperechoic endometrium) and to estrogen therapy if the dose is high enough. However, there is little advantage to increasing the thickness of an endometrium using estrogen that is already 8 to 10 mm thick. Estrogen stimulation with exogenous estrogen in the presence of an already estrogen-primed endometrium will only produce a heavier menses and/or clotting and possibly cramping and may increase the patient's concern regarding her menstrual bleeding problem.

If a developing preovulatory follicle is noted in the ovary that is an appropriate size for the endometrial thickness—for example, a 16-mm (diameter) follicle and a 8-mm three-line endometrium—this pattern can indicate a normally developing cycle in a patient who had been experiencing DUB, but that has spontaneously resolved with development of a normal cycle. A repeat sonographic evaluation will reveal continued follicular development with an increase in the diameter of the follicle (or disappearance of the follicle if ovulation occurs before the repeat sonographic evaluation). A clinical clue that may suggest this scenario would be the report by the patient that she had not experienced any bleeding in the week or so before the sonographic examination. Persistence of a "follicle" without a change in size suggests that the structure is not a normal follicle, but probably is a small functional cyst. A follicular cyst and bleeding may be associated with a three-line endometrium. It must be kept in mind that not only is the imaging technique a dynamic process but that also the anatomy and physiology being imaged may be changing rapidly. Therefore, clinical judgment, as well as knowledge of the physiologic and pathologic possibilities, must be utilized to interpret the sonographic findings properly.

Sometimes a definite diagnosis cannot be made based on a single sonographic evaluation, and a repeat scan will be necessary to correlate accurately the anatomic finding with the clinical problem. For example, two patients in my study who were ovulatory but with low serum progesterone had a three-line endometrium.[1] These patients were experiencing an inadequate luteal phase. In these cases the presence of a three-line sonographic endometrium that is associated with estrogen stimulation but not progesterone correctly reflected the physiology of the bleeding (an estrogen-stimulated endometrium but inadequate progesterone in the luteal phase), but possibly not the patients' ovulatory status.

DUB with an Atypical Poorly Developed Ultrasound Endometrial Pattern The third endometrial image type,

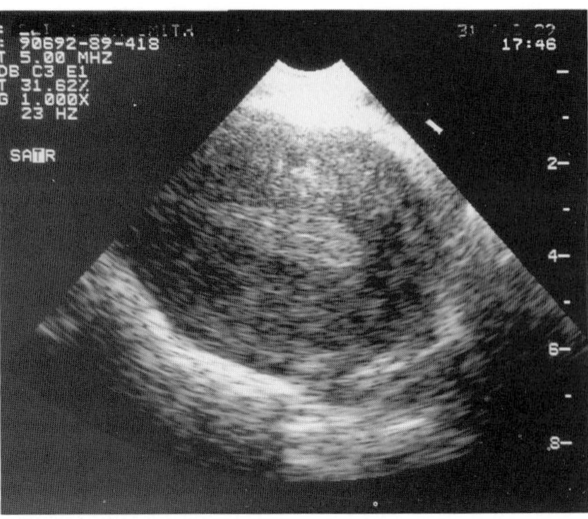

Fig. 11-11. Atypical poorly developed endometrial pattern. This type of pattern is frequently associated with chronic anovulation. This hyperechoic pattern is similar to a luteal phase endometrium, but is "washed out" and less hyperechoic than a well-developed luteal phase endometrium. There is persistence of the endometrial central echo of the endometrial cavity.

which was noted in 17 percent of patients experiencing anovulatory DUB, was an atypical poorly developed pattern. This pattern is characterized by a minimal hyperechoic or pale white endometrial image that is not as hyperechoic or "bright" white as the normal luteal phase endometrium. This pattern is often (but not always) thinner than the normal, well-developed luteal phase endometrium, and the central bright hyperechoic line representing the endometrial cavity is usually visible (Fig. 11-11). This pattern is generally associated with chronic anovulation and/or long term menometrorrhagia. It can also be associated with endometrial hyperplasia.

Office biopsy may be indicated depending on the endometrial thickness and clinical situation. Unfortunately, this pattern can be easily confused with the normal luteal phase endometrium by the novice sonographer. In the occasional case when it is not clear which type of endometrium is present, a serum progesterone, serial scans, endometrial biopsy, and/or the clinical history will generally lead to the appropriate diagnosis. These patients are best treated with a progestational agent to effect a chemical curettage. Some of these patients will have PCOD.

There seem to be significant clinical differences between patients experiencing anovulatory DUB and those experiencing ovulatory DUB. The average duration of bleeding in anovulatory patients was 3.8 months, and the average serum estradiol was 61 pg/ml, in contrast to 2.1 months and 101 pg/ml, respectively, in ovulatory patients.[1] The mean serum estradiol in anovulatory DUB patients was significantly lower than in ovulatory patients ($P = .047$). Therefore, ovulatory DUB tends to be of shorter duration, generally only extending through one to two cycles, and is associated with a significantly higher serum estrogen levels than is anovulatory DUB.

DUB With a Hyperechoic Ultrasound Endometrial Pattern Ovulatory DUB was associated with a typical hyperechoic luteal phase endometrium or a transitional endometrium—an endometrial pattern noted during transition from an estrogen-stimulated follicular (proliferative) endometrium to a luteal phase (secretory endometrium). Traditionally it was assumed that patients with ovulatory DUB were experiencing corpus luteal dysfunction of some type with inadequate or fluctuating estrogen or progesterone levels. However, the exact reason for the bleeding in these patients is a bit harder to discern since almost all of these patients had normal serum progesterone levels and/or a normal secretory endometrium histologically and a normal luteal phase endometrium sonographically. Perhaps, there were fluctuations in hormonal levels that were not detected. The best treatment approach in these patients is also not clear. Possibly, no treatment is necessary since the bleeding in most of these patients is of short duration and only involves one or two cycles. In patients with a very thick endometrium (especially older patients), an endometrial biopsy may be indicated to rule out hyperplasia or endometrial carcinoma (Fig. 11-12).

DUB With a Hyperechoic Thickened Ultrasound Endometrial Pattern A thickened hyperechoic endometrium may be associated with chronic anovulation and DUB. However, this type of endometrium may also be associated with a variety of organic pathologic conditions, such as endometrial carcinoma, endometrial polyps, or submucosal leiomyomas. It must be noted that different categories or classifications can blend together and are not always seen in a "pure form." For example, a patient may be bleeding from chronic anovulation, DUB, and have a thickened endometrium as noted above, with the development of atypia or even early endometrial carcinoma.

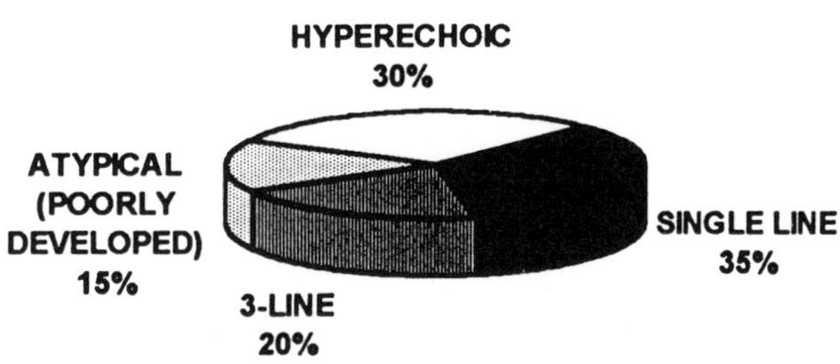

Fig. 11-12. Endometrial patterns in patients with DUB.

PCOD and Menometrorrhagia

As noted above, PCOD may be classified either as an anatomic associated problem, or if the endocrine features and anovulation status are considered the primary features of the syndrome, PCOD patients experiencing bleeding may also be regarded as experiencing anovulatory DUB. In fact, many patients with PCOD who are bleeding abnormally are clinically diagnosed as experiencing DUB. Viewed in this way, about half the patients in my study[1] were experiencing DUB, and in about two-thirds of patients the DUB was anovulatory. The diagnosis of PCOD can be based both on the ovarian enlargement and the increased number of immature follicles noted by ultrasound (see Ch. 18) and the clinical and endocrine findings. Patients with PCOD and menometrorrhagia most commonly have an atypical, poorly developed endometrial ultrasound pattern similar to that noted in some non-PCOD patients experiencing chronic anovulatory bleeding. Patients with PCOD have the longest duration of bleeding (average 7.1 months) compared to patients with ovulatory or anovulatory DUB, which is consistent with the more chronic nature of their hormonal (and anovulatory) dysfunction. The average serum estradiol in PCOD patients in my study was 66 pg/ml.[1]

In summary, transvaginal ultrasound may be of value in patients experiencing DUB by ruling out organic pelvic pathology that may be missed clinically and by confirming more accurately the diagnosis of DUB. It is also helpful in evaluating the endometrial pattern, the ovulatory or anovulatory status of the patient, and the possibility of PCOD. The endometrial pattern may also help suggest a rational approach to therapy, such as the case of estrogen in the anovulatory DUB patient with a thin atrophic endometrium (ultrasound single-line endometrial pattern) or progesterone in a patient with chronic atypical, poorly developed endometrial pattern or a three-line endometrial pattern, or the need for further evaluation in a patient with a thickened hyperechoic endometrium (endometrial biopsy).

REFERENCES

1. Dodson M: The use of transvaginal ultrasound in the diagnosis of the etiology of menometrorrhagia. J Reprod Med (in press)
2. ACOG Technical Bulletin: Amenorrhea. Number 128. May, 1989
3. Franks S: Primary and secondary amenorrhea. Br Med J 294:805, 1987
4. Bonilla-Musoles F, Simon C, Sampaio M, Pellicer A: An assessment of hysterosalpingosonography (HSSG) as a diagnostic tool for uterine cavity defects and tubal patency. J Clin Ultrasound 20:175, 1992
5. Morcos RN, Leonard MD, Smith M et al: Vaginosonographic measurement of endometrial thickness in the evaluation of amenorrhea. Fertil Steril 55:543, 1991
6. Pache TD, Vladimiroff JW, Hop WCJ, Fauser BC: How to discriminate between normal and polycystic ovaries: transvaginal US study. Radiology 183:421, 1992
7. Nesse R, Abnormal vaginal bleeding in perimenopausal women. Am Fam Physician 40:185, 1989
8. Stabile I, Campbell S, Grudzinskas JG: Ultrasonic assessment of complications during the first trimester of pregnancy. Lancet 2:1237, 1987
9. Mantoni M: Ultrasound signs in threatened abortion and their prognostic significance. Obstet Gynecol 65:471, 1985
10. Cashber KA, Christopher CR, Dysert GA: Spontaneous fetal loss after demonstration of a live fetus in the first trimester. Obstet Gynecol 70:827, 1987
11. Stein IF, Leventhal ML: Amenorrhea associated with bilateral polycystic ovaries. Am J Obstet Gynecol 29:181, 1935
12. Benjamin F, Seltzer VL: Excessive menstrual bleeding, menorrhagia, and dysfunctional uterine bleeding. p. 67. In Rosenwaks Z, Benjamin F, Stone M (eds): Gynecology: Principles and Practice. Macmillan, New York, 1987
13. Wall JA, Jacobs WM: Dysfunctional uterine bleeding in the premenopausal and menopausal years. Am J Obstet Gynecol 73:985, 1957
14. Jacobs WM, Lindley JE: Functional uterine bleeding. Am J Obstet Gynecol 71:1322, 1956
15. Bird CC, McEdlin TW, Manalo-Estrella P: The exclusive adenomyosis of the uterus-revised. Am J Obstet Gynecol 112:583, 1983
16. Bohlman ME, Ensor RE, Sanders RC: Sonographic findings in adenomyosis of the uterus. AJR 148:765, 1987
17. Walsh JW, Taylor KJW, Rosenfield AT: Gray-scale ultrasonography in the diagnosis of endometriosis and adenomyosis. AJR 132:87, 1979
18. Siedler D, Laing FC, Jeffrey RB, Wing VW: Uterine adenomyosis — a difficult sonographic diagnosis. J Ultrasound Med 6:345, 1987
19. Henricksen E: Causes of menometrorrhagia. Am J Obstet Gynecol 41:179, 1941
20. Syrop CH, Sahakian V: Transvaginal sonographic detection of endometrial polyps with fluid contrast augmentation. Obstet Gynecol 79:1041, 1992
21. Fedele L, Bianchi S, Dorta M et al: Transvaginal ultrasonography versus hysteroscopy in the diagnosis of uterine submucous myomas. Obstet Gynecol 77:745, 1991
22. Sutherland AM: Histology of the endometrium in "organic uterine bleeding." Lancet 2:742, 1950
23. Smith P, Bakos O, Heimer G, Ulmsten U: Transvaginal ultrasound for identifying endometrial abnormality. Acta Obstet Gynecol Scand 70:591, 1991
24. Forrest TS, Elyaderani MK, Muilenburg MI et al: Cyclic endometrial changes: US assessment with histologic correlation. Radiology 167:233, 1988
25. Kempers RD: Dysfunctional uterine bleeding. Gynecol Obstet 20:1, 1991

12

Other Clinical Problems

Melvin G. Dodson

CERVICAL INCOMPETENCE

Brown et al.[1] have found transvaginal ultrasound superior to transabdominal scanning for evaluating the cervix and lower uterine segments in pregnancy. Transabdominal ultrasound was adequate in 76 percent of patients compared with 83 percent using transvaginal scanning. For transvaginal scans, the transducer was placed 2.5 cm into the vagina with no contact with the cervix. The closed vaginal vault and vaginal fornix provided an adequate acoustic window. The accuracy of both transabdominal and transvaginal sonography in imaging the cervix decreased as gestational age advanced. Cervical length and cervical dilatation were measured as shown in Figure 12-1.

The internal os is located at the level where the uterine vessels can be readily seen lateral to the cervix. The normal lower uterine segment was noted to appear either as a Y configuration, a U or ballooning shape, or a funneling V shape (Fig. 12-2).[1] Ballooning or funneling may indicate an incompetent cervix.

The length of the cervix, its width at the internal os, and the degree of cervical dilatation can be measured (see Fig. 12-1). Changes in cervical length can be observed serially. In the first half of pregnancy, shortening of the cervix or dilatation of the internal cervical os may indicate an incompetent cervix. Later in pregnancy (20 to 36 weeks), cervical shortening and dilatation may herald premature labor.

INTRAUTERINE DEVICE LOCALIZATION AND/ OR PERFORATION

Intrauterine device (IUD) localization and/or perforation may be diagnosed using ultrasound. IUDs are imaged as a hyperechoic density with a shadow within the uterus (Figs. 12-3 and 12-4). Copper-containing IUDs may give a comet tail artifact.

GESTATIONAL TROPHOBLASTIC DISEASE

Gestational trophoblastic disease consists of three recognized pathologic entities: hydatidiform mole, chorioadenoma destruens or invasive mole, and choriocarcinoma.

The characteristic sonographic findings in hydatidiform moles are multiple small cysts, generally less than 15 mm in diameter, representing swollen hydropic villi. These cysts are uniformly distributed in the uterine cavity (Fig. 12-5). Earlier reports frequently described a snowstorm or snowflake appearance in the uterus resulting from multiple echoes from the small cysts of the swollen villi. With higher frequency ultrasound probes, the grapelike dilated villi can be visualized easily.

It is not uncommon for patients with hydatidiform mole to be anemic due to blood loss consistent with the vaginal bleeding noted and/or to iron deficiency secondary to the pregnancy. Anemia may also be caused by bleeding into the uterine cavity or rarely into the abdominal cavity in some cases of invasive moles. Ultrasound may be used to assess the presence of large collections of blood within the uterine or abdominal cavity.

Interestingly, impressive bleeding may be noted at the time of a suction curettage for a hydatidiform mole (even in the absence of any associated coagulation disorder, despite the fact that one of the characteristic histologic findings of a mole is the absence of

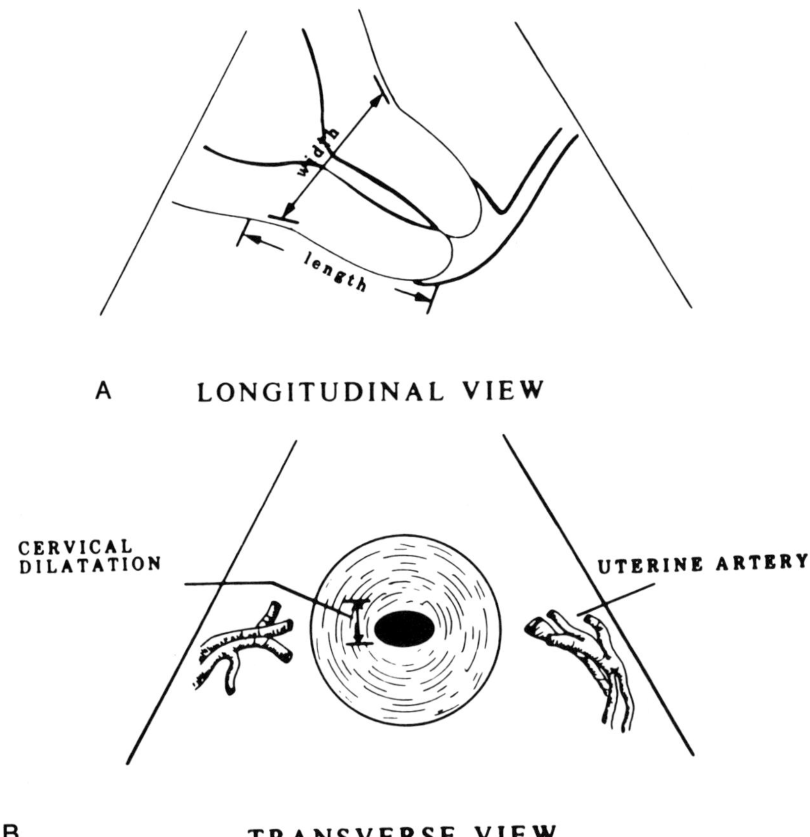

Fig. 12-1. (A) Points of measurement used to obtain the length and width of the cervix in the midline AP-pelvic view. Relationships of uterine arteries to the cervix are also indicated. (B) Cervical dilatation is measured in the trans-pelvic view. (From Brown et al,[1] with permission.)

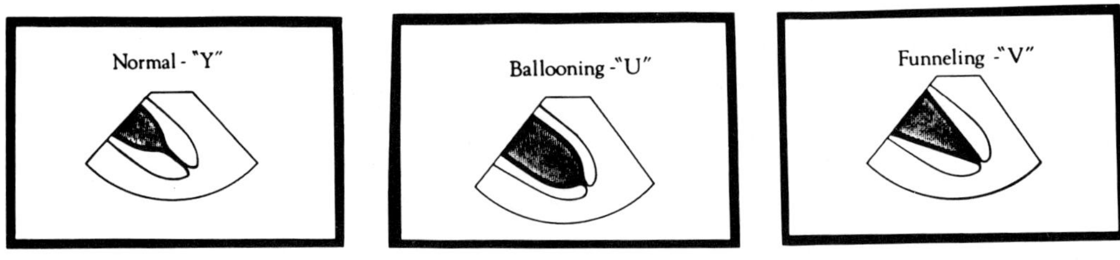

Fig. 12-2. Different configurations of the lower uterine segment. (From Brown et al,[1] with permission.)

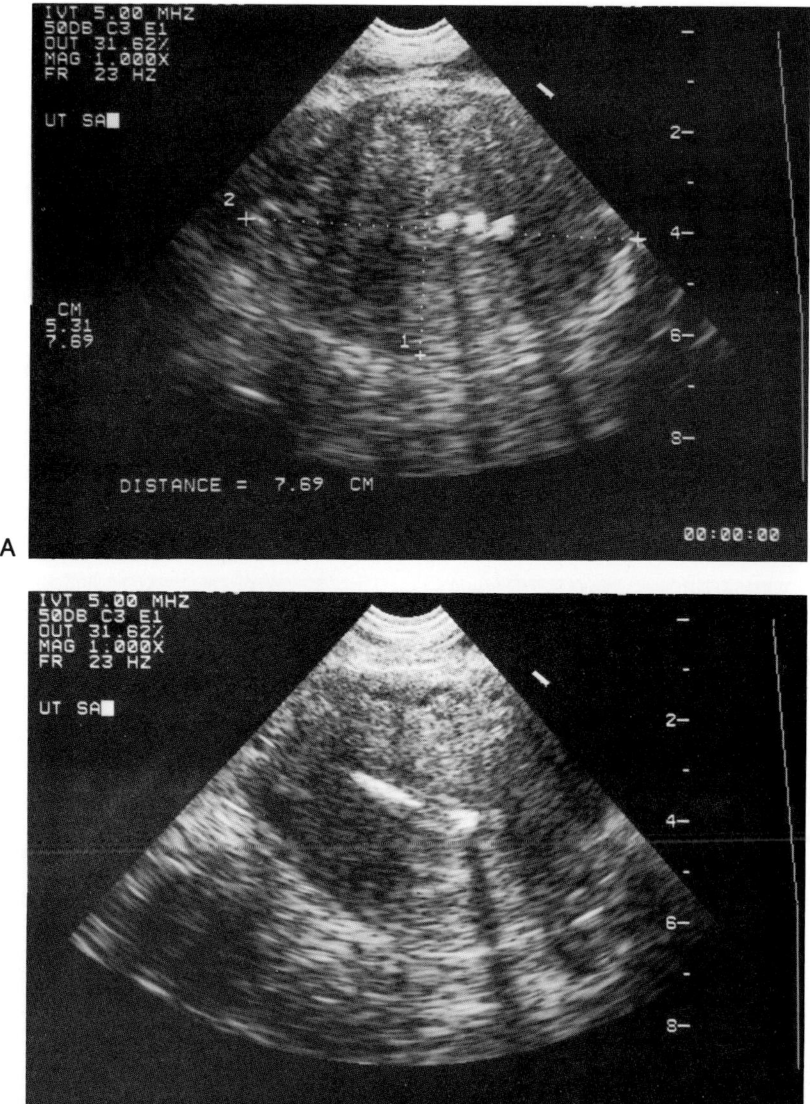

Fig. 12-3. Trans-pelvic (T-pelvic) (**A**) and anterior posterior-pelvic (AP-pelvic) (**B**) images of the uterus showing an IUD in place with shadowing.

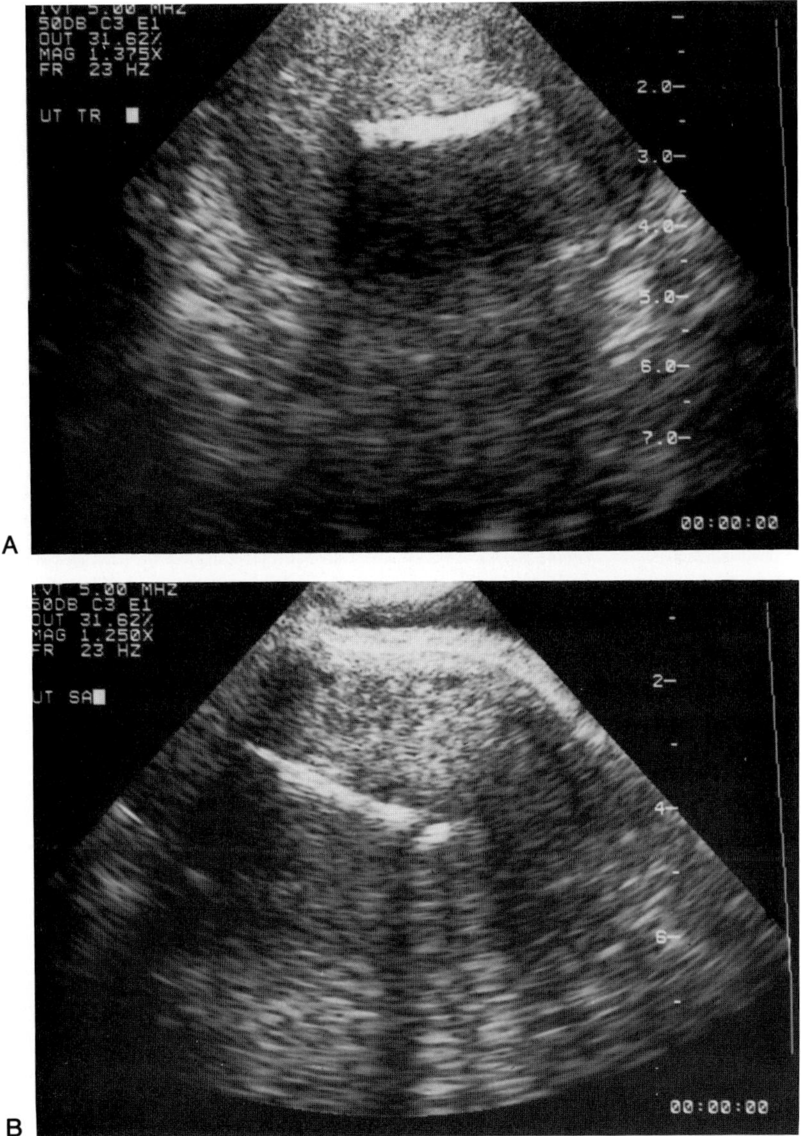

Fig. 12-4. (**A**) Patient with a lost IUD. No IUD string is visible at the cervical os. T-pelvic view of the uterus shows a hyperechoic IUD in the miduterus. (**B**) AP-pelvic view. The IUD is again noted to be positioned in the miduterus within the endometrial cavity.

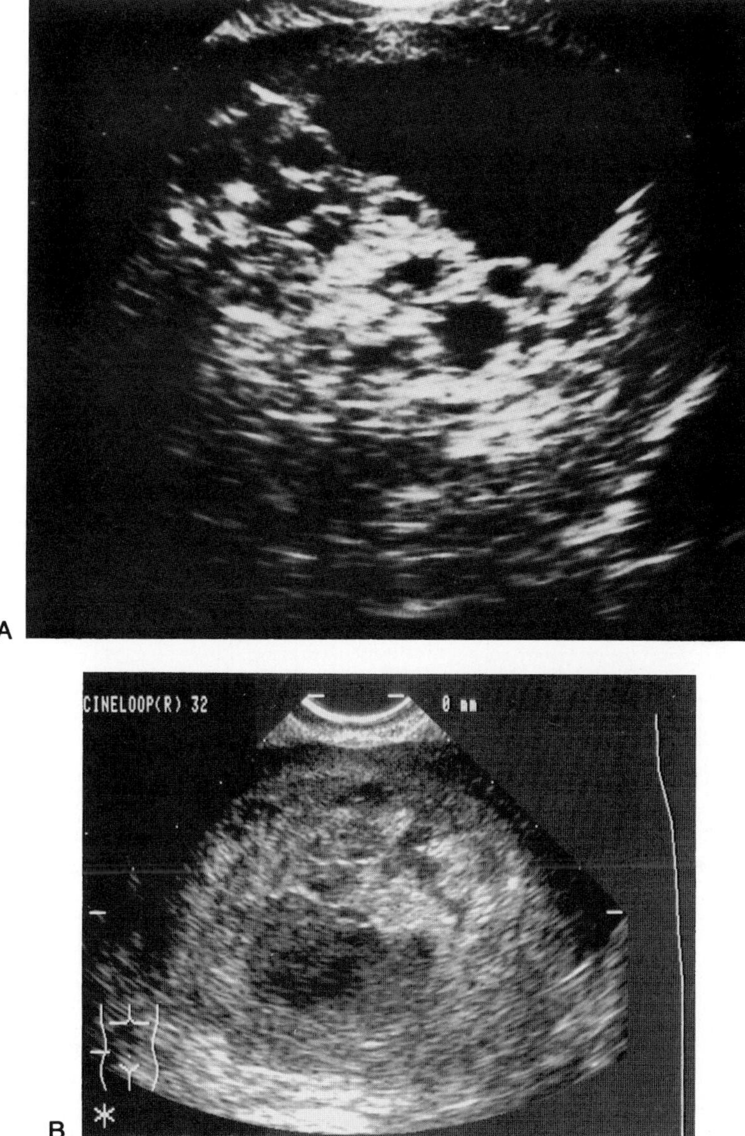

Fig. 12-5. **(A)** T-pelvic view showing a hydatidiform mole with multiple small grapelike vesicles and a large area of blood clot or fluid anteriorly. Note the thin uterine wall anteriorly. **(B)** Twenty-two-year-old white female with a complex mass of hyperechoic and anechoic echogenic material within the uterus. The quantitative B-hCG was 126,969. The patient was 8 weeks, 0 days pregnant by her last menstrual period. Area hyditiform moles may be difficult to diagnose before the characteristic grapelike vesicles can be imaged.

blood vessels to the dilated and cystic villi. I have always attributed this bleeding to the distended uterus and to the fact that oxytoxics are not utilized (to prevent trophoblast embolization) until a significant portion of the mole is removed and the uterus is allowed to contract. However, the last five cases of hydatidiform mole that I have imaged have each had a "high flow area" localized to a small area of the mole, generally, with several significantly dilated vascular structures that seem to represent a vascular pedicle. This vascular pedicle is easily imaged by ultrasound, and has not (to my knowledge) been previously reported. Although some of the bleeding may be due to a dilated uterus and uterine atony, it is clear that generally a significant vascular pedicle is associated with a hydatidiform mole, which can also contribute to the bleeding.

Early moles may not have well developed dilated villi and sonographically may resemble an incomplete abortion. Crade and Weber[2] have correctly diagnosed a mole at 9.5 weeks after conception; however, Woodward and Filly reported on three cases that were not diagnosed correctly in the first trimester utilizing transabdominal ultrasound.[2,3]

Transvaginal ultrasound may also be utilized to localize persistent trophoblastic tissue in the myometrium in patients whose quantitative β-hCG levels rise or persist after a D&C[4].

Theca-lutein cysts of the ovary are found in about 15 percent of cases. The cysts are multiloculated and can be easily imaged by sonography.

More recently, a partial or incomplete mole has been described by Vassilakos et al[5] and later by Szulman and Surti.[6] In the partial mole, fetal parts, membranes, or umbilical cord are often present and the hydropic villi are dispersed among normal villi. The partial mole seems to have less malignant potential than the complete or classic mole. The major ultrasonographic feature that differentiates these lesions is the presence of fetal parts and of recognized placental tissue. Partial moles may be diagnosed by the presence of hydatidiform changes, with swollen villi dispersed among normal placental tissue with a fetus present.[7] A fetus or fetal tissue is never present in a classic mole. The karyotype is generally triploidy. However, even a normal karyotype may be noted.

Hydropic changes have been reported in 20 to 40 percent of placentas from abortions.[8] Such hydropic

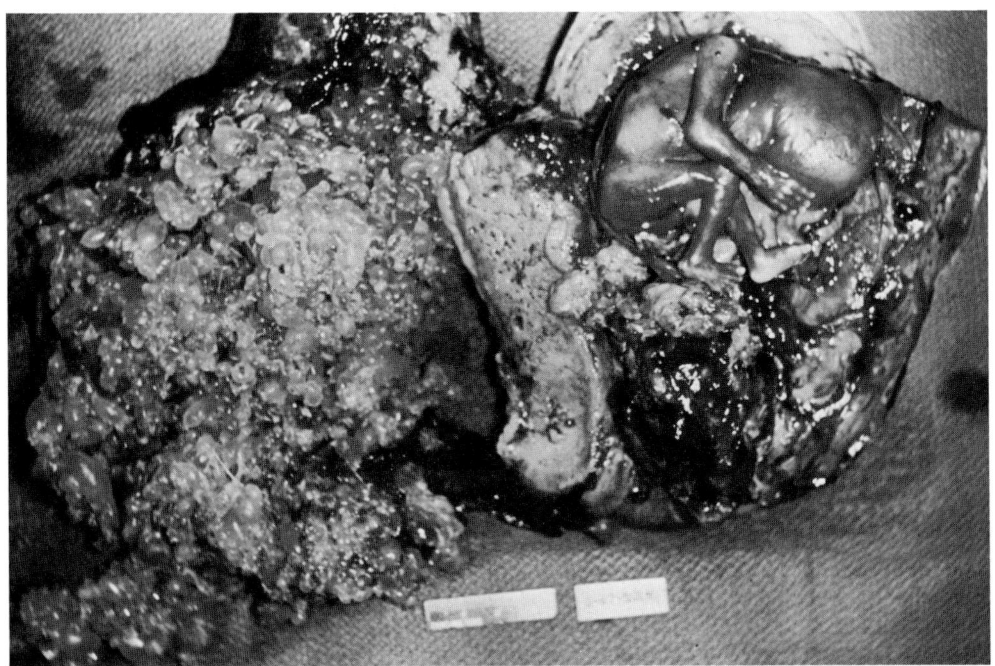

Fig. 12-6. Hydatidiform mole with normal twin in hysterectomy specimen. (Courtesy of Dr. Don Hall, Knoxville, TN.)

degeneration in an abortus may be differentiated from a classic mole by the presence of fetal parts and the inhomogeneous distribution of the cyst, but may be difficult to differentiate from a partial mole. If an area of noncystic placenta is noted, the diagnosis is a partial mole or hydropic degeneration of an abortus. Leiomyomas may also give the appearance of hydatidiform mole, but cyst areas are generally less than 5 mm. Classic hydatidiform mole may also occur in association with a normal "twin" fetus (Fig. 12-6). I have previously estimated a normal fetus-molar pregnancy to occur in about 1 in 10,000 to 1 in 100,000 pregnancies in the United States.[9] Twin hydatidiform mole-normal fetus pregnancies would be characterized by a normal fetus with an area of normal placenta adjacent to an area of grapelike cystic villi (classic mole).

ASHERMAN'S SYNDROME

Asherman's syndrome may occasionally be diagnosed using the transvaginal approach. The endometrium may be noted to have intrauterine irregularities.[10] Although Asherman's syndrome may occasionally be diagnosed or suspected by ultrasound, Asherman's is best diagnosed by hysterosalpingography or hysteroscopy.

ULTRASONOGRAPHY OF DISORDERS OF SEXUAL DEVELOPMENT

The sonographic findings in a variety of complete and incomplete forms of precocious puberty have been reported.[11] In *idiopathic premature thelarche*, defined as breast development before age 7, the ovarian and uterine sizes were comparable using sonography to those of age-matched controls. In children with *precocious puberty*, defined as signs of puberty before age 7 or menarche before age 8, the mean uterine and ovarian volumes were increased. Children with a chronologic age of 6.8 years with precocious puberty had a uterine volume of 11.4 cm^3 and an ovarian volume of 2.8 cm^3. By comparison, control children with a mean chronologic age of 6.7 years had a uterine volume of 2.4 cm^3 and an ovarian volume of 1.1 cm^3. Children with precocious puberty had a much greater number of small ovarian cysts (immature follicles) less than 9 mm in size. Children with *premature pubarche*, defined as pubic hair development before age 8, with no breast development, had ovarian and uterine volumes noted on ultrasound comparable to those of controls. In children with congenital adrenal hyperplasia, the ovarian and uterine volumes were similar to those of age-matched controls. However, the ovaries had more microcysts, and a few had larger cysts than those of normal children. Transabdominal ultrasonography is used in children.

PELVIC ADHESIONS

Pelvic adhesions cannot generally be visualized directly. Adhesions are suggested when the ovary is approximated to the uterus or lateral pelvic wall with no intervening space or when the uterus is deviated toward the pelvic wall. Sometimes the panoramic image obtained using transabdominal ultrasonography with movement of the uterus by the examiner's hand or sponge stick in the vagina allows a better appreciation that the ovary and uterus are adherent to one another. The ovary will be noted to remain adjacent and fixed to the uterus. Sometimes this can also be appreciated when the transvaginal probe tip is used to push or move the uterus or ovary and the ovary and uterus remain closely approximated. With significant adhesions the ovary will remain fixed to the uterus, and the ovary and uterus will move as a unit. No space can be created between them with dislocation of either organ. The knee-chest position and transvaginal sonography can also be used to evaluate the ovary-uterus complex for adhesions. Occasionally, when there is an increase in cul-de-sac fluid, ascites, or after the introduction of fluid in the pelvis, adhesions can be appreciated using sonography. However, despite suggestive evidence of potential adhesions, adhesions per se are rarely visualized.

REFERENCES

1. Brown JE, Thieme GA, Shah DM: Transabdominal and transvaginal endosonography: evaluation of the cervix and lower uterine segment in pregnancy. Am J Obstet Gynecol 155:721, 1986
2. Crade M, Weber PR. Appearance of molar pregnancy

9.5 weeks after conception. J Ultrasound Med. 10:473, 1991
3. Woodward RM, Filly RA, Callen PW. First trimester molar pregnancy: nonspecific ultrasonic appearance. Obstet Gynecol 3:55, 1980
4. Ansbacher R, Hopkins MP, Roberts JA, Randolph JF. Localization of trophoblastic disease with vaginal ultrasonography J Reprod Med. 35:835, 1990
5. Vassilakos P, Riotton G, Kajii T: Hydatidiform mole: two entities: a morphologic and cytogenetic study with some clinical considerations. Am J Obstet Gynecol 127:167, 1977
6. Szulman AE, Surti U: The syndromes of hydatidiform mole. I. Cytogenetic and morphologic correlations. Am J Obstet Gynecol 131:665, 1978
7. Feinberg RF, Lockwood CJ, Salafia C, Hobbins JC: Sonographic diagnosis of a pregnancy with a diffuse hydatidiform mole and coexistent 46,XX fetus: a case report. Obstet Gynecol 72:485, 1988
8. Reid MH, McGahan JP, Oi R: Sonographic evaluation of hydatidiform mole and its look-alikes. AJR 140:307, 1983
9. Dodson MG: New concepts and questions in gestational trophoblastic disease. J Reprod Med 28:741, 1983
10. Mendelson EB, Bohm-Velez M, Joseph N, Neiman HL: Gynecologic imaging: comparison of transabdominal and transvaginal sonography. Radiology 166:321, 1988
11. Salardi S, Orsini LF, Cacciari E et al: Pelvic ultrasonography in girls with precocious puberty, congenital adrenal hyperplasia, obesity, or hirsutism. J Pediatr 112:880, 1988

13

Early Pregnancy

Melvin G. Dodson
Michael Gast

Just 20 short years ago the intrauterine events of early gestation were a mystery to the medical community. The introduction of powerful transabdominal, and subsequently transvaginal sonographic technology, now allows us to both understand and aggressively manage obstetric problems in the first trimester of pregnancy. Assignment of the expected date of confinement (EDC), reassurance about the normalcy of early gestation, and diagnosis of multiple gestation are just a few of the currently routine first trimester uses of vaginal ultrasound.

Among the most challenging and time-consuming problems for the working gynecologist is that of the woman with a positive pregnancy test and vaginal bleeding in the first trimester. Normal pregnancy, spontaneous abortion, and ectopic pregnancy can all present in this fashion. High resolution vaginal ultrasound, when used appropriately by experienced examiners, is the cornerstone in the diagnosis and management of early pregnancy and its disorders. It has come to occupy a central role in the diagnosis of early pregnancy or postabortal vaginal bleeding, use of steroid replacement, early surgical and medical intervention in the ectopic gestation, and genetic study, as well as more unusual indications, such as selective reduction of multiple gestations.

To interpret ultrasonographic images of early pregnancy, it is important to appreciate some aspects of ovulation, fertilization, and early embryonic development that affect when gestational and embryonic developmental markers can be visualized.

OVULATION AND VARIABILITY IN THE TIMING OF FERTILIZATION

Assignment of the EDC and assessment of the normal progression of early pregnancies are important functions of the physician in early pregnancy. Dating of pregnancy and assignment of gestational age may be based on menstrual age (gestational age) or conceptual age (ovulation age). The implications of this process for the diagnoses of post-datism, prematurity, and preterm labor and the fact that assignment of EDC is most accurate when based on first and second trimester landmarks make it critical to assess gestational age carefully using not just one but several gestational landmarks.

Menstrual or gestational age is assigned by calculating the length of gestation from the first day of the last menstrual period (LMP). This method assumes a 28-day menstrual cycle or that ovulation/conception occurs about 14 days before the last normal menstrual flow. Utilizing this method, the duration of normal pregnancy is, on the average, 40 weeks (or 280 days). Menstrual dating is the standard clinical format in which the expected duration of pregnancy is described.

Conceptual age is computed from the estimated time of ovulation. This is the mode of pregnancy dating most commonly used by embryologists to describe developmental phenomena. Using this dating technique, pregnancy lasts a mean of 38 weeks. With the increasing use of artificial insemination, in vitro fertilization (IVF), and other assisted reproductive technologies (ARTs), the precise timing of fertilization is often known, therefore avoiding the modest inaccuracies of menstrual and conceptual dating.

The exact timing of ovulation is critical for many infertility therapies and can have a significant impact on when embryonic structures, such as a gestational sac, yolk sac, or fetus, or fetal cardiac activity can be expected to be imaged using ultrasound. In women with longer menstrual cycles or with frequent anovulatory cycles, ovulation may occur much later in the cycle than expected. For example, a patient with a

35-day menstrual cycle may not ovulate until day 21. Any delay in ovulation and subsequent fertilization will, of course, shift the interval from the LMP when developing embryonic structures would be expected to be imaged ultrasonographically. An anovulatory cycle with a missed menses followed by later ovulation and pregnancy can cause even greater discrepancies. In addition, the patient's recollection of the date of her LMP may be unreliable.

Other variables that may influence the imaging of developmental landmarks include variations in the timing of conception after ovulation. Sperm-oocyte fusion (fertilization) is thought to be possible over a 24-hour period after ovulation. Variations in the rate of embryo development could also potentially result in variations in the imaging of gestational development markers. In addition, the ultrasound equipment utilized and the experience of the sonographer can affect when a particular embryonic development marker will first be imaged. This is particularly true when comparing transabdominal and transvaginal images.

As a generalization, early gestational structures are seen about 1 week earlier using transvaginal ultrasound compared with the transabdominal technique. All these variations must be kept in mind when interpreting ultrasonographic images. The nonvisualization of an intrauterine pregnancy at 5 or even 6 weeks may simply reflect a pregnancy that is less developed than expected because ovulation occurred late in the cycle.

Since transvaginal ultrasonography now allows imaging of gestational sacs as small as 1 to 2 mm and a fetus as small as 2 mm, much if not most of the variability in the temporal sequence of when a particular gestational structure can be measured is due to the actual conception date and/or biologic variability, rather than limitations in the ultrasound imaging capability.

DEVELOPMENTAL LANDMARKS, GESTATIONAL AGE, AND THE LAST MENSTRUAL PERIOD

Although the LMP has classically been used for dating a pregnancy, as noted above, it is only reliable in patients with regular menstrual cycles and only in those patients who ovulated in midcycle. Ultrasound evaluation of fetal size using the crown-rump length (CRL) and gestational sac size; the presence or absence of developmental markers, such as the yolk sac and fetal cardiac activity; and biochemical markers, such as serum beta-human chorionic gonadotropin (hCG) levels and the hCG doubling time, give more objective and probably more reliable evidence of gestational age and normal development. The LMP is a reliable marker for gestational age in a normally developing pregnancy when it is in agreement with sonographic and/or biochemical markers, but may be misleading in the oligo-ovulatory patient or the patient with irregular periods. Therefore, an LMP that is in agreement with the sonographic estimate and hCG levels is reassuring and gives added significance to gestational dating. An LMP not in agreement with these other markers warrants close follow-up with serial evaluation until the gestational age and normal or abnormal status of the pregnancy are evident. Considerable caution must be exercised in using the LMP to determine when a gestational developmental marker should be imaged and in deciding that a pregnancy is abnormal based on the absence of a gestational developmental marker.

VISUALIZATION OF THE GESTATIONAL SAC

The very early morula enters the uterus about 3 days after fertilization.[1] Implantation occurs about 7.5 days after fertilization.[2] Dividing cells of the developing blastocyst separate into an inner cell mass and a single layer of trophoblasts surrounding the blastocyst cavity.[2-4] The embryo hatches from the zona pellucida 4 to 5 days postfertilization (PF), and the zygote attaches to the endometrium on about day 5 PF. The endometrium is generally invaded by day 7 PF. On day 8 PF the amniotic cavity begins to form, and the conceptus is only 0.1 mm. By day 10 PF, the conceptus is completely embedded in the endometrium. The cavity within the developing gestational complex and surrounding the fetus and yolk sac is called the extraembryonic coelom or chorionic cavity.

The chorionic cavity and surrounding trophoblastic shell can be imaged during the sonographic examination (Fig. 13-1).[3] The gestational sac is the first developmental marker that can be imaged. Although a gestational sac could generally be visualized by 6 weeks of gestation using transabdominal ultrasound[5], using transvaginal technology a gestational complex with a gestational sac of 1 to 2 mm has been imaged as early as 4 weeks 2 days from the LMP (Figs. 13-2 and

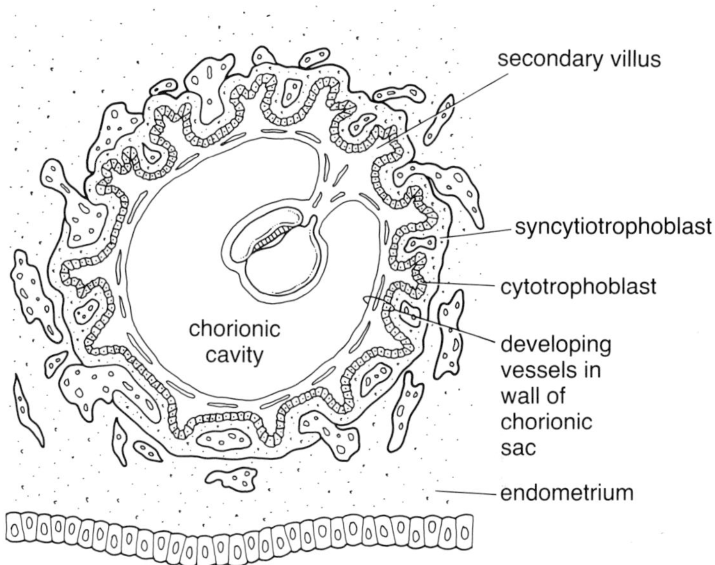

Fig. 13-1. Early development of chorionic villi and embryo, about day 16 (PF).

13-3).[6-8] By imaging very early gestations, Kawakami et al[9] have noted that implantation generally occurs on the ipsilateral uterine wall to the ovulating ovary. de Crespigny et al[6] noted that the gestational sac increased to 2 to 4 mm by 5.0 weeks and was 5 mm by 5.2 weeks. Bernaschek et al[7] also reported the gestational sac to be 5 mm by the fifth gestational week.

A gestational sac of 2-, 5-, 10-, 20-, and 25-mm diameter roughly corresponds to a pregnancy of about 4, 5, 6, 7, and 8 weeks from LMP, respectively (Table 13-1, Fig. 13-4).[7,10,11] The gestational sac volume increases from 1 ml at six weeks to 31 ml at 10 weeks and 100 ml at 13 weeks.[12] However, since the gestational sac is frequently irregular in shape and the

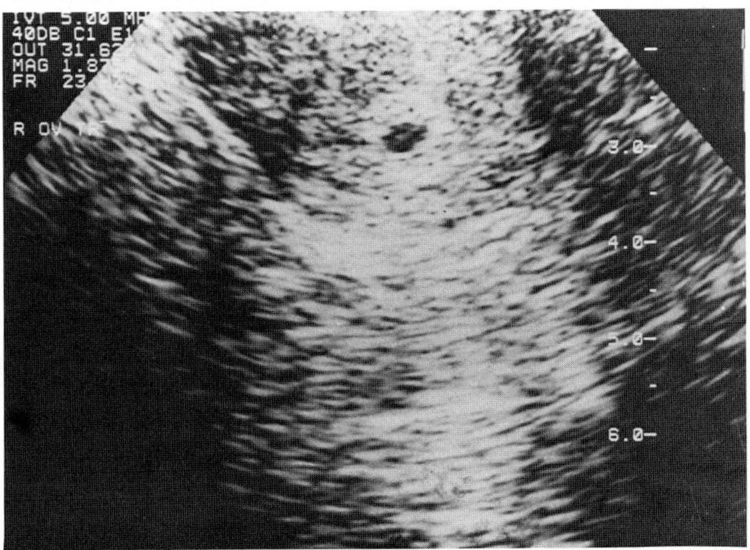

Fig. 13-2. T-pelvic scan of the uterus showing a 2-mm gestational sac at 4.5 weeks of gestation (from LMP). The serum hCG was 789 mIU/ml (2IS), and the progesterone was 42.9 ng/ml. A repeat scan 11 days later revealed a CRL of 7 mm or about 6.3 weeks with fetal cardiac activity present.

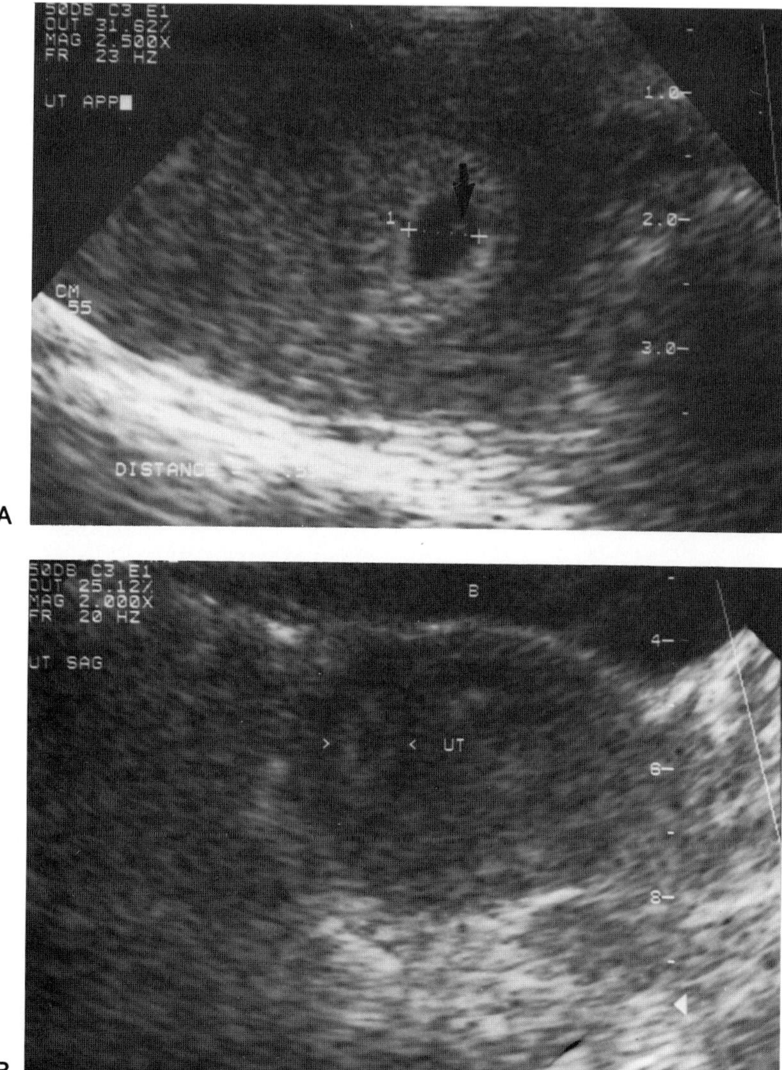

Fig. 13-3. **(A)** Transvaginal anterior posterior-pelvic (AP-pelvic) ultrasound of an early gestational sac 5.5 mm in size consistent with 5 weeks of gestation (from LMP) with a yolk sac present (above cursor line; see arrow). The DDS and good gestational reaction are present. A fetal pole and/or fetal heart activity was not noted. **(B)** Sagittal image of the same patient seen transabdominally. A gestational sac is evident, but the yolk sac is not visualized.

Table 13-1. Gestational Age from LMP with Approximate Sac Size, Gestational Developmental Markers, and Serum hCG

LMP[a]	*Gestational Sac Size (diameter, mm)*	*Gestational Markers*	*β-hCG (21S) (mIU/ml)*	*Range of β-hCG (mIU/ml)*
4 wks 2 days	2	Chorionic sac	141[7]	
5th wk[10]	5[10]	Yolk sac	1,932	1,026–3,636[11]
6th wk[10]	10[10]	Fetus/fetal heart	4,478	2,483–8,075[11]
7th wk[10]	20[10]	Fetal heart	24,060	12,820–45,130[11]

[a] Variations in menstrual cycle length, timing of ovulation, and conception must be considered when using LMP for estimation of when a gestational developmental marker should be imaged.
(Data from Nyberg et al,[10,11] and Bernaschek et al.[7])

method of evaluating the volume is complex, the use of gestational sac volumes is of less value than measurements of crown-rump length (CRL) in estimating gestational age. Robinson[12] has noted that at 12 weeks gestation, the gestational sac volume measurement gives a gestational age estimate with a range of ±9 days compared with ±4 days for the CRL. A quick method for estimating gestational age by sac size in the first 50 to 60 days of pregnancy is: age (day from LMP) = mean sac diameter (mm) + 30.[13]

Goldstein et al[14] noted that it is not always possible to image a very small sac in two planes at right angles. Although most early sacs are round, some are ellipsoid. Therefore, Goldstein et al[14] suggest that a single maximal sac diameter be utilized for measurement rather than using the sac volumes or mean sac diameter when the sac is irregular.

The rate of growth of the gestational sac can also be helpful in evaluating a pregnancy (Table 13-2).[10,15] In a normal pregnancy the sac increases by about 1.2 mm/day. Gestational sac growth in serial scans can be helpful in early diagnosis of an abnormal pregnancy that will eventually abort. Nyberg et al[10] reported that 20 percent of abnormal pregnancies showed no

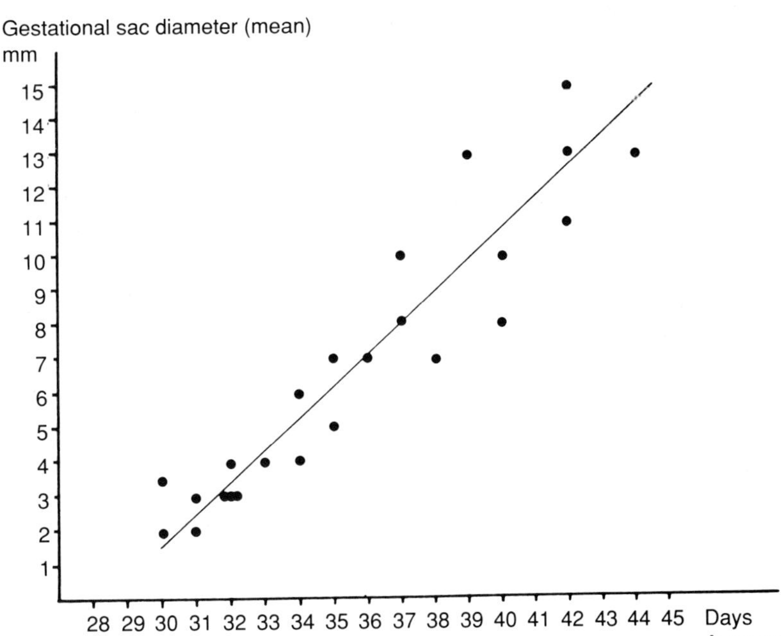

Fig. 13-4. Correlation between gestational sac diameter and LMP. (From Bernaschek et al,[7] with permission.)

Table 13-2. Gestational Sac Growth by Ultrasound

Growth Rate (mm/day)	*Author(s)*
Normal	
1.13[a] (range 0.71–1.75)	Nyberg et al.[10]
1.0	Piiroinen[52]
1.2[b]	Bernard and Cooperberg[15]
Abnormal	
<0.7	Nyberg et al.[10]

[a] From 5 to 11 weeks from LMP.
[b] Longitudinal study.
(Data from Nyberg et al,[10] Bernard and Cooperberg,[15] and Piiroinen[52])

growth of the gestational sac, whereas 53 percent showed growth of less than 0.7 mm/day. Normal growth was noted in 27 percent of abnormal pregnancies. No growth or growth of less than 0.7 mm/day is a poor prognostic sign. Bernard and Cooperberg[15] noted that about one-half of pregnancies without an embryo (blighted ovum) that eventually aborted still showed normal growth of the gestational sac (about 1.1 mm/day); (Table 13-3). Robinson[16] has suggested as a rule of thumb that failure of a gestational sac of 2.5-cm volume to increase in size by 75 percent in 1 week is highly suggestive of a blighted ovum.

THE DECIDUA-TROPHOBLAST REACTION

The quality of the trophoblastic and decidual reaction around the gestational sac can be used as an indicator of the development potential of the pregnancy. Blighted ova that will eventually abort tend to have poorer gestational reactions that may not be continuous around the sac. However, there is considerable variation, and the assessment of the gestational reaction as a prognostic indicator is subjective.[15]

Table 13-3. Gestational Sac Growth in Abnormal Pregnancies

No growth	20%
Abnormal growth (< 0.7 mm/day)	53%
Normal growth	27%

(Modified from Nyberg et al,[10] with permission.)

Double Decidual Sign

Early intrauterine structures are at best difficult to evaluate with precision. Differentiating between endometrial-derived structures, decidualized tissues, early trophoblast, and normal or abnormal early gestational sacs can be critical to the diagnosis of clinical problems in the first days postmenstrually. At 4 to 5 weeks, the endometrial cavity may still be visualized before the decidua capsularis becomes approximated with the decidua parietalis.[14] This anechoic area should not be mistaken for a subchorionic hemorrhage. Obliteration of the endometrial cavity by growth of the embryo produces the double decidual sign (DDS). Described by Nyberg et al[17] as a very early sign of intrauterine pregnancy, the DDS consists of two concentric rings surrounding the gestational sac.[18] The inner ring represents the decidua capsularis, chorionic villi, and chorion and surrounds an anechoic area that is the very early gestational sac; the outer ring represents the decidua parietalis (decidua vera). The anechoic ring between these two layers is the remnant of the obliterated uterine cavity (Figs. 13-5 and 13-6).[18]

Initially, the DDS was thought to be a reliable early sign of intrauterine pregnancy. Nyberg et al[18] had reported a DDS to be present in 98.3 percent of clinically confirmed intrauterine pregnancies. Only one ectopic pregnancy was reported among 60 patients (1.7 percent) with a DDS. Nineteen of 68 patients lacking a DDS were thought to be at risk for ectopic pregnancy. Four of these 19 patients were later noted to have a normal intrauterine pregnancy (21 percent), and 15 (79 percent) had an abnormal pregnancy that subsequently aborted or was terminated.

More recent data suggest that the DDS is a less reliable sign for differentiating an inevitable abortion or ectopic pregnancy from a normally developing pregnancy.[17] A DDS was noted in 92 percent of normal gestational sacs, but was also found in 63 percent of abnormal pregnancies that eventually aborted (compare Fig. 13-6 with Fig. 13-23). A DDS was also thought to be present in two of six (33 percent) ectopic pregnancies. In these cases, the DDS was apparently misdiagnosed as a pseudogestational sac. Therefore, the presence of a DDS, although suggestive of an intrauterine pregnancy and normal development, is certainly not diagnostic.

However, the absence of a DDS suggests a poor ultimate pregnancy prognosis. A patient at high risk for an ectopic pregnancy or with signs or symptoms of an ectopic pregnancy must be observed carefully even if a DDS is thought to be present. Since a true

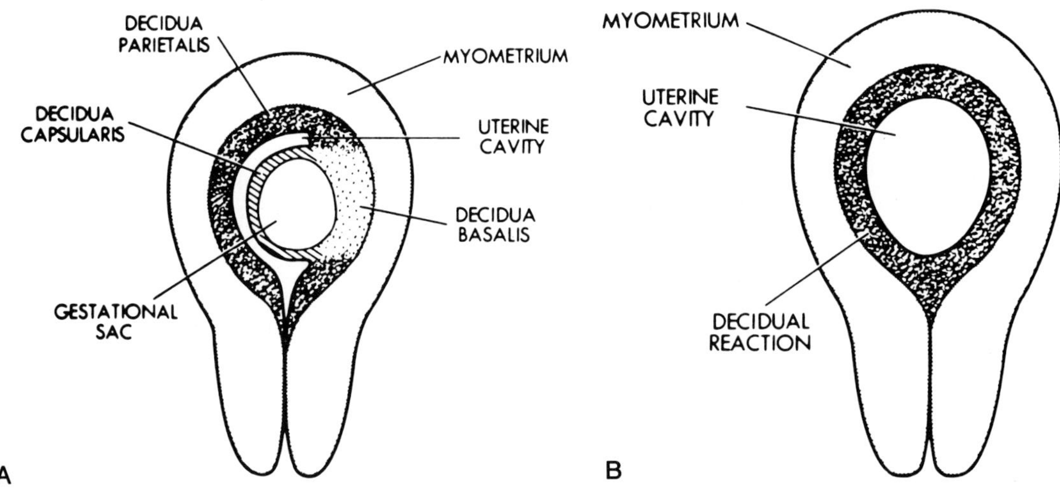

Fig. 13-5. Mechanism resulting in formation of the DDS. (**A**) Growth of an early intrauterine pregnancy after implantation into the endometrium results in the formation of a decidua capsularis overlying the gestational sac and the decidua parietalis separated by the uterine cavity. The decidua adjacent to and beneath the developing gestational sac is the decidua basalis. (**B**) Fluid or blood in the endometrial cavity or a pseudogestational sac associated with an ectopic pregnancy generally does not produce a double layer of decidua separated by an anechoic area representing the uterine cavity. (From Nyberg et al,[18] with permission.)

DDS results from the approximation of the decidua capsularis with the decidua parietalis, the presence of this ultrasound sign in an ectopic pregnancy is probably artifactual or a misdiagnosis, because there is no gestational sac to form a decidua capsularis. However, an alternative explanation for the appearance of a DDS in an ectopic pregnancy might be a subdecidual hemorrhage lifting up some of the decidua above the area of hemorrhage and clot and approximating the decidua from opposite walls of the uterine cavity.

THE ROLE OF THE YOLK SAC IN EARLY PREGNANCY SONOGRAPHY

The yolk sac is attached by a narrow stalk to the fetal umbilicus and floats freely in the chorionic sac (extraembryonic coelom). The yolk sac is initially much larger than the embryo and is the first structure that can be identified accurately within the gestational sac. In fact, during early embryonic development the yolk sac is part of a complex composed of the embryo, yolk sac, and amnion (Fig. 13-7).[2] The yolk sac lies outside the amnion and is connected to the fetus by the vitelline duct (Fig. 13-8). It has a characteristic sonographic appearance consisting of a bright ring-like structure with an internal anechoic area (Fig. 13-9). The yolk sac is visualized by week 5 or 6 of pregnancy from LMP and begins to disappear around week 10 of gestation. It is generally not seen after gestational week 12.[19] Measuring 3 to 8 mm in size, the yolk sac generally attains its greatest size in week 7 and averages about 5 mm in diameter.

The yolk sac is the earliest reliable sign of an intrauterine pregnancy. The presence of a normal yolk sac virtually eliminates the possibility that the gestational sac represents a pseudosac associated with an ectopic pregnancy. The rare exception is that in which an intrauterine pregnancy coexists with an ectopic pregnancy (called a heterotopic pregnancy), which occurs in only 1 of every 30,000 pregnancies.

A gestational sac larger than 20 mm in diameter with no yolk sac or fetus is a presumptive sign of a blighted ovum that will inevitably abort.[15,19,20] Serial sonograms showing disappearance of the yolk sac without growth of the gestational sac also suggest a poor prognosis.[19]

The presence of a yolk sac is not as reassuring in terms of an ultimate good prognosis for the pregnancy as the presence of fetal heart activity. The appearance of a normal yolk sac is associated with a 62 percent

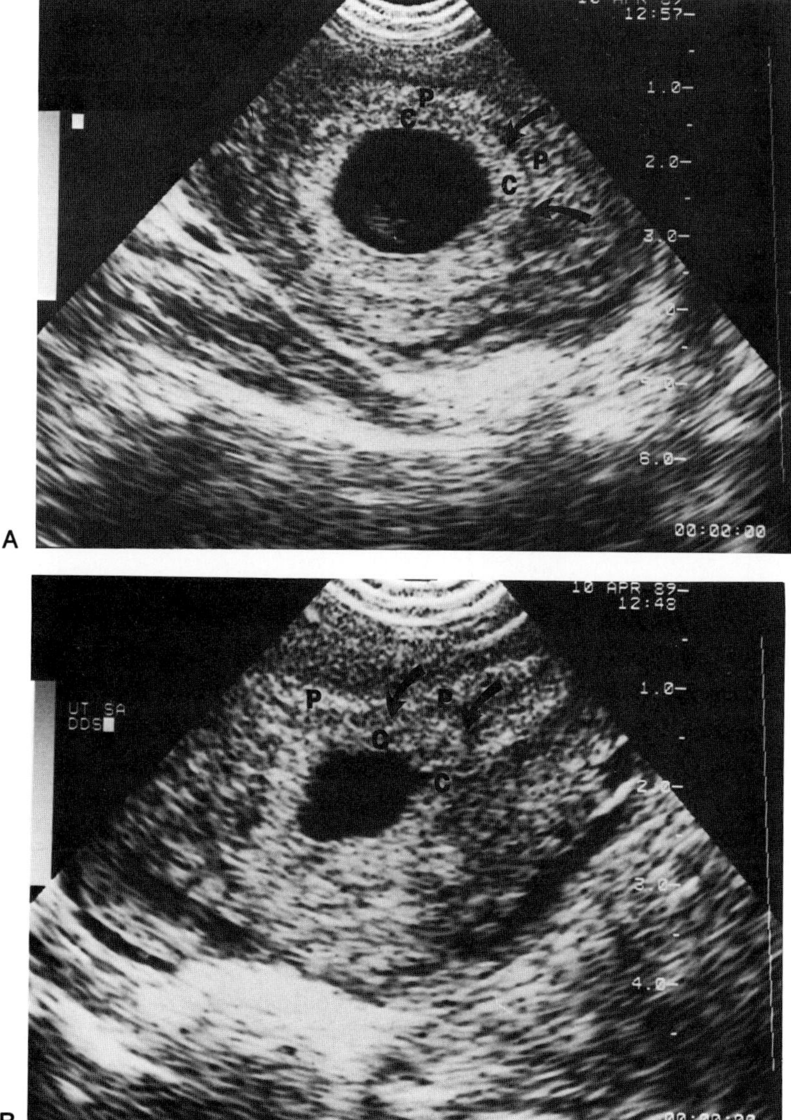

Fig. 13-6. **(A & B)** AP-pelvic views (in different planes) of the uterus with an intrauterine pregnancy at 7 weeks by CRL. Note DDS resulting from fusion of the decidua capsularis (c) with decidua parietalis (vera) (p). The uterine cavity (curved arrows) separates the decidua capsularis and parietalis.

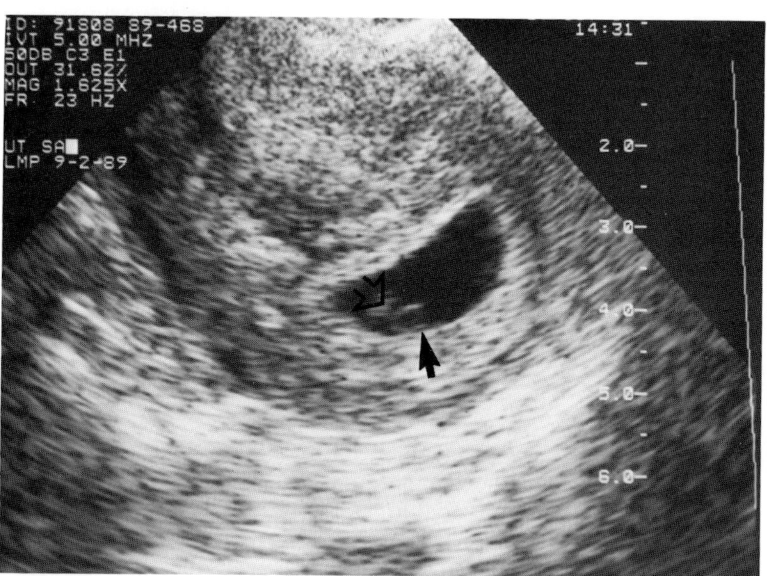

Fig. 13-7. AP-pelvic view of a gestational sac with yolk sac (arrow) and embryo (open arrow). The gestation was 6.5 weeks by LMP with an hCG of 31,380 mIU/ml and a serum progesterone of 36.1 ng/ml.

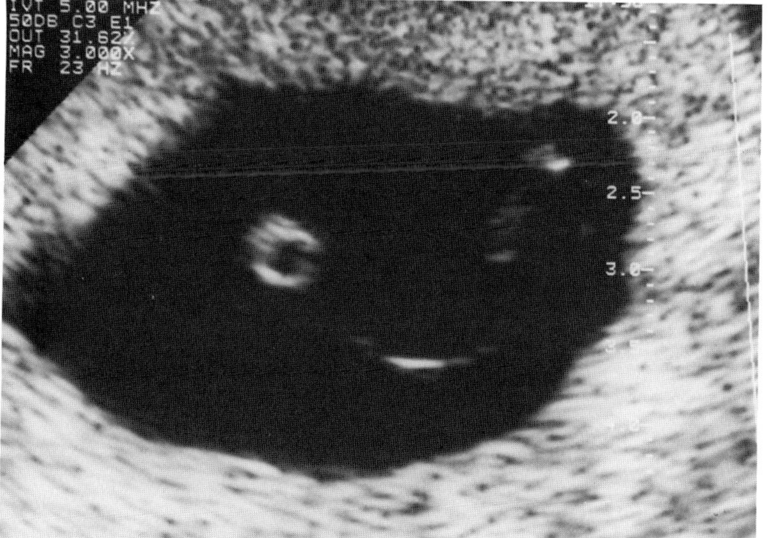

Fig. 13-8. Intrauterine pregnancy at 8.4 weeks by LMP with a gestational sac containing a yolk sac, amnion, and fetus. The yolk sac is outside the amnion. Only a small portion of the fetus is seen in this plane.

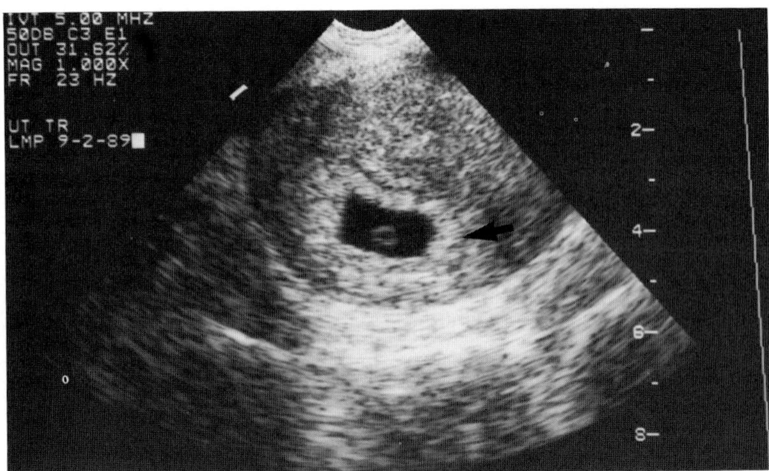

Fig. 13-9. Trans-pelvic (T-pelvic) view of a gestational sac (19 by 10 mm) with a 3.5-mm yolk sac. A well developed decidual reaction and a DDS (arrow points to the obliterated uterine cavity) are present.

incidence of a normal pregnancy.[17] In contrast, for pregnancies with an abnormal outcome, only 16 percent had a yolk sac visualized. Large or abnormal yolk sacs are also associated with a poor prognosis. Pregnancies with a yolk sac with a diameter larger than 10 mm are associated with a 92 percent abnormal outcome (Table 13-4).[21]

THE FETUS AND FETAL CARDIAC ACTIVITY

A fetal pole can often be seen when the fetus is 2 mm in size. The fetal pole can be recognized as a thickened area adjacent to the yolk sac (Fig. 13-10). Fetal cardiac activity can generally be noted almost as soon as the fetus can be recognized as a separate entity.[22] The identification of cardiac activity is particularly important, since about 97 percent of embryos with cardiac activity will progress to become viable babies.[23-25]

Fetal cardiac activity can generally be noted using a 3.5-MHz transabdominal sector transducer by menstrual days 41 to 43 (about 6 weeks of gestation) with a gestational sac of 8 to 16 mm and a CRL of 2 to 4 mm.[26] Early detection of fetal cardiac activity has continued to improve with the introduction of the transvaginal probe. A fetal heart beat should always be present in a normal developing embryo of 4 to 6 mm or at about 6.5 weeks from the LMP (Table 13-5) and as noted above can often be seen in a 2- or 3-mm fetus.

Table 13-4. Yolk Sac

First noted in gestational week 5
Confirms an intrauterine pregnancy
Size varies from 3-8 mm, average is 5 mm
Disappears by gestational week 12
Always present in a normal pregnancy with a 20-mm or greater gestational sac diameter
Large yolk sac (≥ 10 mm) associated with a poor prognosis

AMNION IN EARLY PREGNANCY

The amnion can be imaged as a separate sac in early pregnancy. In imaging performed during the first trimester, the amnion is often found to be detached from the chorion. The two membranes gradually fuse, but this process may extend until gestational week 14 (Fig. 13-11). In multiple gestations it is critical to assess the presence of single or multiple amnions (or discrete gestational sacs) as early as possible, as this task may be considerably more challenging late in gestation.

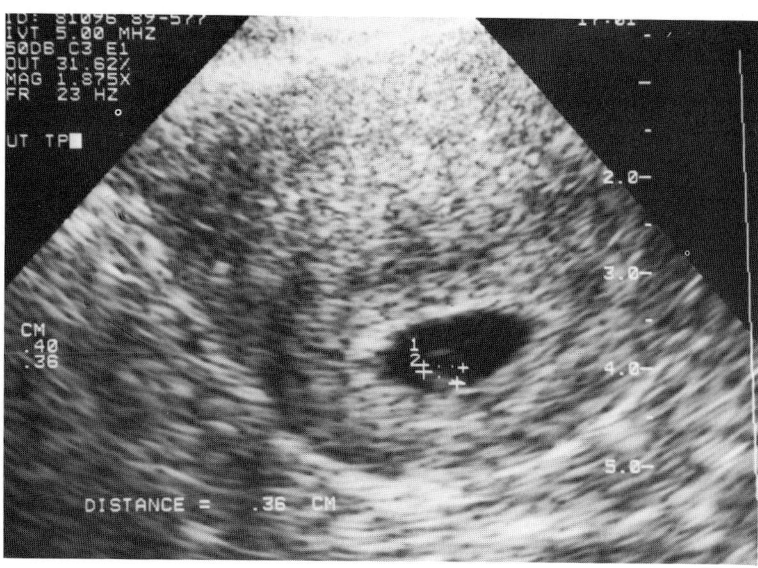

Fig. 13-10. A 20-year-old woman G5 P1 with a history of four previous abortions. The ultrasound examination was performed 6 weeks after her LMP. T-pelvic image of the uterus showing an intrauterine pregnancy with a 4-mm yolk sac (cursor line 1). The fetus measured 3.6 mm (cursor line 2). A fetal heartbeat was noted. Quantitative hCG was 9,842 mIU/ml (2IS). Anticardiolipin IgG and IgM antibody levels were normal. The pregnancy progressed normally.

ADJUNCTS TO EARLY PREGNANCY IMAGING: HUMAN CHORIONIC GONADOTROPIN

In the series of de Crespigny et al[6] of 28 early pregnancies, only three-fourths of the gestational sacs were visualized by 5 weeks 2 days using transvaginal ultrasound. Although ultrasound is not the primary technique for the very early diagnosis of pregnancy, it still allows a diagnosis of an unsuspected pregnancy in a patient in whom an hCG assay has not been performed. For example, pregnancy is occasionally diagnosed by ultrasound in a patient being scanned for an adnexal mass with a normal menstrual history. The mass may represent a corpus luteum cyst and the menses may result from implantation bleeding or may be a threatened abortion with early bleeding at the time of an expected period.

Serum quantitative hCG assays are more sensitive for detecting very early pregnancy than is ultrasound. Sensitive hCG assays can detect pregnancy as early as 8 to 12 days postconception. If conception occurs on day 15 of a 28-day cycle, pregnancy may be diagnosed as early as 5 days before a missed menstrual period. This type of early detection of circulating hCG is now standard in assisted reproductive technology (ART) programs and some infertility practices.

Table 13-5. Ultrasound in Early Pregnancy

Developmental Marker	*Comments*	*Gestational Age*	*Caution*
Gestational sac	May be seen at 1–2 mm size	4 wks, 2 days	May represent a pseudosac
Double decidual sign	Results from approximation of decidua capsularis with decidua vera	5th wk	Present in one-third ectopics, two-thirds abortions
Yolk sac	Confirm intrauterine pregnancy	5th wk	
Gestational sac > 20 mm	Yolk sac should be present	7th wk	No yolk sac—poor prognosis
Embryo	Confirms intrauterine pregnancy	6th wk	No embryo in a 25-mm sac—poor prognosis
Fetal heart	Confirms viability	6th wk	Abortion rate of only 3—7% if fetal heart present

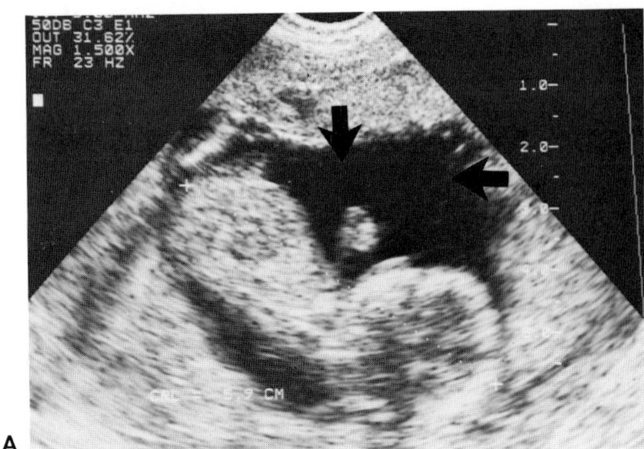

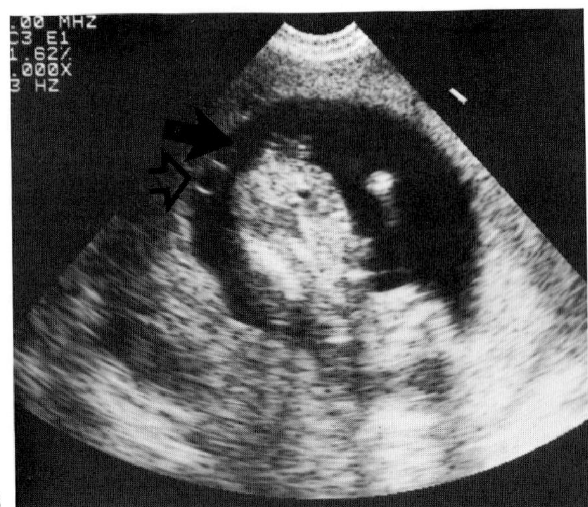

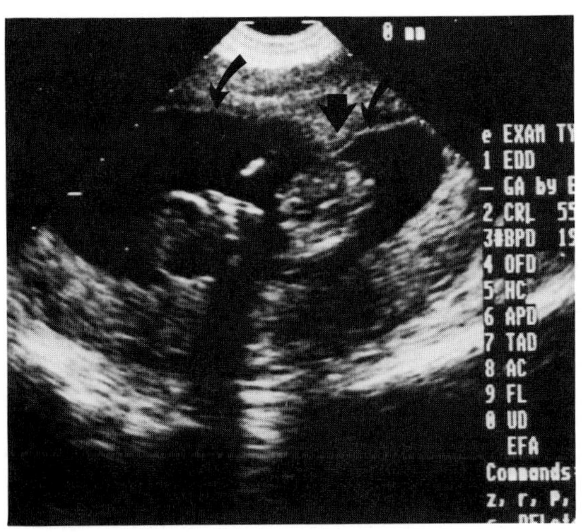

Fig. 13-11. A 27-year-old woman G3 P2. **(A)** A CRL of 5.9 cm correlating with a 12.2-week gestation. Note that amnion has not yet fused with chorion (arrows). **(B)** Same fetus in a different plane. The yolk sac (open arrow) can still be visualized outside of the amnion (arrow). **(C)** Twelve-week gestation showing amnion fusing with chorion (curved arrows). Note the placental cone formed from the chorionic frondosum (arrow).

With the increasing early use of sensitive hCG assays it is also possible to assess the true incidence of very early pregnancy loss. The "chemical pregnancy" is characterized by modest rises in serum hCG values, followed by a rapid return to nondetectable values. The use of ultrasound for diagnosis in these pregnancies is problematic. Administration of hCG as a therapeutic adjunct in ovulation induction regimens precludes serum hCG evaluation as a diagnostic test for early pregnancy until 17 to 18 days after hCG administration.

Qualitative urinary hCG testing has also become a common tool for detecting pregnancy. Home pregnancy testing ELISAs are available at nearly any pharmacy or general store. Office pregnancy test kits with sensitivities of 10 to 25 mIU/ml (Second International Standard [2IS]) now enable quick and reliable diagnosis of early pregnancy and are often used as a screening test before intrauterine office procedures and almost all surgical interventions in reproductive-aged women.

Human Chorionic Gonadotropin Standards

Quantitative serum hCG levels may be a helpful adjunct to vaginal sonography for gestational dating. When interpreting hCG levels, it is very important to

Table 13-6. Recognized hCG Standards

Second International Standard (2IS)
International Reference Preparation (IRP)
Third International Standard (3IS)

appreciate that there have been two commonly used standards for hCG: (1) the Second International Standard (2IS); and (2) the International Reference Preparation (IRP). The IRP is purer and roughly twice as sensitive as the 2IS (actually, 1 mIU/ml 2IS = 2.2 mIU/ml IRP).[7] Therefore, hCG levels of 6,000 to 6,500 using the IRP are equivalent to about 3,000 to 3,250 mIU/ml using the 2IS. This has caused some confusion in the literature regarding the serum hCG levels at which a gestational sac should first be visualized in the uterine cavity using sonography. Recently, the Third International Standard (3IS) has been introduced. The 3IS is equivalent to the IRP and is therefore also twice the 2IS (Tables 13-6 and 13-7). Sonographers interested in the subject should be wary of the literature in this area in terms of hCG standards used. However, despite some of the confusion, the concept of using serum hCG levels as criteria for gestational dating or as a guide for when gestational markers should normally be visualized by ultrasound is quite valid.

Human Chorionic Gonadotropin Discriminatory Zone

The hCG level at which an intrauterine gestational sac should be visualized becomes important in the diagnosis of an ectopic pregnancy or an abnormal pregnancy that will eventually abort. The concept of a discriminatory hCG zone when an intrauterine gestational sac should be imaged using ultrasound is helpful in differentiating patients with inevitable abortions or ectopic pregnancies from patients with normal intrauterine pregnancies. The original description of the hCG level at which an intrauterine pregnancy should be imaged within the uterus (discriminatory zone) was reported by Kadar et al.[27] A serum hCG level of 6,500 mIU/ml (IRP standard) was suggested as the hCG level above which a gestational sac should be visualized in the uterus. Because of the use of the 2IS and the widespread availability of 5- and 7-mHz vaginal transducers, the level of serum hCG that defines the discriminatory zone below which an intrauterine gestational sac should be imaged has continued to decrease since the concept was first introduced by Kadar et al[27] in 1981. Bernaschek et al[7] reported a 2-mm gestational sac at 4 weeks 2 days with a beta-hCG level of only 141 mIU/ml (2IS). However, only two of eight pregnancies in their series were sonographically imaged with beta-hCG levels between 50 and 280 mIU/ml. In all pregnancies with serum beta-hCG levels greater than 300 mIU/ml, a gestational sac was identified (Fig. 13-12). Clinical experience, however, using very low discriminatory zones (300 mIU/ml) is still quite limited.

We feel that an hCG level above 750 mIU/ml (2IS) or 1,500 mIU/ml (IRP) is currently the discriminatory zone at which an intrauterine gestational sac should be imaged in a normal pregnancy by experienced sonographers using transvaginal ultrasound. Lack of visualization of a gestational sac in pregnancy with hCG levels above 750 to 1000 mIU/ml (2IS) on such an examination makes these pregnancies suspicious for extrauterine gestation. A patient with a beta-hCG level of greater than 300 mIU/ml in whom a gestational sac cannot be imaged using transvaginal ultrasound should be rescanned in 2 to 3 days and the serum hCG level repeated. Since in a normal pregnancy the hCG doubles every 2.2 days, a repeat scan after 2 to 3 days should allow visualization of a distinct intrauterine gestational sac.[7]

Failure to visualize the gestational sac or failure of the beta-hCG level to double suggests an abnormal pregnancy, either an inevitable abortion or ectopic pregnancy. Significant decreases in hCG levels suggest an inevitable abortion. Twins may have a higher hCG level for a given gestational age.

In patients desiring to maintain a pregnancy, in the pregnant infertility patient, or when the transvaginal sonography is done by a physician with limited experience, it is prudent to do a repeat evaluation to ensure the correct diagnosis before recommending a dilatation and curettage unless the patient's clinical conditions (vaginal bleeding and/or pain) warrant immediate intervention. In the asymptomatic patient who desires to maintain a pregnancy there is little

Table 13-7. Relationship of hCG Reference Preparation

IRP = 3IS
2IS = IRP/2
2IS = 3IS/2

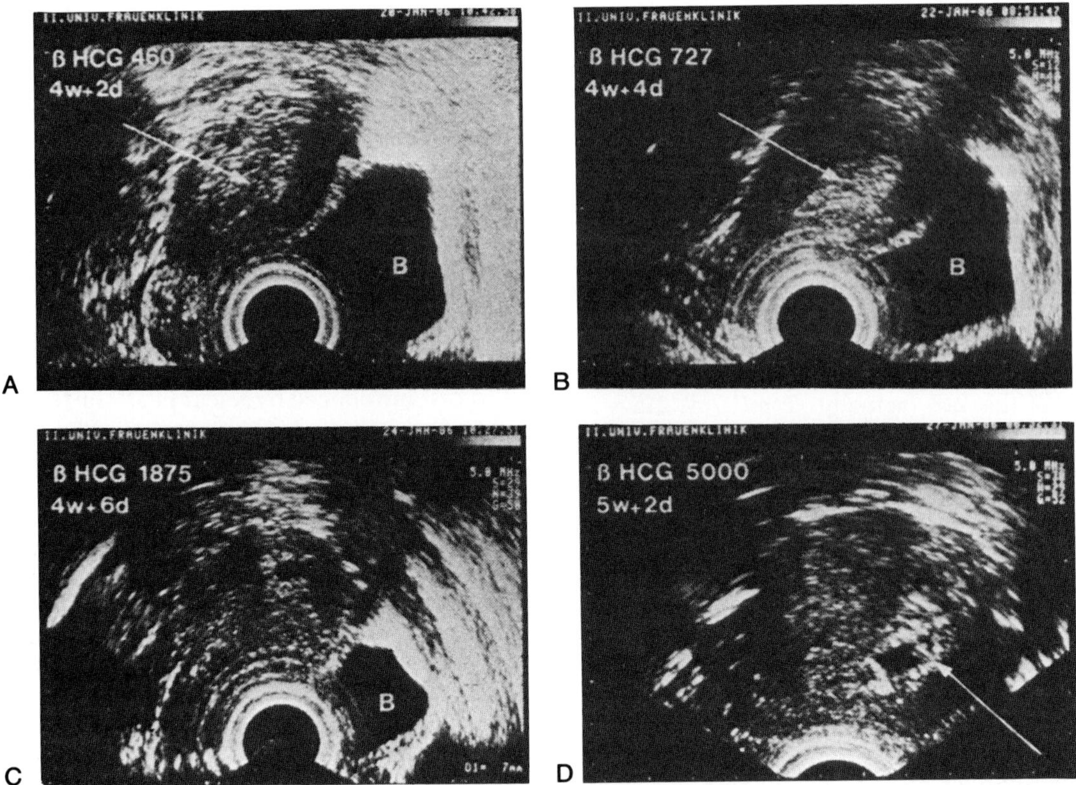

Fig. 13-12. (**A-D**) Four vaginosonographic examinations in the same patient over 7 days demonstrating the growth of the gestational sac. The corresponding beta-hCG values are shown in the upper left corner. Note the first appearance of the fetal pole (arrow) in panel D. B, bladder. (From Bernaschek et al,[7] with permission.)

clinical benefit to performing a D & C for an inevitable abortion based on a single ultrasound and beta-hCG assessment if there is any question regarding the diagnosis. A clear exception is the patient with clinical or ultrasound findings suggestive of an ectopic pregnancy (see Ch. 15).

Although the visualization of an intrauterine gestational sac (especially if a yolk sac is present) confirms an intrauterine pregnancy (Table 13-8), the presence of a complex adnexal mass (noncorpus luteum) imaged on ultrasound suggests an ectopic pregnancy. An adnexal mass is noted in about 80 percent of patients with an ectopic pregnancy.[28] The major confounding finding in these cases is the presence of a corpus luteum. Found in 80 percent or more of early pregnancies, the corpus luteum can appear in many forms, from a sonolucent follicular appearing structure to that of a solid or stippled spherical structure. When in doubt about the nature of an adnexal mass in early gestation, it is best to take a conservative approach to management. Laparoscopy will inevitably confirm the nature of the mass.

Gestational Sac Size and Serum hCG Levels

The relationship between hCG and gestational sac size has been reported by Goldstein et al (Fig. 13-13).[14] They noted that the serum hCG level (using the IRP) increases proportionally with gestation sac diameter from 1,000 mIU/ml at 0.5 cm (about 455 mIU, 2IS) to 6,000 mIU/ml at 1.0 cm (about 2,727 mIU, 2IS). A gestational sac of 0.5-cm diameter corresponds to about 5 weeks of gestation from the LMP. All pregnancies with gestational sacs of 1.0 cm or greater diameter had hCG levels of 6,000 mIU/ml (IRP) or greater. A gestational sac size of 1.0 cm corresponds to a 6-week gestation (Table 13-1).

Table 13-8. Management of Early Pregnancy Using hCG and Transvaginal Ultrasound

hCG mIU/ml (2IS)	Ultrasound	Treatment
<750	No intrauterine sac No adnexal mass	Repeat hCG and ultrasound in 2 days
>750	No intrauterine sac Suspicious adnexal mass	Laparoscopy Rule out ectopic pregnancy
>750	No intrauterine sac No adnexal mass No cul-de-sac fluid	Repeat hCG and ultrasound in 2 days (A) Falling hCG Diagnosis: Incomplete abortion Treatment: Dilatation and curettage (B) Rising hCG Treatment: Laparoscopy Rule out ectopic

These data are reasonably consistent with those of Nyberg et al using the 2IS.[11] Bernaschek et al reported that the correlation of serum hCG and sac size fell closely between the visualization zones of these two workers (Table 13-1).[7] Goldstein et al's lower hCG levels for smaller gestational sac diameters may have resulted from the fact that sac diameter was measured using transvaginal ultrasound in their series,[14] whereas transabdominal ultrasound was used by Nyberg et al.[11] Transabdominal sonography would be less sensitive and probably less accurate, especially for very small diameter sacs.

Goldstein et al,[14] using transvaginal real-time sector scanning, were able to visualize a gestational sac in 98 percent of 197 very early intrauterine pregnancies. There were no false-positives. In the three patients in whom a sac could not be visualized, two had leiomyomas and one had a coexisting intrauterine device (IUD). A gestational sac of 4 mm could always be imaged in their series when the hCG levels were greater than 1,025 mIU/ML (IRP) (about 466 mIU/ml [2IS]), provided that the uterus was normal (no fibroids).

Nyberg et al[13] used the 2IS for hCG and visualized an intrauterine gestational sac in all of their 36 patients when the hCG levels were above 1,000 mIU/ml. Nyberg et al[11,13] have emphasized the importance of using the gestational sac size for any given hCG level to differentiate between normal and abnormal pregnancies.

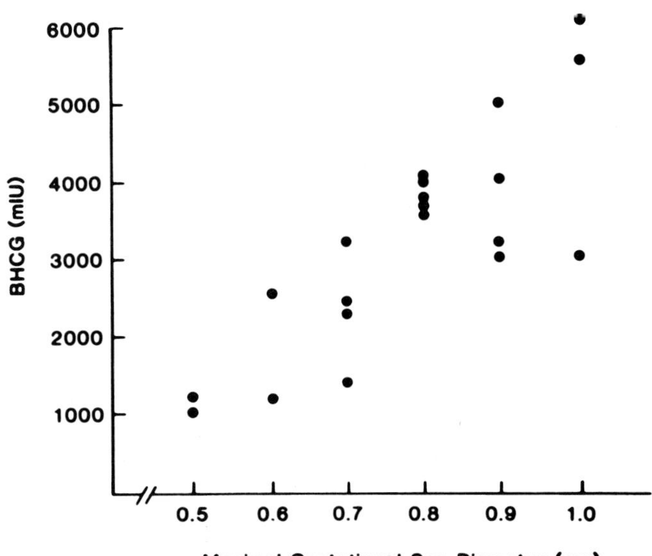

Fig. 13-13. hCG levels (mIU/ml [IRP]) as a function of maximal gestational sac diameter in 20 cases. (From Goldstein et al,[14] with permission.)

SAC SIZE AND FETAL CARDIAC ACTIVITY

Batzer et al,[5] using transabdominal ultrasound, detected fetal heart activity in 100 percent of pregnancies when the gestational sac mean diameter was greater than 30 mm. In 95 percent of pregnancies in this series fetal cardiac activity was detected by the end of gestational week 7 (LMP). This series eliminated some of the uncertainties in dating a pregnancy resulting from variations in menstrual cycle length and timing of ovulation by using the basal body temperature (BBT) nadir as the criterion of ovulation. The studies of Batzer et al,[5] although well done, used transabdominal ultrasound, and the smallest gestational sac noted was 8 mm at 21 days after ovulation. This is about 5 days later than reports of very early gestational sacs of 2-mm diameter using transvaginal ultrasound that can be visualized as early as day 30 from the LMP (Fig. 13-14).

Using high resolution vaginal imaging, Fossum et al[29] detected fetal heart motion between 40 to 50 days post-LMP and at 10,000-15,000 mIU/ml serum hCG concentration (2IS). Martin et al[30] also demonstrated cardiac activity between 5.5 to 7.5 weeks of gestation and at hCG values as low as 4500 mIU/ml. Timor-Trisch et al[31] have stated that failure to visualize fetal heart motion by 6.5 menstrual weeks of gestation is a poor prognostic sign. Batzer et al[32] have subsequently redefined their transabdominal and transvaginal landmarks of early pregnancy. They noted that in 95 percent of early pregnancies studied, the first appearance of the gestational sac was at 24

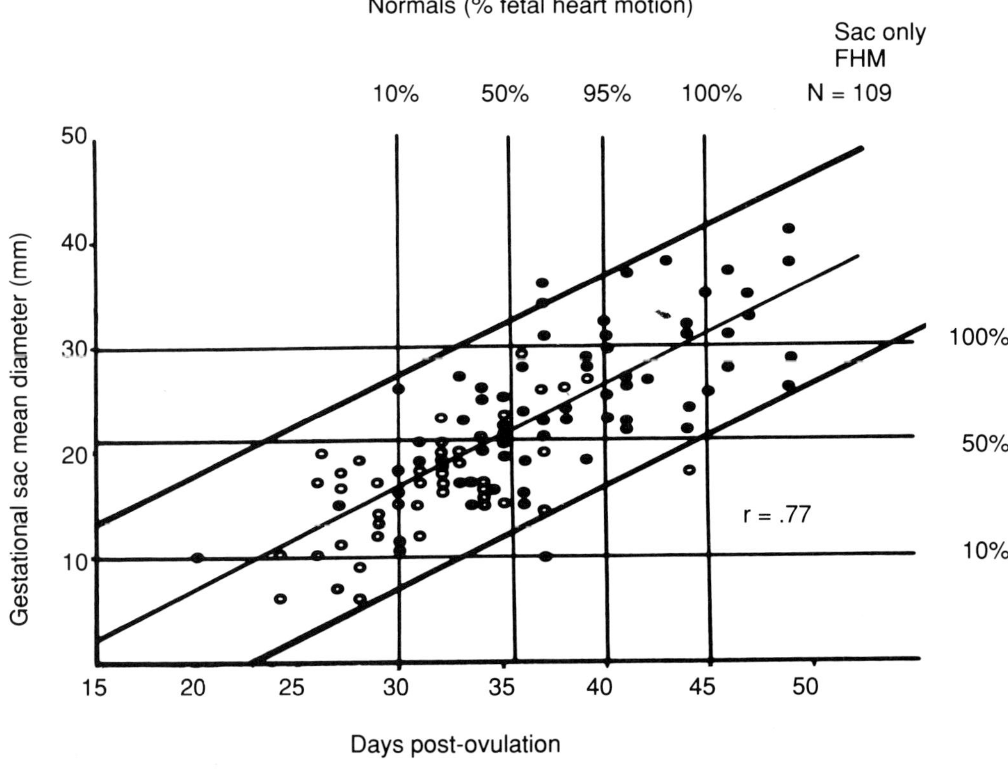

Fig. 13-14. Growth of gestational sac mean diameter during the first 50 days after ovulation in 109 observations (71 pregnancies). The diagonal lines represent the mean $\pm$ 2 standard errors of the mean in these successful pregnancies ($r = 0.77$). Open circles indicate the presence of a gestational sac only, whereas solid circles indicate simultaneous fetal heart motion. The vertical and horizontal grids indicate the increasing percentage of cases in which fetal heart motion was noted, the vertical grid by days after ovulation and the horizontal grid by gestational sac mean diameter. (From Batzer et al,[5] with permission.)

Table 13-9. Basic Mean and 2 Standard Deviation (SD) Values for Each Day of Menstrual Age from 6 Weeks 2 Days to 14 Weeks, and Mean Values After Correction for the Systematic Errors (1 mm + 3.7 percent) of the Technique

Menstrual Maturity (weeks, days)	*CRL (mm)* Mean	*CRL (mm)* 2 SD	*Corrected Regression Analysis (mm, mean values)*
6, 2	7.0	3.3	5.5
6, 3	6.5	1.4	6.1
6, 4	7.0	4.6	6.8
6, 5	6.5	4.2	7.5
6, 6	10.0	2.6	8.1
7, 0	9.3	2.3	8.9
7, 1	10.3	8.0	9.6
7, 2	11.8	5.7	10.4
7, 3	12.8	4.8	11.2
7, 4	13.4	6.7	12.0
7, 5	15.4	3.6	12.9
7, 6	15.4	4.4	13.8
8, 0	17.0	4.9	14.7
8, 1	19.5	5.7	15.7
8, 2	19.4	6.2	16.6
8, 3	20.4	5.0	17.6
8, 4	21.3	3.8	18.7
8, 5	20.9	2.4	19.7
8, 6	23.2	3.6	20.8
9, 0	25.8	6.0	21.9
9, 1	25.4	4.6	23.1
9, 2	26.7	4.4	24.2
9, 3	27.0	2.8	25.4
9, 4	32.5	4.2	26.7
9, 5	30.0	10.0	27.9
9, 6	31.3	5.5	29.2
10, 0	33.0	7.2	30.5
10, 1	33.8	7.6	31.8
10, 2	35.2	7.3	33.2
10, 3	36.0	7.9	34.6
10, 4	37.3	9.7	36.0
10, 5	43.4	7.7	37.4
10, 6	40.1	7.1	38.9
11, 0	46.7	6.1	40.4
11, 1	43.6	7.2	41.9
11, 2	47.5	6.2	43.5
11, 3	48.8	5.9	45.1
11, 4	49.0	9.5	46.7
11, 5	54.0	9.8	48.3
11, 6	56.2	9.5	50.0
12, 0	58.3	9.4	51.7
12, 1	56.8	7.2	53.4
12, 2	59.4	6.6	55.2
12, 3	62.6	8.6	57.0
12, 4	63.5	9.5	58.8
12, 5	67.7	6.4	60.6
12, 6	66.5	8.2	62.5
13, 0	72.5	4.2	64.3
13, 1	69.7	8.5	66.3
13, 2	73.0	15.1	68.2
13, 3	77.0	8.5	70.2
13, 4			72.2
13, 5			74.2
13, 6	76.0	5.7	76.3
14, 0	79.6	7.8	78.3

(Modified from Robinson and Fleming,[33] with permission.)

days postovulation vaginally and 29 days postovulation abdominally. Similarly, detection of fetal heart motion occurred in 95 percent of cases by 32 days transvaginally compared to 38 days abdominally.

CROWN-RUMP LENGTH AND THE SONOGRAPHIC DATING OF GESTATION

The CRL is one of the most accurate methods of estimating gestational age (Table 13-9; Figs. 13-15 and 13-16; see also Fig. 13-11). Robinson and Fleming,[33] whose original transabdominal work was the benchmark of CRL measurement, noted that variations in CRL can be attributed to (1) biologic variations in fetal size, (2) variation in the timing of ovulation and fertilization, and (3) errors in the measurement techniques. Although the CRL, as defined by Robinson, was originally calculated using transabdominal ultrasonography, the current use of transvaginal sonography allows better imaging and potentially more accurate measurements. Goldstein and Wolfson studied 143 viable, singleton pregnancies with 5- or 7.5-mHz

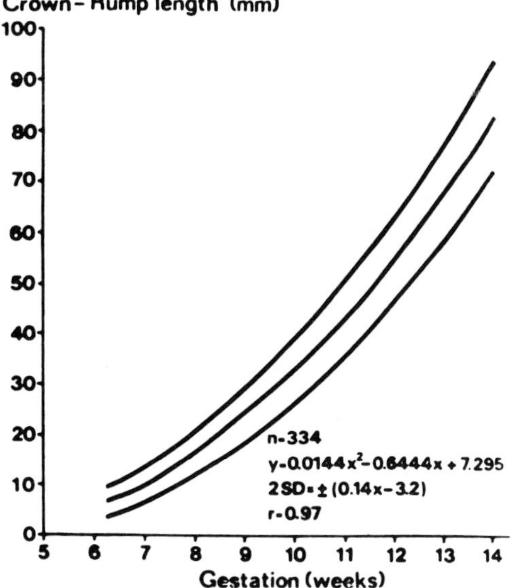

Fig. 13-15. Mean and standard deviation limits derived from 334 CRL measurements by means of a weighted nonlinear repression analysis designed to obtain the curve of best fit. (From Robinson and Fleming,[33] with permission.)

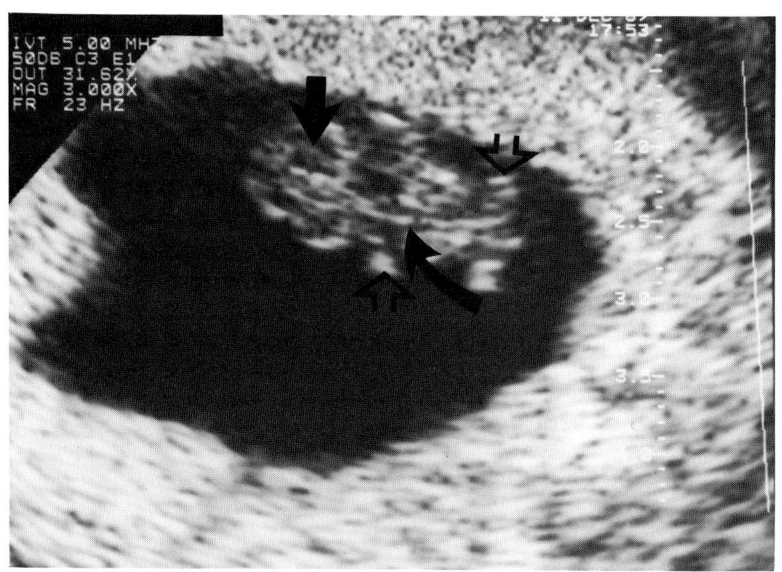

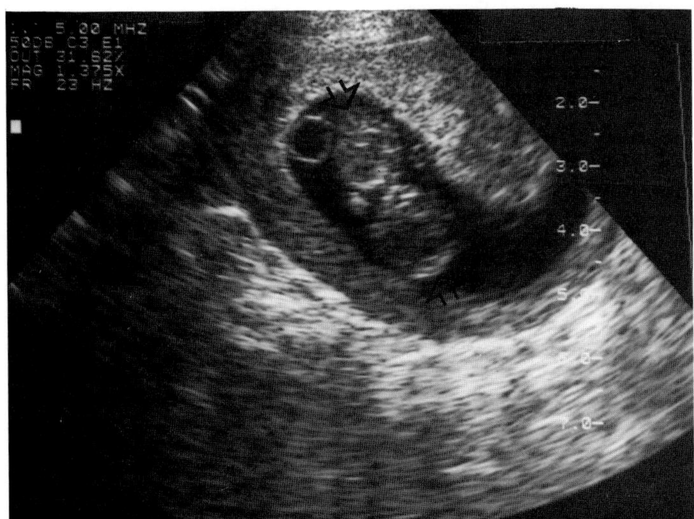

Fig. 13-16. (**A**) Fetus with a CRL of 19 mm correlating with a gestation of 8 weeks (see Table 13-9, corrected mean values). Note the limb buds (open arrows), spine (curved arrow), and ventricular cavity (arrow) in the head. (**B**) CRL of 30 mm (between open arrows) giving a gestational age (from LMP) of 9 weeks 5 days (Table 13-9). Note yolk sac at left in photo.

vaginal transducers.[34] All women in the study had a clear recollection of their LMP. CRL was plotted against LMP for all pregnancies. Regression analysis of the data revealed a linear equation of gestational age (days) = early embryonic size (mm) + 42 with a confidence limit of ±3 days. Daya,[35] by contrast, found a curvilinear (quadratic) relationship between CRL and days of gestation when figured from the date of oocyte retrieval in a group of 94 women undergoing IVF. He found that estimates of duration of gestation were similar to published data over the 40 to 60 mm range of CRL.

Despite some recent misgivings, the CRL remains one of the most accurate current assessments used for gestational dating before 12 weeks and clearly is superior to the biparietal diameter (BPD) measured after 26 weeks of gestation. CRL in the first trimester and BPD in the second trimester have been suggested to be relatively equivalent as predictors of gestational age. In an early series by Drumm,[36] 95 percent of patients delivered within ±12 days of the date of confinement estimated by CRL. However, CRL measurements in the Drumm[36] study were made using a 3.5-MHz linear array transducer. Each patient was scanned by two operators. The mean difference between any two CRL measurements was 1.6 mm, but differences as great as 10 mm were noted.[36]

Kopta et al[37] reported the mean error of the CRL to be 7.73 days using the actual delivery date for comparison. In their study, the BPD done in the second trimester had a mean error of 7.65 days. Seventy-eight percent of patients delivered within 14 days of the date of confinement estimated by CRL. This study used an interesting approach in assessing the accuracy of the CRL by comparing it and the actual delivery date and considering the length of pregnancy to be 280 days (Table 13-10). However, it is not clear whether the accuracy of 7.73 days reflects the biologic variation in the length of pregnancy, the variation in estimates of fetal age based on CRL, or measurement error. Quite probably all these factors contribute to the CRL variability reported.[36,37]

Table 13-10. Delivery (Percentage of Patients) Using CRL for Calculating Estimated Delivery Data[a]

	Days	*Patients (%)*
Kopta et al.[37]	±7	56
	±14	78
Drumm[36]	±6	74
	±12	95

[a]Accuracy calculated using delivery date. (Data from Kopta et al[37] and Drumm.[36])

ULTRASOUND IN THE MANAGEMENT OF FIRST TRIMESTER BLEEDING

Vaginal bleeding occurs in one-third of all pregnancies. About 50 percent of pregnancies experiencing bleeding will ultimately abort spontaneously. In a series of 466 pregnant patients with vaginal bleeding, only 48.7 percent progressed normally beyond 20 weeks of gestation.[23] The remainder had ectopic pregnancy (12.8 percent), hydatidiform mole (0.2 percent), or spontaneous abortion (32.7 percent). Elective termination occurred in 5.6 percent (Table 13-11). Mantoni[24] also studied patients with vaginal bleeding in early gestation. Fetal heart activity was noted in 61 percent of 244 patients. In 9 percent of patients, the ultrasound examination was done too early for diagnosis, and in 30 percent, there was an unsalvageable pregnancy (Table 13-12).

Some of the difference in prognosis in different studies results from the method of case accruement and when pregnant bleeding patients are first scanned. In Mantoni's study,[24] the abortion rate in pregnant patients with bleeding was 35 percent when the first bleeding episode began in weeks 5 to 9, but

Table 13-11. Outcome of Pregnant Patients with Bleeding

	%
Intrauterine pregnancy	
Normal progress beyond 20 weeks	48.7
Elective termination of pregnancy	5.6
Subsequent spontaneous abortion	1.3
Anembryonic pregnancy	14.4
Complete abortion	0.9
Incomplete abortion	8.8
Missed abortion	7.3
Hydatidiform mole	0.2
Extrauterine pregnancy	
Tubal	12.4
Ovarian	0.2
Cornual	0.2

(Modified from Stabile et al,[23] with permission.)

Table 13-12. Ultrasound Findings in Patients with Threatened Abortion ($n = 244$)

Ultrasound Finding	*Patients (%)*
Fetal life detected	61
Inconclusive study	9
Missed abortion	15
Blighted ovum	8
Incomplete abortion	5
Hydatidiform mole	1
Ectopic pregnancy	1

(Modified from Mantoni,[24] with permission.)

was 45 percent if bleeding first began between weeks 10 and 20.

The detection of fetal cardiac activity in a pregnant patient with vaginal bleeding indicates a viable fetus and suggests a good prognosis. When fetal cardiac activity is noted, the risk of spontaneous abortion in the bleeding patient is reduced from about 40 to 50 percent to between 1.3 and 2.6 percent, depending on the gestational age when the fetal heart is first imaged and the method of case accruement, as reported in various studies.[23-25,38-42] In Mantoni's series[24] of 148 patients with fetal heart motion, 19 (1.3 percent) subsequently aborted. In another series, when fetal cardiac activity was first imaged between 8 and 12 weeks, the risk of abortion before 20 weeks of gestation was only 2 percent.[25] In the series of Stabile et al[28] of 406 patients with an intrauterine pregnancy, the subsequent abortion rate when a live fetus was identified was only 2.6 percent.

Fetal bradycardia in the first trimester is associated with a poor prognosis. Laboda et al[44] noted that the fetal heart rate (FHR) increases from an average of 100 beats/minute (bpm) at 5 to 6 weeks of gestation to 140 bpm at 8 to 9 weeks of gestation. All 5 of the 65 pregnancies between 5 and 8 weeks of gestation in which the heart rate was less than 85 bpm ended in a spontaneous abortion. Achiron et al[39] noted similar heart rate changes during study of a cohort of 603 fetuses in very early gestation, noting that FHR increases progressively from 110 beats per minute at a CRL of 3 to 4 mm to 170 beats per minute at a CRL of 15 to 30 mm. The absence of cardiac activity when the fetus is clearly imaged indicates fetal death and inevitable abortion (Fig. 13-17).[41,42]

The presence of a gestational sac without an embryo is more difficult to interpret and may represent a very early viable pregnancy, an abnormal pregnancy, a blighted ovum that will ultimately abort, or even a pseudogestational sac associated with an ectopic pregnancy.[42] A gestational sac diameter of 20 mm without a yolk sac or 25 mm without a fetus is generally associated with a blighted ovum or abnormal gestation that will eventually abort (Fig. 13-18).

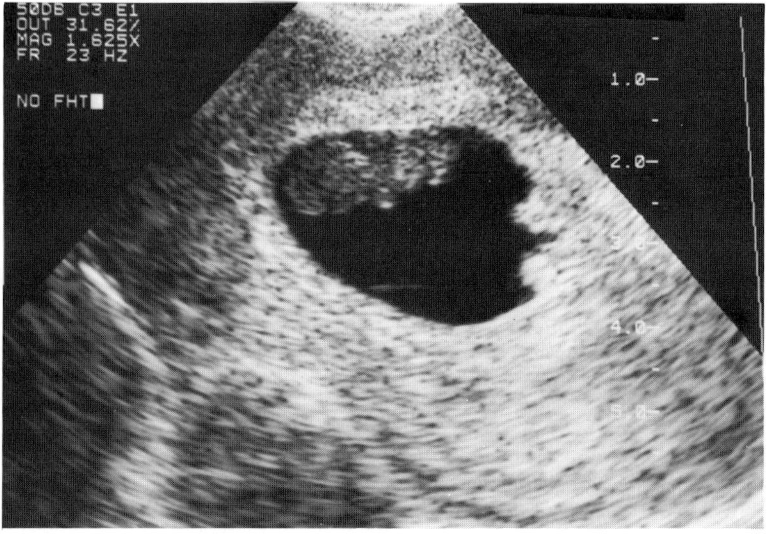

Fig. 13-17. A 32-year-old woman G2 P1 with light vaginal spotting. Quantitative hCG at 6.8 weeks by LMP was 4,524 mIU/ml (2IS), giving an estimated gestational age of 6.4 weeks, which was in agreement with the gestational age by dates. Although the hCG and dates were in general agreement in gestational week 6, by 9.5 weeks by dates the hCG had only increased to 16,990 mIU/ml (2IS). Transvaginal ultrasound at 10.8 weeks by dates showed an intrauterine sac with a 21-mm fetus by CRL (8 weeks 4 days by CRL). No fetal heartbeat was noted. Note the abnormal placenta on the right of photo. Fetal heart activity should be visualized easily in a fetus this size. Before a dilatation and curettage at 11.2 weeks by date, the hCG had fallen to 3,848 mIU/ml (2IS).

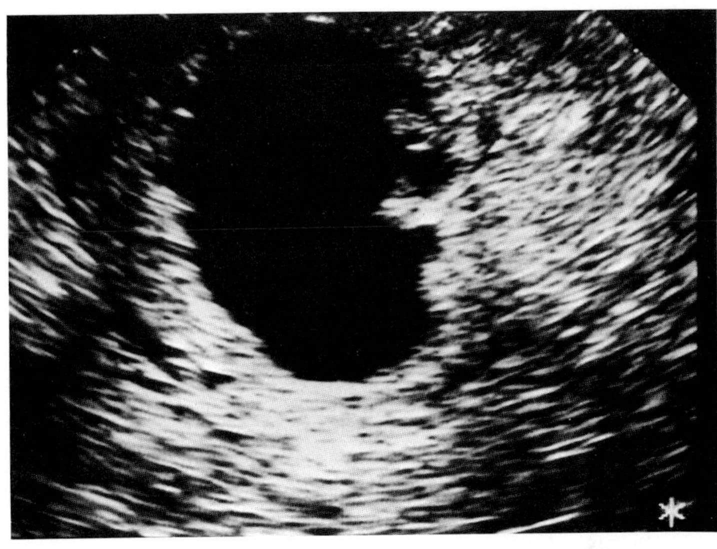

Fig. 13-18. Gestational sac of 38 by 36 mm. The patient was 11 weeks pregnant by dates with an empty sac. Serum hCG was 3,135 mIU/ml (2IS) at 10 weeks of gestation and decreased to 1,380 mIU/ml over the next 5 days. The serum progesterone was low (12.7 ng/ml). A gestational sac larger than 20 mm without a fetus is abnormal. In this image some placental remnants can be seen along the right.

Etiology of Vaginal Bleeding with a Live Fetus

One of the most difficult clinical decisions facing the obstetrician involves the woman at 5 to 10 weeks' gestation with vaginal bleeding. In the past, this condition has carried with it a variety of colorful clinical terms reflecting the possible outcomes of such pregnancies. Missed, threatened, inevitable, incomplete, and complete abortion all related to clinical presentations of the first trimester vaginal bleeder. Today, with high resolution vaginal ultrasound, it is often possible to make a definitive sonographic diagnosis (and prognosis) for this condition.

In the series of Stabile et al[23] of 406 women with vaginal bleeding, a live fetus was noted in 189 patients. Two abnormalities that might account for the bleeding, a second empty gestational sac or a sub-

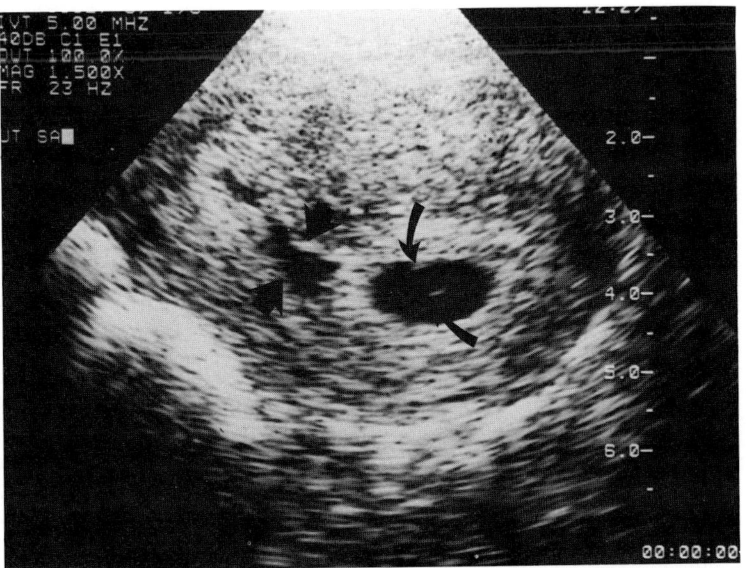

Fig. 13-19. Intrauterine pregnancy with a 4-mm yolk sac at 5 weeks of gestation (curved arrows). Note area of subchorionic hemorrhage (arrows). The patient delivered at term.

chorionic hemorrhage, were identified by sonography in patients with a live fetus. A second empty gestational sac was noted in 16 patients (3.9 percent of total patients; 8.5 percent of patients with a live fetus with bleeding). These cases represent a variant of the vanishing twin syndrome, in which one twin is a blighted ovum. An intrauterine hematoma or retroplacental clot 0.7 to 16 ml in size was noted in 22 cases (5.4 percent of total cases; 8.6 percent of patients with a live fetus with bleeding; (Figs. 13-19 and 13-20). None of these patients subsequently aborted. In Mantoni's series[24] of 244 cases of threatened abortion, there were six cases with intrauterine hematomas (2.5 percent). In two of these six cases, the hematoma was larger than 50 ml and one aborted, whereas the other delivered a 1650-g premature infant. All four patients in whom the hematoma was less than 50 ml had a normal pregnancy.

Dickey et al[43] evaluated 2,116 first trimester pregnancies by abdominal ultrasound and 783 with vaginal imaging. They differentiated subchorionic bleeding from subchorionic fluid collection using color Doppler scanning techniques. In this large series, subchorionic fluid was found equally often in women scanned with vaginal or color Doppler ultrasound and less often with abdominal scanning techniques. Color Doppler revealed subchorionic bleeding (defined as pulsatory fluid motion) in 47 percent of patients with subchorionic fluid collections. Forty-four of 102 women in this study had clinical bleeding or spotting associated with subchorionic fluid collections. Embryonic death occurred equally often in women with and without subchorionic fluid and/or bleeding. Therefore, current data suggest that an intrauterine or subchorionic hematoma in association with a viable fetus does not necessarily predict a poor prognosis when less than 50 ml in size, but may be associated with bleeding in early pregnancy. Other causes of early pregnancy bleeding in the presence of a live fetus included the placenta covering the internal os and the presence of an IUD or a uterine leiomyoma (Table 13-13).

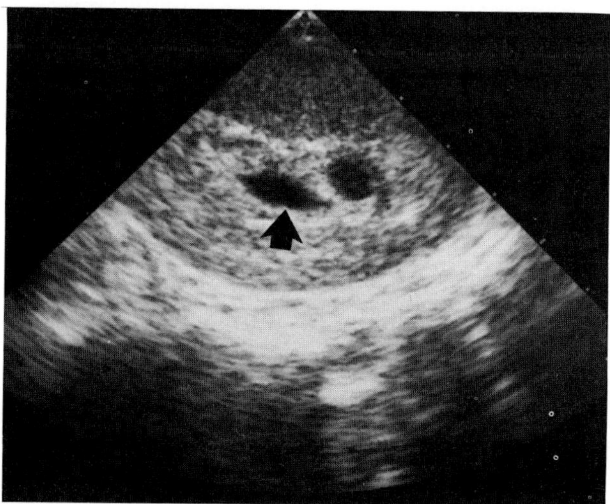

Fig. 13-20. Subchorionic hemorrhage (arrow). The patient spontaneously aborted.

Table 13-13. Causes of Bleeding in Early Pregnancy

Abortion	~50%
Complete	
Inevitable	
Incomplete	
Missed	
Blighted ova	
Threatened abortion	~50%
Subchorionic hemorrhage	
Blighted ovum/normal twin (vanished twin)	
Placenta covering the internal os	
IUD pregnancy	
Leiomyomas	
Size (CRL)/dates (LMP) discrepancy	
Unknown	
Ectopic pregnancy	1%
Gestational trophoblastic disease	1/2,000 (in United States, higher in Asia)

CRL and Fetal Loss

In patients with a reliable menstrual history, fetal growth delay as determined by a discrepancy between the CRL and fetal age by LMP and associated bleeding have been suggested to have a poor prognosis. Five of 12 such patients aborted.[24] However, the reliability of the discrepancy between fetal size and age depends on the accuracy of the LMP and ovulation occurring at midcycle.

Human Chorionic Gonadotropin and Gestational Sac Size

Nyberg et al[11] reported on the relationship between sac size and serum hCG levels in 70 abnormal and 56 normal gestations (Fig. 13-21). In all these cases the gestational sac size was less than 20 mm. In 39 (56 percent) abnormal pregnancies, no gestational sac was noted. In all normal pregnancies a gestational sac

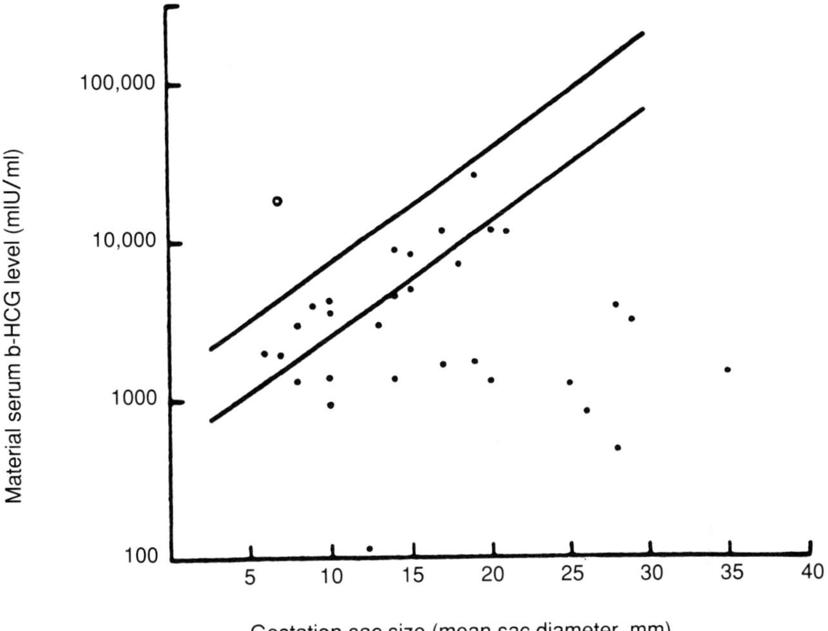

Fig. 13-21. Mean sac diameter compared with serum hCG levels for 31 abnormal gestations. In 20 cases (65 percent), the hCG level was disproportionately low. Only one woman (with a molar pregnancy) had an elevated hCG determination (O). (From Nyberg et al,[11] with permission.)

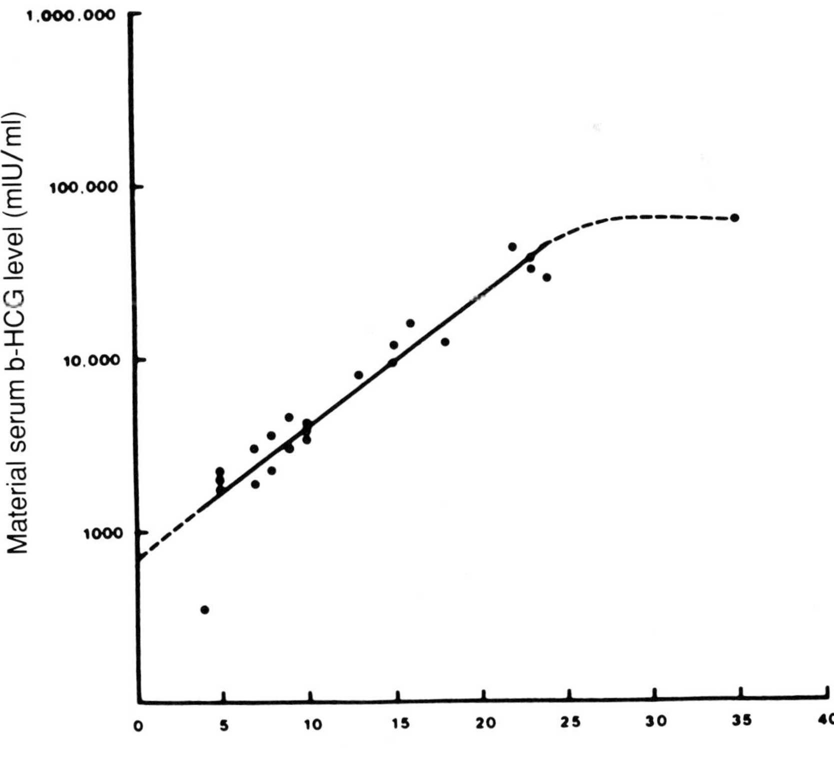

Fig. 13-22. There is a good correlation between maternal serum hCG levels and gestational sac size in early pregnancy. (From Nyberg et al,[13] with permission.)

Table 13-14. Gestational Sac Detection and hCG Levels for Normal and Abnormal Gestations

hCG (mIU/ml [2IS])	*Normal* (n = *56*)		*Abnormal* (n = *70*)	
	No Sac	*Sac*	*No Sac*	*Sac*
<1,800	17	0	35	12
>1,800	0	39	4	19

(From Nyberg et al,[11] with permission.)

was noted when the hCG levels were above 1,800 mIU/ml (2IS); (Table 13-14). In 31 abnormal pregnancies in which a sac was visualized, 20 patients (65 percent) had an hCG level that was disproportionately low for the gestational sac diameter. In this series, no normal pregnancies had an hCG level-gestational sac size discrepancy. After 8 weeks or when the gestational sac is 25 mm, the hCG levels begin to plateau while the gestational sac continues to increase in size (Fig. 13-22).[13] Therefore, hCG: sac ratios cannot be used after week 8 of gestation (or sac sizes greater than 25 mm). Batzer et al[5] found the hCG level-gestational sac mean diameter less useful in predicting an inevitable abortion. Only 7 of 25 observations in abnormal pregnancies fell below the standard error of the mean for successful pregnancies.

Nyberg et al[11] have also emphasized the importance of serial scans to monitor sac growth. A patient with a serum beta-hCG level of 4,500 mIU/ml (2IS) and a 10-mm sac diameter should have a sac of 17 mm 7 days later, and the hCG level should have increased to 14,500 mIU/ml and be a minimum of 7,900 mIU/ml (Table 13-15). Considering a normal sac growth rate, Nyberg et al[10] have suggested that the time interval for a repeat sonograph in which a yolk sac or fetus should be seen can be calculated by the formula: time interval (in days) = 25 − initial mean sac diameter. A patient with a gestational sac of 10 mm at about the sixth gestational week, but without a yolk sac or fetus, would be scanned 15 days later. Failure to demonstrate a yolk sac and a living fetus by that date would indicate an abnormal pregnancy. In practice, we have found that repeating these scans at 1-week intervals adequately balances patient anxiety over the outcome of their pregnancy and the ability to diagnose accurately an abnormal pregnancy. The appearance of normal gestational structures (and especially fetal heart motion) and appropriate interval growth of the sac are good prognostic signs. An abnormally shaped gestational sac or a sac surrounded by a poor gestational reaction suggests a poor prognosis (Fig. 13-23). Serial scans may be repeated weekly until fetal heart motion is detected, or the patient has passed appropriate sonographic landmarks without the reassuring development of fetal structures.

Making a definitive diagnosis of an inevitable abortion is still a challenging clinical situation (Table 13-16). In some cases, current ultrasound techniques or ultrasound combined with biochemical markers, such as beta-hCG, may make a definitive diagnosis possible. In a pregnant patient with bleeding with

Table 13-15. Sac Size Versus hCG Levels for Normal Pregnancies (*n* = 56)

Mean Sac Diameter (mm)	*hCG Level (mIU/ml [2IS])*		
		95% Confidence Limits	
	Predicted[a]	*Lower*	*Upper*
5	1,932	1,026	3,636
6	2,165	1,226	4,256
7	2,704	1,465	4,990
8	3,199	1,749	5,852
9	3,785	2,085	6,870
10	4,478	2,483	8,075
11	5,297	2,952	9,508
12	6,267	3,502	11,218
13	7,415	4,145	13,266
14	8,773	4,894	15,726
15	10,379	5,766	18,682
16	12,270	6,776	22,235
17	14,528	7,964	26,501
18	17,188	9,343	31,621
19	20,337	10,951	37,761
20	24,060	12,820	45,130
21	28,464	15,020	53,970
22	33,675	17,560	64,570
23	39,843	20,573	77,164
24	47,138	24,067	93,325

[a] Log hCG = 2.92/0.073 × MSD (mean sac diameter), R^2 = 0.93, $P < 0.001$ (From Nyberg et al,[11] with permission.)

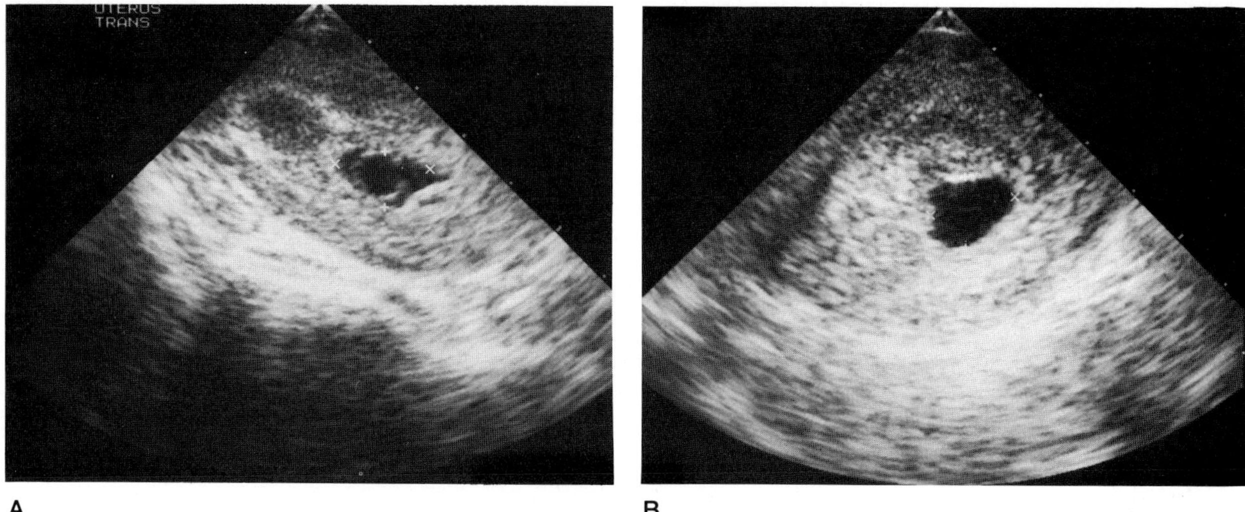

Fig. 13-23. A 15-year-old girl with vaginal bleeding and a positive pregnancy test. (**A**) The ultrasound shows an intrauterine pregnancy with a sac of 14 by 8 mm consistent with a 6-week gestation. A separate sac 8 mm in size is also noted. This sac could represent a yolk sac with oligohydramnios and collapse of the gestational sac around it, or the gestational sac per se with subchorionic hemorrhage. The presence of some gestational reaction (arrows) surrounding the area suggests the former. No fetus is noted. The gestational reaction around the sac is poor. (**B**) Ten days later the "yolk sac" is gone, and the gestational sac has not increased in size. The sac is irregular, and there is a poor gestational reaction. The patient spontaneously aborted the next day.

serum hCG levels less than 750 mIU/ml (2IS), serial quantitative beta-hCG determinations and pelvic transvaginal ultrasound are the best way to differentiate an inevitable or missed abortion from a normal pregnancy resulting from a late ovulation. Serum progesterone may also be useful. A serum progesterone level of less than 10 ng/ml suggests a poor prognosis.

Table 13-16. Criteria Suggesting an Abnormal Gestation

Criterion	*Comment*
LMP > 6 wks (accurate)	No gestational sac
DDS	Poorly formed or incomplete around the gestational sac
Gestational sac	No sac when β-hCG (2IS) ≥ 750 mIU/ml
Yolk sac	Absent (gestational sac > 20 mm)
Embryo	Absent (gestational sac > 25 mm)
Sac growth	≤0.6 mm/day
Yolk sac > 10 mm	Abortion (92%)

VANISHED TWINS

Ultrasound has demonstrated that twins and multiple gestations occur much more commonly than previously appreciated. However, many twins do not progress to term. This phenomenon has been termed the vanished twin syndrome. Landy et al[45] reviewed nine studies that noted a loss of one twin in 53 to 78 percent of multiple pregnancies (vanished twin), as diagnosed sonographically during the first trimester. The vanished twin rate varies with the gestational age at which the diagnosis is made. In a series of 6,690 pregnant women. Levi[46] diagnosed 118 multiple pregnancies sonographically. When the diagnosis was made before gestational week 10, 71.4 percent of the twins vanished. When twins were first diagnosed between weeks 10 and 15, 62.5 percent vanished. After week 15, no vanished twins occurred in 79 cases. These high loss rates are not universally accepted. Wax et al[42] found that only one of 11 women achieving twin pregnancy in an IVF program experienced loss of a second twin. They also noted significant differences in the number of early gestational sacs and liveborn infants in higher level gestations (triplets and quadruplets) in an IVF population. Sulak and Dodson[47] noted histologic evidence of a vanished twin sac, confirming the validity of the sonographic finding in early pregnancy.

In Mantoni's series[24] of 244 patients, there were 3 sets of twins, 3 cases of twin blighted ova, and 12 cases of a blighted ovum and normal pregnancy (5 percent). Only one blighted ovum and normal pregnancy twin combination aborted in this series (8 percent). However, the blighted ovum-normal pregnancy combination seems to predispose to bleeding in early pregnancy.

OLIGOHYDRAMNIOS

Oligohydramnios in early pregnancy has a poor prognosis. Oligohydramnios was noted in two patients before 13 weeks of gestation with bleeding in early pregnancy.[23] One patient aborted at 23 weeks and the other at 25 weeks of gestation. Maternal cytomegalovirus infection and fetal karyotypic abnormalities have been suggested as possible causes for this condition in early pregnancy.[48,49] Dickey et al[49] have looked at the relationship between gestational sac diameter (GSD) and the fetal CRL. Overall, the GSD-CRL difference averaged 11 mm at 37 to 44 days of gestation and 12.4 mm by 58 to 65 days of pregnancy in 539 women scanned between 37 to 65 days from their LMP. A GSD-CRL difference of less than 5 mm occurred in 1.9 percent of these gestations and was associated with a fetal death rate of 80 percent. The fetal loss rate was 26.5 percent when this difference was 5 to 8 mm, and 10.6 percent when the difference was 8 mm or more. There was no association between karyotype and abnormally low GSD-CRL differences.

ULTRASOUND IN INCOMPLETE ABORTION

Transvaginal ultrasound examination may be used to estimate the amount of tissue remaining in the uterus preceding suction curettage for an incomplete abortion (Fig. 13-24). Rulin et al[50] have demonstrated that uterine imaging is a highly reliable test for the management of women thought to have spontaneous complete abortion. In their series, 98 percent of patients thought to have an "empty uterus" by sonographic examination had an uneventful recovery without surgical intervention. In contrast, 69 percent of 13 patients with evidence of retained tissue or a "thickened endometrium" on ultrasound evaluation had chorionic villi present during curettage. Obviously, heavy vaginal bleeding and fever or leukocytosis still remain compelling reasons for intervention in these patients, regardless of sonographic findings. Maternal serum hCG levels are also a helpful diagnostic adjunct in these cases.

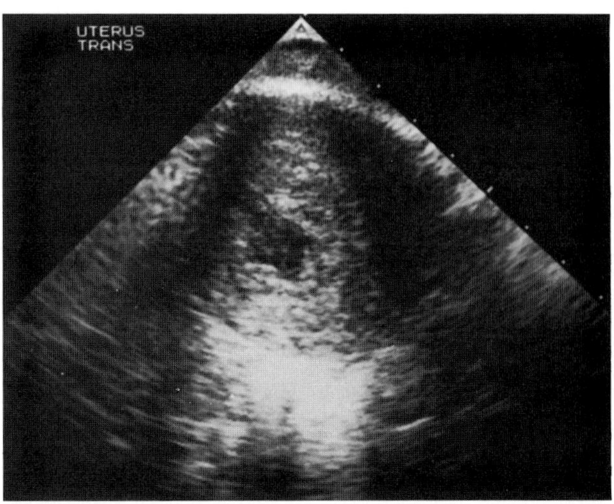

Fig. 13-24. A 19-year-old woman presented in the emergency room with vaginal bleeding and abdominal pain with a positive pregnancy test at 12 weeks 5 days by LMP. The cervical os was open, and tissue was noted in the os that was removed. The uterus was 8 weeks size by clinical examination. Transvaginal ultrasound showed a small anechoic area (T-pelvic view) of 7 by 9 mm, probably representing blood with a thin layer of endometrium about 3 mm thick. Suction curettage yielded only a small amount of tissue as noted on the ultrasound. Although villi were present in the histologic sections of tissue taken from the cervical os in the emergency room before the ultrasound and suction, only decidua with Arial-Stella phenomenon were noted on the tissue from the suction.

Table 13-17. Early Embryonic Development

Fetus	6 weeks
Cardiac activity	6–7 weeks
Bowel herniation into umbilical cord	8 weeks
Ventricular system	8 weeks
Limb buds	8 weeks
Choroid plexus	8–9 weeks

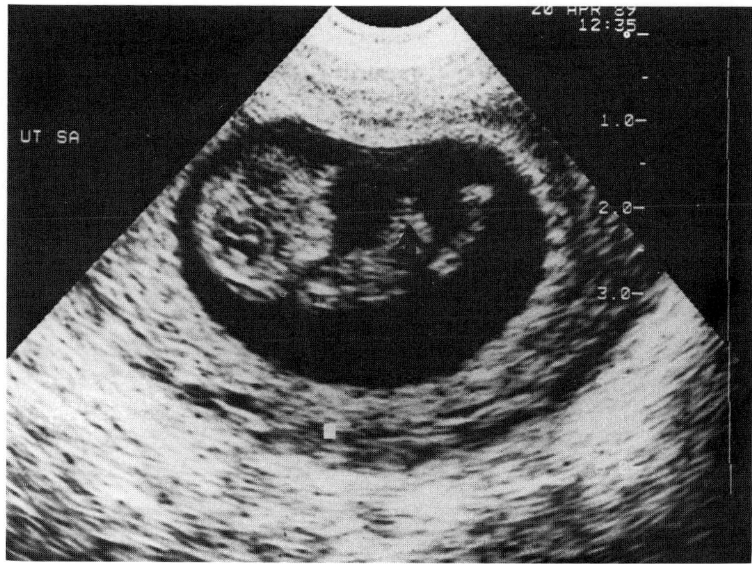

Fig. 13-25. AP-pelvic view of the uterus with a fetus seen in a longitudinal plane at 9.9 weeks showing the physiologic herniation of bowel into the umbilical cord (arrow).

EARLY FETAL DEVELOPMENT

Ultrasound delineation of early embryonic developmental structures and early diagnosis of congenital anomalies are still quite limited. Early gestational structures, such as the yolk sac, amnion, placenta, umbilical cord, and decidua, are consistently imaged, as discussed previously and noted in Table 13-17. The fetus is identified in weeks 5 and 6, with fetal cardiac activity noted almost as soon as the fetus can be identified accurately, generally in gestational week 6. The fetal limb buds and the developing ventricular system in the head are sometimes imaged in gestational week 8 (see Fig. 13-16). The fetal spine is generally seen (see Fig. 13-16). Physiologic herniation of the bowel is characteristically seen between gestational weeks 7 and 10.[51,52] This physiologic herniation should not be mistaken for an omphalocele (Fig. 13-19 to 13-29).

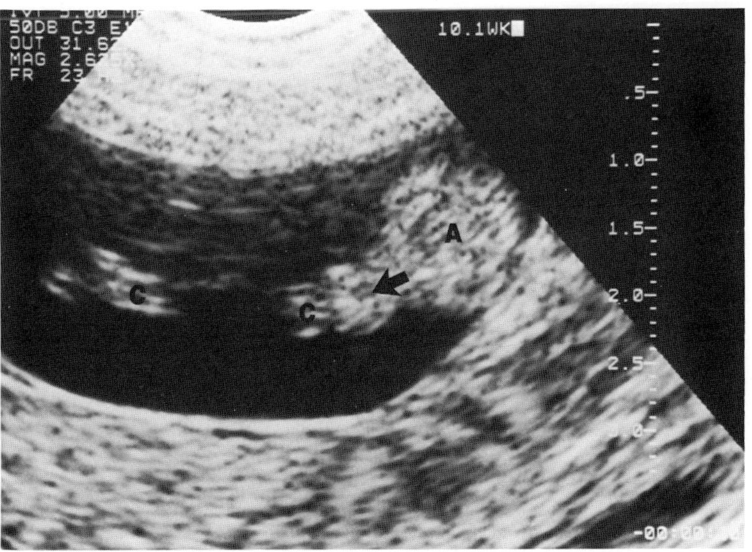

Fig. 13-26. Transverse plane of the fetal abdomen (A) at the level of the umbilical cord (C) insertion at 10.1 weeks of gestation showing the physiologic herniation of the bowel into the base of the umbilical cord (arrow).

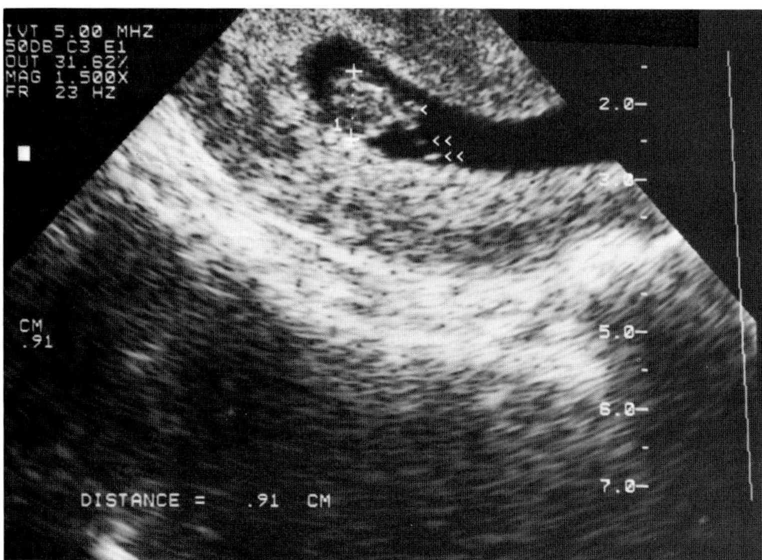

Fig. 13-27. Transverse view of fetal abdomen at 8.3 weeks of gestation (from LMP) showing the physiologic hernia and the umbilical cord (small white arrowheads).

ROUTINE SONOGRAPHS IN EARLY PREGNANCY

Although routine sonography in pregnancy has not been recommended by a National Institutes of Health blue ribbon panel that was convened to consider this possibility, there are still a rather large number of indications for sonography in early pregnancy.

Between one-fourth and one-third of pregnant patients experience bleeding in early pregnancy. Ultrasound is helpful in determining the prognosis and is the diagnostic test of choice for differentiating among an inevitable abortion, a viable intrauterine pregnancy, and a molar pregnancy and to help exclude or diagnose an ectopic pregnancy. Multiple gestations can also be diagnosed during sonographic evaluation in early pregnancy.

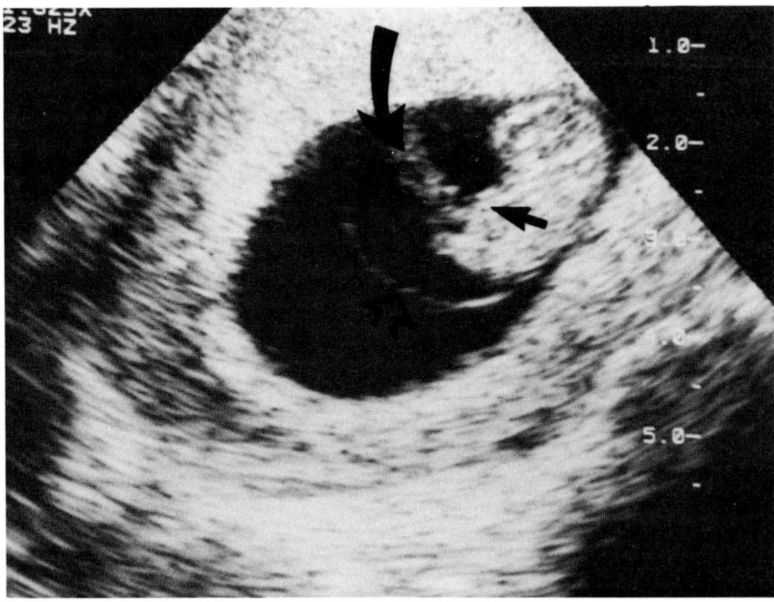

Fig. 13-28. Fetus with CRL of 18 mm or 8.3 weeks of gestation (LMP) with amnion (arrow). Note umbilical cord (curved arrow) and physiologic bowel herniation (open arrow).

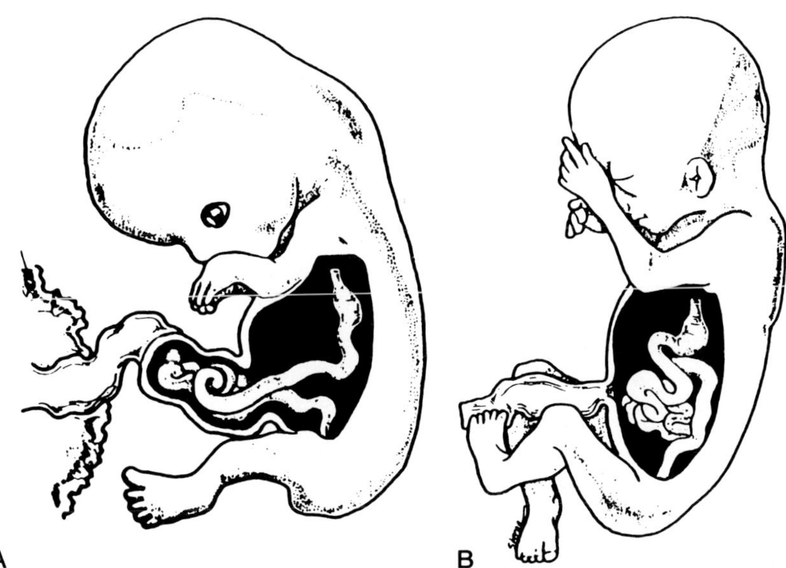

Fig. 13-29. **(A)** Diagram of fetus illustrating fetal bowel herniation into the base of the umbilical cord during early pregnancy. **(B)** Fetus showing normal umbilical cord insertion with return of fetal bowel into the abdominal cavity. (Modified from Cyr et al,[52] with permission.)

Perhaps equally critical is the dating of the gestation. It is well recognized that the LMP is frequently inaccurate. Sonographic landmarks of fetal development have been studied carefully using contemporary, high resolution vaginal technology. The appearance of embryonic or extraembryonic structures, such as gestational and yolk sacs, fetal organ development, and specific patterns of normal growth have permitted the establishment of nomograms that provide a simple and extremely accurate method for pregnancy dating in the first trimester. Ultrasound findings are reported as those of menstrual age, i.e., based upon a 40 week gestation and the presumption of normal menses 14 days before conception. Early pregnancy dating may be of enormous value in the prevention of post-datism, as well as the delivery decisions in women with preterm labor, preterm rupture of the membranes, intrauterine growth retardation, repeat cesarean section, and third trimester vaginal bleeding. Unfortunately, many of the women who would greatly benefit from accurate gestational dating cannot be discerned in advance (Table 13-18).

The question of an early ultrasound for all pregnant women revolves around potential complications and side effects from the sonography and the cost effectiveness of the procedure. The Federal Republic of Germany and several other countries now encourage universal ultrasound evaluation of all pregnancies. Although there has been extensive experience with early ultrasound screening without confirmed complications in humans, theoretic considerations and animal studies still raise the possibility of risks. Despite this continuing debate, the use of ultrasound in early pregnancy has become increasingly popular.

Table 13-18. Pregnancy Complications and Approximate Incidence When Ultrasound Evaluation and/or Accurate Dating Would be of Value

Threatened abortion (abortion)	30% (15%)
Ectopic pregnancy	1%
Molar pregnancy	1/2,000
Multiple gestations	0.9%
Confirmation of dates	
Post-dates	12%
Inaccurate dates	25%
IUGR	5%
Bleeding complications	
Abruptio placentae	1.5%
Placenta previa	0.5%
Repeat cesarean section	10%
Premature labor	8%

REFERENCES

1. Biggers JD: Fertilization and blastocyst formation. p. 223. In Alexander NJ (ed): Animal Models for Research on Contraception and Fertility. Harper & Row, Hagerstown, MD, 1979
2. Moore KL: The Developing Human. 3rd Ed. WB Saunders, Philadelphia, 1982
3. Hertig AT, Rock J, Adams EC: A description of 34 human ova within the first 17 days of development. Am J Anat 98:435, 1956
4. Hertig AT, Rock J: Two human ova of the pre-villous stage, having an ovulation age of about eleven and twelve days respectively. Contrib Embryol 29:129, 1941
5. Batzer FR, Weiner S, Corson SL: Landmarks during the first forty-two days of gestation demonstrated by the beta-subunit of human chorionic gonadotropin and ultrasound. Am J Obstet Gynecol 146:973, 1983
6. de Crespigny LC, Cooper D, McKenna M: Early detection of intrauterine pregnancy with ultrasound. J Ultrasound Med 7:7, 1988
7. Bernaschek G, Rudelstorfer R, Csaicsich P: Vaginal sonography versus serum human chorionic gonadotropin in early detection of pregnancy. Am J Obstet Gynecol 158:608, 1988
8. de Crespigny LC: The value of ultrasound in early pregnancy. Clin Obstet Gynaecol 30:136, 1987
9. Kawakami Y, Yamada K, Andoh K et al: Assessment of the implantation site by transvaginal sonography. Fertil Steril 59:1003, 1993
10. Nyberg DA, Mack LA, Laing FC, Patten RM: Distinguishing normal from abnormal gestational sac growth in early pregnancy. J Ultrasound Med 6:23, 1987
11. Nyberg DA, Filly RA, Duarte Filho DL et al: Abnormal pregnancy: early diagnosis by US and serum chorionic gonadotropin levels. Radiology 158:393, 1986
12. Robinson HP: "Gestation sac" volumes as determined by sonar in the first trimester of pregnancy. Br J Obstet Gynaecol 82:100, 1975
13. Nyberg DA, Filly RA, Mahony BS et al: Early gestation: correlation of hCG levels and sonographic identification. AJR 144:951, 1985
14. Goldstein SR, Snyder JR, Watson C, Danon M: Very early pregnancy detection with endovaginal ultrasound. Obstet Gynecol 72:200, 1988
15. Bernard KG, Cooperberg PL: Sonographic differentiation between blighted ovum and early viable pregnancy. AJR 144:597, 1985
16. Robinson HP: The diagnosis of early pregnancy failure by sonar. Br J Obstet Gynaecol 82:849, 1975
17. Nyberg DA, Laing FC, Filly RA: Threatened abortion: sonographic distinction of normal and abnormal gestational sacs. Radiology 158:397, 1986
18. Nyberg DA, Laing FC, Filly RA et al: Ultrasonographic differentiation of the gestational sac of early intrauterine pregnancy from the pseudogestational sac of ectopic pregnancy. Radiology 146:755, 1983
19. Hurwitz SR: Yolk sac sign: sonographic appearance of the fetal yolk sac in missed abortion. J Ultrasound Med 5:435, 1986
20. Nyberg DA, Mack LA, Harvey D, Wang K: Value of the yolk sac in evaluating early pregnancies. J Ultrasound Med 7:129, 1988
21. Dodson MG: Bleeding in pregnancy. p. 451. In Aladjem S (ed): Obstetrical Practice. CV Mosby, St. Louis, 1980
22. Robinson HP: Fetal heart rates as determined by sonar in early pregnancy. J Obstet Gynaecol Br Commonw 80:805, 1973
23. Stabile I, Campbell S, Grudzinskas JG: Ultrasonic assessment of complications during first trimester of pregnancy. Lancet 2:1237, 1987
24. Mantoni M: Ultrasound signs in threatened abortion and their prognostic significance. Obstet Gynecol 65:471, 1985
25. Cashner KA, Christopher CR, Dysert GA: Spontaneous fetal loss after demonstration of a live fetus in the first trimester. Obstet Gynecol 70:827, 1987
26. Cadkin AV, McAlpin J: Detection of fetal cardiac activity between 41 and 43 days of gestation. J Ultrasound Med 3:499, 1984
27. Kadar N, DeVore G, Romero R: Discriminatory hCG zone: its use in the sonographic evaluation for ectopic pregnancy. Obstet Gynecol 58:156, 1981
28. Burry KA, Thurmond AS, Suby-Long TD, et al: Transvaginal sonographic findings in surgically verified ectopic pregnancy. Am J Obstet Gynecol 168:1796, 1993
29. Fossum GT, Davajan V, Kletzky OA: Early detection of pregnancy with transvaginal ultrasound. Fertil Steril 49:788, 1988
30. Martin CM, Tobler R, McCreary B, et al: Correlation of intact ELISA, human chorionic gonadotropin levels, and sensitive vaginal ultrasound in the early diagnosis of ectopic pregnancy (Abstract). Fifth Meeting of the World Federation for Ultrasound in Medicine and Biology, Washington, DC, October, 1988
31. Timor-Trisch IE, Farine D, Rosen MG: A close look at early embryonic development with the high frequency vaginal transducer. Am J Obstet Gynecol 159:676, 1988
32. Batzer FR, Hasty LA, Corson SL, et al: Redefining landmarks of early pregnancy utilizing transvaginosonography. Am J Gynecol Health 7:18, 1993
33. Robinson HP, Fleming JEE: A critical evaluation of sonar "crown-rump length" measurements. Br J Obstet Gynaecol 82:702, 1975
34. Goldstein SR, Wolfson R: Endovaginal ultrasonographic measurement of early embryonic size as a means of assessing gestational age. J Ultrasound Med 13:27, 1994
35. Daya, S: Accuracy of gestational age estimation by means of fetal crown-rump length measurement. Am J Obstet Gynecol 168:903, 1993

36. Drumm JE: The prediction of delivery date by ultrasonic measurement of fetal crown-rump length. Br J Obstet Gynaecol 84:1, 1977
37. Kopta MM, May RR, Crane JP: A comparison of the reliability of the estimated date of confinement predicted by crown-rump length and biparietal diameter. Am J Obstet Gynecol 145:562, 1983
38. Hertz JB: Diagnostic procedures in threatened abortion. Obstet Gynecol 64:223, 1984
39. Achiron R, Tadmor O, Mashiach S: Heart rate as a predictor of first-trimester spontaneous abortion after ultrasound proven viability. Obstet Gynecol 78:330, 1991
40. Merchiers EH, Dhont M, De Sutter PA et al: Predictive value of early embryonic cardiac activity for pregnancy outcome. Am J Obstet Gynecol 165:11, 1991
41. Stern JJ, Coulam CB: Mechanism of recurrent spontaneous abortion. I. Ultrasonographic findings. Am J Obstet Gynecol 166:1844, 1992
42. Wax MR, Frates M, Benson CB, et al: First trimester findings in pregnancies after in vitro fertilization. J Ultrasound Med 11:321, 1992
43. Dickey RP, Olar TT, Curole DN, et al: Relationship of first-trimester subchorionic bleeding detected by color Doppler ultrasound to subchorionic fluid, clinical bleeding, and pregnancy outcome. Obstet Gynecol 80:415, 1992
44. Laboda LA, Estroff JA, Benacerraf BR: First trimester bradycardia: a sign of impending fetal loss. J Ultrasound Med 8:561, 1989
45. Landy HJ, Keith L, Keith D: The vanishing twin. Acta Genet Med Gemellol 31:179, 1982
46. Levi S: Ultrasonic assessment of the high rate of human multiple pregnancy in the first trimester. J Clin Ultrasound 4:3, 1976
47. Sulak LE, Dodson MG: The vanishing twin: pathologic confirmation of an ultrasonographic phenomenon. Obstet Gynecol 68:811, 1986
48. Chow KK, Vengadasalam D: The predictive value of routine ultrasound in the clinical measurement of early pregnancy wastage (Abst). 12th World Congress on Fertility and Sterility, Singapore, 1986
49. Dickey RP, Olar TT, Taylor SN et al: Relationship of small gestational sac-crown-rump length differences to abortion and abortus karyotypes. Obstet Gynecol 79:554, 1992
50. Rulin MC, Bornstein SG, Campbell JD: The reliability of ultrasonography in the management of spontaneous abortion, clinically thought to be complete: a prospective study. Am J Obstet Gynecol 168:12, 1993
51. Curtis JA, Watson L: Sonographic diagnosis of oomphalocele in the first trimester of fetal gestation. J Ultrasound Med 7:97, 1988
52. Cyr DR, Mack LA, Schoenecker SA et al: Bowel migration in the normal fetus: US detection. Radiology 161:119, 1986
53. Piiroinen O: Studies in diagnostic ultrasound: size of the non-pregnant uterus in women of child-bearing age and uterine growth and foetal development in the first half of normal pregnancy. Acta Obstet Gynecol Scand (suppl.) 46:1, 1975

14

Congenital Anomalies

Rudy E. Sabbagha

The development of transvaginal probes, utilizing high frequency multifocal transducers, has markedly improved ultrasonic imaging of the pelvis and fetal structures, particularly in the interval between 8 and 15 weeks' gestation. In fact, transvaginal ultrasound has been the impetus for the development of sonoembryology—the study dealing with the ultrasonic visualization of fetal anatomic structures as they develop embryologically.

SONOEMBRYOLOGY

Eight to Ten Weeks' Gestation

At 8 weeks' gestation the neural axis appears as a thin line traversing the mid-aspect of the fetal body.[1] However, the diagnosis of spina bifida at this time remains uncertain. The fetal pole is quite clear, and the crown-rump length can be determined.

In the interval of 9 to 10 weeks' gestation the division of the brain into the telencephalon, diencephalon, mesencephalon, metencephalon, and myelencephalon is more apparent sonographically (Fig. 14-1).[1,2] The telencephalon, diencephalon, and mesencephalon develop into the cerebral hemispheres, thalami, and cerebral peduncles, respectively. The myelencephalon develops into the medulla, and the metencephalon into the pons and cerebellum. Interestingly, a nonmagnified view of the fetus from 9 to 11 weeks' gestation is more likely to show an overall uniformly echogenic pattern (Fig. 14-2). At 9 weeks the size of the fetal head surpasses that of the yolk sac,[1] and the biparietal diameter measures approximately 12 mm.[2] Visualization of the limb buds is also possible.

The posterior contour of the fetus including any nuchal translucency becomes evident. Presence of a nuchal translucency assumes significance in relation to fetal abnormalities (see the section, External Body Defects). The physiologic midgut hernia is also seen[3,4]; it appears as a hyperechogenic thickening of the cord at its abdominal insertion (Fig. 14-3).[4] At this point it should be emphasized that, under normal circumstances, the midgut may not completely retract into the abdominal cavity until the end of the 13th pregnancy week[3,4] (see section, Gastrointestinal Tract). The genitalia are still not apparent and are best imaged at 15 to 16 weeks' gestation.

Ten to Twelve Weeks' Gestation

By 10 weeks' gestation the embryo is termed a fetus. In the interval between the 10th and 11th pregnancy weeks the telencephalon develops into the cerebral hemispheres, and the falx, ventricles, choroid plexus, and cisterna magna can be identified (Fig. 14-4). By the 11th to 12th pregnancy week, ossification of the spine and skull occurs, allowing clearer sonographic demarcation of the neural canal and calvarium.[2] The cerebellum becomes visible by the 11th to 12th pregnancy week.[2]

The fingers also begin to form. However, clear visualization of the fingers even from the 12th to the 14th pregnancy weeks is not only a difficult task to achieve but can also be time consuming to accomplish.

Twelve to Fourteen Weeks' Gestation

The extraembryonic coelom becomes obliterated, but the yolk sac may still be visible during this time. The four-chamber heart may be visible in a larger

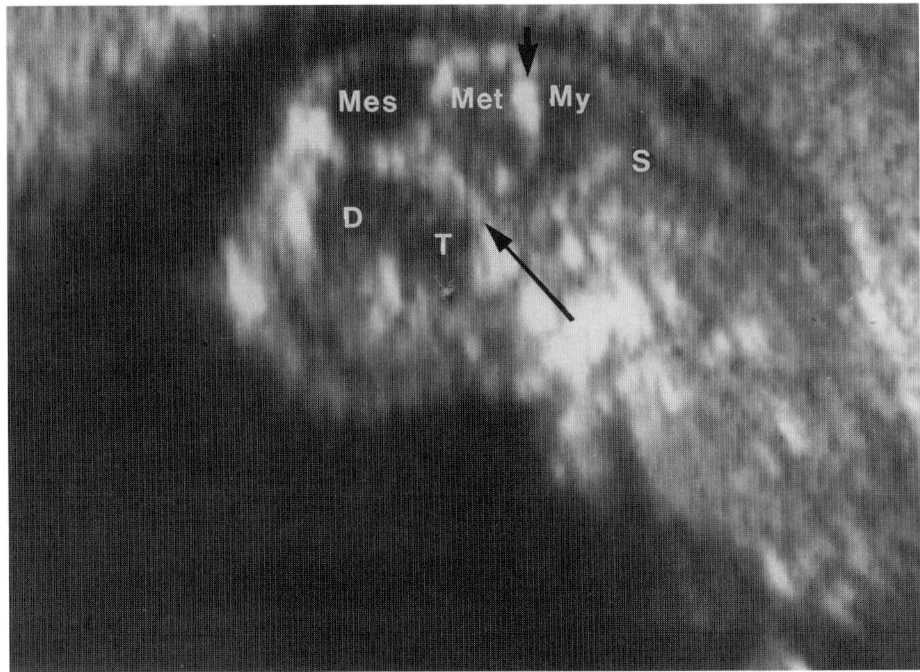

Fig. 14-1. Magnified profile of 10-week fetus showing the five mildly hypoechoic brain compartments. T, telencephalon; D, diencephalon; Mes, mesencephalon; Met, metencephalon; My, myelencephalon. (From Timor-Tritsch and Rottem,[1] with permission.)

percentage of fetuses, and the central nervous system can be imaged in sagittal, transverse, and coronal planes. The kidneys and bladder can also be seen in this interval. The frequency of imaging various anatomic planes between 10 to 14 weeks' gestation is shown in Table 14-1.

Fourteen to Sixteen Weeks' Gestation

The face, lungs, diaphragm, stomach, bowel, liver, and bladder are imaged in a larger proportion of fetuses during this time (Table 14-1).

ROLE OF TRANSVAGINAL ULTRASOUND

Presently, transvaginal ultrasound is *not* used as a screening examination for the diagnosis of congenital anomalies for the following reasons:

- Inability of the ultrasonographer to visualize specific anatomic features consistently. As a result, the definitive presence or absence of an anomaly may remain uncertain.
- Frequent prolongation of the time necessary to arrive at a diagnosis, which is attributed to the limited ability of the examiner to angle the transducer sufficiently to obtain the desired targeted anatomic plane. In fact, scanning by transvaginal ultrasound is usually performed in a random manner, and its success is dependent on how the fetus moves and what structures are visualized during such motion. In this regard, videotaping the study allows for subsequent frame by frame evaluation.
- The need to perform repeated scans to arrive at a definitive diagnosis or to confirm a suspicious finding.
- Insufficient studies to enable the definition of the sensitivity and specificity of transvaginal ultrasound.

Despite the drawbacks in the use of transvaginal ultrasound as a screening method in the diagnosis of congenital anomalies, the procedure is necessary in these specific situations:

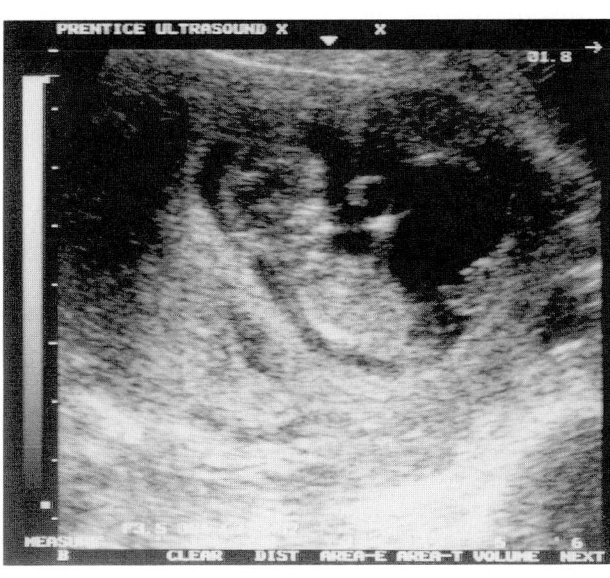

A

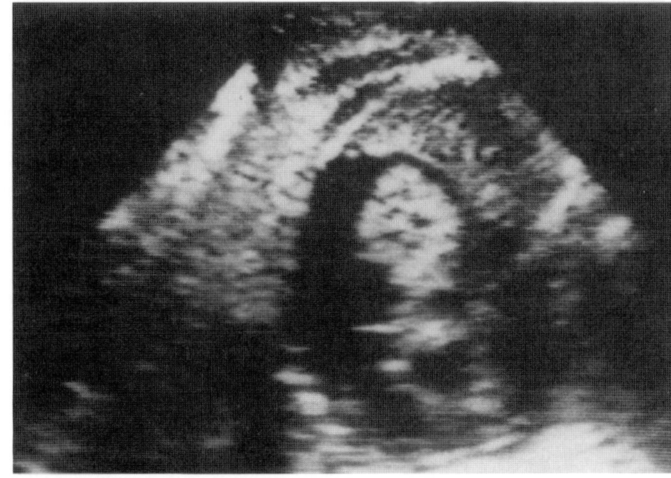

B

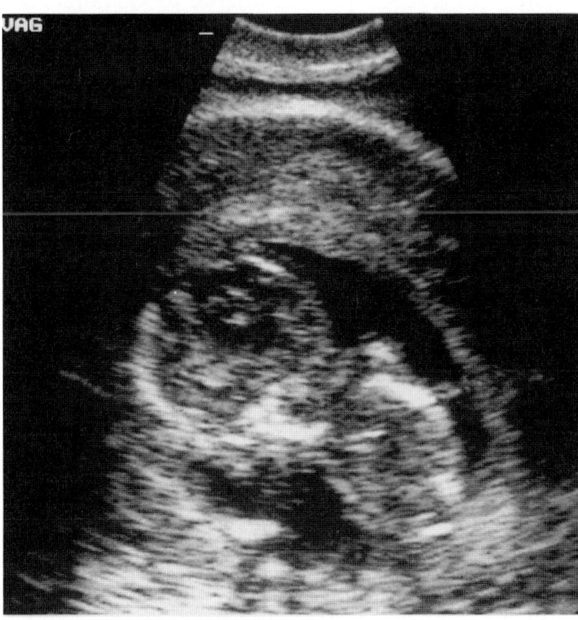

C

Fig. 14-2. Comparison of the echopattern of three fetuses by transvaginal sonography. **(A)** A nonmagnified profile of an 11-week fetus shows the brain to be uniformly echogenic; grossly the head is only slightly larger than the trunk. **(B)** The image of a 10+-week fetus in triplet pregnancy shows one large single ventricle (lower aspect of fetal pole) as in holoprosencephaly. **(C)** The profile of an asymmetrically growth-retarded fetus showing a markedly small abdomen in comparison to head size. The head circumference corresponded to menstrual dates (13 weeks), but the abdominal circumference was equivalent to only 11 weeks' gestation.

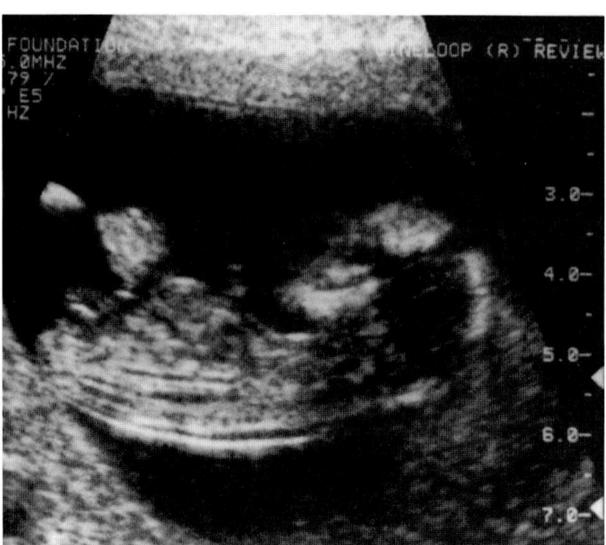

Fig. 14-3. Longitudinal view of 13-week fetus showing midgut herniation. (From Finley et al,[17] with permission.)

- When there is a history of a previous major defect,
- When the sonographer is unable to visualize adequately a low fetal head or one positioned in an occiput anterior or posterior position
- Multiple pregnancy,
- Need to undergo pregnancy reduction from, for example, five to two fetuses or to undergo a cervical cerclage procedure for an incompetent cervix
- Evaluation of other anomalies.

History of Major Congenital Anomaly

A history of a previous major fetal abnormality generates a great deal of parental anxiety in subsequent pregnancies. In such cases, normal findings by transvaginal ultrasound between 12 to 14 weeks' gestation will bring emotional relief to the parents—at least until such time that a detailed targeted scan is performed at approximately the 20th pregnancy week. The early diagnosis of an abnormality allows for appropriate counseling and the development of a management plan suitable to the prospective parents. The following congenital anomalies may be diagnosed by transvaginal ultrasound in the first trimester of pregnancy.

Central Nervous System

Congenital anomalies of the central nervous system (CNS) occur in approximately 3 in 1,000 births. Although transvaginal ultrasound has made it possible to visualize a specific CNS defect by 12 to 14 weeks' gestation, there is a paucity of data regarding its accuracy in the diagnosis of subtle CNS anomalies. A review of the sequential appearance of fetal neural structures would be helpful in understanding transvaginal images during the first trimester of pregnancy (Table 14-2).[2]

Anencephalus/Exencephalus The primary defect results from absence of the telencephalon and midbrain in association with maldevelopment of the frontal, parietal, and occipital bones.[2] Diagnosis by transvaginal ultrasound is now possible by 11 weeks' gestation (Fig. 14-5).[2] The frog-eye appearance of the face in exencephalus is so characteristic that it can no longer be mistaken for a normal cephalic pole, as was the case with abdominal ultrasound (Fig. 14-5).[2,5]

Microcephalus does not develop until the second or third trimester of pregnancy and cannot be diagnosed by first trimester transvaginal ultrasound.[6]

Hydrocephalus By 11 weeks' gestation the lateral ventricles normally extend to the inner parietal bones and are completely filled by the uniformly echogenic choroid plexus (see Fig. 14-4). However, the frontal aspects of the lateral ventricles remain relatively translucent. Early hydrocephalus results in compression of the choroid plexus and exaggeration of the translucency in the frontal horns (Fig. 14-4). Any deviation from the normal appearance of the choroid plexus is reason to ultrasonically reevaluate the fetus at a later gestational age. Other major CNS anomalies can also be diagnosed, including holoprosencephaly (Fig. 14-2).

Choroid plexus cysts are associated with an increase in the frequency of aneuploidy, particularly trisomy 18.[7] However, there are no data regarding early diagnosis of this entity by transvaginal ultrasound.

Dandy-Walker Malformation This malformation results in dilatation of the area occupied by the cisterna magna (Fig. 14-6). The transverse diameter of the cisterna magna, extending from the vermis to the inner aspect of the occipital bone, remains constant from 14 to 35 weeks' gestation—mean value = 5 mm (2 SD ± 6 mm).[8] In Dandy-Walker malformation there is aplasia or hypoplasia of the cerebellum. In addition the fourth ventricle is dilated and is displaced into the area of the cisterna magna, distending its cystic appearance.[9]

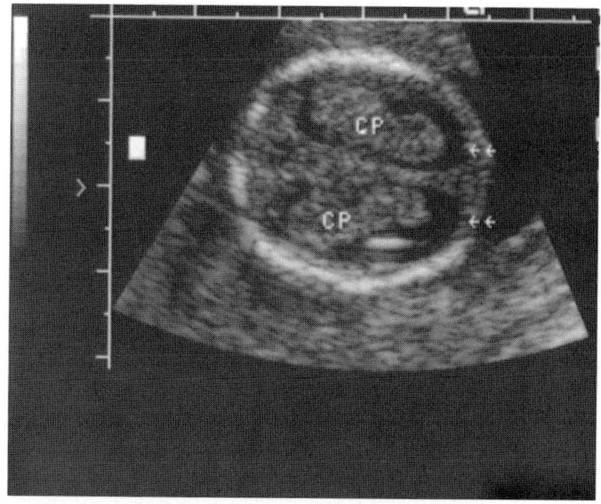

A

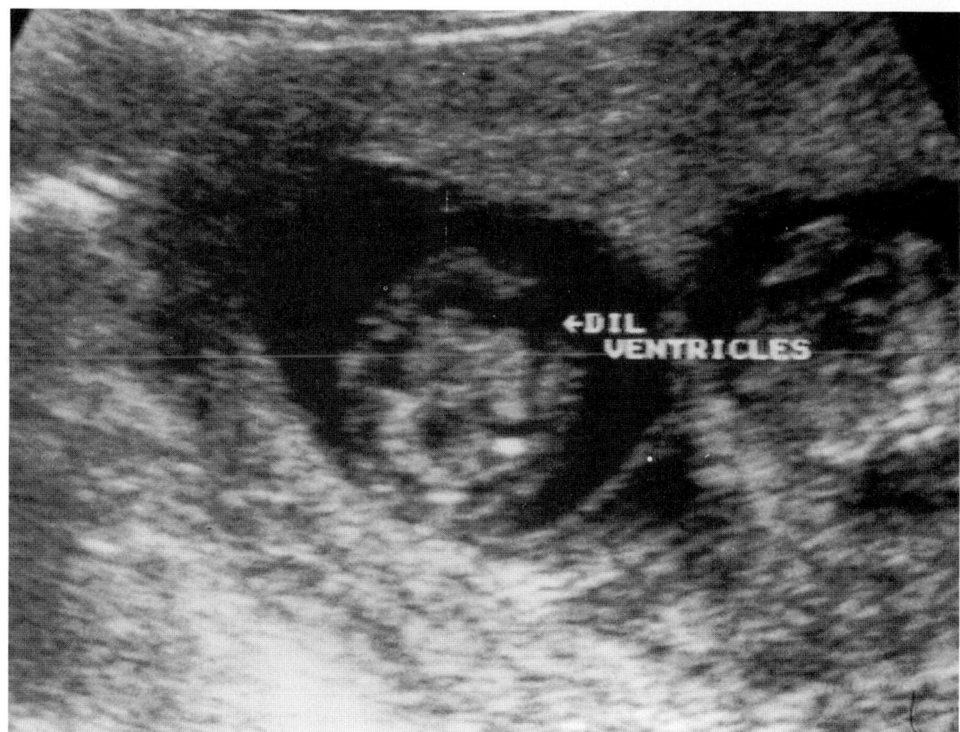

B

Fig. 14-4. Transvaginal scan of fetal head at 14+ weeks' gestation. **(A)** Transverse scan of fetal head shows choroid plexus (CP) filling the lateral ventricles. Note how the lateral ventricular wall reaches the inner aspect of the parietal bone posteriorly. The frontal horns appear somewhat large and are hypoechoic (arrows). **(B)** Transverse scan of fetal head with mild early hydrocephalus showing compression of the choroid plexus and a hypoechoic space between the lateral ventricular wall and the inner aspect of the parietal bone. Note how the frontal horns (arrow) appear more dilated than in Fig. A.

Table 14-1. Frequency In Which Specific Fetal Anatomic Structures Are Visualized By Transvaginal Sonography From Approximately 10 to 14 Weeks Gestation[a]

Gestation (weeks)	<10	10-12	12-14	>14
Patients	19	34	65	26
Four chamber	–	13 (37)	44 (68)	21 (81)
Head	–	13 (37)	43 (66)	16 (62)
Spine	–	5 (15)	28 (43)	8 (31)
Stomach	2 (10)	19 (56)	62 (95)	24 (92)
Kidneys	–	5 (15)	38 (58)	14 (54)
Bladder	3 (16)	14 (42)	52 (80)	23 (88)

[a] Percentages are shown in brackets. Study included 150 low risk pregnancies and utilized Acuson equipment and a 5-MHz transducer.
(Adapted from Johnson et al,[36] with permission.)

The abnormality occurs by 6 weeks' gestation, but may be detected using transvaginal ultrasound between 11 to 12 pregnancy weeks; that is, the interval when the cerebellum is normally visible (Table 14-2).[2]

The differential diagnosis of dilated cisterna magna includes aneuploidy, infection with human immunodeficiency virus, and arachnoid cyst.[6,9]

Fetal Spine Although the fetal spine is visualized by 8 weeks' gestation ossification does not occur until the 11th to 12th pregnancy week.[2] At this time the vertebral bodies can be visualized. Splaying of the spine is characteristic of spina bifida (Fig. 14-7).[1] Again, there are no data to indicate how accurate the diagnosis would be or whether a small spina bifida can also be detected readily. Meningocele has also been diagnosed in the first trimester of pregnancy.[2]

Table 14-2. Sequential Appearance of Fetal Neural Structures During the First Trimester

	Menstrual Age (Weeks)							
Structure	*6*	*7*	*8*	*9*	*10*	*11*	*12*	*13*
Cephalic pole		—	—	—	—	→		
Univentricular system		—	—	→				
Falx cerebri				—	—	—	→	
Biventricular system					—	—	→	
Choroid plexus					—	—	→	
Thalamus						—	→	
III ventricle						—	→	
Corpus callosum						—	→	
Cerebral peduncles						—	→	
Pons							→	
Cerebellum							→	
Cerebellar tentorium							→	
Hippocampus							→	
Posterior fossa (cisterna magna)							→	
IV ventricle							→	
Cerebral arteries						—	→	
Corpus striatum							→	
Calvarial skeleton								→
Spinal skeleton								→

(From Achiron and Achiron,[2] with permission.)

Cardiac System

Adequate evaluation of the heart by transvaginal ultrasound at 14 weeks' gestation is only possible if all cardiac views are obtainable, including the four chamber (4-CH), the left ventricular outflow tract (LVOT), the right ventricular outflow tract (RVOT), great vessel view, short axis view, and aortic arch. Frequently, however, only the 4-CH plus one or two other views can be obtained in a 15- to 20-minute interval (Fig. 14-8).

In the second trimester of pregnancy difficulty in imaging the heart by abdominal sonography is related to early gestational age, maternal adipose tissue thickness less than or equal to 2 cm, and a history of previous pelvic surgery.[10] These factors increase the absorption of sound and deflect the sound beam, resulting in fewer returning echoes. DeVore and associates[10] showed that the probability of imaging the 4-CH view in a pregnant woman at 16 weeks, with a 2 cm thick adipose tissue and a pelvic scar, is 55 percent.[10] By comparison, rescanning at 21 weeks' gestation increases this probability to 90 percent.[10]

With transvaginal ultrasound, gestational age at the time of the cardiac scan is the most important factor affecting image resolution (Table 14-1). Therefore, Johnson and associates[11] used a 5-MHz probe to examine the role of transvaginal ultrasound in the early detection of heart disease. They examined 270 and 32 pregnant women at low and high risk for cardiac defects, respectively. The scan time for each patient was

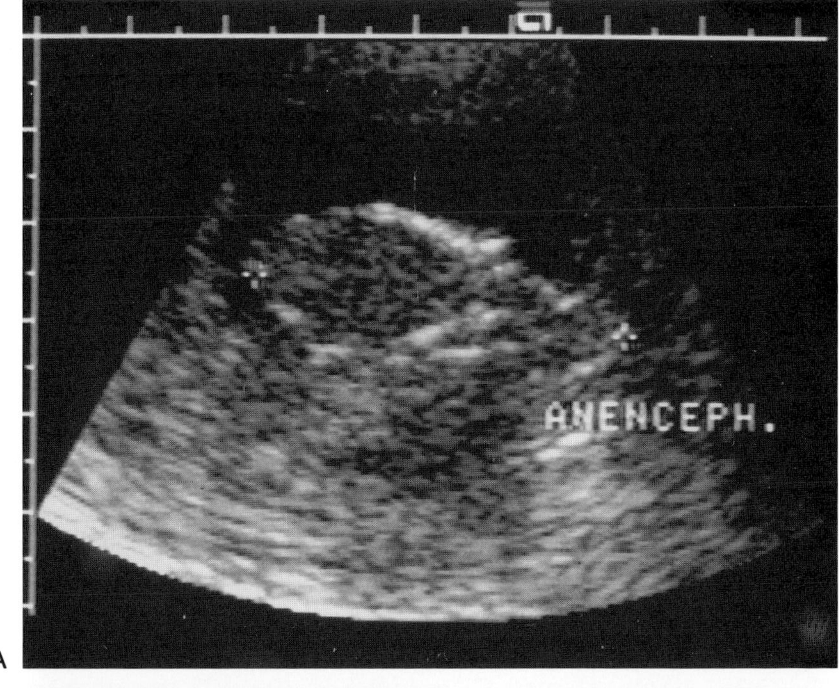

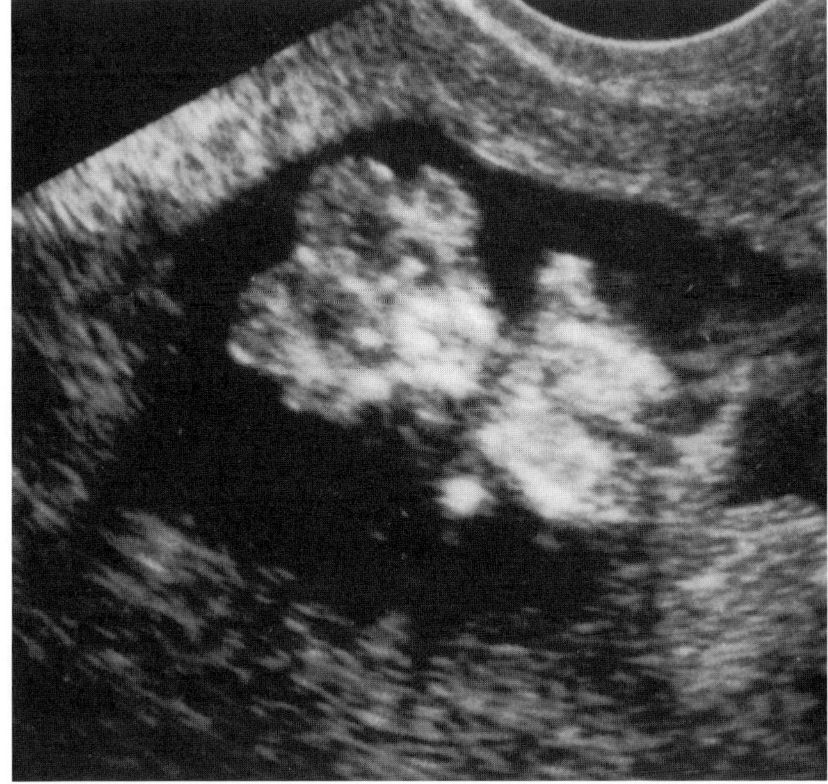

Fig. 14-5. (**A**) Transvaginal scan of anencephalic fetus with absence of fetal cranium on right side of image. (**B**) Frog-like appearance of fetus with exencephaly. (From Nishi and Nakano,[5] with permission.)

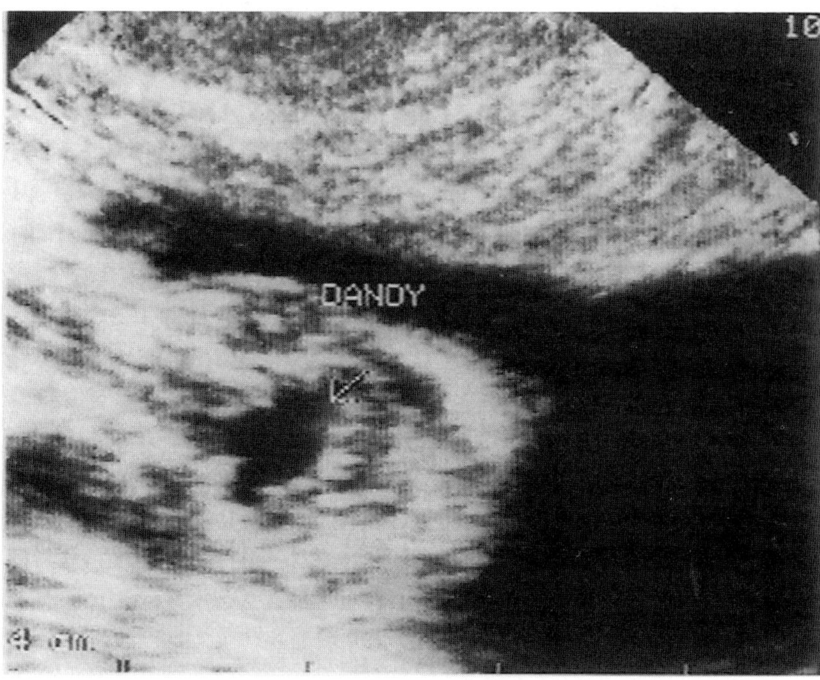

Fig. 14-6. Transvaginal scan of fetus at 12 weeks gestation shows a dilated hypoechoic interface in the area of the cisterna magna (arrow) as in Dandy-Walker malformation. (From Achiron and Achiron,[2] with permission.)

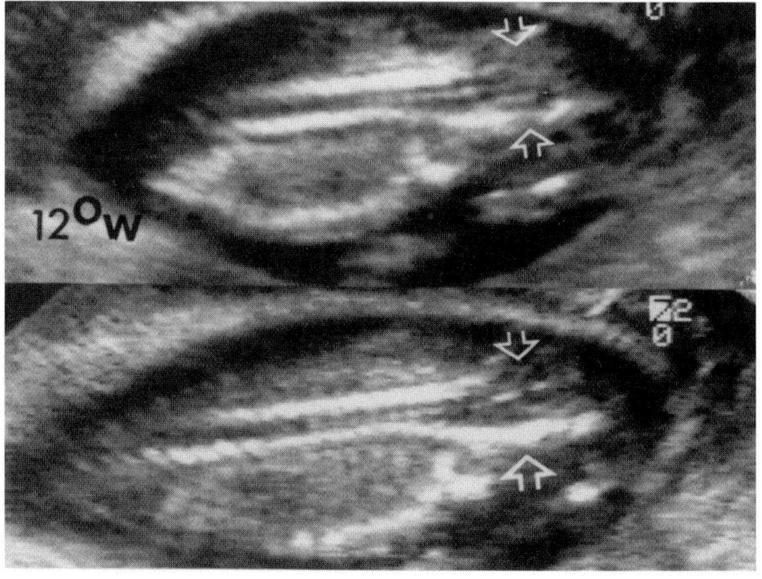

Fig. 14-7. Transvaginal scan of 12-week fetus showing ossification of the spine and splaying in the lower aspect (arrows) consistent with spina bifida. (From Timor-Tritsch and Rottem,[1] with permission.)

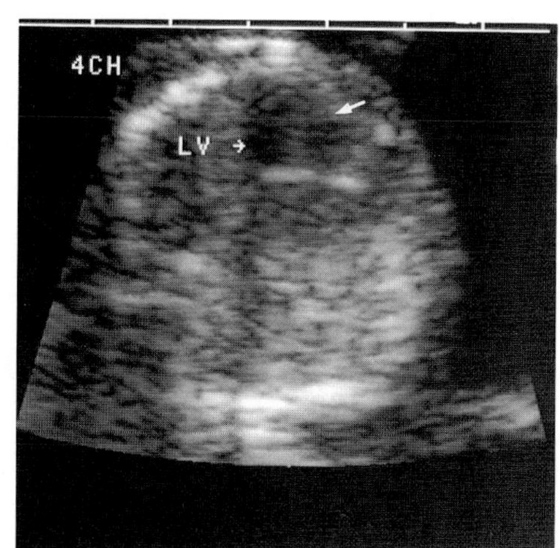

A

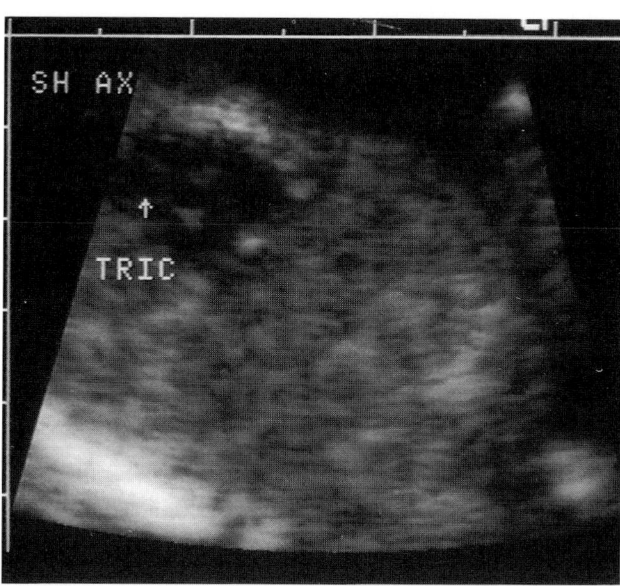

B

Fig. 14-8. Transvaginal scan of a normal fetal heart at 14+ weeks' gestation. **(A)** Four-chamber heart view: the left ventricle (LV, arrow) appears normal; the right ventricle is normal in size and shows the moderator band (arrow). The atrioventricular valves appear normal. The interventricular septum is complete. The atria are of normal size, but the foramen ovale is not visualized. **(B)** Short axis view. The tricuspid valve is on the left side of the image (arrow); the right ventricular outflow tract and pulmonary valve are seen clockwise from the arrow and extend over the aorta (circle in center).

preset at 10 minutes; they reasoned that transvaginal ultrasound would not be useful as a screening study if it required a longer time. However, they videotaped all cardiac scans and reviewed them later. They showed that full cardiac anatomy could not be assessed in 46 percent of fetuses at 14 weeks' gestation (Table 14-3). Their ability to visualize the 4-CH view and the outflow tracts at different gestational intervals is shown in Tables 14-4 and 14-5.

Table 14-3. Number of Cases in Which a Full Cardiac Anatomy was Possible

Gestational Age (Weeks)	*n*	*Full Cardiac Anatomy (%) (Four-Chamber and Great Vessels)*
10	26	—
11	33	—
12	51	16 (31)
13	61	26 (43)
14	39	18 (46)
15	4	2 (50)
16	1	—

(From Johnson et al,[11] with permission.)

Cardiac imaging by transvaginal ultrasound may be improved if longer time is spent videotaping the scan. Although Bronshtein and associates[12] discovered heart defects in 47 of 12,793 pregnant women examined by transvaginal ultrasound over a 5-year period,

Table 14-4. Number of Cases in Which the Three- or Four-Chamber View was Possible

Gestational Age (Weeks)	*n*	*Four-Chambers Visualized (%)*
6	1	—
7	2	—
8	16	—
9	26	—
10	26	7 (27)
11	33	19 (58)
12	51	36 (71)
13	61	45 (74)
14	39	28 (72)
15	4	3 (75)
16	1	1 (100)

(From Johnson et al,[11] with permission.)

Table 14-5. Number of Great Vessels–Aorta, Pulmonary Artery and Pulmonary Veins–Demonstrated

Gestational Age (Weeks)	*n*	*Aorta (%)*	*Pulmonary Artery (%)*	*Pulmonary Veins (%)*
6	1	—	—	—
7	2	—	—	—
8	16	—	—	—
9	26	—	—	—
10	26	1 (4)	3 (12)	—
11	33	8 (24)	7 (21)	—
12	51	30 (59)	21 (41)	3 (6)
13	61	38 (62)	31 (51)	7 (11)
14	39	22 (56)	22 (56)	7 (18)
15	4	3 (75)	2 (50)	—
16	1	1(100)	—	—

(From Johnson et al,[11] with permission.)

Table 14-6. Prevalence of Congenital Heart Defects by Diagnosis

Diagnosis	*Gestational Age (wk)**	*N (%)*
Ventricular septal defects	12.6	22 (47%)
Isolated	14	2 (4%)
+Overriding aorta	12.6	10 (21%)
+Other anomalies	14	10 (21%)
Asymmetrical chambers (total)	11.8	13 (28%)
Hypoplastic left heart	11.8	6 (13%)
Ebstein anomaly	14	3 (6%)
Other	12	4 (9%)
Common atrioventricular canal	12	6 (13%)
Cardiomyopathy	14	6 (13%)
Transposition of great arteries	15	4 (9%)
Single ventricle	12	2 (4%)
Coarctation of aorta	15	3 (6%)
Other†		7 (15%)

* Earliest gestational age at which the diagnosis was made.
† Includes dextrocardia, ectopic heart, "five ventricles" (conjoined twins), pulmonary hypoplasia (two cases), aortic stenosis, and microcalcifications.
(From Bronshtein et al,[12] with permission.)

they did not describe the time it took them to complete different scans. Further, 95 percent of the scans were performed between 14 and 16 weeks' gestation. In their study they used a 6.5-MHz vaginal probe. They were able to visualize the 4-CH view and the outflow tracts in the majority of fetuses and detected a number of significant abnormalities (Table 14-6). Importantly, they showed that the rate of aneuploidy in fetuses with cardiac defects plus other malformations was 37 percent. They also indicated that 23 percent of cardiac lesions would have been missed if the 4-CH were the only view obtained. However, there was a discrepancy between the ultrasound diagnosis and pathologic results in 15 fetuses.

Pulmonary System

Accurate diagnosis of types II and III cystadenomatoid malformation (CAM) of the lungs (pulmonary cysts less than 1 cm and less than 0.5 cm, respectively) has been reported by transabdominal sonography as early as 16 to 17 weeks' gestation.[13,14] However, there is a paucity of data regarding diagnosis by transvaginal ultrasound from the 13th to the 14th pregnancy week. In CAM the embryologic insult arresting cellular development between the bronchioles and the alveoli occurs before the seventh week of gestation.[15] Thus, early diagnosis by transvaginal ultrasound is theoretically possible. In CAM type I the cystic lesions are large, but the prognosis is favorable. In CAM types II and III, hydrops secondary to cardiac and mediastinal compression is frequently present and is directly responsible for adverse fetal outcome. Fetal hydrops can be recognized readily by transvaginal ultrasound as early as 9 weeks' gestation (see section, External Body Defects). The detection of hydrops may result in early detection of CAM by transvaginal ultrasound. Spontaneous regression of the abnormality has been reported in a few cases, particularly in type I disease. The differential diagnoses include lung sequestration and diaphragmatic hernia. In appropriately selected cases, in utero resection has been successful in preventing placentomegaly and hydrops.[16]

Gastrointestinal Tract

Anterior Wall Defects Development of the anterior abdominal wall depends on the fusion of the lateral folds during the fourth embryonic week.[3] Failure of fusion leads to the formation of an omphalocele, an echogenic-appearing mass protruding into the umbilical stalk of the abdominal wall (Fig. 14-3).[17] However, the diagnosis of omphalocele should not be made before the 13th pregnancy week because physiologic bowel herniation may be normally present until that time.[3,4]

Abnormality in the return of bowel may be associated with the development of GI abnormalities. Finley and associates[17] reported a case in which there was delayed return of the gut at 13 weeks' gestation, the ultrasonic image being consistent with herniation of bowel, rather than an abdominal wall defect. Subsequently, the cord insertion appeared normal, but at 20 weeks' gestation dilatation of the bowel became apparent. At birth the neonate had midgut volvulus, bowel obstruction, and gangrene of the small intestine. In contrast, Bromley and Benacerraf[18] reported a case in which an omphalocele apparent at 15+ weeks' gestation resolved naturally at term.[18]

The early diagnosis of omphalocele is important because the condition is associated with an increase in the frequency of other congenital anomalies and aneuploidy. Although it is known that herniated bowel alone is more likely to be associated with chromosomal abnormalities than is herniated bowel plus liver,[19] the distinction between these two possibilities may not be possible by first trimester transvaginal ultrasound. At this time it is also not clear whether gastroschisis can always be differentiated from omphalocele by transvaginal ultrasound.

Hyperechogenic Bowel In some cases hyperechogenic bowel (HB) may be a normal ultrasonic finding. However, the condition may be associated with an increased frequency of aneuploidy, intestinal obstruction or atresia, intrauterine growth retardation, infection with cytomegalovirus, and cystic fibrosis.[20] Using abdominal ultrasound it is possible to visualize HB as early as the 16th pregnancy week.[20] However, diagnosis by transvaginal ultrasound in the first trimester has not been reported.

Renal Anomalies

The frequency of visualization of the kidneys and bladder by transvaginal ultrasound in the first trimester is shown in Table 14-1. However, abnormalities, such as posterior urethral valve (PUV), pelviectasis, and ureteropelvic junction (UPJ) dilatation, have not been reported that early. Early diagnosis is likely to lead to evaluation of fetal karyotype, particularly in the presence of pelviectasis, and the possibility of early intervention in PUV abnormality.

External Body Defects: Nuchal Translucency

Frequently a nuchal translucency or thickening measuring 2.5 mm to 3.0 mm is visualized by transvaginal ultrasound from 9 to 14 weeks gestation. The translucency or hypoechoic area is covered by a thin membrane and is situated in the posterior aspect of the occipital, nuchal, or upper thoracic area (Fig. 14-9).[21] Although the presence of septation/s within the translucency is more likely to represent cystic hygroma (Fig. 14-9), the exact etiology cannot be determined by transvaginal ultrasound in the first trimester

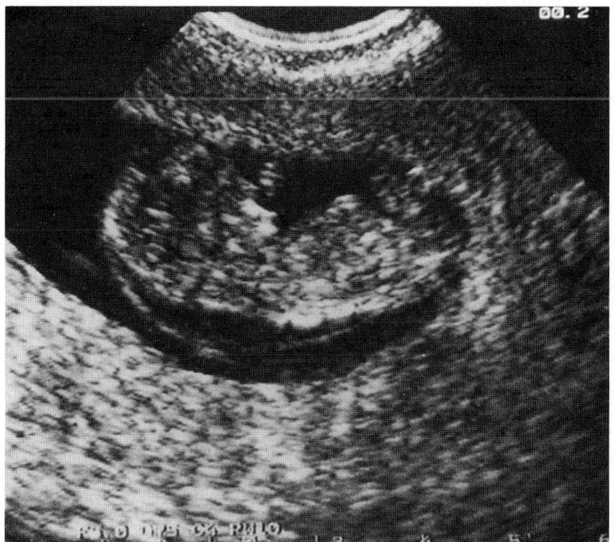

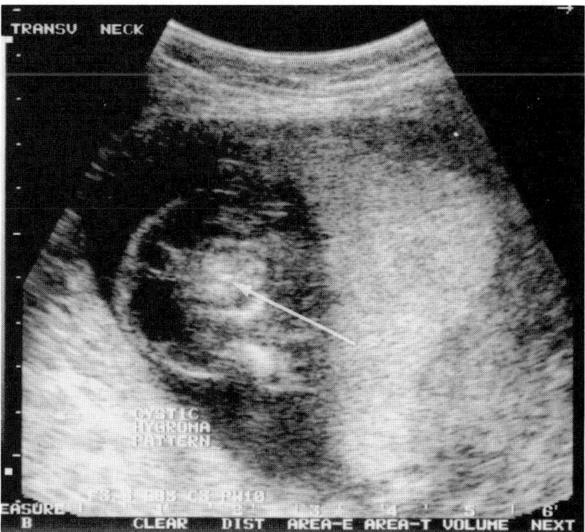

Fig. 14-9. (**A**) Occipital-thoracic translucency in 10+-week fetus. (**B**) Cross-section of neck in a fetus with cystic hygroma. Note the spine (arrow) and hypoechoic area with septation surrounding the neck. (Fig. A from Ville et al,[21] with permission.)

Table 14-7. Outcome of Fetuses with Nuchal Cystic Hygromata or Nuchal Translucency

	Cystic Hygromata (n = 56)		*Nuchal Translucency (n = 29)*	
	n	%	*n*	%
Abnormal karyotype	16	29	8	28
Hydrops	4	7	—	—
Termination	15	27	8	28
Intrauterine death	1	2	—	—
Normal karyotype	40	72	21	73
Other defects	10	18	—	—
Hydrops	6	11	—	—
Termination	9	16	—	—
Neonatal death	1	2	—	—
No other defect	30	54	21	73
Hydrops	1	2	—	—
Termination	1	2	—	—
Neonatal death	1	2	—	—
Normal infant	23	41	16	55
Ongoing pregnancy	5	9	5	18

(From Ville et al,[21] with permission.

Table 14-9. Associated Anomalies in 10 of the 40 Chromosomally Normal Fetuses with Nuchal Cystic Hygromata

Facial cleft
Micrognathia, low-set ears, intrauterine growth retardation, and pulmonary hypoplasia
Choanal atresia and atrioventricular septal defect
Flexion contractures of the fingers and knees
Pulmonary artery stenosis
Multiple pterygia with documented family history
Micrognathia and pulmonary artery stenosis
Short limbs and exomphalos
Micrognathia, low-set ears, cleft lip, diaphragmatic hernia and digital anomalies
Renal dysplasia

(From Ville et al,[21] with permission.)

of pregnancy. Nonetheless, the differential diagnosis includes nuchal thickening secondary to aneuploidy, cystic hygroma, and a normal finding.

The largest series to date has been reported by Ville and associates (Table 14-7).[21] Importantly, none of the fetuses without septations within the translucent neck area had monosomy X, whereas 4 of 56 believed to have cystic hygroma had Turner's syndrome (Table 14-8). Ten of the fetuses with cystic hygroma and normal karyotype had other associated anomalies (Table 14-9); furthermore, six of such fetuses developed hydrops. Importantly, hydrops can be readily visualized by transvaginal ultrasound as early as 9 weeks' gestation.

In a review of the literature encompassing 71 fetuses with nuchal thickening, Shulman and associates[22] found an abnormal karyotype in 52.9 percent. In their study of 32 cases diagnosed by transvaginal ultrasound in the first trimester of pregnancy, the proportion of monosomy X to autosomal aneuploidy was 26.6 percent. By contrast, Chervenak and associates[23] found a 73.3 percent rate of monosomy X in 15 cases of cystic hygroma diagnosed in the second trimester of pregnancy. Importantly, in the presence of nuchal translucency, the presence or absence of septations did alter the rate of chromosomal abnormalities, as previously reported by Bronshtein and associates.[24]

Interestingly, a large number of first trimester fetuses with nuchal translucency and normal karyotype show no phenotypic evidence of cystic hygroma at birth. This can be attributed to resolution of the obstruction between the lymphatic and venous channels in the neck or development of an alternative route connecting the lymphatic and venous systems.[23]

Table 14-8. Cytogenetic Results in 56 Fetuses with Nuchal Cystic Hygromata and 29 with Nuchal Translucency

	Fetal Karyotype						
	46XX	*46XY*	*45X*	*47XXX*	*Trisomy 21*	*Trisomy 18*	*Trisomy 13*
Cystic hygromata	21	19	4	1	5	6	0
Nuchal translucency	11	10	0	0	4	3	1

(From Ville et al,[21] with permission.)

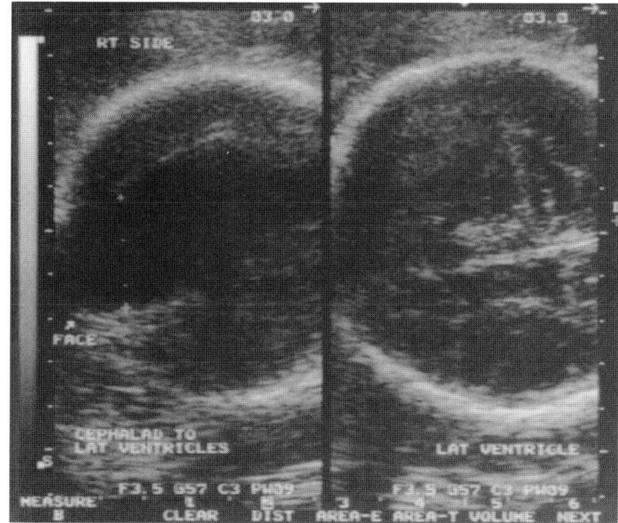

Fig. 14-10. **(A)** Image on left shows poor resolution of fetal brain anatomy by abdominal scan because of an abdominal scar. **(B)** In the right image of the fetal head the falx and lateral ventricles are clearly seen with transvaginal ultrasound.

Poor Visualization of Fetal Head

Poor visualization of the fetal head by abdominal sonography may result from maternal obesity, thick scar formation in the suprapubic area, and a low lying fetal head (Fig. 14-10).[9] In such cases the use of transvaginal ultrasound is more likely to allow imaging of brain anatomy, including the ventricular system (Fig. 14-10).[25]

Using transvaginal ultrasound, Monteagudo et al[25] were able to produce parasagittal and coronal images of the fetal head (Fig. 14-11). Nomograms of the various normal measurements were also published (Figs. 14-12 to 14-15).[25]

Evaluation of Multiple Pregnancy

When multiple pregnancy is diagnosed by early vaginal ultrasound, further evaluation by 10 weeks' gestation is essential to examine the number of fetuses, the

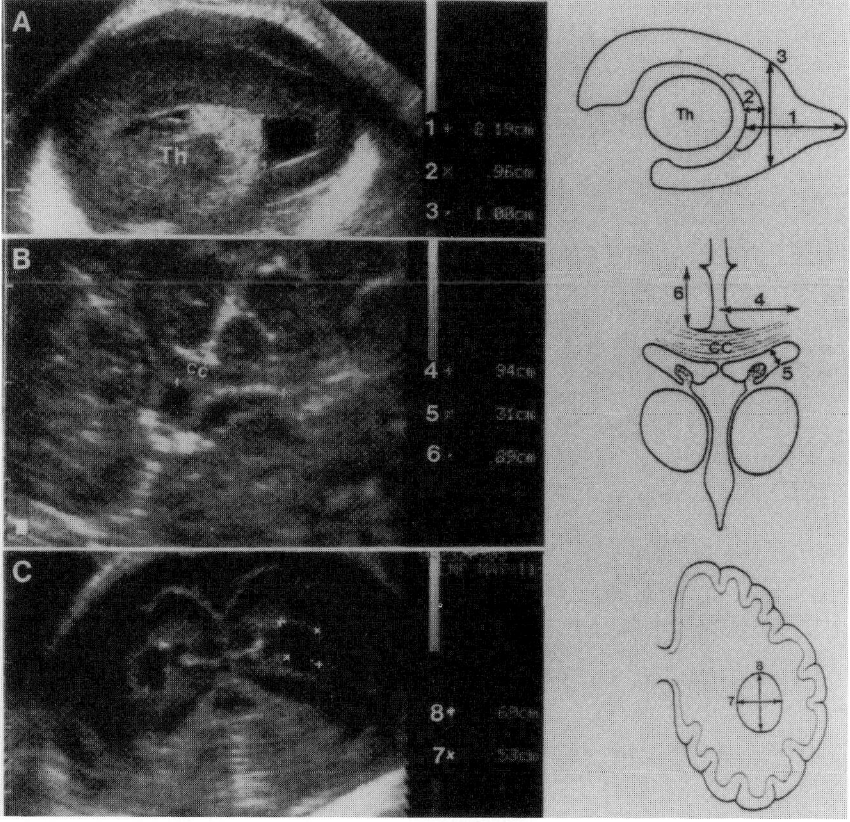

Fig. 14-11. Transvaginal images of the brain. **(A)** Longitudinal image of head showing thalamus (Th), length of ventricle, 1, height of ventricle, 2, thickness of choroid plexus, 3. **(B)** Midcoronal view of the head showing corpus callosum (CC), middle to upper edge of the lateral ventricle, 6; depth of lateral ventricle, 4. **(C)** Occipital coronal section showing width of occipital horn, and height of occipital horn, 8. (From Monteagudo et al,[25] with permission.)

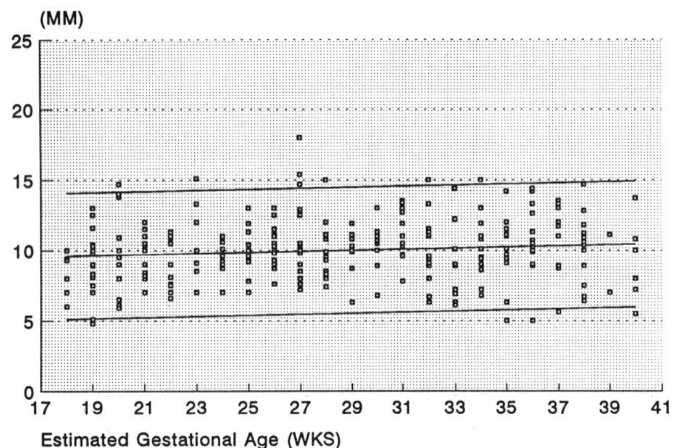

Fig. 14-12. Scattergram and confidence intervals for choroid plexus thickness. (From Monteagudo et al,[25] with permission.)

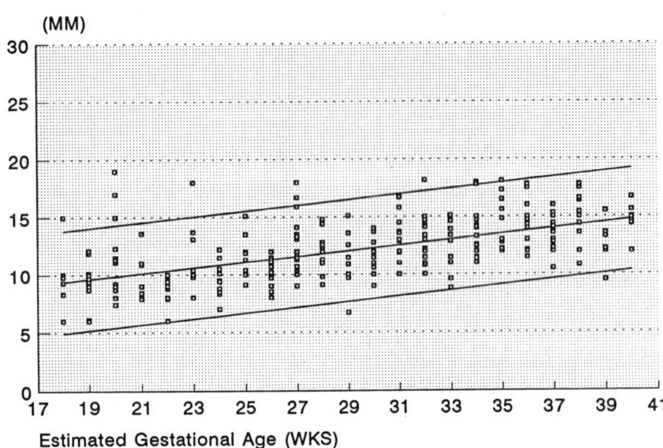

Fig. 14-14. Scattergram and confidence intervals for midline to upper edge of lateral ventricle. (From Monteagudo et al,[25] with permission.)

relative size of the fetuses, (Fig. 14-16) chorionicity (Fig. 14-16), and fetal abnormalities (Fig. 14-17). Recently, Zucchini and associates[26] diagnosed twin reversed arterial perfusion (TRAP) syndrome at 9 weeks' gestation (Fig. 14-17). In this abnormality arterial pressure in one of the monochorionic monoamniotic twins exceeds the other. Thus, blood flow is reversed in the recipient twin, and deoxygenated blood in the umbilical arteries perfuses the lower extremities. As a result, varying degrees of upper body reduction anomalies occur, including acardia (Fig. 14-17). Fetal edema and hydrops are recognizable in the first trimester of pregnancy (Fig. 14-17).

Conjoined twinning occurs once in every 50,000 births. The most common type is chest union or thoracopagus, representing 40 percent of cases.[27] The frequency of the other combinations include omphalopagus in 34 percent, pygopagus or attachment at the buttocks in 18 percent, and ischiopagus or the joining of the ischiums in 6 percent. Conjoined twins have been diagnosed as early as 8 to 10 weeks' gestation.

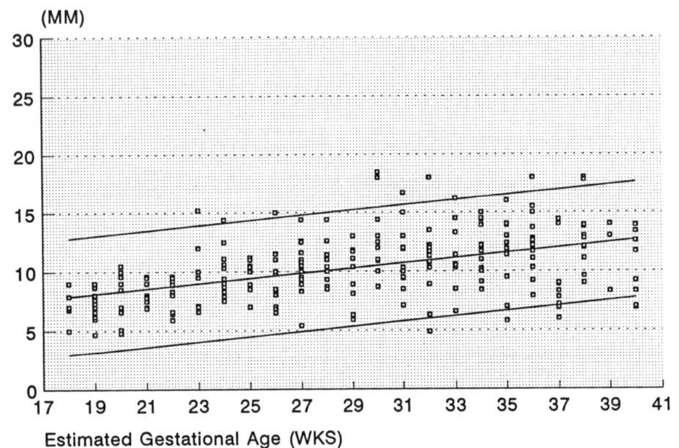

Fig. 14-13. Scattergram and confidence intervals of occipital horn height. (From Monteagudo et al,[25] with permission.)

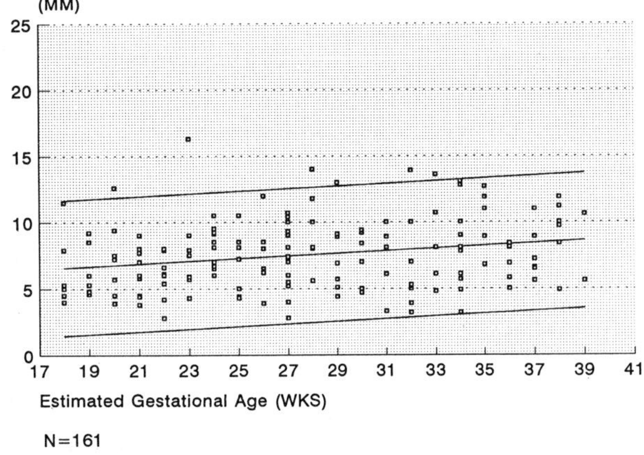

Fig. 14-15. Scattergram and confidence intervals for height of occipital horn. (From Monteagudo et al,[25] with permission.)

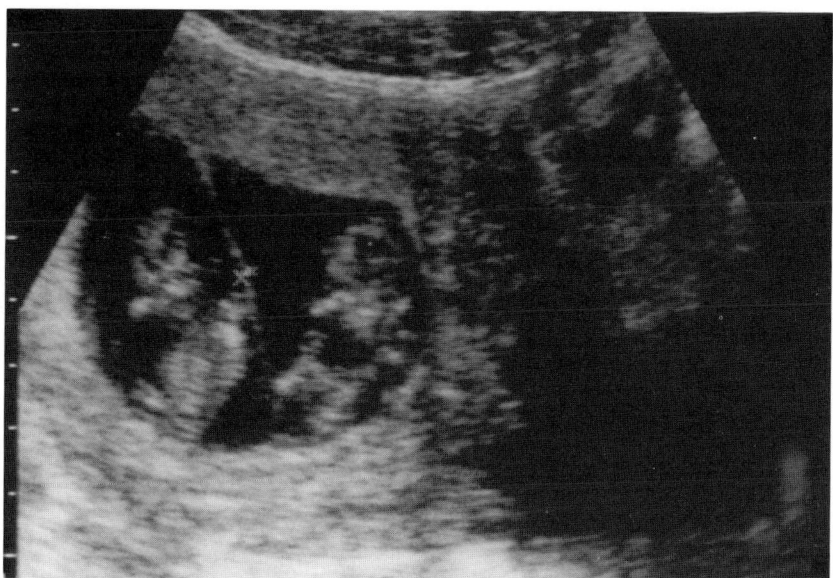

Fig. 14-16. Transvaginal image of twin fetuses at 10+ weeks' gestation showing similar growth, normal anatomy, and a membrane thicker than 2 mm, suggesting dichorionic diamniotic twins.

Such early diagnosis will ensure appropriate parental counseling.

Transvaginal Ultrasound Before Pregnancy Reduction or Cervical Cerclage

In women who elect to reduce pregnancy—for example, from quadruplets to singleton or twin gestation—it is essential to evaluate fetal anatomy by the 10th pregnancy week. In this way the pregnancy can be maintained for those fetuses who exhibit normal anatomic features and growth parameters (Fig. 14-3). Growth parameters of the head and abdominal circumferences have been derived by transvaginal ultrasound (Tables 14-10 and 14-11).[29] Comparison of the head and body circumferences to these tables helps in determining whether early fetal growth retardation is present (Fig. 14-3). If present, fetal karyotype should be determined to rule out chromosomal abnormality as the etiologic factor.[30]

If cervical cerclage is indicated, evaluation of fetal anatomy is essential before the procedure. In such cases the discovery of a major anomaly may obviate the need for surgery or dictate further study, including assessment of fetal karyotype.

Table 14-10. Conversion Table for Head Circumference Measurements (in centimeters) to Menstrual Age.[a]

Menstrual Age (weeks + days)	*Head Circumference (cm)*	*Menstrual Age (weeks + days)*	*Head Circumference (cm)*
8 + 5	3.53	11 + 4	6.49
8 + 6	3.68	11 + 5	6.64
9 + 0	3.82	11 + 6	6.78
9 + 1	3.97	12 + 0	6.93
9 + 2	4.12	12 + 1	7.08
9 + 3	4.27	12 + 2	7.23
9 + 4	4.42	12 + 3	7.38
9 + 5	4.56	12 + 4	7.52
9 + 6	4.71	12 + 5	7.67
10 + 0	4.86	12 + 6	7.82
10 + 1	5.00	13 + 0	7.97
10 + 2	5.16	13 + 1	8.12
10 + 3	5.30	13 + 2	8.26
10 + 4	5.45	13 + 3	8.41
10 + 5	5.60	13 + 4	8.56
10 + 6	5.75	13 + 5	8.71
11 + 0	5.90	13 + 6	8.86
11 + 1	6.04	14 + 0	9.00
11 + 2	6.19	14 + 1	9.15
11 + 3	6.34	14 + 2	9.30

[a] 95% confidence interval is ±4.8 days
(From Lasser et al,[29] with permission.)

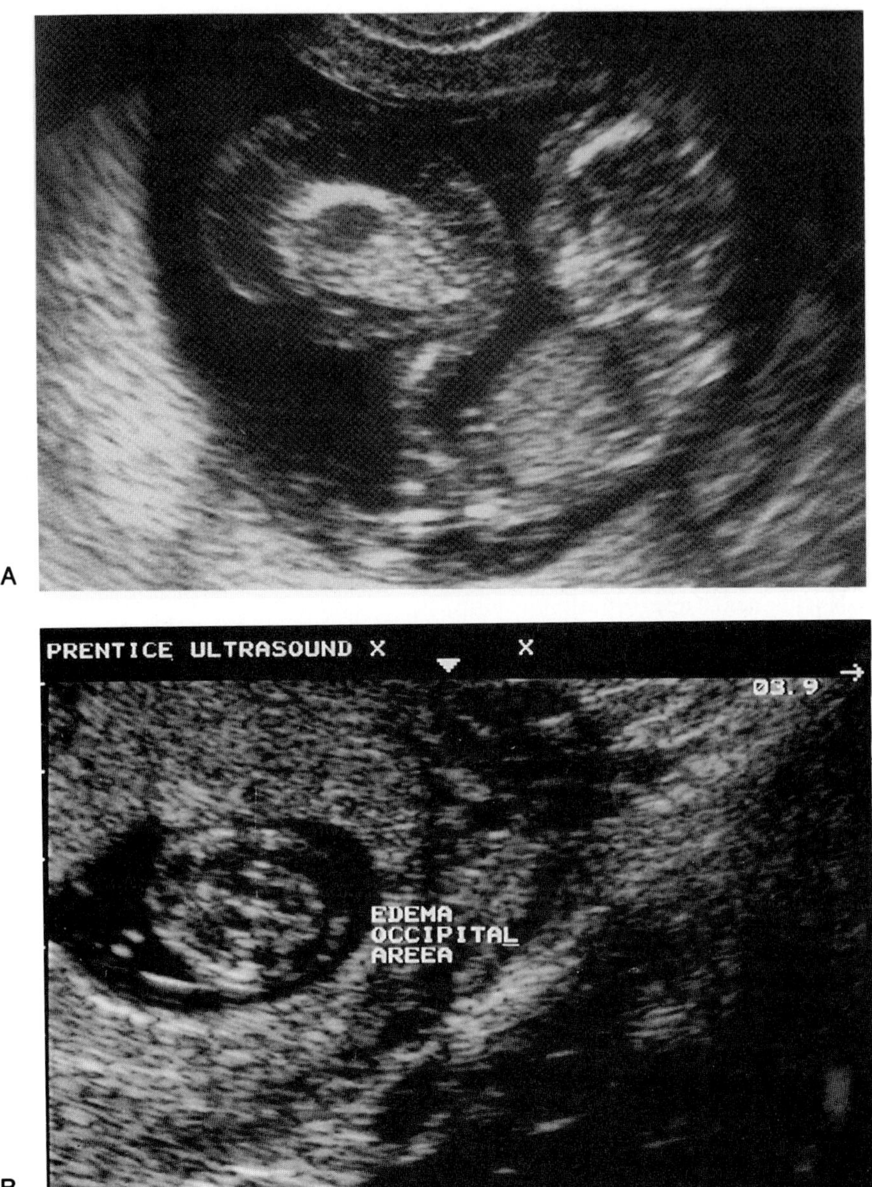

Fig. 14-17. **(A)** Transvaginal image of 9-week twin pregnancy with one acardiac twin on left side. Note marked hydrops in the acardiac twin. **(B)** Transverse scan of occipital area in 12-week fetus with hydrops. (Fig. A from Zucchini et al,[26] with permission.)

Table 14-11. Conversion Table for Abdominal Circumference Measurements (in centimeters) to Menstrual Age.[a]

Menstrual Age (weeks + days)	*Abdominal Circumference (cm)*	*Menstrual Age (weeks + days)*	*Abdominal Circumference (cm)*
8 + 5	3.09	11 + 4	4.91
8 + 6	3.17	11 + 5	5.02
9 + 0	3.24	11 + 6	5.14
9 + 1	3.32	12 + 0	5.26
9 + 2	3.40	12 + 1	5.38
9 + 3	3.47	12 + 2	5.51
9 + 4	3.56	12 + 3	5.64
9 + 5	3.64	12 + 4	5.77
9 + 6	3.72	12 + 5	5.90
10 + 0	3.81	12 + 6	6.04
10 + 1	3.90	13 + 0	6.18
10 + 2	3.99	13 + 1	6.32
10 + 3	4.08	13 + 2	6.47
10 + 4	4.18	13 + 3	6.62
10 + 5	4.27	13 + 4	6.78
10 + 6	4.37	13 + 5	6.93
11 + 0	4.48	13 + 6	7.09
11 + 1	4.58	14 + 0	7.26
11 + 2	4.69	14 + 1	7.43
11 + 3	4.80	14 + 2	7.60

[a] 95% confidence level is ±6 days
(From Lasser et al,[29] with permission.)

Other Anomalies

The face is fully developed by 12 to 13 weeks' gestation. Early detection of cleft lip and cleft palate has been reported.[31] With transvaginal ultrasound it has also been possible to diagnose sacral agenesis in the pregnancy interval of 9 to 17 weeks[32]; club foot, rocker bottom foot, and diaphragmatic hernia at 16 weeks' gestation[31]; and hydranencephaly and holoprosencephaly at 11 and 14 weeks' gestation, respectively.[33-35]

REFERENCES

1. Timor-Tritsch IE, Rottem S: Normal and abnormal fetal anatomy in the first 15 weeks of pregnancy using transvaginal ultrasound. p. 353. In Sabbagha RE (ed): Ultrasound Applied to Obstetrics and Gynecology. 3rd Ed. JB Lippincott, Philadelphia, 1994
2. Achiron R, Achiron A: Transvaginal ultrasonic assessment of the early fetal brain. Ultrasound Obstet Gynecol 1:336, 1991
3. Moore KL. The Developing Human. WB Saunders, Philadelphia, 1988
4. Schmidt W, Yarkoni S, Crelin ES, Hobbins JC: Sonographic visualization of physiologic anterior abdominal hernia in the first trimester. Obstet Gynecol 69:911, 1987
5. Nishi T, Nakano R: First-trimester diagnosis of exencephaly. J Ultrasound Med 13:149, 1994
6. Chervenak FA, Isaacson G, Sabbagha RE, Monteagudo A: Anomalies of the head and spine. p. 381. In Sabbagha RE (ed): Ultrasound Applied to Obstetrics and Gynecology. 3rd Ed. JB Lippincott, Philadelphia, 1994
7. Platt LD, Carlson DE, Medearis AL et al: Fetal choroid plexus cysts in the second trimester of pregnancy: a cause for concern. Am J Obstet Gynecol 164:1652, 1991
8. Mahony BS, Callen P, Filly R, Hoddick K: The fetal cisterna magna. Radiology 153:773, 1984
9. Sabbagha RE: Targeted imaging for fetal anomalies: clues to reaching a correct diagnosis. Obstet/Gynecol Rep 2:142, 1990
10. DeVore GR, Medearis AL, Bear MB et al: Fetal echocardiography: factors that influence imaging of the fetal heart during the second trimester of pregnancy. J Ultrasound Med 12:659, 1993
11. Johnson P, Sharland G, Maxwell D, Allan L: The role of transvaginal sonography in the early detection of congenital heart disease. Ultrasound Obstet Gynecol 2:248, 1992
12. Bronshtein M, Zimmer EZ, Gerlis LM et al: Early ultrasound diagnosis of fetal congenital heart defects in high-risk and low-risk anomalies pregnancies. Obstet Gynecol 82:225, 1993
13. Sherer DM, Abramowicz JS, Metlay LA et al: Nonimmune fetal hydrops caused by bilateral type III congenital cystic adenomatoid malformation of the lung at 17 weeks' gestation. Am J Obstet Gynecol 167:503, 1992
14. Chou MM, Lee HHS, Lee YH et al: Early prenatal diagnosis of type III bilateral congenital cystic adenomatoid malformation of the lung. Ultrasound Obstet Gynecol 2:126, 1992
15. Stocker JT, Madewell JE, Drake RM: Congenital cystic adenomatoid malformation of the lung: classification and morphologic spectrum. Hum Pathol 8:155, 1977
16. Harrison MR, Adzick NS, Jennings RW et al: Antenatal intervention for congenital cystic adenomatoid malformation. Lancet 336:965, 1990
17. Finley BE, Burlbaw J, Bennet TL, Levitch L: Delayed return of the fetal midgut to the abdomen resulting in volvulus, bowel obstruction, and gangrene of the small intestine. J Ultrasound Med 11:233, 1992
18. Bromley B, Benacerraf BR: Transient omphalocele. J Ultrasound Med 12:688, 1993
19. Benacerraf BR, Saltzman DH, Esteroff JA, Frigoletto FD: Abnormal karyotype of fetuses with omphalocele: prediction based on omphalocele contents. Obstet Gynecol 75:713, 1990
20. Hogge WA, Hogge JS, Boehm CD, Sanders RC: In-

creased echogenicity in the fetal abdomen: use of DNA analysis to establish a diagnosis of cystic fibrosis. J Ultrasound Med 12:451, 1993

21. Ville Y, Lalondrelle C, Doumerc S et al: First-trimester diagnosis of nuchal anomalies: significance and fetal outcome. Ultrasound Obstet Gynecol 2:314, 1992
22. Shulman LP, Emerson DS, Felker RE et al: High frequency of cytogenetic abnormalities in fetuses with cystic hygroma diagnosed in the first trimester. Obstet Gynecol 80:80, 1992
23. Chervenak FA, Isaacson G, Blakemore KJ et al: Fetal cystic hygroma. Cause and natural history. N Engl J Med 309:822, 1983
24. Bronshtein BR, Rottem S, Yoffe N, Blumenfeld Z: First-trimester and early second-trimester diagnosis of nuchal cystic hygroma by transvaginal sonography: diverse prognosis of the septated from the nonseptated lesion. Am J Obstet Gynecol 161:78, 1989
25. Monteagudo A, Timor-Trisch IE, Moomjy M: Nomograms of the fetal lateral ventricles using transvaginal sonography. J Ultrasound Med 5:265, 1993
26. Zucchini S, Borghesani F, Soffriti C et al: Transvaginal ultrasound diagnosis of twin reversed arterial perfusion syndrome at 9 weeks' gestation. Ultrasound Obstet Gynecol 3:209, 1993
27. Wilson DA, Young GZ, Crumley CS: Antepartum ultrasonographic diagnosis of ischiopagus: a rare variety of conjoined twins. J Ultrasound Med 2:281, 1983
28. Lopez-Zeno JA, Mota J, Sabbagha RE: Multiple gestation. p. 255. In Sabbagha RE (ed): Ultrasound Applied to Obstetrics and Gynecology. 3rd Ed. JB Lippincott, Philadelphia, 1994
29. Lasser DM, Peisner DB, Vollebergh J, Timor-Trisch I: First-trimester fetal biometry using transvaginal sonography. Ultrasound Obstet Gynecol 3:104, 1993
30. Nicolaides K, Shawwa L, Brizot M, Snijders R: Ultrasonographically detectable markers of fetal chromosomal defects. Ultrasound Obstet Gynecol 3:56, 1993
31. Rottem S, Bronshtein M: Transvaginal sonographic diagnosis of congenital anomalies between 9 weeks and 16 weeks, menstrual age. J Clin Ultrasound 18:307, 1990
32. Baxi L, Warren W, Collins MH, Timor-Trisch I: Early detection of caudal regression syndrome with transvaginal scanning. Obstet Gynecol 75:486, 1990
33. Bronstein M, Rottem S, Timor-Trisch IE: Early detection of fetal anomalies. p. 307. In Timor-Trisch IE, Rottem S (eds): Transvaginal sonography. 2nd Ed. Elsevier, New York, 1991
34. Yue-Shan L, Fong-Ming CH, Chi-Hong L: Antenatal detection of hydranencephaly at 12 weeks menstrual age. J Clin Ultrasound 20:62, 1992
35. Rottem S, Bronshtein M, Thaler I, Brandes JM: First trimester transvaginal sonographic diagnosis of fetal anomalies. Lancet 1:444, 1989
36. Johnson P, Sharland G, Chita S et al: Vaginal ultrasound and early confirmation of fetal anatomy, abstracted. Ultrasound Obstet Gynecol, suppl. 114:84, 1991

15

Ectopic Pregnancy

Melvin G. Dodson

The incidence of ectopic pregnancies is 0.5 to 1.0 percent, with 97.5 percent occurring in the fallopian tubes, 0.7 percent in the ovary, and the remaining 1.8 percent occurring somewhere else in the abdominal cavity.[1] The importance of early diagnosis of ectopic pregnancies is reflected by the fact that they account for about 10 percent of maternal deaths. Although this text is concerned mainly with the use of ultrasound, it is important to appreciate the role of ultrasound in the total scheme, and in proper perspective, in the diagnosis of an ectopic pregnancy, as well as the ability to use other information, such as quantitative human chorionic gonadotropin (hCG) values in interpreting the ultrasound findings (or vice versa).

The first step in the diagnosis of an ectopic pregnancy is a high degree of suspicion in any patient who has abnormal vaginal bleeding, a missed or late period, pelvic pain, pelvic tenderness, or an adnexal mass. In addition, signs or symptoms of cardiovascular instability, such as dizziness, fainting, shortness of breath, anemia, and/or hypotension, should raise the suspicion of an ectopic pregnancy. Even a history of a normal menstrual period does not rule out an ectopic or even intrauterine pregnancy, since abnormal bleeding or implantation bleeding at the expected time of a period may be mistaken for a normal menstrual period. Therefore, evaluation for an ectopic pregnancy should be undertaken even in a patient with a supposed normal menstrual period if other signs and symptoms of an ectopic pregnancy, as noted above, are present. Ectopic pregnancy should also be considered in any pregnant patient with a history of predisposing factors for an ectopic pregnancy.

PREDISPOSING FACTORS

Predisposing factors for ectopic pregnancy include a variety of conditions affecting normal tubal function, such as a history of pelvic inflammatory disease, peritubular adhesions from surgery or infection, previous tubal surgery, congenital anomalies of the tube, or endometriosis. A history of infertility is more common in patients with an ectopic pregnancy than the general population. Repeat ectopic pregnancies account for about 10 percent of all ectopic pregnancies, and 0.5 percent follow tubal sterilization.[1]

Transmigration of the ovum has been suggested as an important etiologic factor in ectopic pregnancies. The corpus luteum has been noted on the opposite side of the ectopic pregnancy in 13 to 23 percent of patients, suggesting transmigration of the ovum.[1] The frequent contralateral relationship between the corpus luteum and an ectopic pregnancy should be kept in mind when an ectopic pregnancy is suspected. Berry et al[2] ultrasonically studied 24 patients with an ectopic pregnancy. In one-third, ovulation was contralateral to the side (right versus left) of the ectopic pregnancy as determined by ultrasonic demonstration of a corpus luteum; in one third, ovulation was ipsilateral; and in one-third, a corpus luteum could not be determined. Therefore, imaging of a corpus luteum gives no help in terms of localizing an ectopic pregnancy (same side versus opposite side).

SIGNIFICANT SYMPTOMS

Symptoms of an ectopic pregnancy include (1) a missed menstrual period, which is reported by three-fourths of patients; (2) abnormal vaginal bleeding, which will be noted by one-half to three-fourths of patients; (3) pelvic pain, which is present in 95 percent of patients; (4) shoulder pain, which may occur secondary to blood irritating the diaphragm (Danforth's sign); and (5) vascular instability characterized by fainting, dizziness, lightheadedness, or a rapid heart rate, which may be noted in patients with a ruptured ectopic pregnancy and significant intra-abdominal bleeding.[1] About 10 percent of patients with an ectopic pregnancy are in vascular shock at the time of the diagnosis, and about 60 percent have 500 ml or more of free blood in the peritoneal cavity at the time of surgery.[1,3] The work-up of a patient in vascular shock should be limited to those procedures that can be readily accomplished while the patient is on her way to the operating room. Generally, a serum pregnancy test, complete blood count and type, and cross match for blood can be sent to the laboratory while the patient is being stabilized, an intravenous line started, and the operating room prepared. Ultrasound is not necessary for diagnosis for a patient in vascular shock with a positive pregnancy test and other signs or symptoms of an ectopic pregnancy. The ultrasound room is not the place to evaluate a patient with vascular instability secondary to intra-abdominal bleeding. If there is any question regarding the diagnosis, and the patient's clinical condition will allow, a culdocentesis can be done in the operating room before laparotomy. Nonclotting blood confirms a hemoperitoneum (see discussion below).

DIAGNOSIS

Presently, there are four tests used to confirm or eliminate the diagnosis of a suspected ectopic pregnancy: (1) hCG, (2) ultrasound, (3) culdocentesis, and (4) laparoscopy. More recently, the determination of serum progesterone has also been noted to be of value. In the past 10 years, the use of sensitive pregnancy tests, quantitative hCG assays, and high frequency transvaginal ultrasound has had a major impact on the approach to diagnosis and especially early diagnosis of an ectopic pregnancy. Before the development of these very sensitive pregnancy tests, 50 percent of patients with ectopic pregnancies had negative pregnancy tests. The sensitivity of transabdominal ultrasound for the diagnosis of an ectopic pregnancy was also poor in the past, and a negative examination was not reliable. As a consequence, culdocentesis and laparoscopy were the major diagnostic modalities for ectopic pregnancy. In the not too distant past, pregnancy tests and ultrasound were so unreliable that it was quite common to perform a laparoscopy on patients with suspicious clinical findings who were not pregnant or on patients with an early intrauterine pregnancy. Currently, the considerably increased sensitivity of pregnancy tests, the use of quantitative pregnancy tests, and the use of transvaginal ultrasound with high resolution, high frequency probes have made these modalities the first line of diagnostic tests for an ectopic pregnancy, with laparoscopy now reserved for confirmation and treatment (Fig. 15-1).

Human Chorionic Gonadotropin

The first step in the diagnosis of an ectopic pregnancy is the confirmation of pregnancy using a sensitive hCG assay. Although I have seen two ectopic pregnancies in patients with negative serum hCG tests, this is extremely unusual and generally represents an ectopic pregnancy that has spontaneously aborted out of the fimbrial end of the fallopian tube or a pregnancy in which the chorionic villi have become nonviable but the ectopic pregnancy complex has persisted. Pregnancy can now almost always be confirmed or ruled out by a sensitive hCG assay. Current serum assays can be done in a matter of minutes in any physician's office or in the emergency room with a sensitivity down to 10 to 15 mIU of hCG per ml (2IS). The physician should be aware of the sensitivity of the hCG assay used, since there can be considerable variability in different assays. Pregnancy tests with sensitivities much above 15 mIU/ml (2IS) are not reliable in eliminating the potential of an ectopic pregnancy. The difference between the use of the International Reference Preparation (IRP) and the Second International Standard (2IS) should also be kept in mind. The 2IS gives results about one-half those of the IRP (see Ch. 13).

It is also important to note the units used in reporting beta-hCG values. Beta-hCG is often reported in milli-International Units per milliliter (mIU/ml), but may be reported as International Units per liter (IU/L), which will give the same numeric values and actual concentrations of beta-hCG as mIU/ml, since both the numerator and denominator (values) are multiplied by 1,000. However, sometimes beta-hCG is reported as mIU/L, which will obviously give numeric values 1,000 times larger than mIU/ml. Sometimes manufacturers of pregnancy test kits report the beta-hCG sensitivity of their tests in International Units per milliliter (IU/ml). This, of course, gives a very small numeric value and makes the test kit appear more sensitive. Not noting the units used can be a trap for the unwary. A value of 100 mIU of serum

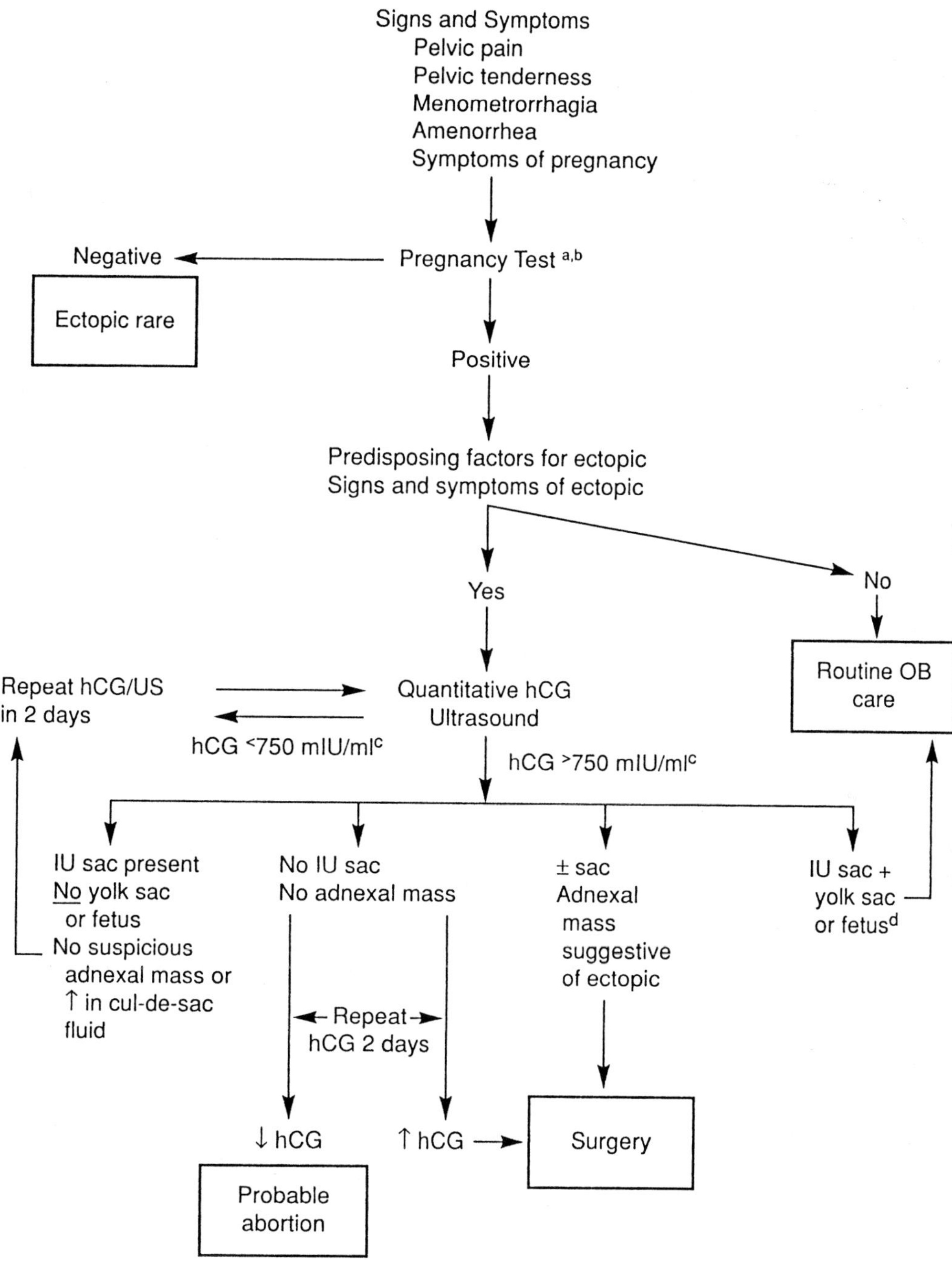

[a]Minimum sensitivity of 10-25 mIU/ml (2IS)
[b]Patient with symptoms of vascular instability (shock) with a probable ectopic pregnancy; should have an IV started and taken immediately to surgery.
[c]Second International Standard (2IS)
[d]Combined intrauterine pregnancy and ectopic - 1 in 30,000 pregnancies except IVF

Fig. 15-1. Diagnosis of ectopic pregnancy.

hCG per ml would therefore be 0.1 IU/ml, and the test would appear very sensitive, if the units are not noted. Although the difference is quite obvious when considered, I have found few technicians, residents, or unfortunately even attending physicians who know the sensitivity and type of reference preparation used as the test standard when discussing a positive pregnancy test or the units or standards used when discussing a quantitative hCG level. These differences are critical for accurate diagnosis and management of an ectopic pregnancy.

Quantitative hCG levels and serial measurements have become important factors in evaluating the status of a pregnancy. Although ectopic pregnancies have been reported with hCG levels as low as 15 mIU/ml (2IS), this is uncommon and reflects a very early ectopic pregnancy, an ectopic pregnancy that has aborted out of the end of the tube, or one in which the trophoblastic tissue is no longer viable and the hCG level is decreasing. There is a direct correlation between hCG levels and the mass of viable cyto/sync-tiotrophoblast cells present. An ectopic pregnancy rarely ruptures when the mass of trophoblastic tissue is small and the serum hCG concentration is very low. Rupture is rare when the hCG level is below 1,000 mIU/ml (2IS). As a benchmark, the hCG level in a normal pregnancy at the time of a missed menstrual period (day 28 from last menstrual period [LMP] or 13 to 14 days after ovulation) is 50 to 300 mIU/ml (2IS).[4] The gestational complex at that time is less than 1 mm in size. hCG levels can be used to date a normal pregnancy and to determine when gestational structures should be visualized using ultrasound. This has been termed the discriminatory hCG zone.

However, the hCG level above which an intrauterine pregnancy should be visualized has continued to decrease (see discussion in Ch. 13 and below). Using transvaginal ultrasonography, an intrauterine gestational sac should be imaged in normal pregnancies when the quantitative hCG is greater than 750 mIU/ml (2IS). In patients in whom an intrauterine gestational sac is not identified during a transvaginal sonographic examination, there is no adnexal mass, and the quantitative hCG is less than 750 mIU/ml (2IS), a repeat quantitative hCG and ultrasound should be done in 2 days.

Ultrasound

In patients with a positive pregnancy test and signs or symptoms of an ectopic pregnancy or predisposing factors for an ectopic pregnancy, an ultrasound should be done to localize the gestation.

The potential of an ectopic pregnancy can generally be eliminated when a viable intrauterine pregnancy is visualized on ultrasound. An intrauterine pregnancy will be imaged in about one-half of the patients with a positive pregnancy test and signs or symptoms suggestive of an ectopic pregnancy. In one study, an ectopic pregnancy was confirmed in almost one-half of the remaining patients.[5] The coexistence of an intrauterine pregnancy and an ectopic pregnancy (heterotopic pregnancy) has been reported to occur in about 1/30,000 pregnancies.[1] However, the heterotopic pregnancy rate is higher with in vitro fertilization (IVF) when multiple ova are transferred or with ovulation induction when multiple follicles develop. In a series of 204 pregnancies resulting from ovulation induction using clomiphene citrate or human menopausal gonadotropin, two heterotopic pregnancies were reported (1/100).[6] In both cases, the patients presented with pain, but no abnormal vaginal bleeding. Most patients with ectopic pregnancies will have both pain and abnormal vaginal bleeding. The absence of vaginal bleeding in these cases of ectopic pregnancy was suggested to have resulted from the presence of the viable intrauterine pregnancy. In both cases, the ectopic pregnancy was surgically removed and the normal intrauterine pregnancy progressed to term.

An intrauterine gestational sac can frequently be visualized by week 5 after the LMP using transvaginal ultrasound. Even in pregnancies in which a viable embryo cannot be identified within the gestational sac in the uterus, identification of a yolk sac is reliable evidence of an early intrauterine pregnancy and excludes the possibility of an ectopic pregnancy (except heterotopic pregnancies as noted above).

Unfortunately, visualization of an anechoic area within the endometrial cavity can be mistaken for an intrauterine gestational sac. A pseudogestational sac has been reported in up to 10 to 20 percent of patients with an ectopic pregnancy.[7] It appears as an anechoic area in the endometrial cavity and may represent a blood clot (Fig. 15-2).Nyberg et al[8] noted a pseudogestational sac in 13 percent of 48 ectopic pregnancies. A yolk sac was not seen in any of six pseudogestational sacs. Rempen[9] reported a pseudogestational sac in 3 of 21 (14 percent) ectopic pregnancies. However, the sac had an abnormal shape and was easily distinguished from a true gestational sac.[9] A well-developed gestational reaction surrounding a pseudosac is usually absent. However, small pseudosacs may be harder to differentiate (Fig. 15-3).

In addition to eliminating the possibility of an ectopic pregnancy by visualizing an intrauterine yolk

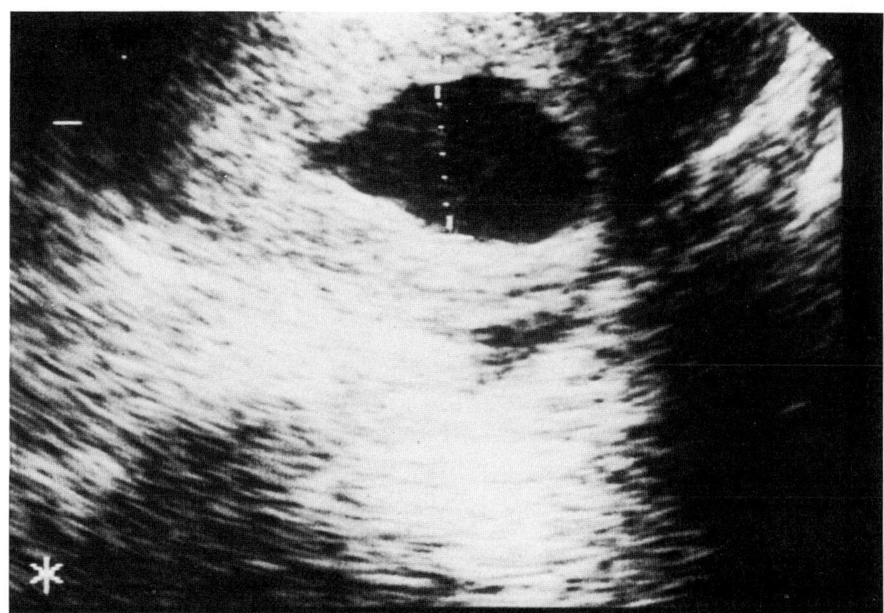

Fig. 15-2. Pseudosac in the uterus probably representing blood in a patient with an ectopic pregnancy. The sac is irregular with a poorly developed decidua with no evidence of the double decidual sign. The sac is 17 mm with no evidence of a fetus or yolk sac.

sac or fetus (except with heterotopic pregnancy), an ectopic pregnancy may be diagnosed by imaging a fetus, gestational sac, or cardiac activity in the adnexa. More commonly, an ectopic pregnancy is suspected when no sac is noted in the uterus and a complex mass is noted in the adnexa. Generally, an adnexal mass can be appreciated in patients with an ectopic pregnancy using transvaginal ultrasonography. In a series of 22 ectopic pregnancies published by Shapiro et al,[10] an adnexal mass was identified in 50 percent of patients using transabdominal imaging techniques and in 91 percent of patients using transvaginal ultrasound. The

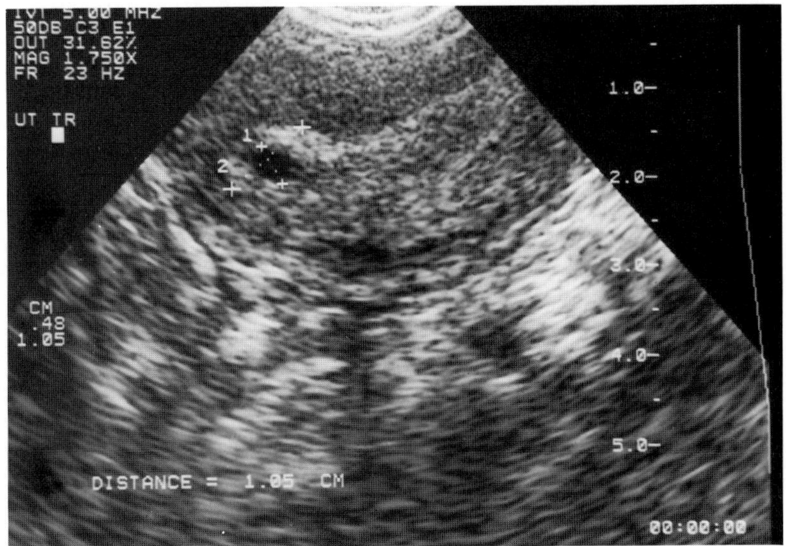

Fig. 15-3. T-pelvic view of the uterus in a patient with a positive pregnancy test, vaginal bleeding, and pain. There is an anechoic area of 0.48 cm in the fundus that appears to be an early intrauterine pregnancy. The quantitative hCG was 117 mIU/ml, and the serum progesterone was 27.2 ng/ml. This is a pseudogestational sac. The patient had an ectopic pregnancy.

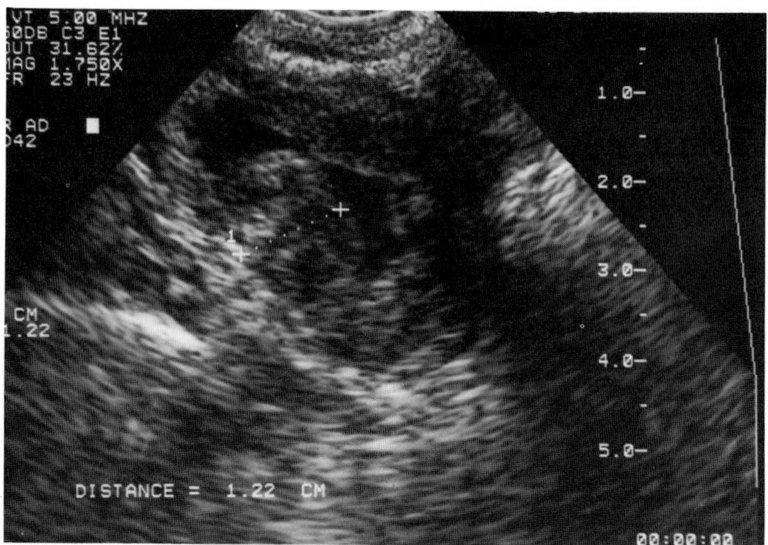

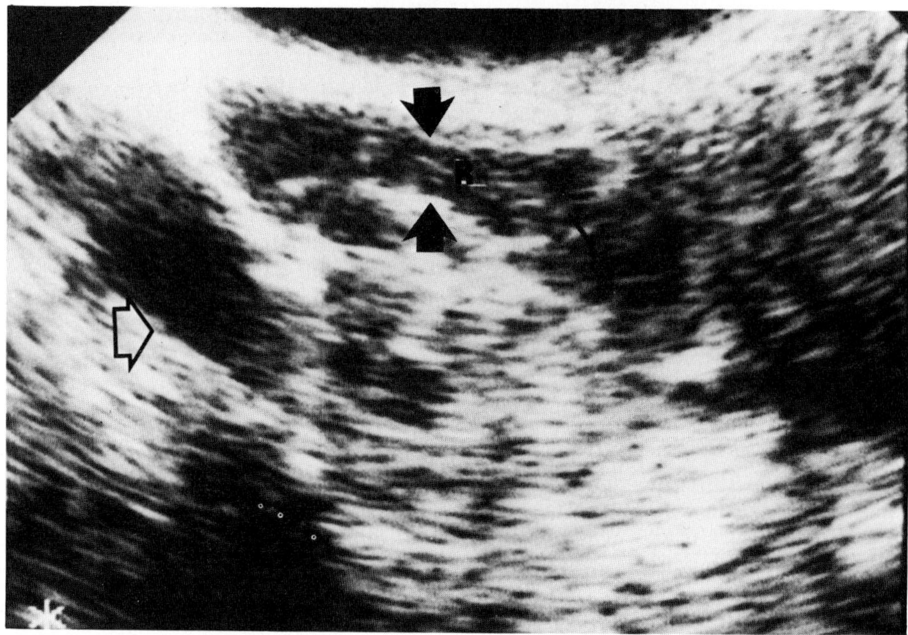

Fig. 15-4. **(A)** Trans-pelvic (T-pelvic) view of the right adnexa. The right tube is dilated 1.22 cm and is surrounded by free peritoneal fluid. **(B)** T-pelvic image of thickened right tube (dark arrows) representing an ectopic pregnancy. The iliac vein is to the left (open arrow). The uterus is on the right of the photograph.

sonographic appearance of an ectopic pregnancy in the adnexa may take four forms: (1) a gestational sac with fetus with or without a discernible fetal heartbeat, (2) an empty gestational sac, (3) a thick echogenic band surrounding a small hypoechoic area giving the appearance of a donut, and (4) a diffuse echogenic mass within the fallopian tube (Fig. 15-4).[9] In Shapiro et al.s series,[10] the hCG titers in patients in whom an ectopic adnexal mass was identified ranged from 35 to 45,800 mIU/ml (IRP), and the average size

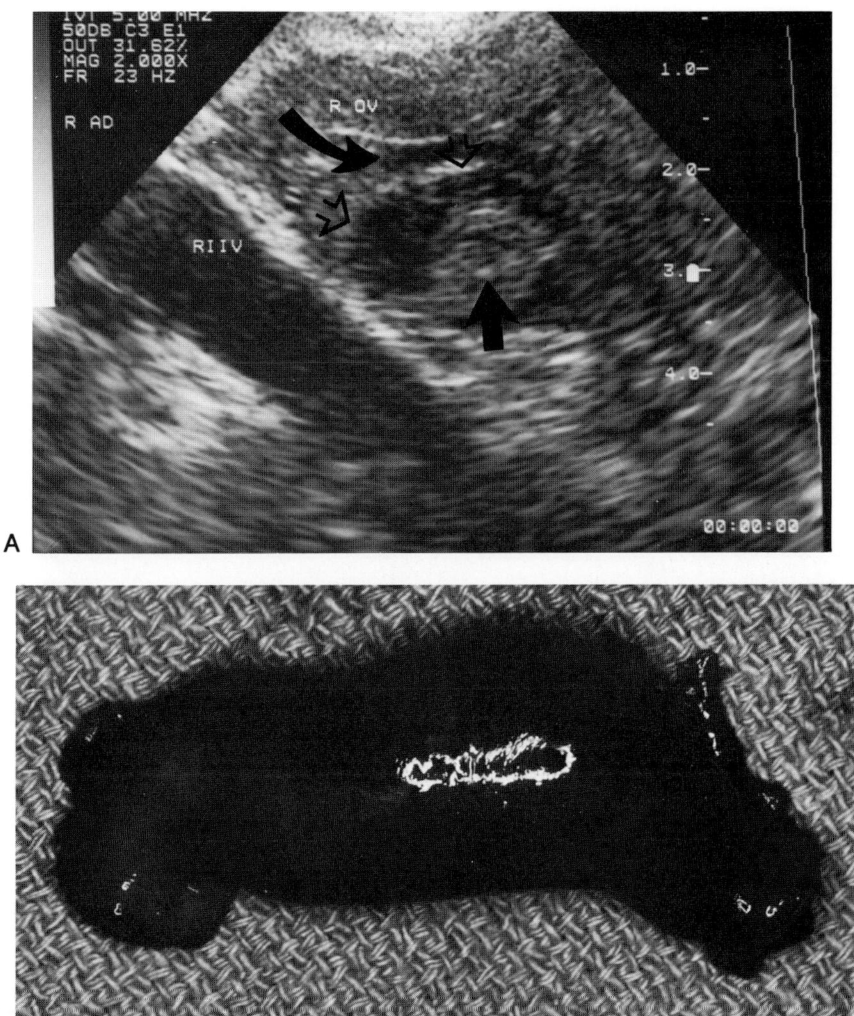

Fig. 15-5. (**A**) T-pelvic view of the uterus showing the donut sign consisting of the tubal wall (open arrows) with a hyperechoic blood clot within the tube (arrow) surrounded by an anechoic area probably representing liquified clot and fluid. There is a small amount of fluid seen outside the tube (curved arrow). The right ovary (ROV) and right internal iliac vein (RIIV) are labeled. The hyperechoic clot is 1 cm in diameter. The donut measures 2.41 by 1.74 cm. hCG was 169 mIU/ml, and the serum progesterone was 6.9 ng/ml. (**B**) Tube with ectopic pregnancy after surgical removal. *(Figure continues.)*

of the ectopic pregnancy identified by transvaginal ultrasound was 3.5 ± 0.57 cm.

Rempen[9] noted an adnexal mass in 19 of 21 (90 percent) patients with an ectopic pregnancy. In 15 of these 21 patients (71 percent), the adnexal mass had a donut-like appearance (Fig. 15-5). The donut wall was 2 to 8 mm thick. Sometimes the donut may be surrounded by an inhomogeneous mass of low amplitude echoes representing a hematoma or free blood in the peritoneal cavity. Generally, the mass is filled with fluid. In almost one-fourth of patients, a fetus with fetal cardiac activity was noted. Less commonly (20 percent), the adnexal mass appeared as a complex solid or cystic mass caused by a hematoma and/or a ringlike gestational sac. In 10 percent, no adnexal mass was visualized by Rempen[9] in an initial sonographic evaluation. An ovarian cyst, representing a corpus luteum, may be present in over two-thirds of

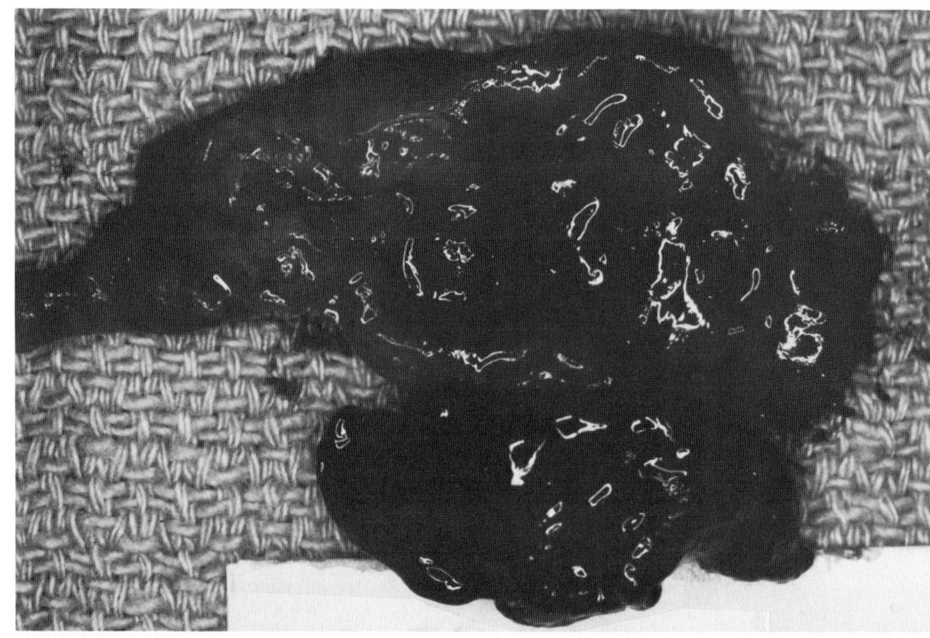

C

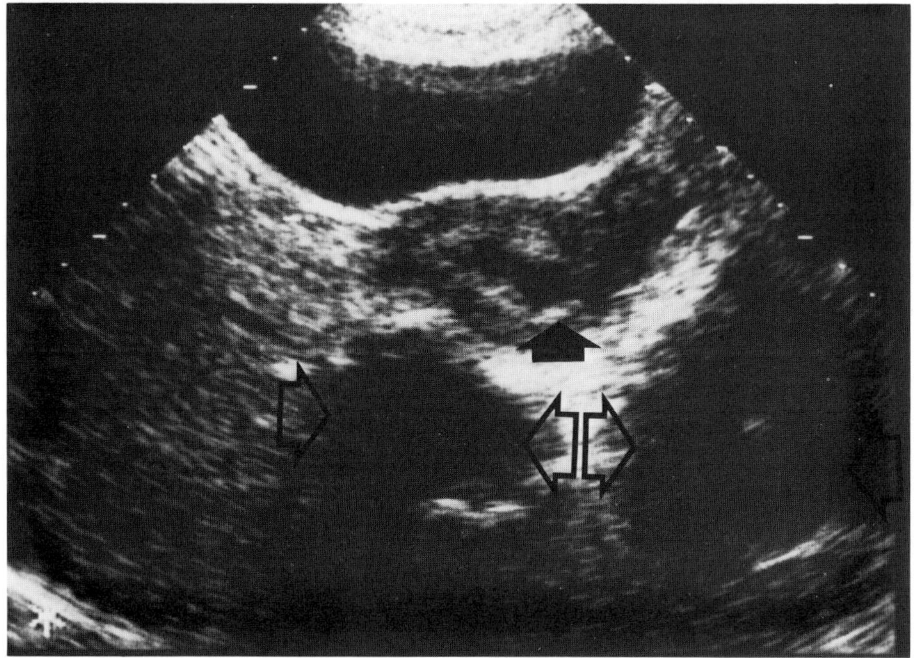

D

Fig. 15-5 *(Continued)*. **(C)** Tube opened showing the clot within the tube. Histologic section showed a blood clot and chorionic villi. **(D)** Transabdominal view of two large blood clots in the pelvis after rupture of an ectopic pregnancy (open arrows). Note the pseudosac in the uterus (arrow). The transabdominal technique gives a more panoramic view.

patients. A corpus luteum should not be confused with an ectopic pregnancy. Corpus luteal cysts (greater than 1.5 cm) are also present in two-thirds of patients with intrauterine gestations.

A correct diagnosis of an ectopic pregnancy was possible in 86 percent of cases on the initial scan reported by Rempen and in 95 percent of cases when follow-up sonographic examinations were included.[9] A false-positive diagnosis of an ectopic pregnancy was made in 1 of 383 intrauterine pregnancies, giving a specificity of ultrasound diagnosis of 99.7 percent.

Although on transvaginal ultrasound examinations most patients will be clearly noted to have either an intrauterine pregnancy or an ectopic pregnancy, there still remain a few patients in whom an intrauterine pregnancy cannot be confirmed and an ectopic pregnancy cannot be excluded. Most of these patients are between 4 and 6 weeks of gestation from the LMP in what might be called the gestational blind spot, since the pregnancy sometimes cannot be localized by ultrasound imaging. With transvaginal ultrasound this blind spot has generally been narrowed to the period between a missed period (28 days from the LMP) and the end of week 5 with a normal pregnancy (day 35). However, because of the biologic variation in the timing of ovulation and other factors, the time interval from the LMP to the imaging of gestational anatomic markers can occasionally be longer. The quantitative hCG is used to confirm the true gestational age. The findings of a positive pregnancy test with an hCG greater than 750 mIU/ml (2IS), pelvic pain, and bleeding between weeks 4 and 6 and no intrauterine gestational sac imaged by sonography are very suspicious of an ectopic pregnancy. However, an early pregnancy that has aborted with collapse of the early gestational sac may present similarly. A patient presenting with a suspicious adnexal mass would suggest an ectopic pregnancy. A repeat quantitative hCG study in 24 to 48 hours is quite helpful in patients without an intrauterine gestational sac and no adnexal mass or evidence of blood in the cul-de-sac. If the hCG is rising and above 750 mIU/ml (2IS), laparoscopy should be performed despite the lack of visualization of an ectopic pregnancy on the ultrasonographic examination. However, most patients with a falling hCG level will have aborted (a few may have even had a tubal abortion).

Some patients with ectopic pregnancies have falling hCG levels. However, it is not clear at this time whether all patients with ectopic pregnancies, falling hCG levels, and no adnexal mass (by transvaginal ultrasound) require surgery. Additional studies are needed, particularly in cases where hCG levels are low and continue to fall. There are some risks in delaying laparoscopy under these circumstances, and careful clinical judgment is required. However, as noted above, in most patients with an ectopic pregnancy, an adnexal mass can be imaged. Probably the most common reason that an ectopic pregnancy is not imaged using ultrasound is that the mass is quite small and therefore has less risk of immediate rupture.

Serum Progesterone

Serum progesterone levels are significantly lower in patients with ectopic pregnancies and abnormal pregnancies compared with those in a normal pregnancy. Even in normally developing pregnancies, there is relatively little increase in the serum progesterone levels from 5 to 10 weeks of gestation. Using a progesterone value of 20 ng/ml (63 nmol/L) or higher, progesterone determination was 92 percent sensitive and 84 percent specific in predicting a normal pregnancy. Serum progesterone had a positive predictive value of 90 percent and a negative predictive value of 87 percent in discrimination between a normal and a complicated pregnancy.[11] Yeko et al[12] used a progesterone level of less than 15 ng/ml as a discriminatory value. All patients ($n = 28$) with an ectopic pregnancy had serum progesterone levels below 15 ng/ml, and all normal intrauterine pregnancies had serum progesterone levels above 15 ng/ml. In patients with abnormal intrauterine pregnancies, 94 percent had serum progesterone concentrations between 15 and 20 ng/ml. The discriminatory serum progesterone level did vary depending on the manufacturer of the progesterone assay. Combining a quantitative hCG assay with ultrasound and progesterone determination increases the potential for prediction of an abnormal pregnancy, an incomplete or inevitable abortion, or an ectopic pregnancy (Table 15-1).

Culdocentesis

A culdocentesis may be helpful in the presence of a large amount of cul-de-sac fluid and/or the suspicion of blood clots suggestive of a ruptured ectopic pregnancy in a patient with a positive pregnancy test and the absence of an intrauterine gestational sac. Likewise, the absence of any fluid or minimal fluid after a careful transvaginal ultrasound evaluation indicates

Table 15-1. Findings Suggestive of an Ectopic Pregnancy

	Ultrasound Findings	*Comments*
Intrauterine pregnancy noted	Gestational sac	10-20% of ectopic pregnancies have an intrauterine pseudogestational sac
		Sac larger than 20 mm with no fetus suggests a blighted ovum or ectopic pseudosac
	Double decidual sign	Found in one-third of ectopic pregnancies
	Yolk sac	Confirms intrauterine pregnancy
	Fetus	Confirms intrauterine pregnancy
		Fetal cardiac activity = viable fetus
No intrauterine pregnancy	Uterus	hCG $>$ 750 mlU/ml
		Progesterone $<$ 15 ng/ml
	Adnexa	Presence of an adnexal mass: 91%
		Donut sign: 71%
		Complex mass: 20%
		Fetus: 25%
		Caution: Corpus luteal cyst is very common and should not be mistaken for ectopic pregnancy
	Cul-de-sac	Blood clots
		Cul-de-sac fluid in 81% of ectopic pregnancies
		Caution: There is frequently cul-de-sac fluid in early pregnancy (22%)

that an ectopic pregnancy, if present, has not ruptured. In a series by Rempen,[9] cul-de-sac fluid was noted in 81 percent of patients with an ectopic pregnancy, but in only 22 percent of normal pregnancies.

Lawson[13] reported fluid in the cul-de-sac in 23 percent of patients with an ectopic pregnancy using ultrasonography. Free blood has been noted in the cul-de-sac in 83 to 97 percent of patients using needle aspiration of the cul-de-sac in four different studies.[14-17] However, these are older studies in which the ectopic pregnancy was generally diagnosed late. Ultrasound can be particularly useful in quickly evaluating for the presence of fluid or blood in the pelvis.

Laparoscopy

Occasionally, despite recent advances in ultrasonography and quantitative hCG assays, a diagnostic laparoscopy will still be needed to make a definitive diagnosis of an ectopic pregnancy. Early diagnosis using sensitive pregnancy tests, quantitative hCG assays, and transvaginal sonography may also allow laparoscopic salpingotomy with removal of an ectopic pregnancy by laparoscopy or laparoscopic salpingectomy.

Diagnosis and management of patients with a suspected ectopic pregnancy and the proper use of laparoscopy involve good clinical judgment based on the history and physical findings and a detailed knowledge of the use and limitation of such laboratory tests as the quantitative hCG and serum progesterone and ultrasound imaging of the pelvis.

REFERENCES

1. Dodson MG: Bleeding in pregnancy, p. 451. In Aladjem S (ed): Obstetrical Practice. CV Mosby, St. Louis, 1980
2. Berry SM, Coulam CB, Hill LM, Breckle R: Evidence of contralateral ovulation in ectopic pregnancy. J Ultrasound Med 4:293, 1985
3. Pagano R: Ectopic pregnancy—a seven year survey. Med J Aust 2:586, 1981
4. Bernaschek G, Gudelstorfer R, Csaicsich P: Vaginal sonography versus serum human chorionic gonadotropin in early detection of pregnancy. Am J Obstet Gynecol 158:608, 1988
5. Mahony BS, Filly RA, Nyberg DA, Callen PW: Sonographic evaluation of ectopic pregnancy. J Ultrasound Med 4:221, 1985
6. Berger MG, Taymor ML: Simultaneous intrauterine and tubal pregnancies following ovulation induction. Am J Obstet Gynecol 113:812, 1972
7. Nyberg DA, Laing FC, Filly RA et al: Ultrasonographic differentiation of the gestational sac of early intrauterine pregnancy from the pseudogestational sac of ectopic pregnancy. Radiology 146:755, 1983

8. Nyberg DA, Mack LA, Harvey D, Wang K: Value of the yolk sac in evaluating early pregnancies. J Ultrasound Med 7:129, 1988
9. Rempen A: Vaginal sonography in ectopic pregnancy. J Ultrasound Med 7:381, 1988
10. Shapiro BS, Cullen M, Taylor KJW, DeCherney AH: Transvaginal ultrasonography for the diagnosis of ectopic pregnancy. Fertil Steril 50:425, 1988
11. Buck RH, Joubert SM, Norman RJ: Serum progesterone in the diagnosis of ectopic pregnancy: a valuable diagnostic test? Fertil Steril 50:752, 1988
12. Yeko TR, Gorrill MJ, Hughes LH et al: Timely diagnosis of early ectopic pregnancy using a single blood progesterone measurement. Fertil Steril 48:1048, 1987
13. Lawson TL: Ectopic pregnancy: Criteria and accuracy of ultrasonic diagnosis. Am J Roentgenol Radium Ther Nucl Med 131:153, 1978
14. Webster HD, Jr, Barclay DL, Fischer CK: Ectopic pregnancy—a seventeen-year review. Am J Obstet Gynecol 92:23, 1965
15. Johnson EM, Schoenbucher AK: Ectopic pregnancy: a five-year study (128 cases) at William Beaumont General Hospital—some unusual features as related to war brides. Milit Med 125:633, 1962
16. Helvacioglu A, Long EM, Jr, Yang SL: Ectopic pregnancy: an eight-year review. J Reprod Med 22:87, 1979
17. Gilstrap LC III, Harris RE: Ectopic pregnancy: a review of 122 cases. South Med J 69:604, 1976

16

Urogynecology

Melvin G. Dodson

Transvaginal ultrasound is being increasingly utilized to evaluate both the anatomy and the physiologic function of the lower female urinary tract. The bladder is readily visualized during transvaginal ultrasound and, in conjunction with the uterus, can serve as an anatomic landmark for orientation in the pelvis. The bladder volume can be calculated, and the residual post-voiding urine volume can be estimated accurately. Large residual urine volumes after voiding suggest urinary retention and overflow incontinence, whereas a small bladder volume in a patient who symptomatically feels "full" is consistent with interstitial cystitis or chronic infection, especially in association with a thickened bladder wall. Pathologic conditions, such as tumors, ureterocele, and even occasionally infections, can be diagnosed by ultrasound. Unusual bladder content, such as blood, bladder stones, or occasionally pus, can be visualized. Transvaginal ultrasound is now being utilized by some clinicians as part of the urodynamics evaluation for stress urinary incontinence.

The urethra can be imaged, hypermobility of the position of the bladder neck in response to increased intraabdominal pressure consistent with stress urinary incontinence can be noted, and the degree of motility can be measured. Funneling of the bladder neck can also be imaged by real-time ultrasound. Diverticula of the urethra can be diagnosed.

Although the ureters are generally not visualized, they can be imaged when dilated or when there are urethral stents as noted in Figure 16-1. The use of transvaginal ultrasound for evaluating the female urinary tract is a rapidly developing area. This chapter reviews some of the common areas where ultrasound technologies are being utilized.

URINARY BLADDER

The urinary bladder is a prominent pelvic structure that can be imaged easily during the transvaginal pelvic ultrasound examination. During the sonography examination, there is a tendency to regard the bladder as a prominent but rather boring structure because of the low incidence of abnormalities noted. However, the bladder should not be ignored and should be imaged and evaluated carefully during every complete pelvic ultrasound examination.

The bladder wall is 3 to 6 mm thick (Fig. 16-2). However, it may be thickened secondary to chronic infection, surgery, or radiation (Fig. 16-3). Many sonologists have the patient empty her bladder before the ultrasound examination to make the bladder wall appear thicker. However, doing so limits the evaluation of the bladder. Performing the transvaginal ultrasound examination with a moderate amount of urine in the bladder (not enough to make the patient uncomfortable) allows better assessment of the bladder. When evaluating bladder wall thickness, and especially if measurements are being made, the posterior bladder wall should not be utilized because it is generally approximated against the anterior uterine surface. It is sometimes difficult to determine where the bladder wall stops and the uterus begins. The bladder wall often appears much thicker adjacent to the uterus than in other areas. This is particularly true when the gain on the ultrasound machine is turned up.

Bladder Volume

Bladder volume may be calculated using the transabdominal technique by ultrasonographically mea-

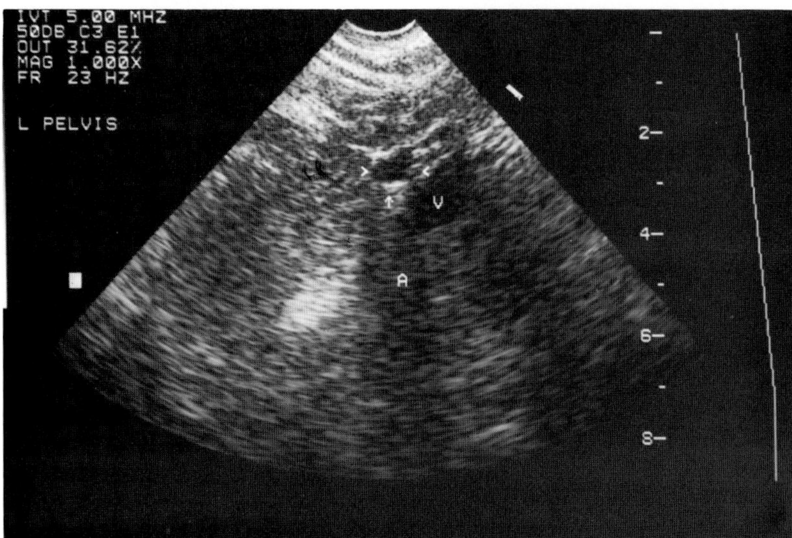

Fig. 16-1. Ureter (between arrows) and stent (arrow). Note the internal iliac vein (V). The plastic ureteral catheter is casting a shadow (A). The ureter is dilated.

suring the bladder width, height, and depth ($V_c = w \times h \times d$), shown in Figure 16-4, and using McLean and Edell's linear regression relationship $V_i = (V_c - 3.14)/2.17$, as shown in the graph shown in Figure 16-5.[1] Roughly, the calculated volume is twice the acute volume. Using transabdominal ultrasonographic measurements, McLean and Edell reported a correlation coefficient of 0.987 between the calculated and actual urinary volume (Fig. 16-6).

Transvaginal ultrasound is also reasonably accurate in estimating urine volume. Haylen reported a ± 15 percent accuracy in measuring urine volume over 50 ml using the transvaginal ultrasound technique.[2] The bladder was measured in two diameters in the AP-pelvic plain (height and depth) and the volume calculated using the equation: Volume $= 5.9 \times (h \times d) - 14.6$ ml. In another study by Haylen, the mean residual urine volume in 53 women without urinary symptoms was 4.5 ml with the upper limits of normal of 10 ml.[3] Most normal women (85 percent in Haylen's study) empty their bladder completely during voiding. The average bladder capacity for a woman is 400 to 500 ml.

It is important to at least take note of the residual urine volume in patients who have voided just before their examination. Estimates of post-void urinary volume can give valuable clinical information and should be provided to the primary care physician, if the sonologist is not providing care to the patient. A persistent increased post-voiding residual urine volume may predispose the patient to recurrent urinary tract infections and/or may be associated with an anatomic abnormality, such as a cystocele or an undiagnosed neurologic problem. In patients with urinary tract symptomatology, such as frequency, dysuria, straining to void, hesitancy, incontinence, or the sensation of incomplete bladder emptying, it is important to perform a complete ultrasound examination of the bladder. Performing the examination with a symptomatically full bladder with measurements of the bladder volume as noted above gives a reasonable estimate of the bladder capacity (without catheterization). A large bladder capacity may be noted in patients with an atonic bladder and overflow incontinence. A careful inspection of the bladder wall and contents may be done followed by voiding and an estimate of the post-void urinary residual.

Chronic cystitis, tumors, or interstitial cystitis may decrease the bladder capacity[4] and/or thicken the bladder wall. Thickening of the bladder wall can also be seen after radiation therapy or surgery. Bladder trabeculations and mucosal irregularities can be seen by sonographic imaging after chronic infection or interstitial cystitis. Bladder diverticula may be noted as anechoic structures adjacent to and communicating with the bladder.[5]

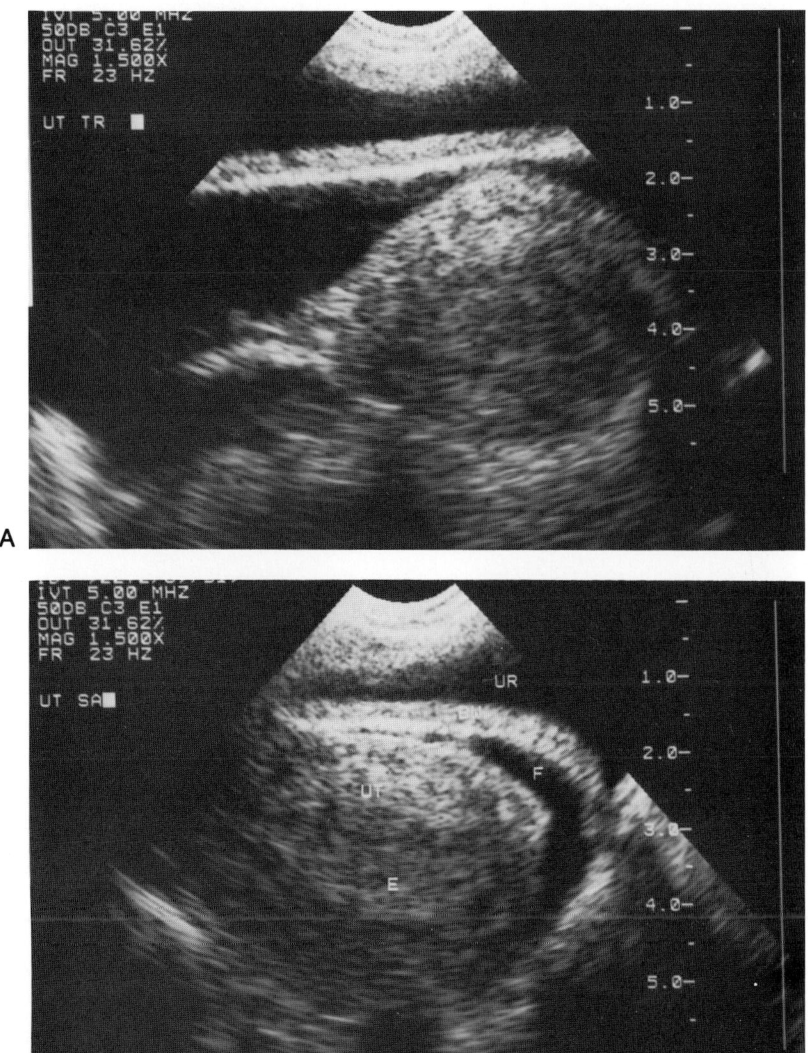

Fig. 16-2. (A) T-pelvic view of uterus and bladder. Note increased peritoneal fluid outlining the uterus and right broad ligament. The bladder wall is clearly outlined by the urine in the bladder and the increased peritoneal fluid. **(B)** AP-pelvic view with the anterior uterine contour and bladder wall outlined by peritoneal fluid. BW, bladder; UT, uterus; E, endometrium; F, peritoneal fluid; UR, urine.

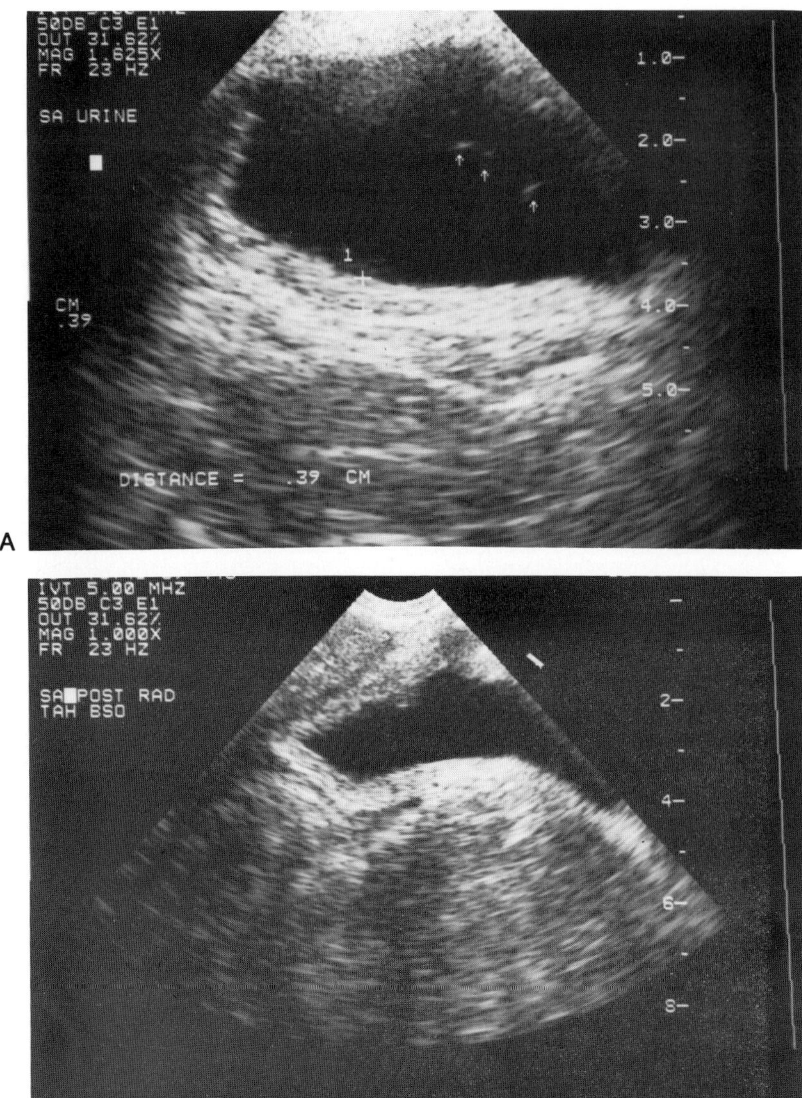

Fig. 16-3. A 47-year-old woman 7 weeks after vaginal hysterectomy and anterior colporrhaphy for menometrorrhagia and stress incontinence. **(A)** Transvaginal ultrasound examination shows thickened bladder wall (3.9 mm) probably secondary to healing after surgery. A stream of urine from the ureteral orifice created turbulence in the bladder, which can be seen as a series of hyperechoic echoes in the bladder (arrows). The urinalysis and culture were normal without evidence of infection. However, care must be taken in measuring the posterior bladder wall, which may appear artifactually thickened because of enhancement. **(B)** AP-pelvic view of bladder after a total abdominal hysterectomy, bilateral salpingo-oophorectomy, and radiotherapy. Bladder wall is thickened. It is important to recognize that the bladder wall thickness varies considerably between the empty and full bladder.

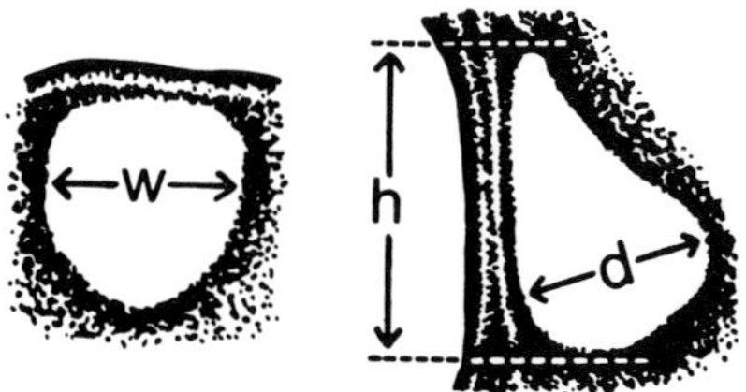

Fig. 16-4. Width *(w)* is obtained from the transverse scan exhibiting the greatest transverse diameter. A midline longitudinal scan yields both height *(h)* and depth *(d)*; the latter is taken as the longest chord in the anterior posterior plane. The calculated volume (V_c) is the product of the three dimensions: $V_c = w \times h \times d$. (From McLean and Edell,[1] with permission.)

Bladder Content

Fluid levels resulting from severe infection may sometimes be noted in the bladder. Blood in the bladder after hemorrhage into the urinary tract may result in blood-fluid levels. Infections may also occasionally produce a fluid-fluid interface that can be imaged by ultrasound. *Candida albicans* cystitis has been reported in 3 of 800 consecutive bladder sonographs and was characterized by a movable echo differentiable fluid-fluid interface.[6] All three patients reported by Goodling[6] had thickening of the bladder wall, pseudomycelia on Gram stain of the urine, and positive cultures for *C. albicans*. The fluid-fluid level is thought to result from the aggregation of the pseudomycelia producing a sludgelike layer that can be imaged as an echo dense fluid layer separate from the urine filling the bladder.

In bullous cystitis, small cystic areas may be seen in the bladder wall. Chronic cystitis may be noted secondary to indwelling catheters. Bladder stones may be noted as hyperechoic structures with posterior acoustic shadowing. Generally, bladder stones will shift position within the bladder with changes in position of the patient.

Bladder Carcinoma

Carcinoma of the bladder comprises 3 percent of all neoplasms, but is one of the most common tumors of the urinary tract.[7] There are 38,000 new cases and 10,000 deaths each year in the United States from bladder cancer. The most common presenting symptom is painless hematuria noted in 60 percent of cases. Excretory urograms have an accuracy of about 70 percent in diagnosing bladder tumors.

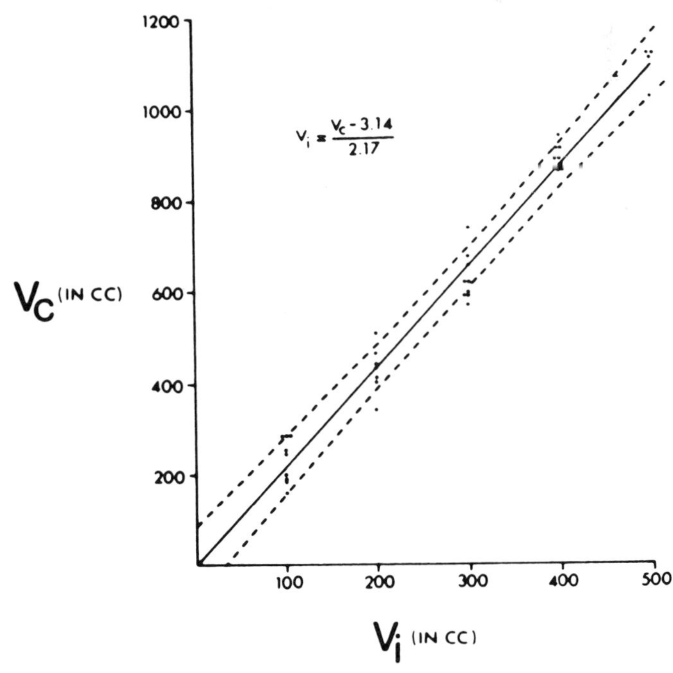

Fig. 16-5. Computed volumes (V_c) are plotted against the volumes of instilled saline (V_i). The calculated linear regression yields the relationship $V_i = (V_c - 3.14)/2.17$, with a correlation coefficient of 0.987. Dashed lines show the 95 percent confidence limits. (From McLean and Edell,[1] with permission.)

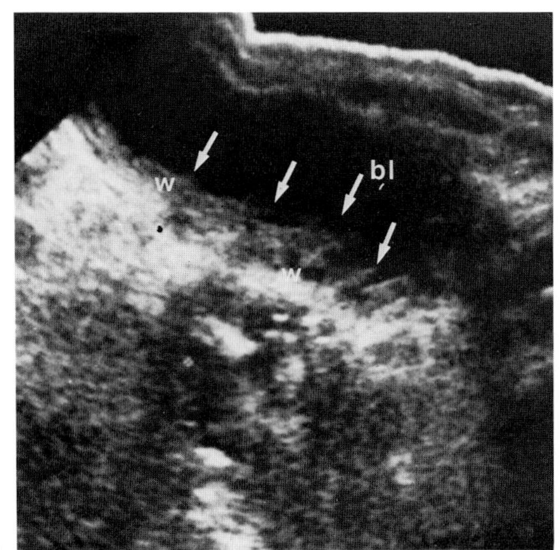

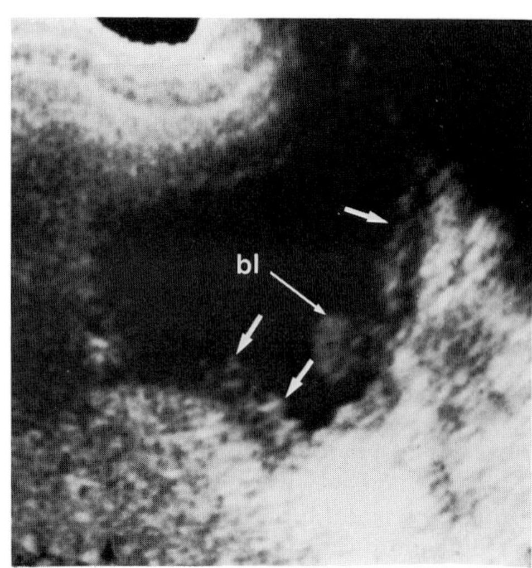

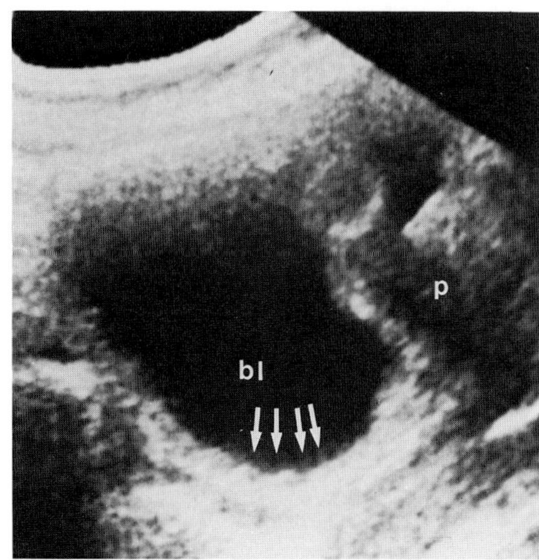

Fig. 16-6. **(A)** Transverse transabdominal bladder sonogram in a patient with bladder outlet obstruction and hematuria receiving constant Foley catheter drainage shows papillary thickening of the mucosa of the posterior wall of the bladder simulating a bladder neoplasm (arrows). Catheter cystitis was proven by cystoscopy. bl, bladder; w, bladder wall. **(B)** Parasagittal transabdominal scan of the urinary bladder (bl) in a patient with long-standing symptoms of bladder outlet obstruction shows mucosal thickening (short arrows) and an echogenic polypoid lesion (long arrow) simulating a neoplasm. Severe bladder trabeculation with no tumor was proved by cystoscopy. **(C)** Parasagittal transabdominal bladder scan shows numerous 1.5-mm bladder lesions (arrows) located in the trigone in a patient with bladder outlet obstruction secondary to an enlarged prostate (p). Bladder trabeculation was proved by cystoscopy. bl, bladder. (Original photographs courtesy of Dr. M. M. Abu-Yousef, Iowa City, IA.) (From Abu-Yousef et al,[4] with permission.)

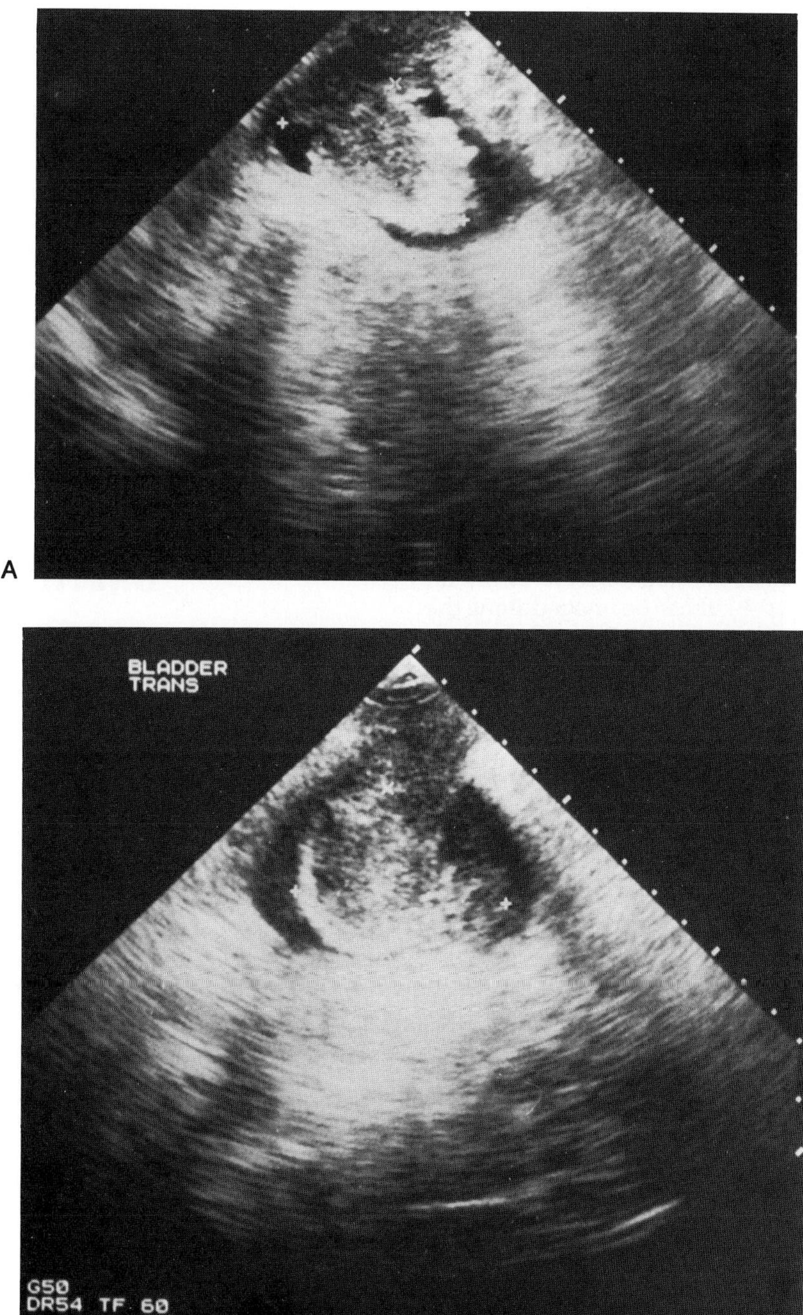

Fig. 16-7. AP-pelvic (**A**) and T-pelvic (**B**) views of bladder demonstrating a large squamous cell carcinoma of the bladder.

Bladder tumors may be imaged as polypoid or exophytic projections into the bladder lumen, irregular surface projections, or bladder wall thickening secondary to tumor infiltration (Fig. 16-7).[4] Itzchak et al[7] detected only 33.3 percent of bladder tumors using ultrasonography when tumors were smaller than 0.5 cm. However, the diagnosis rate was 83.3 percent for tumors larger than 1 cm and 95 percent for tumors larger than 2 cm. Infiltrating tumors may be harder to diagnose. False-positive diagnosis may occur due to bladder trabeculations and catheter cystitis (see Fig. 16-6).

URETERS

The ureters are generally not identified as separate structures along the lateral pelvic wall unless they are dilated. However, occasionally with careful imaging, the ureter can sometimes be seen adjacent to the internal iliac vein (Fig. 16-8). It can be imaged along the lateral pelvic wall when cannulated with a stent (Fig.16-9). Although the ureters are difficult to identify along the lateral pelvic wall, they can almost routinely be visualized as they enter the bladder lateral and posterior to the urethra (Fig. 16-10). Urine can be seen (as a periodic "jet" of turbulence) entering the bladder at the point of entrance of the ureters (see Fig. 16-3). The location of the ureters (and urethra) is often confusing to new sonologists because they are imaged at the top of the screen (in the trans-pelvic plane), rather than at the bottom. Although the ureters enter the base of the bladder, they are imaged at the top of the screen because the ultrasound transducer tip is generally placed in the anterior cul-de-sac in the vagina and the initial sound bang is actually at the level or below the bladder base, depending on how the transducer is being angled. Turbulence from urine entering the bladder is also noted at the top of the screen if the initial sound bang is at the top. In fact, to image the bladder base, ureters as they enter the bladder, and the proximal urethra, is is necessary to direct the transducer tip anteriorly by pushing the transducer handle toward the floor.

URETHRA

The urethra is easily imaged as it enters the bladder in both the AP-pelvic and trans-pelvic plains. (Fig. 16-11). In the T-pelvic plain, the ureter is noted to run vertically on the screen and is imaged above the bladder (Fig. 16-11).

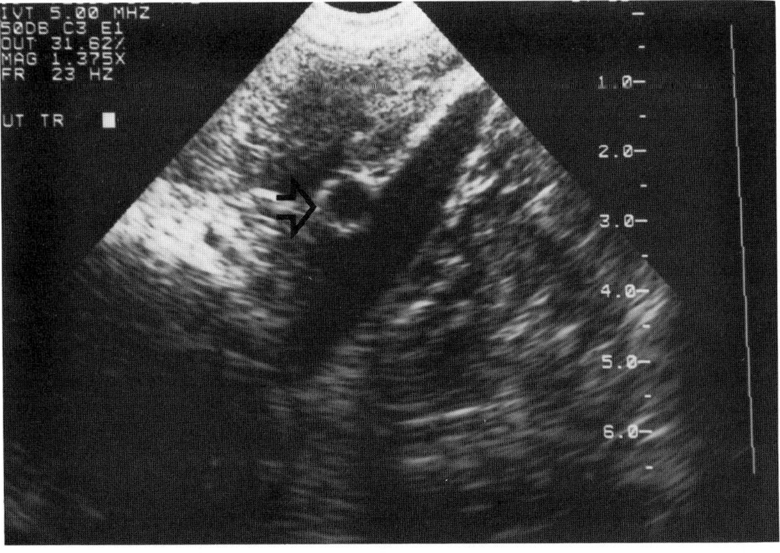

Fig. 16-8. T-pelvic view of the left pelvic wall. Internal iliac vein is noted with the ureter adjacent and superficial. The uterus is to the left of the vein (open arrow).

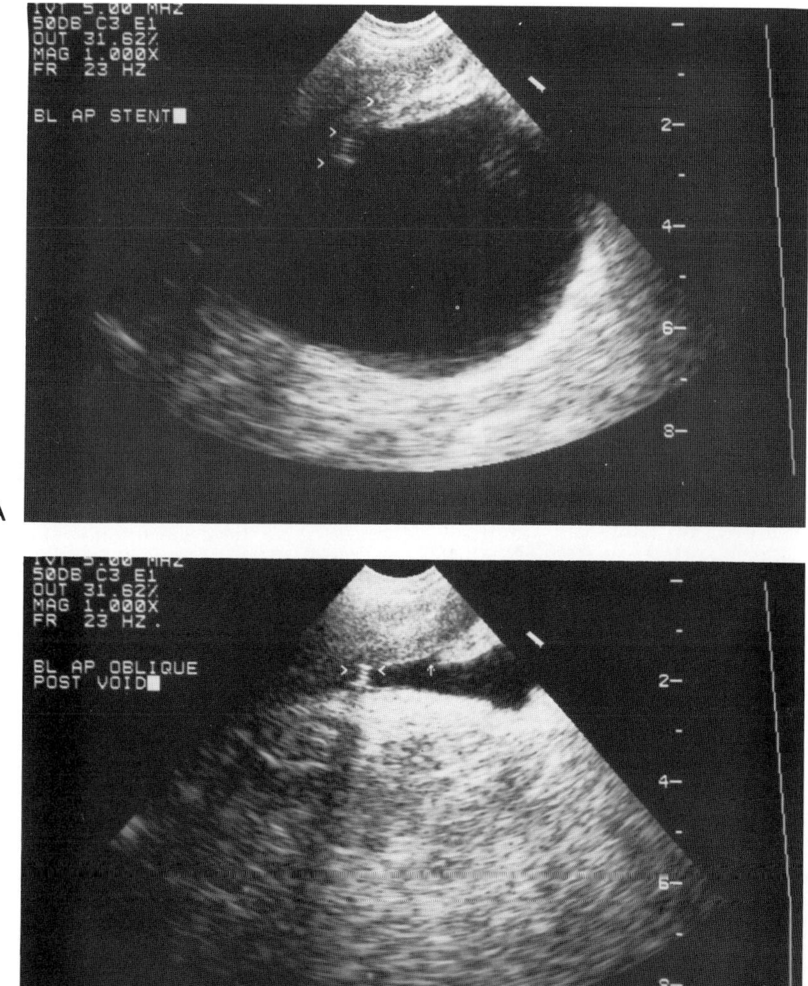

Fig. 16-9. (**A**) AP-pelvic view showing a stent in the left ureter protruding into the bladder. The small white arrowheads delineate the stent and area of the ureteral orifice and the ureter as it penetrates through the detrusor muscle of the bladder. (**B**) AP-pelvic and somewhat oblique view showing the stent in the ureter (arrowheads) and urethra (small arrow) after emptying the bladder.

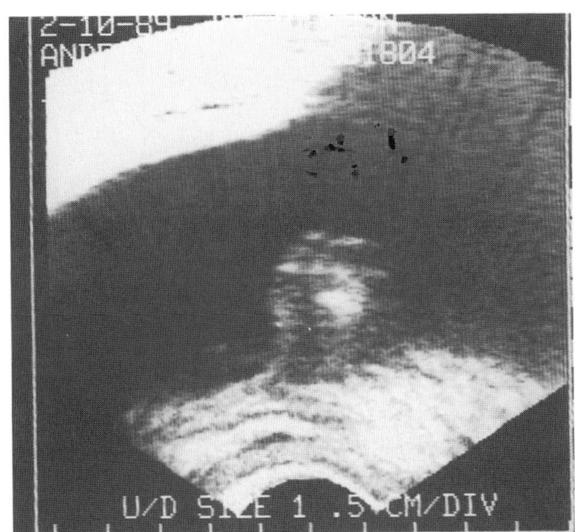

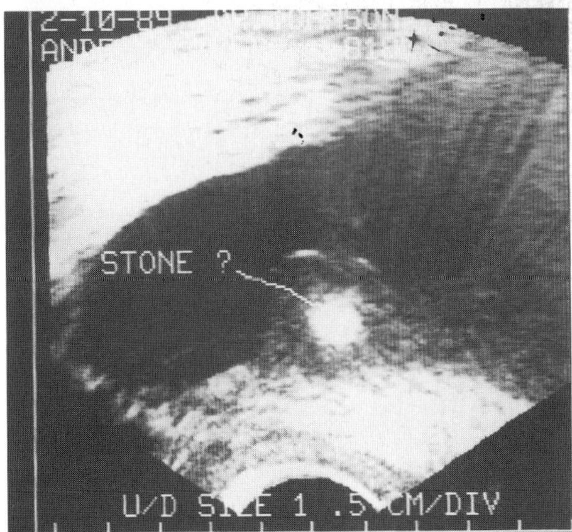

Fig. 16-10. A 48-year-old woman was referred for evaluation of recurrent urinary tract infection associated with microhematuria. Her infections were characterized by urgency, urgency incontinence, worsening of her stress incontinence complaints, and lower abdominal cramping pain. She had no fever or gross hematuria, but she had a constant urge to void. Transvaginal endosonography demonstrated a mass on her bladder base with a central, bright, shadowing echo source compatible with a stone in a ureterocele. IVP ultimately confirmed left hydronephrosis with a 11 × 8 mm distal ureteral calculus impacted in an orthotopic ureterocele or a pseudoureterocele. The stone was extracted cystoscopically after a generous ureteral meatotomy. (From Johnson et al[10] with permission.)

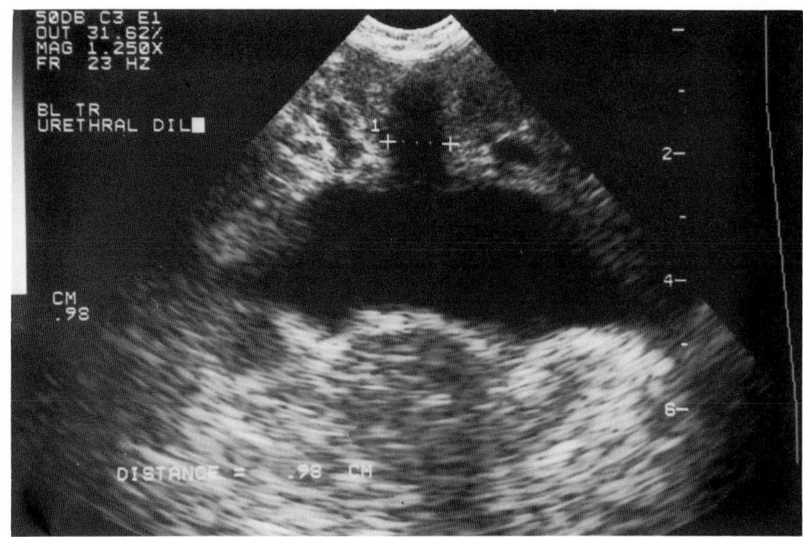

Fig. 16-11. T-pelvic view of the bladder showing the urethra. Parts of the ureters in the detrusor can be seen on each side.

Diverticula

Diverticula of the urethra occur in from 1 to 6 percent of the general population and frequently produce symptoms of dysuria, hematuria, dyspareunia, and incontinence.[8] The classic findings of dribbling after voiding, the presence of a periurethral mass, and the ability to express pus from the urethra are symptoms of a urethral diverticulum. Approximately 20 percent of patients are asymptomatic.

Although diverticula of the female urethra are generally diagnosed using double-balloon urethrography, voiding cystourethrography, or urethroscopy, they can be readily diagnosed using transvaginal ultrasound.[3] Lee and Keller first described the sonographic appearance of diverticula in 1977.[9] Diverticula are generally imaged as a cystic structure adjacent to the urethra with or without septa and internal echoes (debris; Figs. 16-12 and 16-13). Although double-balloon urethrography has been the diagnostic method of choice with an accuracy of 90 percent, Keefe et al[8] noted that sonography could achieve visualization equal to that of contrast radiography and was better for judging the spatial relationship of the diverticulum to the urethra. Double-balloon urethrography is often uncomfortable or painful, whereas sonography is very well tolerated. Considering the quoted incidence of urethral diverticula, transvaginal ultrasound offers the potential for more frequent diagnosis provided the sonologist takes the time to image the urethra. Other periurethral masses, such as abscesses and tumor, can also be imaged (Figs. 16-14 and 16-15).

Ureterocele

A ureterocele is a cystic dilatation of the terminal portion of the urethra. These cystic dilatations involve the intravesical submucosal ureter and can be noted on real-time transvaginal ultrasound to "balloon" out periodically, fill with urine, and deflate slowly as urine is emptied into the bladder. The ureterocele may not be visualized between peristaltic contractions of the ureters. The ureterocele may then be noted to fill over a 5- to 10-second period, forming a cyst-like structure in the bladder. Stones may form in a ureterocele (Fig. 16-16).

PELVIC KIDNEY

A pelvic kidney may occasionally be present and is imaged as a pelvic mass. The outline of the kidney (pelvic mass) is imaged readily, producing a specular reflection. The kidney cortex generally produces a homogeneous isoechoic reflection; however, the renal pelvis is imaged as a hyperechoic echo with the characteristic anatomic pattern of the collecting system. Figure 16-17 shows a pelvic kidney diagnosed by transvaginal ultrasound.

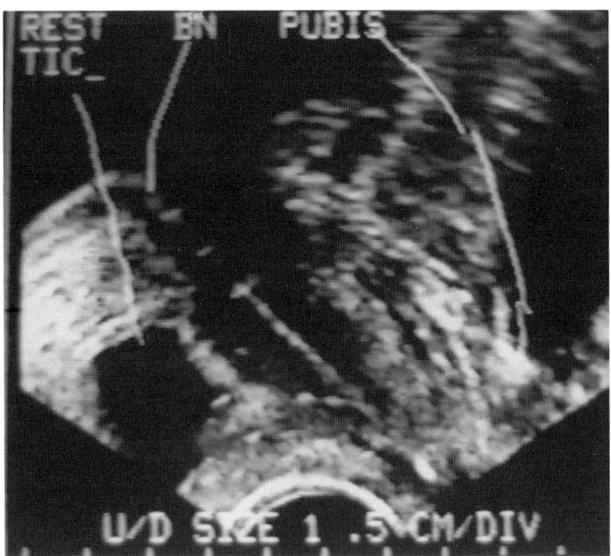

Fig. 16-12. Urethral diverticulum in a 41-year-old woman with stress urinary incontinence and chronic pyuria and dysuria. Cultures grew $<$10,000 *E. coli.* Transvaginal endosonography demonstrated both hypermobility of the bladder neck and a urethral diverticulum that was not easily palpable. She was successfully treated by resection of the diverticulum and a raz needle suspension of the bladder neck. (From Johnson et al,[10] with permission.)

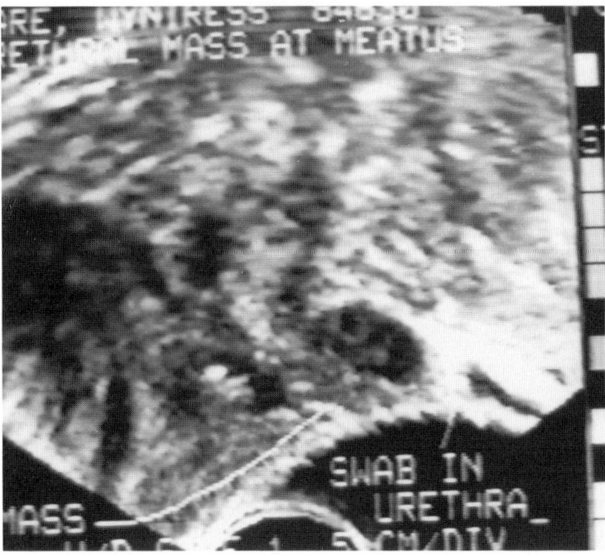

Fig. 16-13. A 41-year-old woman complained of urgency, urge incontinence, and a sense of poor emptying with nocturia two times a night. Pelvic exam revealed a 1.5 cm mass that was rubbery adjacent to the distal urethra. It was extrinsic to the urethra and did not appear to be a caruncle. Transvaginal endosonography demonstrated the mass, which appeared to have a central hyoechoic cavity with a very thick wall. Nothing could be expressed from the mass into the urethra, and it did not change its appearance sonographically after massage. It was resected with complete resolution of her voiding symptoms. Pathologic study revealed a benign mass called an epithelial cyst with a very thick wall. There was no neoplastic change. Despite the lack of demonstrated connection with the urethra, this entity may represent a variation on urethral diverticulum. (From Johnson et al,[10] with permission.)

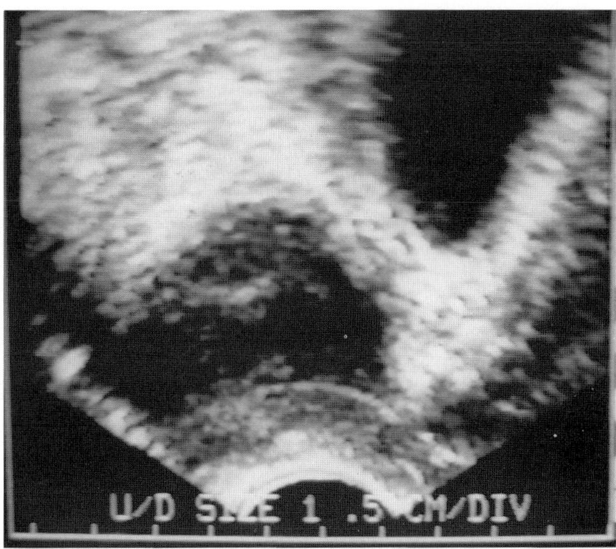

Fig. 16-14. A fleshy, slightly tender mass was found on routine examination in this 28-year-old nulliparous female. She was referred with a presumptive diagnosis of a urethral diverticulum. She had experienced the recent onset of urgency with two episodes of urgency incontinence and had first felt the mass 5 days before her exam. Ultrasound showed a mass with mixed internal echogenicity more compatible with a tumor than a diverticulum. Urine culture grew staph aureus after pyuria was noted on the urinalysis. Scheduled for elective resection 48 hours hence, the patient represented 18 hours later with fever, chills and an obviously fluctuant, tender mass. This was opened, drained and exteriorized with the redundant abscess wall resected. Four weeks after surgery, all irritative voiding symptoms resolved and her urinary control was normal. (From Johnson et al,[10] with permission.)

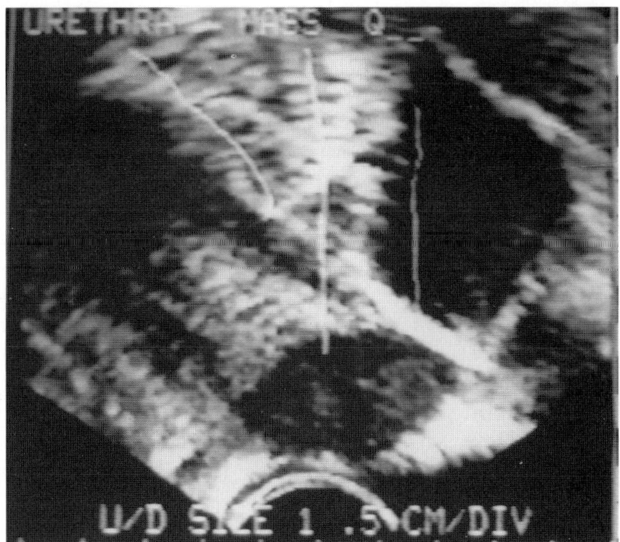

Fig. 16-15. Transvaginal ultrasound demonstrating a tissue density mass adjacent to the distal urethra that was obstructing the flow of urine. The mass was resected and all voiding symptoms resolved. (From Johnson et al,[10] with permission.)

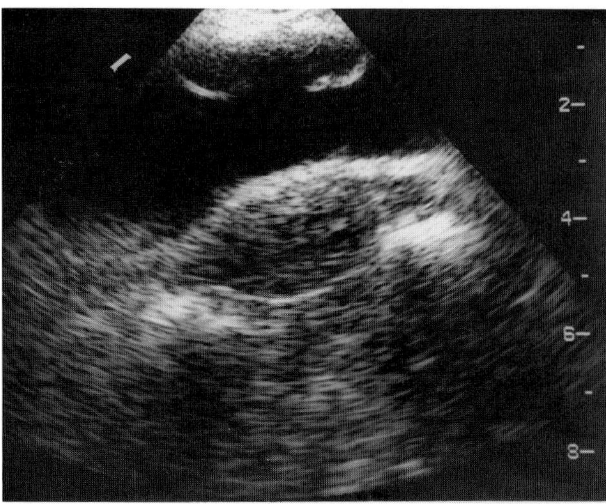

Fig. 16-16. Note bilateral ureteroceles "ballooning" into the bladder. In real time, they could be seen filling over a few minute period, and then rapidly disappearing as urine was emptied into the bladder. The uterus is below the bladder. (From Johnson et al,[10] with permission.)

SONOGRAPHIC URODYNAMICS

Genuine stress incontinence is generally associated with the anatomic findings of posterior rotational movement of the bladder to a dependent position below the pubic bone in response to an increase in intra-abdominal pressure or Valsalva's maneuver.[11] Transvaginal ultrasound can be utilized to dynamically image the bladder neck and posterior urethra, evaluate their normal anatomic relationship to the symphysis, and evaluate any changes during coughing or straining.[12] Ultrasound evaluation of bladder neck function allows a dynamic evaluation and may be recorded on videotape for documentation and future comparisons.

Funneling of the bladder neck may also be noted in association with stress incontinence. Using transvaginal ultrasound Quinn et al[12] identified opening of the bladder neck during coughing in 78 percent (18/23) of patients with primary stress incontinence and in 78 percent (12/14) with recurrent stress incontinence.

Johnson et al[10] studied 279 patients with stress incontinence using transvaginal ultrasound. The patients' were studied in dorsolithotomy position with a full bladder. A calcium alginate swab lubricated with lidocaine jelly was placed in the urethra to allow precise localization of the urethra. The distance between the pubic bone and bladder neck at rest and during a Valsalva's maneuver was measured using electronic calipers. Abnormal bladder neck descent of more than 1 cm was noted in 97 percent (271 patients) with stress incontinence. The average bladder neck descent in patients with no stress incontinence was 0.32 cm. Only 11 percent of patients without stress incontinence had a bladder neck excursion greater than 1 cm, whereas only one patient with stress incontinence failed to demonstrate bladder neck hypermobility of more than 1 cm (Figs. 16-18 and 16-19). Ultrasound also may be used postoperatively to follow patients with stress incontinence after surgical correction. In the Johnson et al[10] series, the average bladder neck descent of 89 patients studied after surgery was only 0.21 cm compared to 1.67 cm before surgery (Fig. 16-20).

Although cystometry, with measurement of the pressure-volume relationship of the bladder and the ability to measure intravesical and abdominal pressure simultaneously, is the method of choice for diagnosing uninhibited detrusor contractions and diagnosing an unstable bladder, it is possible to observe wavelike uninhibited detrusor contractions and opening and/or closing of the bladder neck using ultrasound (Fig. 16-21).[13,14] It is not uncommon to have an unstable bladder in association with stress incontinence. However, Johnson et al[10] noted considerable improvement or cure in 74 percent of patients with an unstable bladder with bladder neck hypermobility after surgical correction.

Kil et al[15] used transvaginal ultrasound to study 60 patients after three bladder neck suspension operations (Gittes, Stamey, and Burch) for stress incontinence and compared the ultrasound findings to urodynamics evaluation. The bladder was filled (400 to 500 ml), and the transvaginal probe was inserted only 1 to 2 cm into the vagina. The pubic symphysis served as an anatomic reference point in the pelvis. The position of the bladder neck in relation to the symphysis was calculated in two directions. Using ultrasound evaluation, no correlation was noted between the absolute position of the bladder neck and postoperative continence. However, the rotational angle in incontinent patients were significantly larger (Fig. 16-22). Patients with intrinsic urethral dysfunction may demonstrate an open immobile bladder neck and urethra with an unfillable bladder that empties passively in response to even small increases in intra-abdominal pressure (Fig. 16-23). The importance of determining the bladder capacity and post-void residual urinary volume has already been emphasized, and is par-

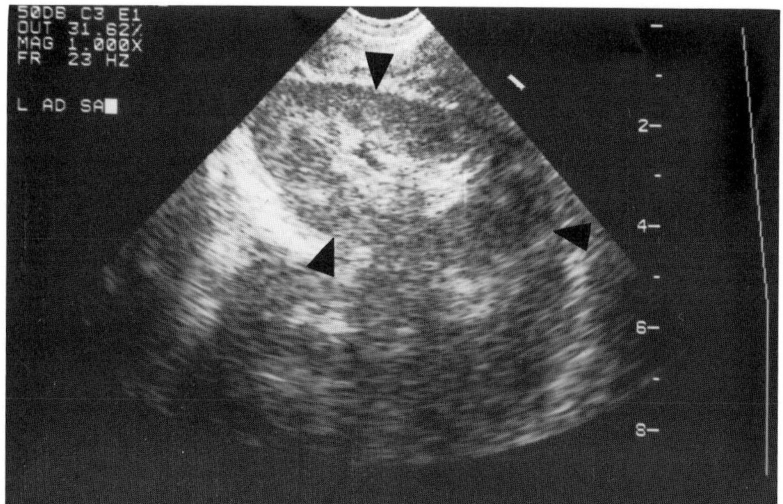

A

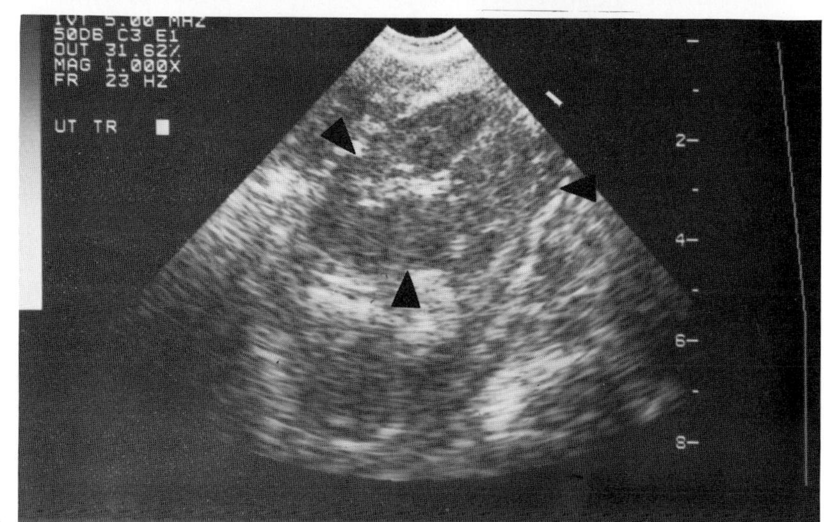

B

Fig. 16-17. A 41-year-old woman G4 P3 referred for evaluation of a left adnexal mass. **(A)** AP-pelvic view shows a pelvic kidney. Note the hyperechoic collecting system. **(B)** T-pelvic view of pelvic kidney. The kidney is outlined by arrowheads. (From Johnson et al,[10] with permission.)

ticularly critical in patients with incontinence (Fig. 16-24).

It is not clear that every patient needs the extensive evaluation sometimes included under the concept of urodynamic testing. It is important when evaluating a patient for stress incontinence to demonstrate clinically both the incontinence during stress maneuvers and the anatomic defect. It is also important to ensure that the patient does not have a very large bladder capacity with overflow incontinence or the very small contracted bladder, since surgical repair of these misdiagnosed conditions can be disastrous. Surgical repairs for stress incontinence can produce a degree of urethra-vesical angle "obstruction" that can further aggravate the problem of patients with a neurogenic bladder and overflow incontinence or patients with a contracted bladder after interstitial cystitis or chronic infection.

Recognition of the "lead pipe or drainpipe urethra," an ectopic ureter or genitourinary fistula, is also important. The more common clinical problem is differentiating the patient with an unstable bladder from one with genuine stress incontinence. Although bladder contractions can be recognized by ultrasound evaluation, additional studies will be necessary to determine the real value of ultrasound in the diagnosis of the unstable bladder. However, as noted by Johnson et al,[10] many patients with an unstable bladder

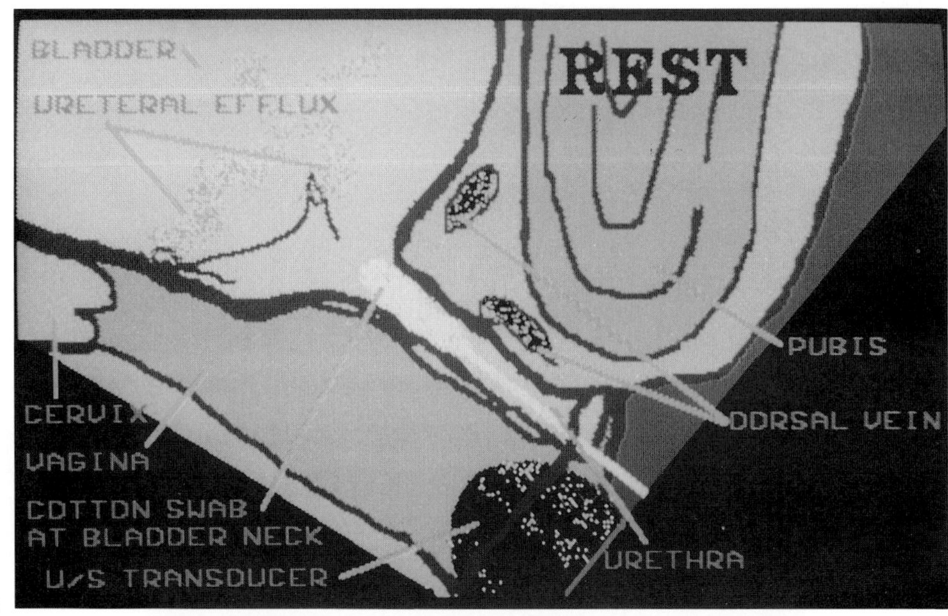

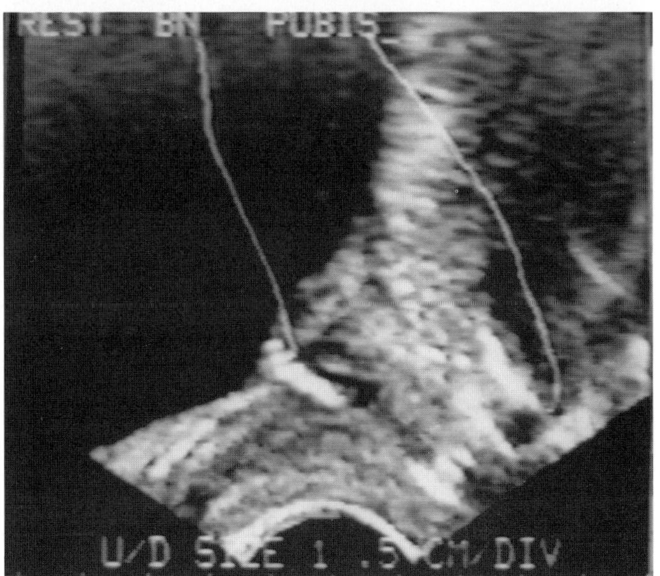

Fig. 16-18. **(A)** Diagram showing the relationship of the bladder neck and os pubis. The ultrasound transducer is illustrated. A calcium alginate urethral swab is illustrated in the uterus. **(B)** Transvaginal ultrasound of a patient with stress urinary incontinence at rest. (From Johnson et al,[10] with permission.)

A

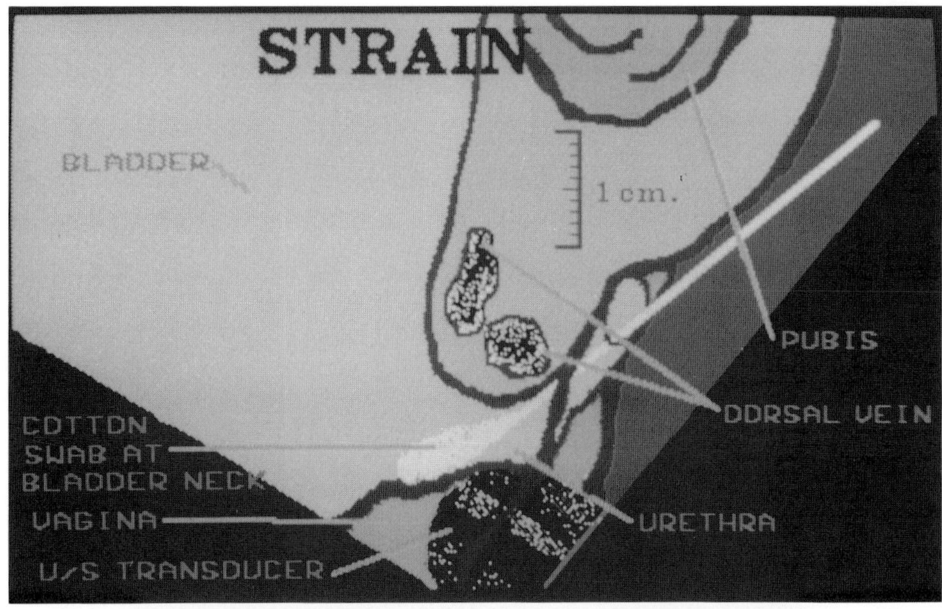

B

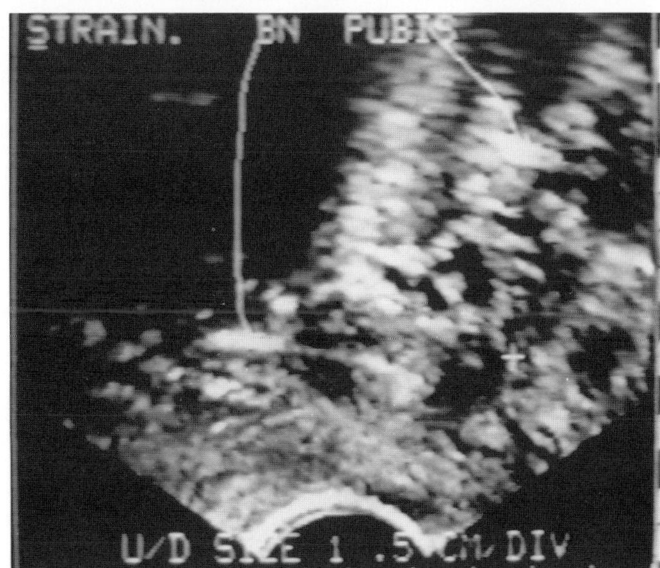

Fig. 16-19. (**A**) Diagram of a transvaginal ultrasound showing abnormal bladder neck descent exceeding 1 cm during a Valsalvas maneuver illustrating hypermobility of the bladder neck. The vertical distance between the bladder neck and the inferior margin of the pubic bone is measured. (**B**) The image is frozen at the point of maximum bladder neck descent during the Valsalva's maneuver.

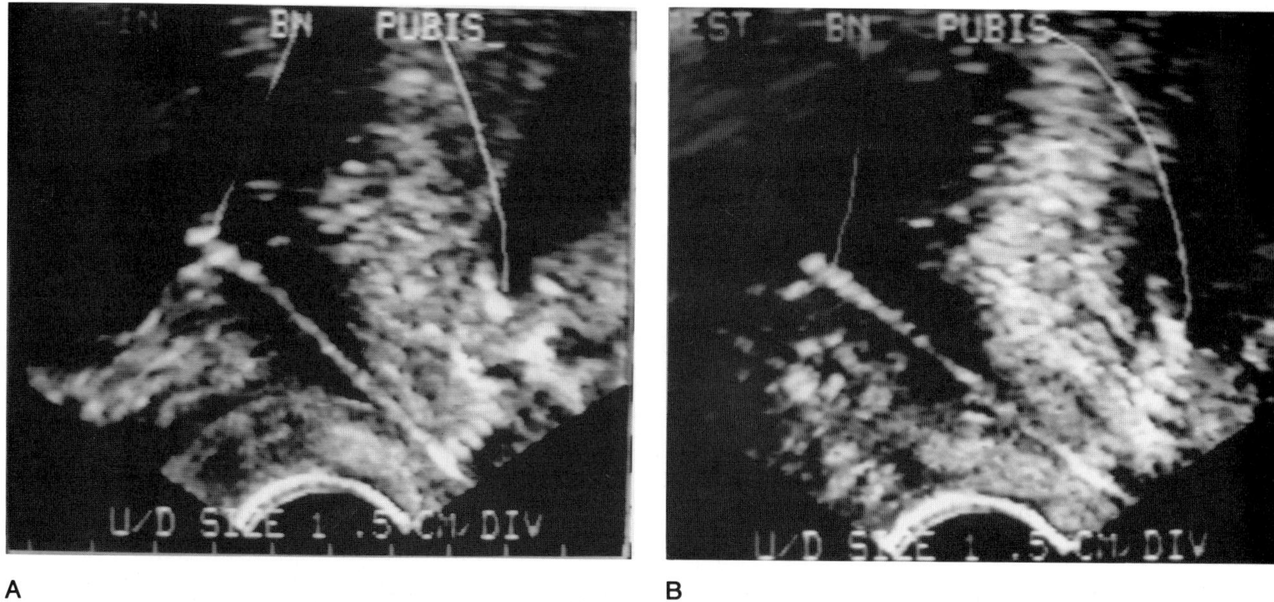

Fig. 16-20. Transvaginal ultrasound image of the bladder neck (BN) at rest after a bladder neck suspension. B) No apparent descent is noted with a Valsalva's maneuver. (From Johnson et al,[10] with permission.)

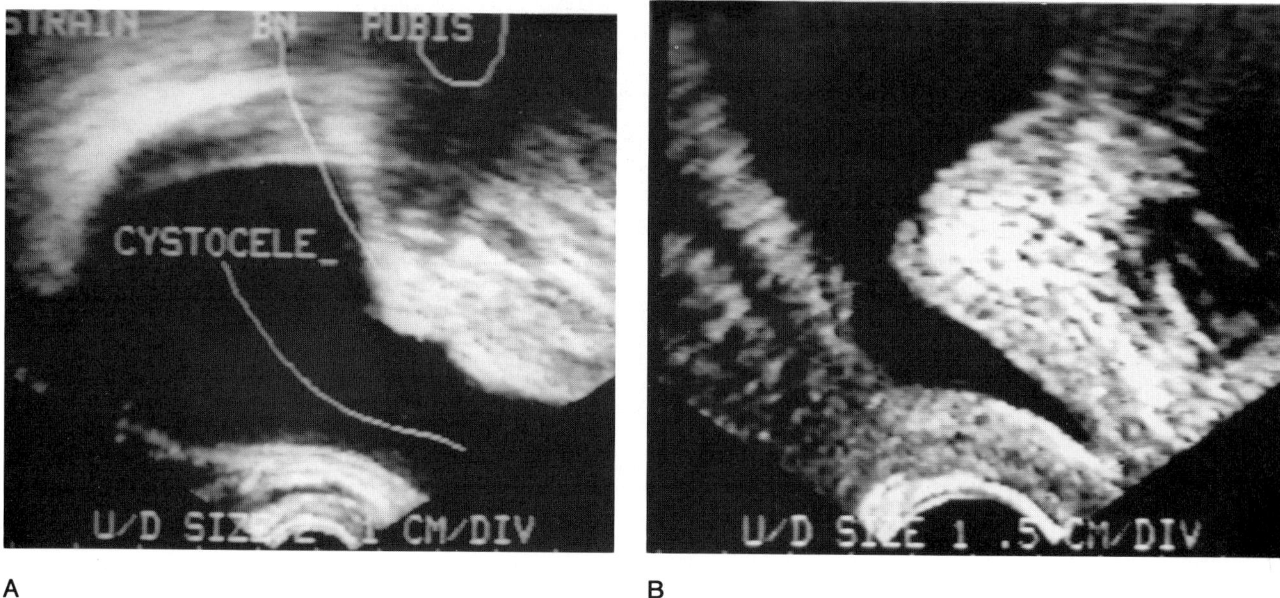

Fig. 16-21. (**A**) Cystocele protruding through the vaginal introitus anterior to the transvaginal transducer during a Valsalva's maneuver. BN, bladder neck. (**B**) Cough-induced unstable detrusor contraction with bladder evacuation simulating genuine stress urinary incontinence. (From Johnson et al,[10] with permission.)

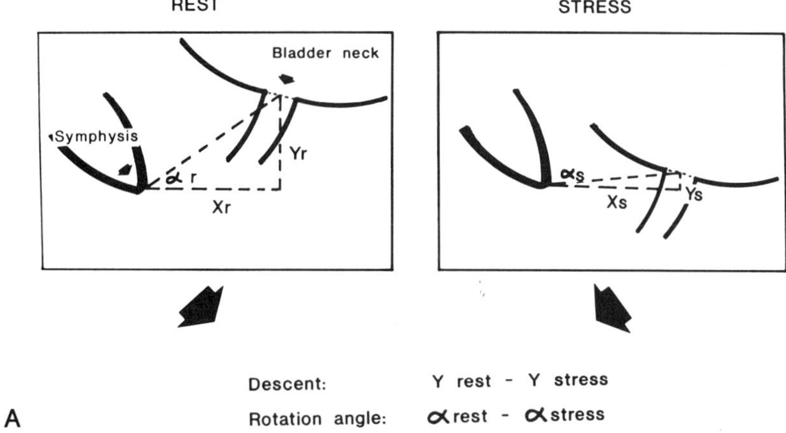

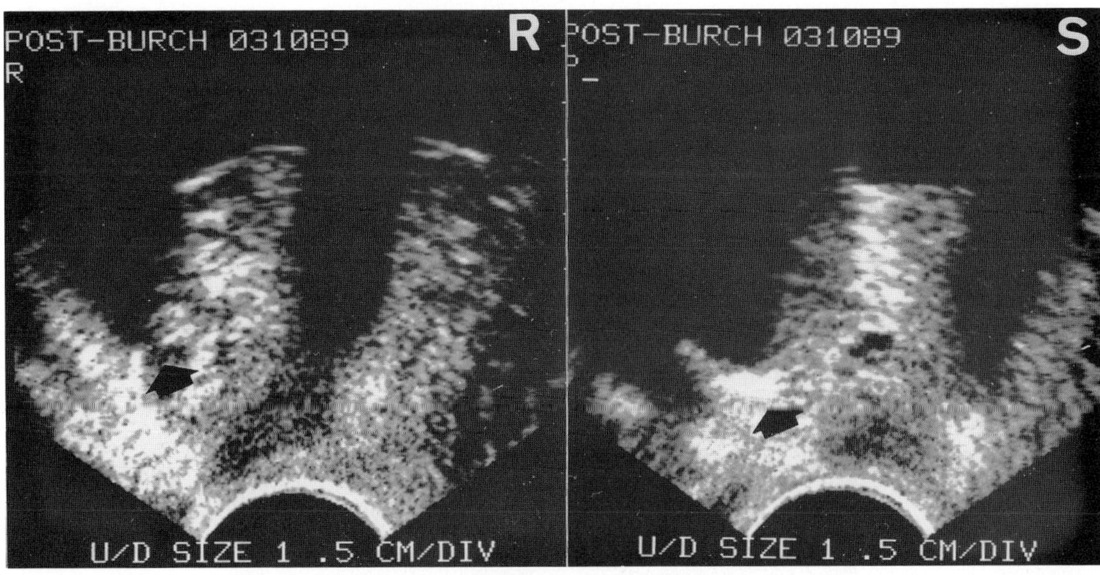

Fig. 16-22. (**A**) Diagram illustrating a method of measurement of descent of the bladder neck. The pubic symphysis serves as a reference point. The position of the bladder neck in relation to the pubic symphysis is calculated in two directions (x and y) during rest and during stress. The angle is calculated. To obtain valid measurements the position of the bladder neck before and after stress should differ by more than 5 percent. (**B**) Ultrasound showing the bladder neck during rest (R) and during stress (S) in a continent patient after a Burch colposuspension. The arrow indicates the symphysis pubis. *(Figure continues.)*

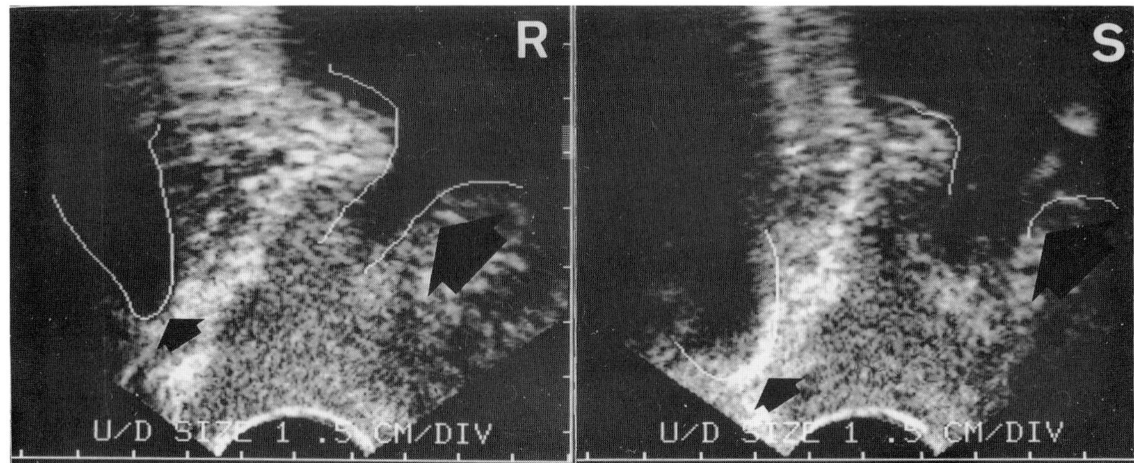

Fig. 16-22 *(Continued)*. (C) Ultrasound of continent patient after a Stamey suspension during rest (R) and during stress (S). Small arrow marks the symphysis pubis, and the large arrow marks the bottle neck. (From Kil et al,[15] with permission.)

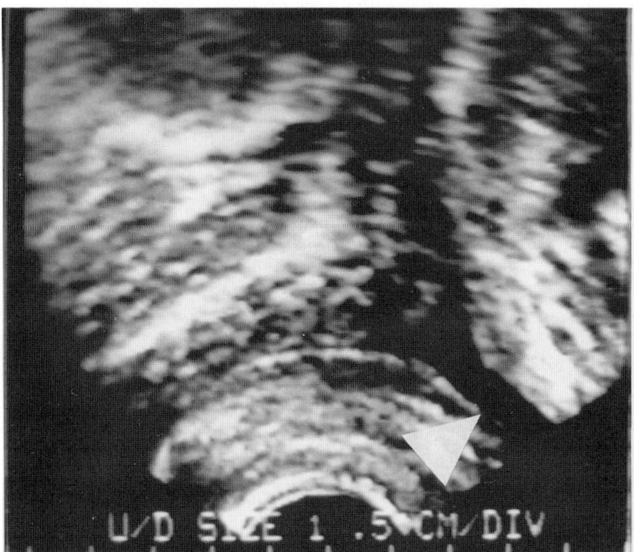

Fig. 16-23. Incontinence due to intrinsic urethral dysfunction in a 56-year-old woman who has had three unsuccessful bladder neck suspensions. The bladder cannot accumulate any volume with leakage of urine occurring under the stress of gravity or deep breathing. (From Johnson et al,[10] with permission.)

A

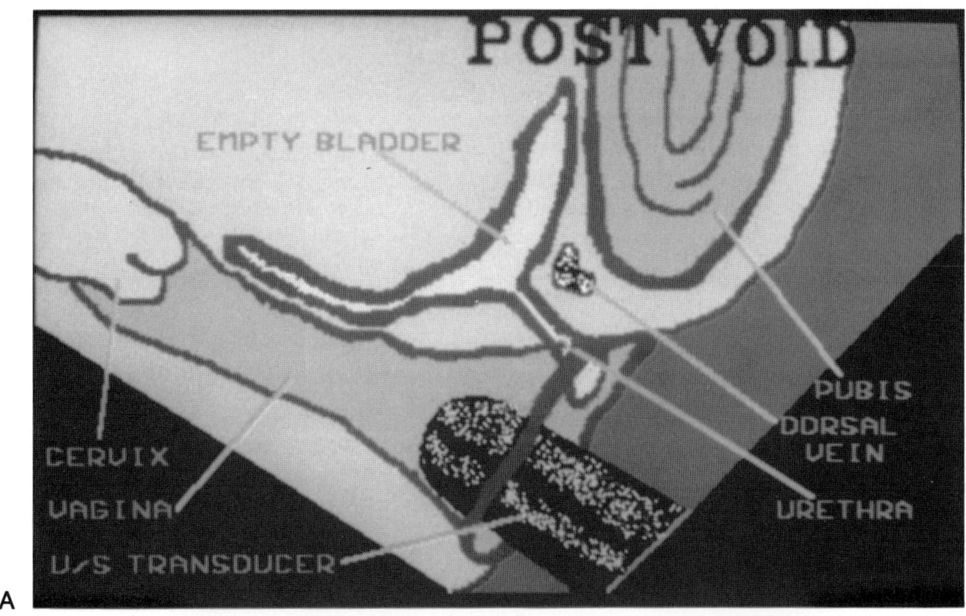

B

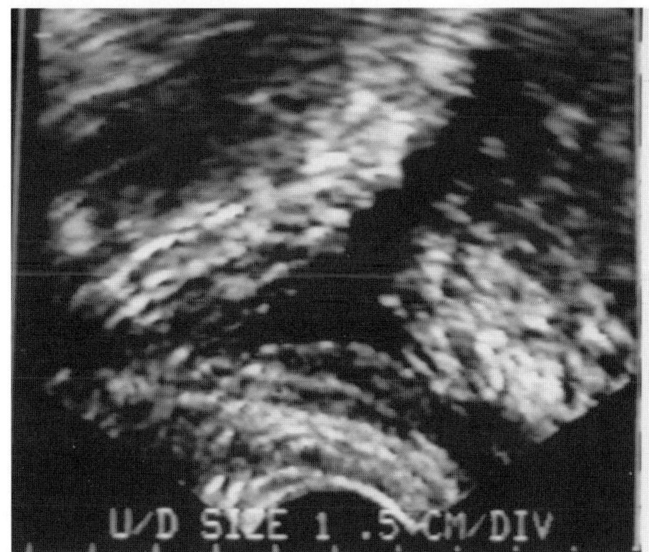

Fig. 16-24. (**A**) Diagram showing the bladder after voiding in relation to the symphysis pubis. (**B**) Ultrasound image illustrating the same anatomy. The bladder is empty after voiding. (From Johnson et al,[10] with permission.)

will be improved by surgical repair provided there is a demonstrable anatomic component with confirmed bladder neck hypermobility and associated genuine stress incontinence.

The use of ultrasound in the evaluation of incontinence is a new and evolving area. However, despite the fact that a considerable amount of diagnostic information can be obtained from the ultrasound evaluation of the bladder and proximal urethra in patients with stress incontinence, it should be utilized in conjunction with a thorough history, physical examination, and other diagnostic techniques as warranted to confirm the diagnosis of stress incontinence.

REFERENCES

1. McLean GK, Edell SL: Determination of bladder volumes by gray scale ultrasonography. Radiology 128:181, 1978
2. Haylen BT: Verification of the accuracy and range of transvaginal ultrasound in measuring bladder volume in women. Br J Urol 64:350, 1989
3. Haylen BT: Residual urine volume in a normal female population: application of transvaginal ultrasound. Br J Urol 64:347,1989
4. Abu-Youssef MM, Narayana AS, Franken EA, Jr, Brown RC: Urinary bladder tumors studied by cystosonography. Radiology 153:223, 1984
5. Rifkin MD, Needleman L, Kurtz AB et al: Sonography of nongynecologic cystic masses of the pelvis. AJR 142:1169, 1984
6. Goodling GAW: Sonography of *Candida albicans* cystitis. J Ultrasound Med 8:121, 1989
7. Itzchak Y, Singer D, Fischelovitch Y: Ultrasonographic assessment of bladder tumors. I. Tumor detection. J Urol 126:31, 1981
8. Keefe B, Warshauer DM, Tucker MS, Mittelstaedt CA: Diverticula of the female urethra: diagnosis by endovaginal and transperineal sonography. AJR 156:1195, 1991
9. Lee TG, Keller FS: Urethral diverticulum: diagnosis by ultrasound. AJR 128:690, 1977
10. Johnson JD, Lamensdorf H, Hollander IN, Thurman AE: Use of transvaginal endosonography in the evaluation of women with stress urinary incontinence. J Urol 147:421, 1992
11. Fellows GJ: Dynamic ultrasonography for voiding dysfunction. Urol Clin North Am 16:809, 1989
12. Quinn MJ, Beynon J, Mortenson NJ, Smith PJ: Transvaginal endosonography: a new method to study anatomy of the lower urinary tract in urinary stress incontinence. Br J Urol 62:414, 1988
13. Tanagho EA, Stoller ML: Urodynamics: cystometry and urethral closure pressure profile. pp. 164–170. In Ostergard D, Bent AE (eds): Gynecologic Urology and Urodynamics: Theory and Practice. 3rd Ed. Williams & Wilkins, Baltimore, 1980
14. Bhatia NN, Thomas S: Ultrasound in urogynecology. pp. 197–205. In Ostergard D, Bent AE (eds) Gynecologic Urology and Urodynamics: Theory and Practice. 3rd Ed. Williams & Wilkins, Baltimore, 1980
15. Kil PJ, Hoekstra JW, van der Meijen Apm et al: Transvaginal ultrasonography and urodynamic evaluation after suspension operations: comparison among the Gittes/Stamey and Burch suspensions. J Urol 146:132, 1991

17

Invasive Techniques

Melvin G. Dodson

The use of ultrasound to image pelvic structures has led to the development of an increasing number of invasive ultrasound diagnostic and therapeutic techniques (Table 17-1). The high image resolution provided by transvaginal ultrasound coupled with the use of saline or other fluids allows detailed visualization and evaluation of such structures as the endometrial cavity, and to some extent the fallopian tubes. Recently the development of sonographic contrast media and the combined use of Doppler and color flow have resulted in improved accuracy in the diagnosis of endometrial pathology and patency of the fallopian tubes. (see Ch. 20)

Transvaginal ultrasound has been used to guide or confirm catheter placement to allow tubal cannulization for corneal obstruction and tubal embryo transfer and transcervical GIFT. The use of a needle guide attached to the transvaginal transducer allows very accurate ultrasound direction and placement of needles. Transvaginal ultrasound needle aspiration of follicles has become the most common technique for ovum recovery for assisted reproductive technologies, such as in vitro fertilization, zygote tubal transfer, and the like. Transvaginal ultrasound-guided aspiration of ovarian cysts and hydrosalpinx and drainage of tubo-ovarian abscesses are becoming important adjunct techniques in properly selected patients. Chorionic villus, early amniocentesis, biopsy, and embryo reduction may be done utilizing transvaginal ultrasound (Table 17-1).

SONOSALPINGOGRAPHY

Hysterosalpingography (HSG) under fluoroscopic imaging and chromotubation under direct laparoscopic visualization have been the primary techniques for evaluation of tubal patency. The endometrial cavity has generally been evaluated by HSG or hysteroscopy and histologically by D&C or endometrial biopsy.

HSG is an excellent technique, but has the disadvantage of x-ray exposure and the potential of allergic reactions to the radio-opaque dye. Laparoscopy has the disadvantages of requiring general anesthesia and a surgical incision, and it is expensive. Complications are relatively uncommon, but can be serious. The advantages of laparoscopy are that the entire pelvis can be visualized and evaluated for endometriosis, pelvic adhesion, etc. in addition to evaluating tubal patency.

HSG, laparoscopy, and hysteroscopy are all valuable diagnostic procedures, and each technique can be utilized to provide inpatient clinical information. However, sonographic evaluation of the pelvic organs and contrast sonosalpingography are developing into very useful diagnostic and therapeutic tools that provide important diagnostic information. Although contrast sonosalpingography is the most comparable to HSG, and can be used for some of the same clinical indications, it has several important differences, advantages, and disadvantages. Sonosalpingography may be considered the technique of choice for evaluating the endometrial cavity, tubes, and tubal patency in patients who are allergic to radiographic contrast agents. There is, of course, no x-ray exposure with sonosalpingography and no risk of allergic reaction (when normal saline is utilized as the distention fluid). Sonosalpingography is at least as good if not superior to HSG for evaluating the endometrial cavity. Sonographic evaluation of the endometrium, myometrium, ovaries, and pelvis is clearly superior to HSG, which yields little information about these structures (see below). HSG remains the technique of choice in evaluating tubal patency. However, it is much more invasive and expensive, and it truly is not comparable.

Table 17-1. Invasive Transvaginal Ultrasound Guided Techniques

Sonosalpingography
Catheter placement for tubal catheterization/recannulization
Follicular aspiration for assisted reproductive technologies
Embryo/gift tubal transfer
Ovarian cyst aspiration/cytology
Drainage of tubo-ovarian abscesses
Early amniocentesis
Transvaginal ultrasound directed chorionic villus biopsy
Embryo reduction

Laparoscopy should be utilized when there is a clinical indication to evaluate the pelvis in addition to evaluating tubal patency.

Sonographic evaluation of the myometrium and ovaries is clearly superior to that provided by HSG. HSG evaluation of the myometrium is generally limited to lesions that impinge upon or distort the endometrial cavity. Evaluation of follicular development and ovulation can be an important added piece of diagnostic information obtained by ultrasound at the time of sonosalpingography (see Ch. 7 and 18).

Sonographic Contrast Media

Two types of sonographic contrast media have been utilized: (1) saline or other fluids (Dextran 60) that give an anechoic or hypoechoic image and may be utilized to distend the endometrial cavity or may be dynamically visualized while moving through the fallopian tubes or in the cul-de-sac and (2) echogenic contrast media. Generally, saline and other similar fluid media allow distension of the uterine cavity with reasonably good evaluation of endometrial thickness, any irregularities of the endometrial wall, or the presence of polyps or leiomyomas protruding into the endometrial cavity. Aqueous contrast media also provide some information on tubal patency, but are not accurate enough to be recommended as a replacement for HSG at this time. When the tubes are patent and the fluid medium enters the pelvis and collect in the pelvis and cul-de-sac, adhesive pelvic bands may be outlined.

One promising echogenic contrast medium consists of stabilized microbubbles and is imaged sonographically as a hyperechoic fluid, giving something of the impression of a radiographic contrast media. Experience with two different microbubble media have been reported. Albunex (Molecular Biosystems, San Diego, CA) consists of human albumin-encapsulated microbubbles produced by sonication. The diameter of the microspheres range from below 1 μ to 15 μ with a mean value of 4.5 μ.[1] This sonographic contrast medium has been utilized in echocardiac studies.[2] All injections were well tolerated. However, safety studies have not been reported, and this agent has not yet been utilized in hysterosalpingography. Another echocontrast agent consists of a saccharide microparticle suspension (SH U 454, Echovist). Safety has been reported in toxicologic and pharmaceutical studies in animals by Fritsch et al.[3] Good tolerance has been reported in echocardiographic studies in over 2,000 patients. Deichert et al have reported on the use of SH U 454 in hysterosalpingographic contrast sonography (discussed below).[4] SH U 454 (Echovist) comes as a two-vial system. One vial contains 3 g of galactose microparticles, and the other vial contains 13.5 ml of 20 percent galactose diluted solution. After mixing and vigorous shaking, a milky echogenic suspension of galactose microparticles and micrometer-sized air bubbles is obtained.

Sonographic Evaluation of Tubal Patency

Schlief and Deichert have reported on the use of SH U 454 (Echovist, Schering, Berlin) for evaluation of tubal patency.[5] A balloon catheter was utilized to introduce the contrast material. Volumes of 1 to 2 ml of media were injected while imaging with a transvaginal transducer in different pelvic plains. An average of 10 ml of contrast material was utilized, with a maximum of 30 ml in individual cases. A sensitivity using B-mode scanning of 88 to 90 percent was noted in the diagnosis of tubal patency, with a specificity of 100 percent. The supplementary use of Doppler techniques improved the diagnostic accuracy to a sensitivity of 91 to 92 percent with a specificity of 100 percent. The predictive value of a positive test was 1.0; however, the predictive value of a negative examination was only 0.5 to 0.7. The criteria for the diagnosis of tubal patency included the demonstration of a steady flow of contrast media in the tube for at least 10 seconds, the accumulation of contrast media in the pouch of Douglas, or the presence of a Doppler flow signal for at least 10 seconds during perturbation.

Tubal flow of contrast material produced a noisy Doppler signal.

Sonographic Evaluation of the Endometrial Cavity

Even without the use of contrast agents, ultrasound has been utilized very successfully to evaluate the endometrial cavity. The endometrium changes sonographically throughout the menstrual cycle, correlating with the histologic changes noted in response to cyclic changes in follicular development and estrogen and progesterone stimulation (see Ch. 6).

However, the use of a contrast fluid, such as saline, may improve visualization of the endometrial cavity and allow more detailed imaging of the endometrium. Bonilla-Musoles et al studied 76 patients using saline solution or Dextran 60 as a distension media.[6] The procedure was done on an outpatient basis without anesthesia and with an empty bladder. A vaginal disinfectant was used, and the patients were given oral ampicillin prophylactically. A Schultze cannula connected to a 50 ml syringe was utilized to introduce distention media. Approximately 5 ml of distension medium was introduced slowly to distend the endometrial cavity. Additional fluid was injected until resistance was noted, or the uterine cavity was imaged adequately.[1] Sonosalpingography was more sensitive but less specific than HSG or hysteroscopy in the diagnosis of uterine cavity pathology (Table 17-2). As might be expected, sonosalpingography was the most effective method for evaluating the myometrium. It could not be done in 2 of 76 patients, one because of pain and one because of cervical stenosis.

HSG also provides reasonable diagnostic information regarding the endometrial cavity in terms of the cavity size and leiomyomas projecting into the endometrial cavity or distorting the cavity, and the presence of endometrial polyps can often be diagnosed. However, HSG has the disadvantages noted above of exposure to x-ray and allergic reactions to the radiopaque dye utilized. Hysteroscopy is probably the gold standard for endometrial evaluation, but is more invasive. Hysteroscopy and HSG give almost no information regarding the myometrium per se and no diagnostic information regarding the ovaries.

Table 17-2. Diagnostic Evaluation of the Uterine Cavity

	Ultrasound	*HSG*	*Hysteroscopy*
Sensitivity	96%	83%	90%
Specificity	98%	100%	100%

(Data from Bonilla-Musoles et al.[6])

Tubal catheterization at the time of hysteroscopy is rapidly becoming an important technique for confirming the diagnosis of tubal obstruction, but is not a primary diagnostic tool. Tubal cannulization should be reserved for the evaluation or treatment of patients with tubal obstruction diagnosed by other techniques, such as HSG, sonosalpingography, or laparoscopy.

Infection and Antibiotic Prophylaxis

All four techniques—HSG, hysteroscopy, laparoscopy, and sonosalpingography—utilized to evaluate the endometrial cavity and fallopian tubes are invasive and have an associated risk of iatrogenic pelvic infections. Although this risk is relatively small, prophylactic antibiotics are frequently utilized after HSG and sonosalpingography. Interestingly, most clinicians do not give prophylactic antibiotics after laparoscopy or hysteroscopy. Perhaps this is because laparoscopies and hysteroscopies are frequently done for indications other than infertility, and since the infection rate is quite low, antibiotic prophylaxis is justifiably not considered necessary. However, there are important arguments for the use of prophylactic antibiotics in all of these procedures when hydrotubation or instrumentation of the tube is being done. Any manipulation (by injection of fluid) or instrumentation of the tube, especially when access is gained by way of the vagina/cervix, may increase the risk of infection by transporting bacteria into the tubes. The tubes are particularly delicate structures that are easily damaged by infections. Since the indication for procedures for evaluating tubal patency is almost invariably infertility, infections although uncommon can be disastrous and can result in infertility, which is the very problem for which the patient is being evaluated.

TUBAL CATHETERIZATION AND RECANNULIZATION

Proximal obstruction of the fallopian tubes is present in about 15 percent of patients whose infertility is due to a tubal factor. Previously, it was treated by tubal microsurgery or IVF. Recent data indicate that proximal obstruction is frequently due to amorphous intraluminal debris or minimal adhesions that are potentially treatable by catheter cannulization of the fallopian tubes with relief of the obstruction.[7] Tubal recannulization has been done under fluoroscopic or hysteroscopic observation. However, ultrasound may also be used to guide and confirm catheter placement.

Cannulization is generally performed between day 8 and 12 of the menstrual cycle in order to avoid the thickened endometrium present in the luteal phase. Prophylactic antibiotics are frequently utilized. Doxycycline, 100 mg two times per day for 5 days beginning before cannulization, or ampicillin 500 mg four times per day, are two common regimens. Placement of a cannula into the tube often produces a very localized lateral pelvic pain.[7] The procedures may be performed under general anesthesia. However, several investigators have utilized preoperative analgesia, such as pethidine 50 mg, diazepam 10 mg, and atropine 0.5 mg IM.[7] Nubain (DuPont pharmaceuticals, Manati, Puerto Rico), phenergan 25 mg IM, and a variety of other regimens have also been utilized (Table 17-3)[8].

Several different tubal cauterization sets are now available commercially. Generally a cervical cannula is used to allow access to the uterine cavity. Stern et al utilized a double-balloon system manufactured by C.R. Bard[9] to hold the cannula in place. One balloon is within the uterine cavity, and the other balloon is approximated against the cervix. This catheter system may also be utilized for hysterosalpingography or sonosalpingography. A curved guide catheter is then passed through the cervical cannula toward the tubal ostium. While visualizing the tube using transvaginal ultrasound, a flex guidewire is passed through the guide catheter through the occluded portion of the tube. The wire may have to be moved back and forth to achieve passage through the obstruction. After recannulization is achieved, the guidewire is removed, and saline is injected with flow through the tube as monitored by ultrasound and color Doppler to confirm tubal patency. Stern et al were able to achieve transcervical catheterization in 90 percent of patients with patency in 88 percent.[9]

Table 17-3. Analgesic Premedication for Tubal Cannulization

Drug	*Route*	*Dose*
Naproxen sodium (Anaprox)	po	550 mg
Ibuprofen (Motrin)	po	800 mg
Nubain plus	IM	20 mg
phenergan	IM	25 mg
Diazepam (Valium) plus[a]	po, IM	10 mg
pethidine or	IM	50 mg
hydroxyzine hydrochloride (Vistaril) or	IM	50 mg
promethazine hydrochlorid (Phenergan) or	IM	25 mg
meperidine hydrochloride (Demerol)	IM	50 mg

[a] Atropine may be added intramuscularly at a dose of 0.4 mg.

Lisse and Sydow have reported on a catheter system developed in cooperation with Labotect (Gottingen, Germany) that consists of a flexible catheter guide cannula with a ball-shaped tip.[7] A tubal catheter is inserted through the guide cannula. The distal 6 cm of the tubal catheter has an outer diameter of 0.6 mm and an inner diameter of 0.3 mm. A 0.38-mm guidewire can be placed into the tubal catheter. Tubal patency is confirmed by hydrotubation under ultrasound imaging. Lisse and Sydow were able to catheterize 91 percent of 34 tubes, with patency in at least one tube in 84 percent of patients. Within 6 months of recannulization 32 percent of patients achieved an intrauterine pregnancy. Unfortunately, reevaluation of those patients who did not achieve a pregnancy in 6 months revealed that 43 percent of the treated tubes had reoccluded.

Maroulis and Yeko have utilized the Jansen-Anderson intratubal transfer set (no. K-JITS-572900, William Cook Company, Spencer, IN) and a tactile technique with ultrasound confirmation of correct catheter placement.[10] The Teflon cannula and curved metallic obturator are introduced into the endometrial cavity and pointed in the direction of the fallopian tube. The obturator is removed and then advanced until resistance is noted. A 3 French Teflon catheter is passed through the cannula with a 0.007-cm guidewire. The guidewire is used to probe the proximal portion of the tube. Once the obstruction is passed, the 3 French catheter is advanced over the guidewire. The guidewire is removed, and fluid is injected under ultrasound imaging.

ULTRASOUND-GUIDED ASPIRATION OF OVARIAN CYSTS

Transvaginal sonographically directed needle aspiration of ovarian or adnexal cystic masses has been suggested as an alternative to surgical exploration or laparoscopic cyst aspiration or removal. Ultrasound-guided aspiration of follicles is currently the most common approach for obtaining ova for in vitro fertilization. A needle guide is attached to the transvaginal transducer, and an electronically generated line is projected onto the scanning screen of the probable needle tract, allowing very accurate needle placement during real-time sonographic imaging. Even follicles as small as 15 mm in diameter can generally be aspirated without difficulty.

This technique was rapidly applied to the aspiration of ovarian cysts. Several investigators have reported that cytologic evaluation of aspirated ovarian cyst fluid is an accurate and reliable diagnostic technique for ovarian cancers and that adequate specimens can be safely obtained from ovarian or adnexal cysts by transvaginal-guided needle aspiration. With an adequate specimen the predictive value of a benign cytologic evaluation of cyst fluid for ovarian malignancy has been suggested to be 95 percent.[11] In addition, sonographic evaluation of ovarian masses based on sonographic morphology (without cytology) has been reported to have a 91 percent accuracy in distinguishing benign from malignant lesions.[11]

Definition of an Ovarian Cyst

Before beginning any discussion of the advantages, disadvantages, indications, and contraindications of needle aspiration of ovarian cysts, it is important to have a clear understanding of what constitutes an ovarian cyst. Although the readers might assume that the answer is trivial, I frequently see patients with a diagnosis of an ovarian cyst who in fact have a normal developing follicle. Developing or preovulatory follicles and multiple small immature follicles are part of the normal physiologic function of the ovary and should not be mistaken for an ovarian cyst. It is also common to find normal follicles of 2.5 to even 3.0 cm in diameter. Occasionally a developing follicle becomes even larger before ovulating. I have noted normal follicles that have developed to 3.5 cm in ovulation induction cycles with spontaneous ovulation at mid cycle. The mislabeling or misdiagnosis of a normally developing follicle as an ovarian cyst by sonographic evaluation leads to unnecessary concern by the patient and occasionally unnecessary medical intervention.

Small (generally less than 10 mm in diameter) follicles are also part of the normal physiology of the ovary. These small anechoic areas are present throughout the menstrual cycle. In fact, the absence of any immature follicles is abnormal and suggests that the patient may be anovulatory or experiencing premature ovarian failure or menopause, depending on her age. The absence of any immature follicles in the ovary is normal only in the postmenopausal patient (see Ch. 7).

Although there is no absolute diameter that separates a normally developing follicle from an ovarian cyst, it is unusual for a normal follicle to increase in size to 4 cm or greater. Therefore, I generally use a size of 4 cm to separate a cyst from a normal follicle, with the realization that such a size criterion may occasionally include a "normal" but large follicle and that some nepotistic cysts or endometriomas will be less than 4 cm. The real distinction between a cyst and a normal follicle must be based on its biologic nature and behavior, rather than any absolute size criterion. A normal follicle increases in size over a period of several weeks and then disappears (ovulates). Likewise, an anechoic area in the ovary that is only 2.5 to 3.0 cm that does not change size over time (for example 4 weeks) is not behaving biologically like a normal follicle and may legitimately be diagnosed as a cyst. I have had the experience of imaging a small cyst (about 3 cm in diameter) that persisted on serial sonographic evaluations over 4 months and did not change in size. The cyst was surgically removed with a histologic diagnosis of a serous cystadenocarcinoma.

An ovarian cyst is an abnormal fluid collection. However it is important to recognize that the most common "fluid collections" in the ovary are normal immature follicles or developing or preovulatory follicles. Sometimes it is difficult or impossible to differentiate a normal follicle from a cyst at one sonographic imaging session. What may cause even more difficulty is the fact that the most common cysts in the ovary are functional cysts that arise from follicles or corpus lutea after ovulation. These cysts are benign and will resolve spontaneously. They do not need treatment. When necessary, the distinction can generally be made by serial sonographic evaluations. Functional cysts are self limiting and generally resolve spontaneously in 8 to 10 weeks. For other ultrasound criteria of ovarian cancers, see Chapter 7.

Cyst Cytology

There is considerable variation in the reported accuracy of cytologic evaluation of cyst fluid. Granberg et al[12] reported a specificity of 100 percent and a positive predictive value of 100 percent from an evaluation of 49 ovarian cysts. However, the sensitivity in detecting a malignancy was only 33 percent, with a negative predictive value of only 77 percent. Other studies have reported the accuracy of cytologic evaluation of ovarian cysts to be about 60 percent.[12] Cytology seems to be very specific, and a positive cytologic evaluation certainly warrants surgical removal of the cyst. Unfortunately, considering the relative poor sensitivity of cytology at least at the present time, a negative cytologic evaluation does not provide reassurance that a malignancy is not present. In Granberg et al's[12] study two of three malignancies were missed by cytology. It should also be borne in mind that most of the studies reported come from larger teaching hospitals, often with pathologists with special expertise in cytology. The results of cytologic evaluation of aspirated ovarian cysts in the community hospital in the absence of pathologists with special training is unlikely to match even the poor sensitivity reported. Probably the major concern regarding the low sensitivity of cytology in patients with ovarian cancer is the delay that will result before definitive therapy is instituted in patients with a negative cytology.

In addition, cytology is even poorer in diagnosing the much more common benign neoplasms, such as the serous and mucinous cystadenomas. Although these tumors are benign and the consequence of misdiagnosis is of much less concern, it is clearly not easier to diagnose them. These neoplasms, although benign, should be removed surgically. There is no evidence that aspiration of these neoplasms is of any benefit, and there have now been numerous reports of "recurrences" of these neoplasms months later after aspiration.

Accuracy of Sonography in Predicting the Malignant Character of Ovarian Cysts

Using a morphologic scoring system to discriminate between benign and malignant ovarian tumors in 812 cases, Kurjak and Predanic[13] reported a 92 percent sensitivity and 96 percent specificity, with a positive predictive value of 80 percent and a negative predictive value of 98 percent (see Ch. 20). The overall accuracy of sonographic evaluation of ovarian morphology was 97 percent.[13] Granberg et al[12] noted a 100 percent sensitivity and negative predictive value of transvaginal ultrasound imaging in diagnosing the malignant character of ovarian cysts; however, the sensitivity was only 82 percent, and the predictive value of a positive test was only 73 percent.

There are some useful clinical generalizations regarding ovarian morphology:

Solid areas, wall nodularity or papillation, thick septa, and large cysts (over 10 cm) are more commonly associated with malignancy. Unilocular cysts without internal echoes or wall nodularity are frequently benign.

The more stringent the morphologic criteria utilized for diagnosis (such as even small solid areas within the cyst or minimal wall nodularity or irregularities), the greater the sensitivity in diagnosing malignant tumors and the poorer the specificity. For example, in the Granberg et al[12] study noted above, all of the malignant tumors were diagnosed correctly; however, 6 of 34 benign tumors were diagnosed incorrectly as malignant. The use of morphologic sonographic criteria for the evaluation of ovarian cysts provides considerable diagnostic information and a marked improvement in the ability to recognize malignant tumors. In fact, sonographic evaluation is currently the most accurate method available for predicting malignancy and the method of choice for ovarian cancer screening. However, the technique is not accurate enough utilizing current techniques and criteria to categorize all cysts accurately.

The most appropriate utilization of ultrasound is in screening, in selecting patients at high risk for malignancy who should be treated by immediate surgical intervention, and in separating those patients who are at relatively low risk for malignancy who may be followed by serial sonographic evaluation. Persistence of a cyst (longer than 8 to 12 weeks) indicates pathology, but not necessarily malignancy.

ULTRASOUND-GUIDED ASPIRATION OF OVARIAN FOLLICLES IN ASSISTED REPRODUCTIVE TECHNOLOGIES

A detailed review of the development of ultrasound-guided aspiration of ovarian follicles as applied to IVF and other assisted reproductive technologies is provided in Chapter 19. A variety of imaging and aspiration routes have been utilized. However, most of the approaches utilized in the past that played an important part in the early development of sonographic follicular aspiration, such as transabdominal sonographic imaging with transabdominal needle aspiration or transabdominal sonographic imaging with transvaginal or periurethral needle aspiration, are not commonly used today. The use of a transvaginal probe for transvaginal sonographic imaging and of a needle guide that may be attached to the transducer to allow aspiration of follicles via the vagina is clearly the current technique of choice.

REFERENCES

1. Schlief R: Ultrasound contrast agents. Current Oper Radiol 3:198,1991
2. Feinstein SR, Cheirif J, Ten Cate FJ et al: Safety and efficacy of a new transpulmonary ultrasound agent: initial multicenter clinical results. J Am Coll Cardiol 16:316, 1990
3. Fritsch T, Hilmann J Kampfe M et al: SH U 508, a transpulmonary echocontrast agent: initial experience. Invest Radiol 25:160, 1990
4. Deichert U, Schlief R, Van de Sandt M, Daume E: Transvaginal hysterosalpingo-contrast sonography for the assessment of tubal patency with gray scale imaging and additional use of pulsed wave Doppler. Fertil Steril 57:62, 1992
5. Schlief R, Deichert U: Hysterosalpingo-contrast sonography of the uterus and fallopian tubes: results of a clinical trial of a new contrast medium in 120 patients. Radiology 178:213, 1991
6. Bonilla-Musoles F, Simon C, Sampaio M, Pellicer A: An assessment of hysterosalpingosonography (HSSG) as a diagnostic tool for uterine cavity defects and tubal patency. J Clin Ultrasound 20:175, 1992
7. Lisse K, Sydow P: Fallopian tube catheterization and recannulization under ultrasonic observation: a simplified technique to evaluate tubal patency and open proximally obstructed tubes. Fertil Steril 56:198, 1991
8. Gleicher N, Pratt DE, Parrilli M, Treatment of tubal disease by hysterosalpingography and selective salpingography. p. 33. In Gleicher N (ed): Tubal Catheterization. Wiley-Liss, New York, 1992
9. Stern TL, Peters AJ, Coularn CB: Transcervical tuboplasty under ultrasonographic guidance: a pilot survey. Fertil Steril 56:359, 1991
10. Maroulis GB, Yeko TR: Treatment of cornual obstruction by transvaginal cannulation without hysteroscopy or fluoroscopy. Fertil Steril 57(5): 1136, 1992
11. Meire HB, Farrant P, Guha T: Distinction of benign from malignant ovarian cysts by ultrasound. Br J Obstet Gynaecol 85:893, 1978
12. Granberg S, Norstrom A, Wikland M: Comparison of endovaginal ultrasound and cytological evaluation of cystic ovarian tumors. J Ultrasound Med 10:9, 1991
13. Kurjak A, Predanic M: New scoring system for prediction of ovarian malignancy based on transvaginal color Doppler. J Ultrasound Med 11:631, 1992

18

Ovulation Induction

Melvin G. Dodson

Anovulation and ovulatory dysfunction are important factors in the etiology of infertility in about 25 percent of infertile women. Serial ultrasounds are an excellent technique for evaluating ovulation and diagnosing anovulation and may be helpful in the diagnosis of polycystic ovarian disease (PCOD). These examinations are useful in monitoring patients undergoing ovulation induction using Clomid (clomiphene citrate), Pergonal (gonadotropins), or gonadotropin releasing hormone (GnRH). In addition, the correct prediction or timing of ovulation is critical for infertility therapies, such as intrauterine insemination, artificial or therapeutic insemination using donor sperm, and the timing of intercourse during ovulation induction therapies.

DIAGNOSIS OF ANOVULATION

Several methods may be utilized to evaluate a patient for anovulation, including basal body temperature (BBT) measurements, midluteal phase serum progesterone, serial luteinizing hormone (LH) assays, and serial ultrasounds.

BBT measurements have been the most commonly used method for assessing and timing ovulation and diagnosing anovulation in the past. They have the advantage of being inexpensive and noninvasive. However, BBT measurements are only a very indirect measure of progesterone production and therefore a very indirect and crude evaluation of ovulation. Also, BBT charting is only as accurate as the particular patient involved. Some patients produce very accurate records; others much less so. Quagliarello and Arny[1] compared BBT with serial urinary LH measurements and found BBT measurements to be relatively inaccurate in precisely predicting the day of the LH surge. The BBT correctly predicted the day of the urinary LH surge in only 18 to 30 percent of patients. In addition, BBT was only accurate to within 1 day on each side of the LH surge in 57 to 70 percent of patients.

A midluteal phase progesterone determination is a good method of more directly assessing progesterone production by the corpus luteum after ovulation. Serum progesterone levels above 2.5 ng/ml suggest ovulation. However, serum progesterone levels greater than 10 ng/ml or even 15 ng/ml are thought to correlate better with adequate corpus luteal function and adequate hormonal support of the luteal phase endometrium.

There are now several home LH urinary assay kits available. These LH kits are helpful in diagnosing anovulation and timing ovulation by assaying for the LH surge.

Ultrasound, particularly transvaginal ultrasound, allows the monitoring of follicular development, including the number, size, location (right or left ovary), and progressive growth of follicles, as well as confirmation of ovulation. In addition, pelvic sonographic monitoring of ovulation allows the diagnosis of the luteinized but unruptured follicle (LUF) syndrome, dysfunctional cyst formation, and PCOD. By imaging the endometrium, information can also be obtained regarding estrogen production and luteinization of the endometrium by progesterone. Serial ultrasound monitoring of follicular development and ovulation is called a folliculogram.

Anovulation is characterized by the lack of development of any follicles, failure to develop a dominant follicle, development of a follicle but failure to ovulate (LUF syndrome), empty follicle syndrome (no ovum and cumulus oophorus within the follicle), or asynchrony (or dys-synchrony) between follicular de-

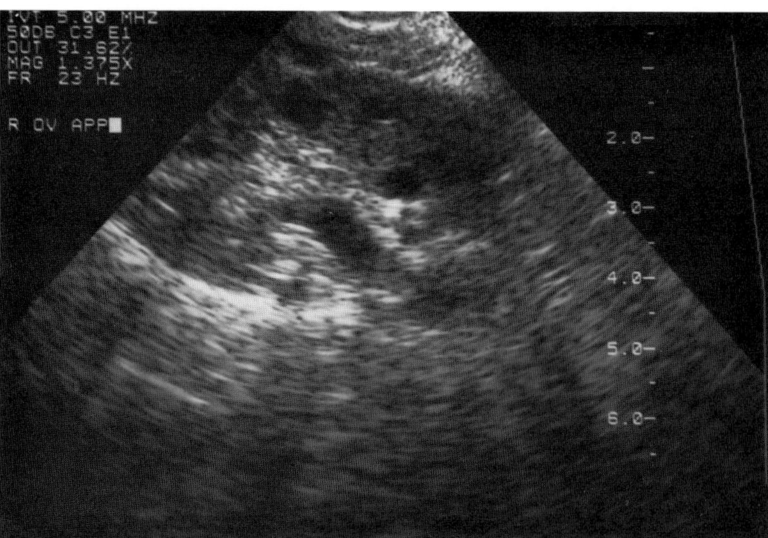

Fig. 18-1. Right ovary showing several nonovulatory follicles. These small (< 10 mm in diameter) follicles can be seen throughout the menstrual cycle.

velopment and the temporal cyclic hormonal changes and endometrial development. Anovulation has been reported to occur in 7 percent of cycles, but in some patients with hypothalamic pituitary dysfunction or PCOD, anovulation may be chronic and persistent. It may be associated with amenorrhea, irregular menses, or occasionally even regular periods resulting from periodic dysfunctional bleeding.

FOLLICULAR DEVELOPMENT

Under the influence of follicle stimulating hormone (FSH) released by the anterior pituitary gland in response to pulsatile GnRH during the early part of the menstrual cycle, a few follicles undergo progressive development each month. Granulosa cells in developing follicles secrete increasing amounts of estrogen and follicular fluid, and the follicles increase in size. As follicular stimulation progresses, one or occasionally two follicles will continue to develop into the dominant follicle(s). Many of the early developing follicles do not progress past the 10 to 14 mm diameter stage of development before they degenerate. This cohort of small nonovulatory follicles destined not to develop and to undergo atrophy has been described in detail by Bomsel-Helmreich et al.[2] They may appear and disappear throughout the normal menstrual cycle. Therefore, it is normal to image a few developing follicles in the ovary throughout the cycle, including the luteal phase or during menses (Fig. 18-1). However, primordial and preantral follicles are too small to be imaged.

There is no consensus on what these small (less than 10 mm) developing follicles should be called. I prefer the term "immature follicle" to differentiate them from developing preovulatory follicles, which are larger and will show progressive growth and generally eventually ovulate. Pache et al[3] noted five immature follicles per ovary in women with regular menstrual cycles.

Hackeloer et al[4] noted a linear increase in the size of the dominant follicle through a normal menstrual cycle. Developing follicles destined to ovulate increase in size 2 to 3 mm/day and reach a maximum diameter of 16 to 33 mm before ovulation.[5] There is a 2± mm interobserver error and a 3± mm error between observers in ultrasound follicular diameter measurements, with the largest measurement errors occurring in the largest follicles.[6] Significantly more follicles are imaged when using the transvaginal probe than with the transabdominal sector or linear transducer.[7]

O'Herlihy et al[8] and Kerin et al[9] noted a good correlation between follicular volume estimated by ultrasound and laparoscopy-measured volume calculated using the volume of aspirated follicular fluid. There is also a good correlation ($R = 0.968$) between follicular diameter and serum estradiol (E_2) levels.[4] As the diameter of the dominant follicle increases, E_2 increases.

Selection of the dominant follicle is thought to occur by cycle days 5 to 7, but is not apparent sonographically until cycle days 8 to 12.[9] Other antral follicles of the developing cohort will generally undergo atresia and will not exceed 14 mm in diameter. However, in 5 to 11 percent of natural cycles, two dominant follicles may develop, but generally in opposite ovaries. Identification of the dominant follicle that will eventually ovulate can be made 4 days before ovulation in only 6 percent of cycles, but this follicle can be identified 2 to 3 days before ovulation in almost all patients. Bomsel-Helmreich et al[2] have suggested that it is possible to separate potentially ovulatory follicles from nonovulatory follicles by size alone as early as 3 days before the LH surge.

PREDICTING OVULATION

A small echogenic mass that is thought to represent the cumulus oophorus may sometimes be noted projecting into the follicle. Visualization of the cumulus oophorus has been reported in 80 percent of follicles greater than 17 mm in diameter. One report has suggested that ovulation will occur within 36 hours after visualization of the cumulus.[10] Kerin et al[9] noted an echogenic area suggesting the cumulus in 23 percent of follicles greater than 18 mm in diameter. Mendelson et al[11] reported a poorly defined echogenic focus adjacent to the follicular wall in 11 of 28 women who conceived during ovulation induction. These follicular structures imaged by ultrasonography were interpreted to be the cumulus oophorus. However, Zandt-Stastny et al[12] have challenged this view and have noted that the cumulus oophorus is only 100 to 150 μ in size and would not be expected to be visualized by sonography. They have suggested that structures imaged in follicles thought to represent the cumulus oophorus are artifacts.[12] This controversy has not yet been resolved (Fig. 18-2).

After the LH surge, the theca tissue becomes hypervascular and edematous, and the granulosa cell layer begins to separate from the theca layer. This separation is appreciated sonographically as a line of decreased reflectivity around the follicle. In 1983 Picker et al[13] suggested that this sonographic sign means impending ovulation within 24 hours.

Jaffe and Ben-Aderet[14] in 1984 described the same sign, which they called a "double contour," and suggested that it occurs a few hours before ovulation. In a later study by Jaffe et al,[15] the double contour sign was noted less than 4 hours after the LH peak and occurred in all patients within 8 hours of the LH peak (Fig. 18-3A). Most follicles (64 percent) had collapsed 4 hours after the appearance of the double contour sign, and all had collapsed within 8 hours. The double contour appears 27.4 hours after the E_2 peak, but with a larger variation (from 16 to 44 hours) than after the LH peak. Again, these changes were not visualized in the study by Zandt-Stastny et al.[12] I have found the double contour sign to be a common finding in mature follicles. However, follicles with a double contour sign have been observed for several days before ovulation has occurred (Fig. 18-3B).

Within 6 to 10 hours before ovulation, separation and folding of the granulosa cell layer produce a crenation or irregularity of the lining of the follicle.[13] This has also been suggested as a sign of impending ovulation (Table 18-1).

Unfortunately, even though several sonographic signs have been described to precede ovulation, there is currently no sonographic sign that predicts exactly when ovulation will occur; the signs only give evidence that the time of ovulation is nearing. Although it is known that ovulation will generally occur when the dominant follicle reaches a size of 16 to 33 mm in diameter, the variation in maximal follicular diameter before ovulation extends the time of ovulation over a 10-day or greater period (Figs. 18-4 and 18-5).[5,15]

The mean peak diameter before ovulation reported by Kerin et al[9] was 23.6 ± 0.4 mm. However, there is considerable variation in follicular size at the time of ovulation. Hamilton et al[5] reported on 158 cycles and noted an average diameter of 21.8 ± 3.2 mm before ovulation, but the maximum diameter ranged from 16 to 33 mm (Fig. 18-5).

Based on follicular diameters, a 14-mm follicle can ovulate from 1.25 to 7 days later. Because of the variation in the slope of individual follicular growth curves, Hamilton et al[5] found a single sonographic measurement of follicular size as accurate as serial measurements in predicting ovulation. A table of predictive intervals was calculated for follicles from 14 to 25 mm (Table 18-2).[5]

Using Hamilton et al's data,[5] a follicle with a 20-mm diameter can ovulate from 0.75 to 3.75 days later in 80 percent of patients. Even a large 25-mm follicle may still not ovulate for several days in some patients (Table 18-2). For clinical purposes for timing of artifi-

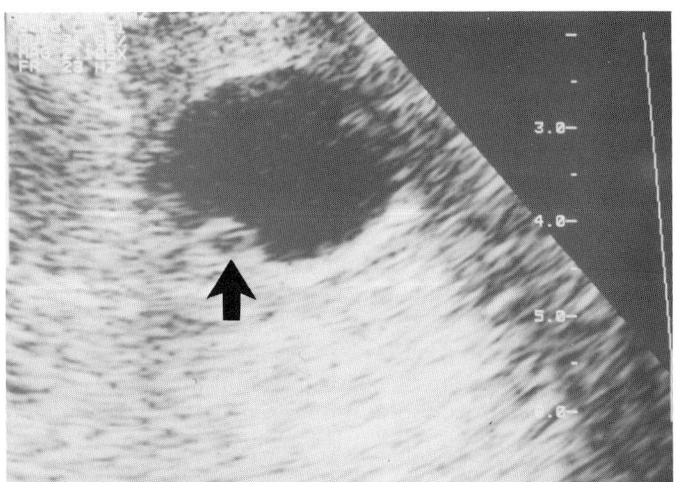

A

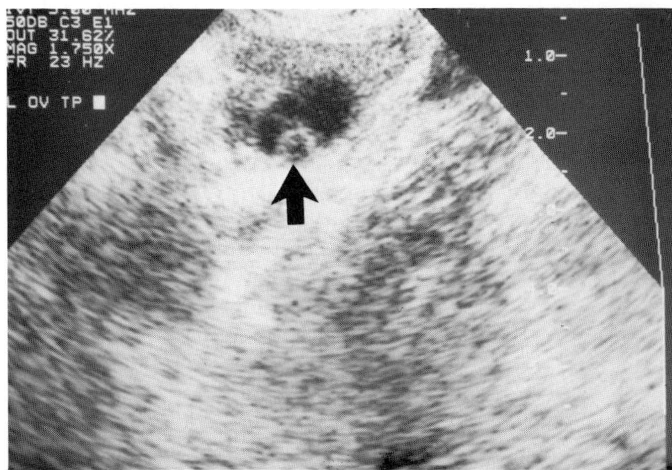

B

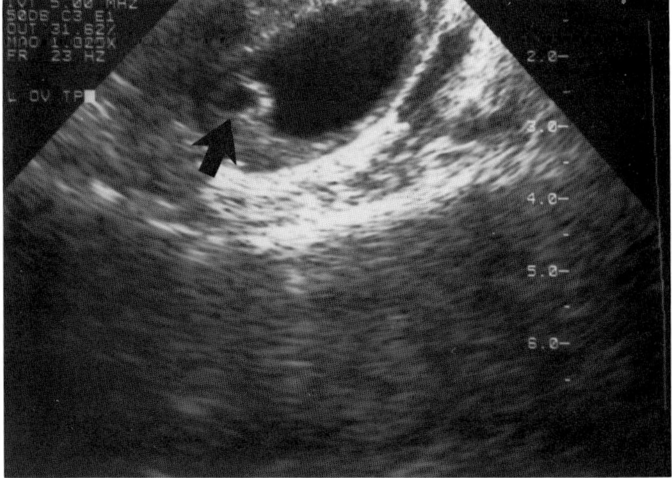

C

Fig. 18-2. Several investigators have reported imaging the cumulus oophorus within a follicle. (A–C) Three follicles with structures resembling those suggested to be the cumulus oophorus. However, these structures are 4 to 6 mm in size, and the cumulus is only 100 to 150 mm in size. *(Figure continues.)*

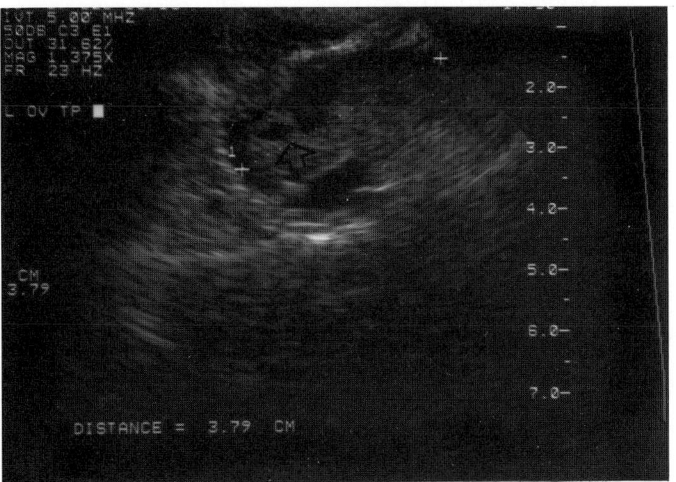

D

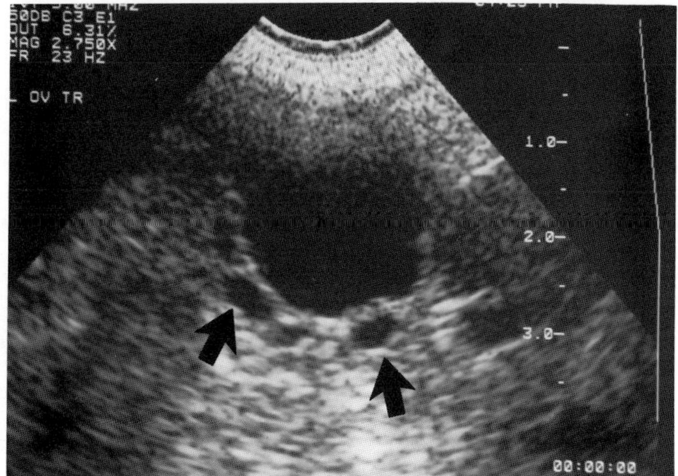

E

Fig. 18-2 *(Continued)*. **(D)** The follicle imaged in panel **C** after ovulation. Note the collapse of the follicle. The cumulus-like structure is slightly collapsed, but has not disappeared. Clearly, the cumulus-like structure has not been expelled from the follicle after ovulation. **(E)** Two small anechoic areas probably representing nonovulatory follicles adjacent to a growing follicle. These small nonovulatory follicles are very similar in appearance to the cumulus-like structures in panels **A**, **B**, and **C**. The structures being described as the cumulus oophorus may represent small Bomsel-Helmreich nonovulatory follicles that protrude into a developing graafian follicle similar to those noted in panel **E**. The ovary in panel **B** was removed 2 days after these photographs were taken. Histologic sections revealed two separate corpus lutea. The cumulus-like structure was a corpus luteum clearly separate from the larger follicle that had also formed into a corpus luteum. This suggests that the cumulus-like structure was, in fact, a separate small follicle.

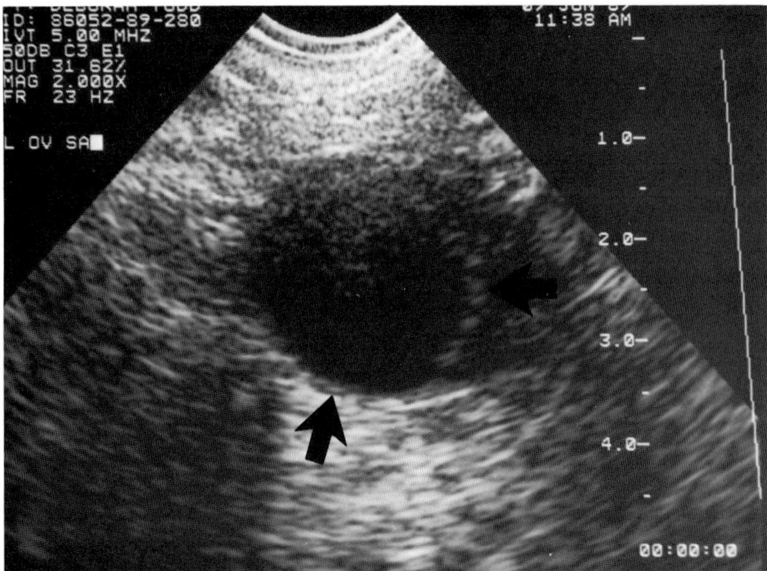

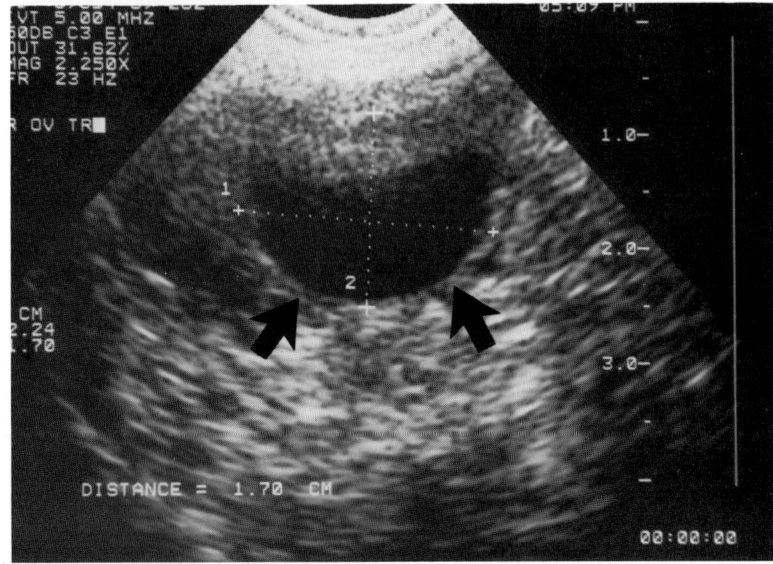

Fig. 18-3. (A) Trans-pelvic (T-pelvic) image of the left ovary showing the follicle wall and double contour sign of a mature follicle on day 16 of a normal menstrual cycle. The follicle is 2.3 cm in diameter. **(B)** A 2.3- by 1.7- cm follicle in the right ovary with a double contour sign (arrow). The patient ovulated 2 days later.

Table 18-1. Potential Signs of Impending Ovulation

Presence of a dominant follicle (usually > 16 mm)
Anechoic area, double contour, around the follicle (possible ovulation within 24 h)
Separation and folding of the follicle lining (ovulation within 6-10 h)
Thickened follicular endometrium (> 6 mm)

cial insemination or postcoital tests, a simplified timetable was suggested as shown in Table 18-3.[5] Multiple inseminations were recommended. These recommendations were based on the time span in which sperm are thought to be capable of fertilization and the predictability of ovulation based on follicular diameter.

Bryce et al[16] compared the values of FSH, LH, E_2, and follicular size in predicting ovulation. Although FSH was noted to rise on the day of ovulation, a dou-

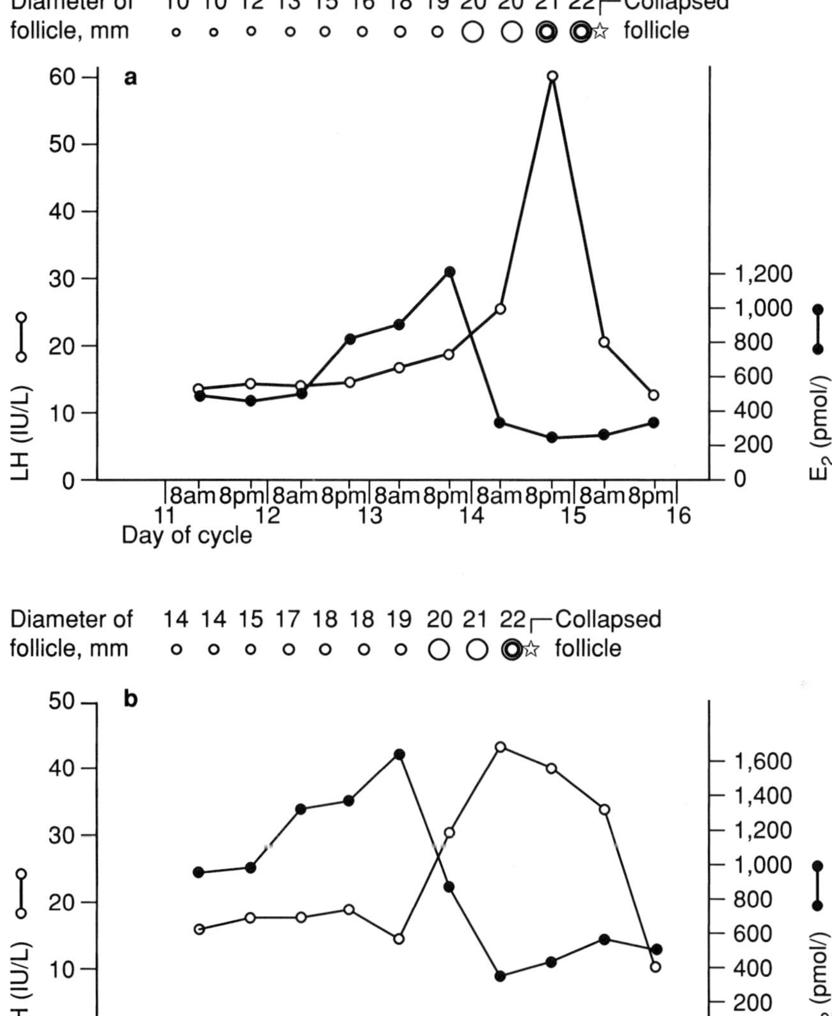

Fig. 18-4. Two cycles showing the relation between the appearance and collapse of the dominant follicle and the LH and estradiol peaks. (From Jaffe et al,[15] with permission.)

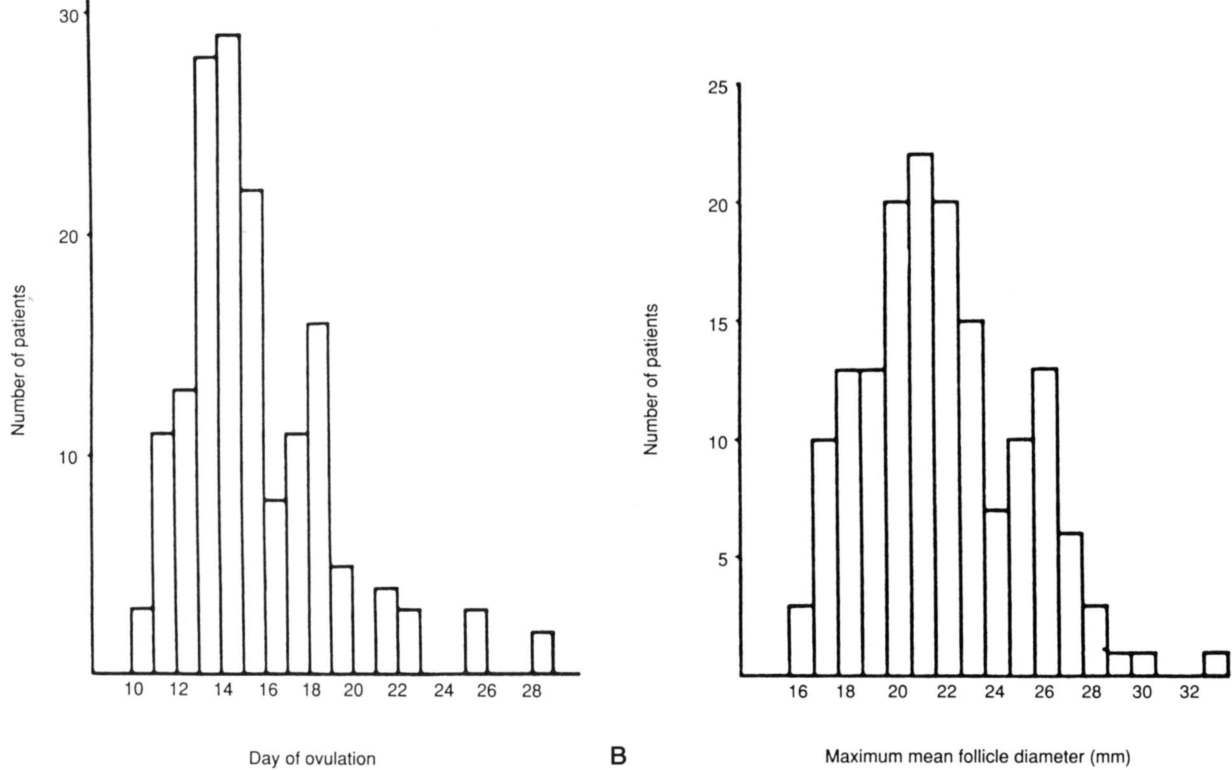

Fig. 18-5. (A) Frequency distribution of the day of the cycle on which ovulation took place in 158 spontaneous menstrual cycles of 158 infertility patients. (B) Frequency distribution of the maximum mean preovulatory follicle diameter in 158 spontaneous menstrual cycles of 158 infertility patients. (From Hamilton et al,[5] with permission.)

Table 18-2. Different Percentiles (In Days) of the Prediction Interval in Which Ovulation Will Take Place, Arranged According to the Various Mean Follicle Diameters

Mean Follicle Diameter (mm)	*Percentiles (days)*				
	10th	*25th*	*50th*	*75th*	*90th*
14	1.25	1.50	2.75	5.25	7
15	1	1.50	2.75	4.75	6.25
16	1	1.50	2.50	4	5.50
17	1	1.25	2.50	3.75	5
18	1	1.25	2	3.25	4.50
19	1	1.25	2	3	4
20	0.75	1	1.75	2.75	3.75
21	0.75	1	1.50	2.50	3.25
22	0.75	1	1.50	2.25	3.25
23	0.50	0.75	1.25	2.25	2.75
24	0.50	0.75	1.25	2	2.75
25	0.50	0.75	1.25	2	2.75

(From Hamilton et al,[5] with permission.)

bling of basal levels was not noted in 7 of 14 patients (50 percent) who ovulated. LH was noted to begin to rise 2 days before ovulation. However, if a doubling of the lowest LH level of the cycle was used as the criterion for ovulation, 4 of 17 women (29 percent) did not fulfill this ovulatory criterion. Likewise, if E_2 levels

Table 18-3. Advised Time to Perform Artificial Inseminations or Postcoital Tests According to the Mean Follicle Diameter Recorded

Mean Follicle Diameter (mm)	*Advised Time for Artificial Insemination or Postcoital Test*
14-16	1, 3, and 5 days later
17-20	1 and 3 days later
≥ 21	0 and 2 days later

(From Hamilton et al,[5] with permission.)

Table 18-4. Mean Time to Ovulation in 14 Women Predicted by FSH, LH, E_2, and Follicle Diameter

Criterion for Ovulation Prediction	*No. of Women Who Failed to Meet Criterion (%)*	*Mean Time to Ovulation for Rest of Women (Days ± 1 Standard Deviation)*
FSH, doubling of cycle low	7 (50)	0.3 ± 0.5
LH, doubling of cycle low	4 (29)	0.7 ± 0.7
E_2, ≥ 800 pmol/L	3 (21)	1.9 ± 0.9
Maximum follicle diameter ≥ 18 mm	0	2.5 ± 1.5
Maximum follicle diameter ≥ 20 mm	0	1.4 ± 1.2
Maximum follicle diameter ≥ 22 mm	2 (14)	0.9 ± 0.8

(Modified from Bryce et al,[16] with permission.)

are used as a criterion for ovulation, an E_2 of 800 pmol/L was not met by 3 of 14 patients who ovulated. The ultrasound finding of a follicle of 20 mm or greater was the best predictor of ovulation. However, ovulation occurred 1.4 ± 1.2 days later. Therefore, the use of this criterion still spreads the predicted time of ovulation over about 2.4 days. When an even larger follicular diameter (22 mm or greater) is used as a criterion for impending ovulation, 2 of 14 women (14 percent) ovulated before reaching the criterion, and the mean time to ovulation still ranged over 1.6 days (0.9 ± 0.8 days; Table 18-4).[16]

Recently, flow velocity waveforms have been noted within a developing follicle at the time of the LH surge, and flow velocity waveforms were noted from the endometrium on the day of follicular rupture.[17] Although very preliminary, it has been suggested that intrafollicular vascularization or angiogenesis detected by Doppler ultrasound might be used to predict ovulation.

CONFIRMING OVULATION

Sonography does seem to be very reliable in confirming ovulation once it has occurred. Disappearance of the follicle is noted in 91 percent of cases after ovulation, and a decrease in follicle size occurs in another 9 percent (Fig. 18-6).[12] Another sign of ovulation that is occasionally seen is a change in follicular shape with increased echogenicity. Other signs suggesting that ovulation has occurred are the appearance of cul-de-sac fluid, particularly when it was not present in a previous scan, or the development of intrafollicular echoes suggesting the formation of a hemorrhagic corpus luteum (Fig. 18-6). Confirmation of ovulation is discussed in Chapter 7.

One strategy of timing ovulation for artificial insemination, intrauterine insemination, or intercourse is to wait until the dominant follicle disappears, confirming that ovulation has occurred. Since current estimates suggest that the oocyte is fertilizable for up to 24 hours after ovulation, insemination immediately after disappearance of the follicle would allow fertilization generally within 24 hours of ovulation if sonographic scans are done daily (depending on how long after the sonogram ovulation occurs).

However, there are, as yet, no good controlled data to indicate that ultrasound timing of ovulation significantly improved the pregnancy rate over other techniques or is cost- effective for this indication. However, folliculograms do give considerable information about follicular development, side of ovulation, cyst formation, and confirmation of ovulation and allow the diagnosis of some ovulatory problems and the monitoring of ovulatory therapies that cannot be done using other current methodologies.

ENDOMETRIUM

During Follicular Development

The endometrium may also be helpful in evaluating follicular development, since E_2 produced by the developing follicle stimulates thickening of the endometrium. Endometrial thickening of 6 mm or greater generally correlates with a serum E_2 level of 200 pg/ml or greater and is generally associated with a developing follicle of 14 mm or greater diameter. How-

A

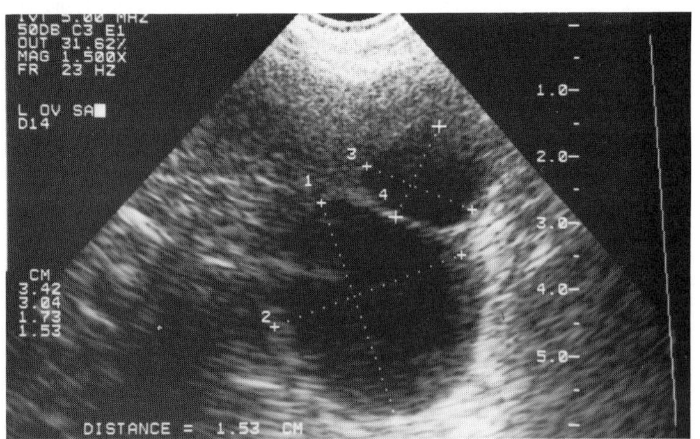

B

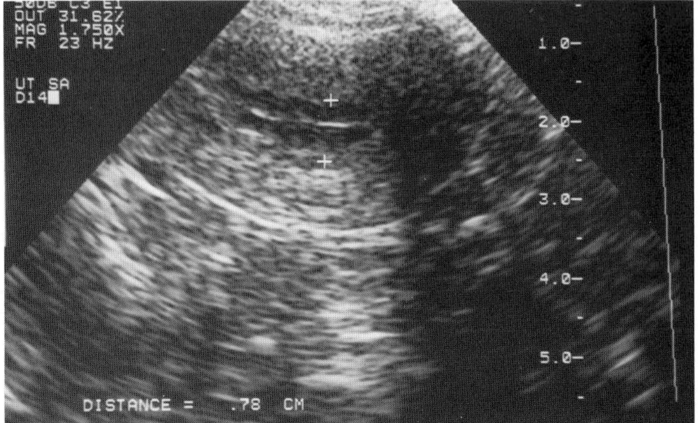

C

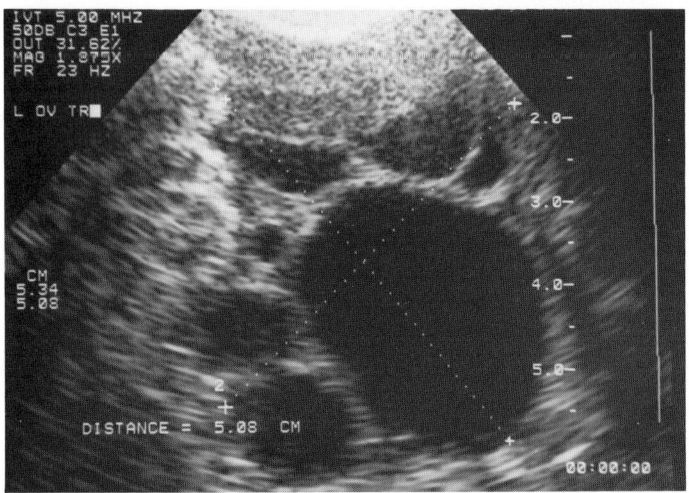

Fig. 18-6. A 25-year-old woman G0 with a 3-year history of infertility. The patient's husband had a sperm density of 34 million/ml with 80 percent motility. The hysterosalpingogram was normal. The FSH was 4.8 mIU/ml, and the LH was 4.2 mIU/ml. Prolactin and dehydroepiandrosterone sulfate were normal. Midluteal phase progesterones were 0.3 and 2.4 ng/ml in two different months. She had been treated with several cycles of clomiphene citrate, increasing to 150 mg/day on cycle days 5 to 9. **(A)** A 34 by 30 mm follicle and a 17 by 15 mm follicle were noted in the left ovary on day 14. **(B)** The endometrium (anterior posterior-plane [AP-pelvic]) was follicular and 7.8 mm thick. **(C)** By day 17, a large 37 by 28 mm follicle and a 20 mm, 19 mm, 17 mm, and several other small follicles were noted. *(Figure continues.)*

Fig. 18-6 *(Continued)*. **(D)** The large follicle and several small follicles collapsed between cycle days 18 and 19. **(E)** A large pocket of cul-de-sac fluid measuring 62 by 20 mm was present in the cul-de-sac on day 19 of the cycle after ovulation. CX, cervix, BO, bowel. The serum progesterone was 17.9 ng/ml. **(F)** A hemorrhagic corpus luteal cyst formed. Note presentation of large amount of peritoneal fluid (F) outlining the left ovary. The serum progesterone level 10 to 11 days after ovulation in that cycle was 139 ng/ml. *(Figure continues.)*

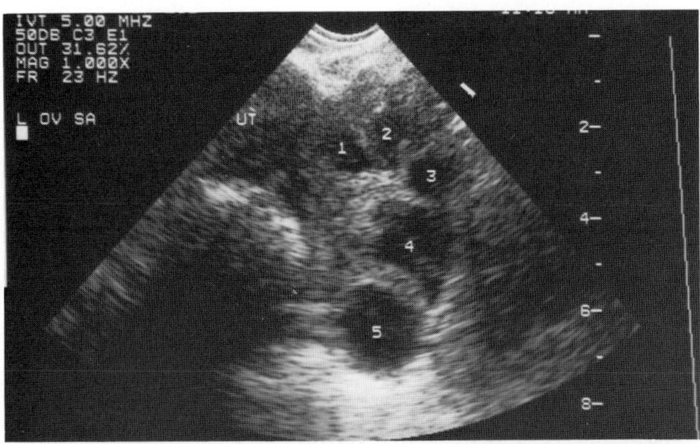

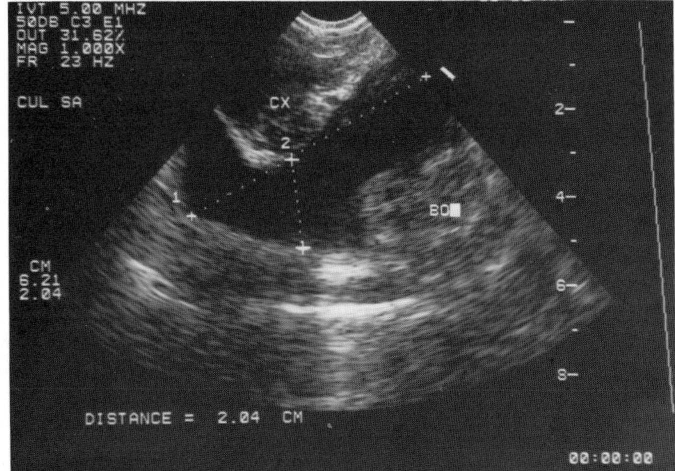

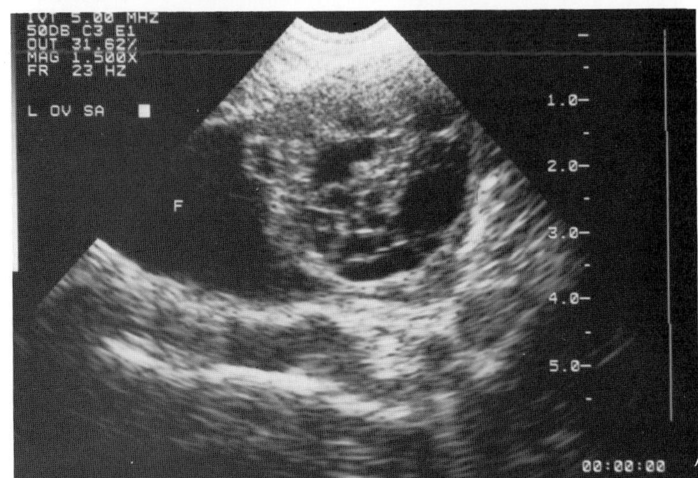

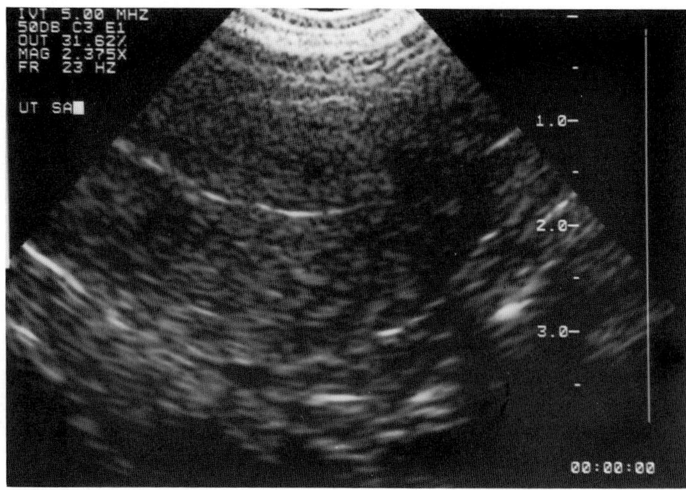

Fig. 18-6 *(Continued)*. (G) The endometrium on day 21 (2 to 3 days after ovulation) is beginning to show signs of luteinization (AP-pelvic view). The central hyperechoic area of the endometrial cavity is still noted, but the endometrium is becoming hyperechoic. Although the central hyperechoic echo of the endometrium cavity is still present, the three-line sign is no longer evident, and the endometrium is becoming hyperechoic. This is a transitional endometrium.

ever, serum E_2 levels correlate poorly with the ultimate endometrial thickness. Within 1 to 2 days before ovulation, some posterior enhancement may occasionally be noted, but not to the extent produced by a fully developed secretory endometrium after ovulation. Gonen et al[18] noted a correlation between endometrial thickness the day after human chorionic gonadotropin (hCG) administration and the subsequent pregnancy rate in an in vitro fertilization (IVF) program. Patients who achieved a pregnancy had a thicker endometrium (8.6 mm) than patients who did not achieve pregnancy (7.1 mm). However, there was no difference in the endometrial thickness on cycle day 10 or in the E_2 levels, despite the statistically significant difference in endometrial thickening after hCG administration.

Cervical mucus may be imaged by ultrasound during ovulation induction or during a normal ovulatory cycle as an anechoic area filling the endocervical canal. This is a normal finding and should not be mistaken for a cervical mass. Hill et al[19] noted cervical mucus in 5 percent of ovulation induction cycles with clomiphene citrate (CC) and hMG; however, the degree of cervical mucus production did not correlate with serum estradiol levels.[1]

After Ovulation

The endometrium may also be used to suggest ovulation, since the characteristic finding of a sonographic luteal endometrium requires at least 1.5 ng of progesterone per ml. After ovulation, the three-line sign is lost, the halo around the endometrium disappears, and the endometrium becomes hyperechoic with posterior enhancement. The persistence of a sonographic follicular endometrium suggests that ovulation has not yet occurred. Unfortunately, there is a poor correlation between sonographic thickness of a luteal endometrium and progesterone levels above 1.5 pg/ml.[20] Therefore, a sonographic luteal phase endometrium may be present despite low serum progesterone. However, a well developed luteal phase endometrium generally confirms ovulation.

ANOVULATORY CYCLES

The Ovary in Anovulatory Cycles

In an anovulatory cycle, ultrasound imaging of the ovaries will reveal either a lack of any follicular development, particularly in the hypogonadotropic hypogonadal patient (World Health Organization [WHO] type I) or the presence of a few nonovulatory immature (less than 11 mm) follicles. A dominant follicle larger than 16 mm in diameter will not develop. A cyst may also be associated with an anovulatory cycle (see discussion below). Anovulatory patients with PCOD often have enlarged ovaries (greater than 8 cm^3 in volume) with multiple small subcapsular follicles less than 10 mm in diameter. However, normal-sized ovaries do not rule out PCOD (see discussion of PCOD below). Anovulation can be diagnosed when serial scans do not reveal the development of a follicle.

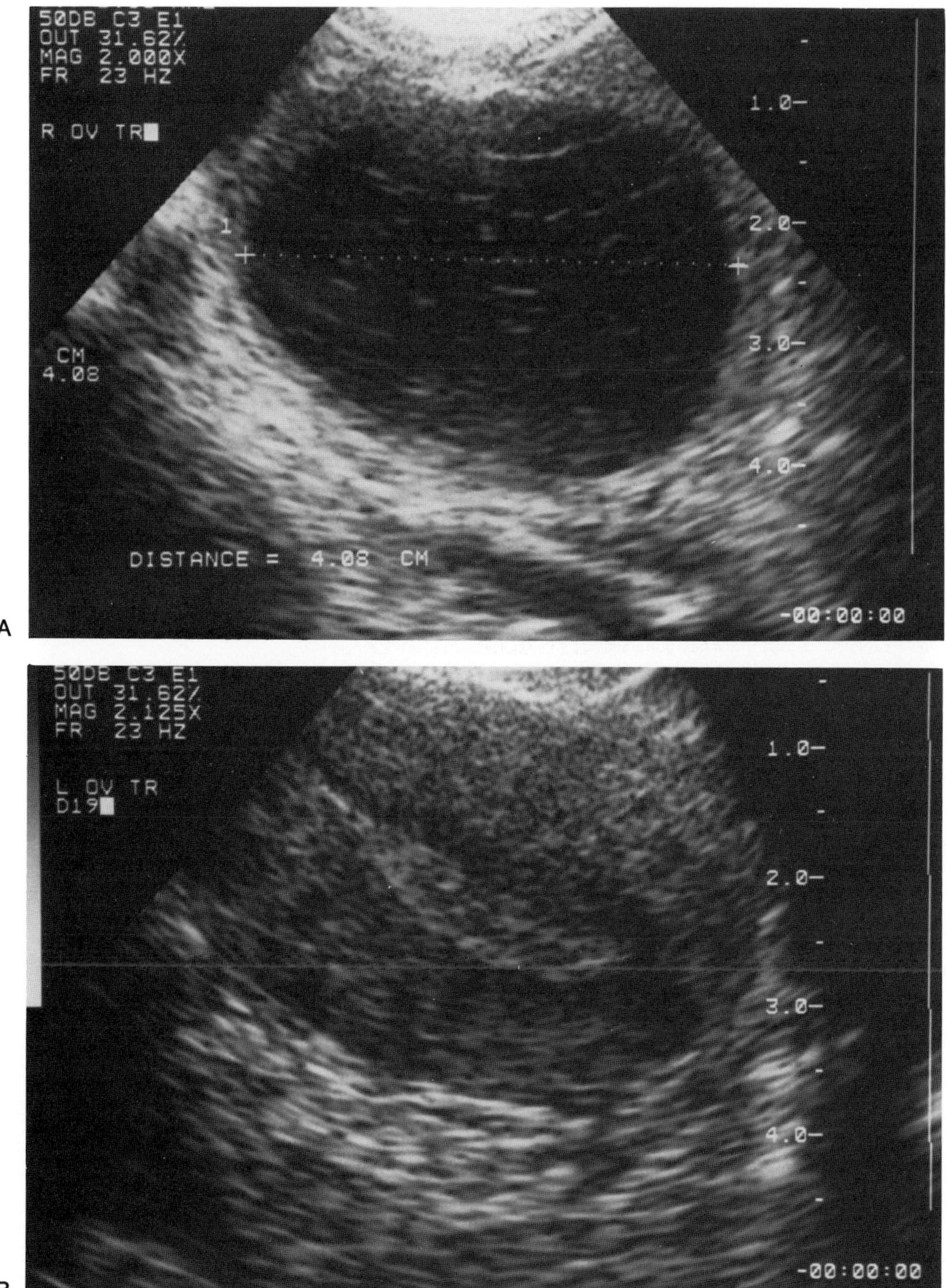

Fig. 18-7. **(A)** T-pelvic view of the right ovary showing a 4-cm corpus luteal cyst on day 19 of a menstrual cycle. Note the internal echoes consistent with blood. **(B)** AP-pelvic view of the uterus showing a luteal-phase endometrium in the same patient. *(Figure continues.)*

Occasionally, several sonographic examinations and clinical evaluations may be necessary to arrive at a correct diagnosis. For example, a patient with a history of menstrual periods every 37 to 40 days and a 12- to 14-mm anechoic area in the ovary suggesting an early developing follicle on day 20 of a menstrual cycle may still be ovulatory. Serial sonographic scanning may reveal progressive enlargement of the follicle at a rate of 1 to 4 mm per day with thickening of the follicular endometrium, with eventual ovulation and disappearance of the follicle on days 23 to 26 of the cycle and development of a characteristic luteal phase endometrium.

In contrast, the presence of a 2.5- to 3.0-cm anechoic area in the ovary during the follicular phase that does not enlarge during serial sonographic examinations, persists throughout the cycle, and is associated with a resting or follicular ultrasound endometrial pattern may represent an anovulatory cycle with a corpus luteal or follicular cyst persisting from the previous cycle, a small endometrioma, or a neoplasm in the ovary. A small (less than 5 cm) simple cyst only rarely represents a neoplasm. An anechoic area in the ovary that does not progress or increase in size and ultimately disappears is not a normal follicle (see discussion of ovarian cysts in Ch. 7). Even a small anechoic or cystic ovarian structure that persists for longer than 8 to 12 weeks rarely represents a functional cyst and certainly does not represent a normal follicle. Persistent ovarian masses warrant further investigation.

A mature corpus luteum is noted sonographically in about 50 percent of patients after ovulation.[9] If pregnancy does not occur, the corpus luteum generally degenerates and disappears just before menstruation. Corpus luteal cysts may be 4 to 6 cm in diameter and occasionally even larger, but are more commonly 2.5 to 3 cm in diameter. They may persist for 4 to 12 weeks and may be responsible for suppressing normal follicular development until they resolve (Fig. 18-7).

Care must be taken to ensure that the first folliculogram is performed early in the cycle, since a few patients will ovulate by day 12. An ultrasound done on day 13 or 14 in a patient who ovulates early would not note a developing follicle since ovulation had already occurred. However, the presence of a sonographic

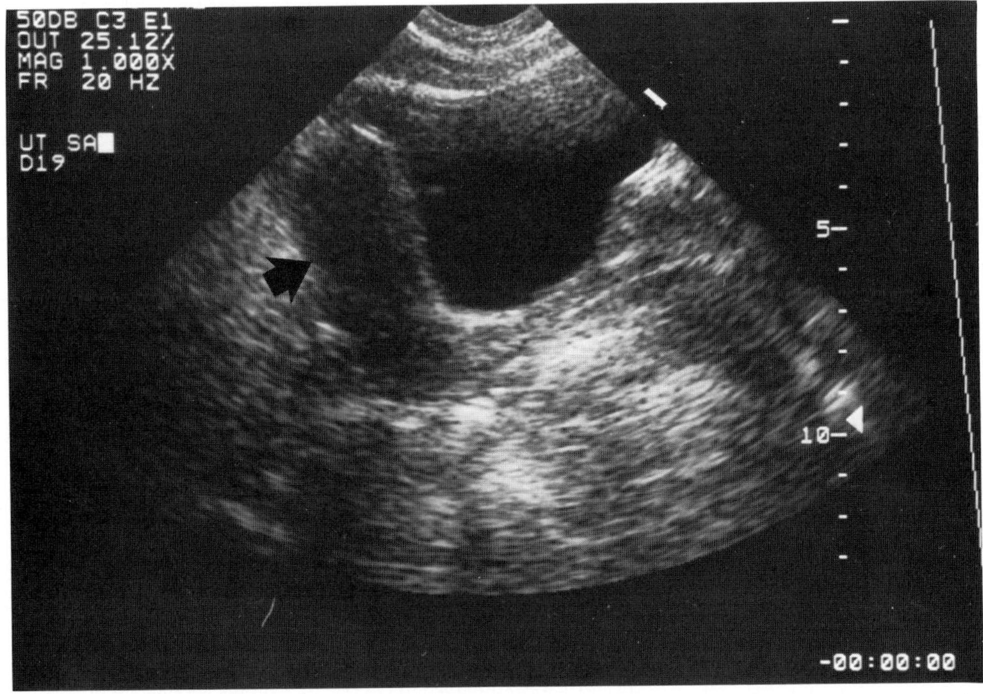

Fig. 18-7 *(Continued).* (C) Comparison sagittal view of the uterus (arrow) obtained using the transabdominal full bladder technique. The endometrium cannot be adequately evaluated.

luteal phase endometrium in a patient first scanned on day 13 or 14 of her cycle would suggest that the patient ovulated earlier in the cycle, that she has taken exogenous progesterone, or that she had a corpus luteal cyst from a previous cycle that has resolved but menses has not yet occurred. Endometrial hyperplasia may appear as a thick luteal phase endometrium. If a small developing follicle is noted early in the cycle, serial scanning should note progressive development of the follicle and eventually evidence of ovulation, such as disappearance of the follicle.

The Endometrium in Anovulatory Cycles

Patients with hypogonadotropic hypogonadism and low endogenous estrogen levels or type I anovulation (WHO classification) do not withdraw to a progesterone challenge. These patients invariably have a single hyperechoic straight-line endometrium. Some may have no endometrial echo that can be visualized. However, the reverse is not always true. A patient with amenorrhea and a single-line or resting endometrium on ultrasound may still withdraw to a progesterone challenge, indicating some low level estrogen stimulation (Fig. 18-8). Therefore, ultrasound may be helpful in confirming a resting endometrium and lack of ovulation, but a resting straight-line endometrium does not guarantee that a patient will not withdraw to a progesterone challenge. A straight-line or resting endometrium is, of course, also noted in a normally menstruating and ovulating patient on days 3 to 7 of her cycle.

The presence of a characteristic ultrasound follicular endometrial pattern with the three-line sign, lack of posterior enhancement, and an anechoic halo with amenorrhea reflects at least some moderate estrogen stimulation. These patients generally menstruate after a progesterone challenge and would be classified as having WHO type II anovulation. Therefore, an amenorrheic patient with a well developed follicular endometrium will generally withdraw and menstruate after a progesterone challenge, whereas a patient with a resting or single-line endometrium may or may not withdraw and menstruate after progesterone. Lack of the characteristic ultrasound findings of an ultrasound luteal phase endometrial pattern during the luteal phase of the cycle, as estimated by the

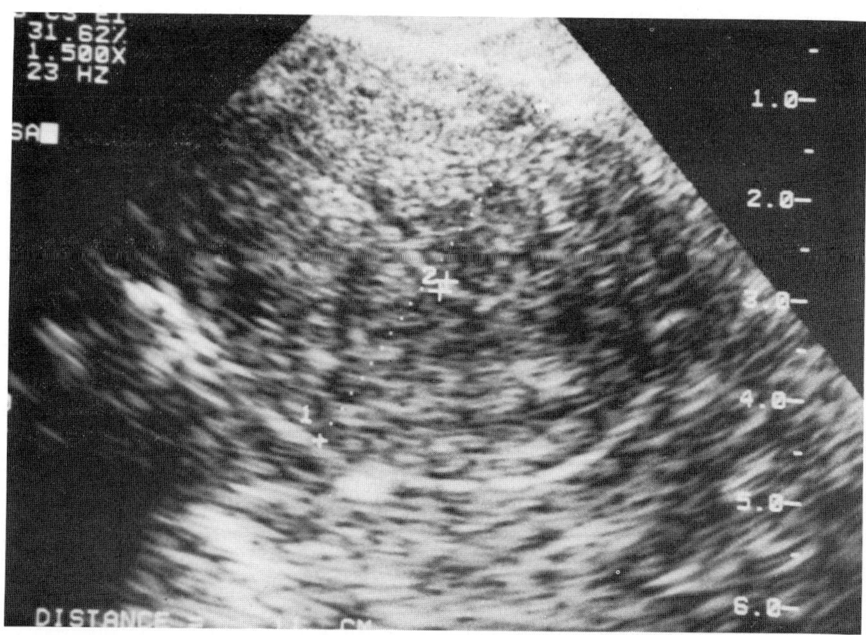

Fig. 18-8. A 49-year-old woman with a history of amenorrhea for 4 months followed by three normal menstrual periods. Sonogram done on day 29 of her cycle. AP-pelvic view shows a single-line endometrium. FSH was 50.2 mIU/ml and LH was 60.5 mIU/ml, suggesting the beginning of menopause.

last menstrual period, suggests a serum progesterone level of less than 1.5 ng/ml, anovulation, or a patient with a long cycle who ovulates late in the cycle.

POLYCYSTIC OVARIAN DISEASE (PCOD)

PCOD was first described in 1935 by Stein and Leventhal.[21] It is a complex endocrine disorder classically characterized by clinical, anatomic, and endocrinologic abnormalities. The common clinical findings suggesting PCOD are oligomenorrhea, amenorrhea or menometrorrhagia, hirsutism, obesity, and infertility. Bilateral enlarged ovaries with a thickened cortex secondary to subcapsular fibrosis and multiple small subcapsular cysts are the common anatomic findings of PCOD. Common endocrine findings are an elevation in serum LH, an increased LH/FSH ratio of 3 or greater, and/or elevated serum testosterone and/or androstenedione.

The diagnosis of PCOD is generally made by clinical and/or endocrinologic findings and is sometimes confirmed by laparoscopic visualization and biopsy of the ovaries. However, ultrasound can now be used to help detect the characteristic anatomic findings associated with PCOD, such as ovarian enlargement and the presence of small subcapsular cysts (Fig. 18-9). Among 863 patients screened using sonography, a diagnosis of PCOD (defined anatomically by ovarian enlargement and small cysts) was found in 2.5 percent (Fig. 18-10).[22] Swanson et al[22] sonographically imaged multiple (6 to 16) small cysts with a diameter of 2 to 6 mm in patients with PCOD. These small cysts were generally located in the ovarian cortex (subcapsular), but were sometimes distributed throughout the ovarian parenchyma. The ovaries were increased in size in patients with PCOD, with a mean ovarian volume ($V = 1/2 \times \text{length} \times \text{width} \times \text{thickness}$) of 12.5 cm^3 and a range from 6 to 30 cm^3 in 22 patients.[22] This can be compared with a mean ovarian volume of 4.0 cm^3 with an upper limit of normal of 5.7 cm^3 reported by Sample et al.[23] Jaffe et al[24] found a mean ovarian volume, measured by ultrasound, of 16.88 cm^3 with a range from 8.30 to 29.37 cm^3 in five patients with PCOD. Four of their five patients also had multiple 5-mm subcapsular cysts. However, this study defined the PCOD population using only the anatomic criterion of ovarian enlargement.

El Tabbakh et al[25] reported on 20 patients with PCOD diagnosed by clinical criteria and noted that three-fourths had enlarged ovaries with a mean volume of 15.46 cm^3. The other one-fourth had normal-sized ovaries despite meeting the clinical criteria for PCOD. Hann et al[26] used endocrine parameters to define PCOD and noted normal-sized ovaries in 29 percent of patients. The remaining 71 percent of PCOD patients had enlarged ovaries, and three different sonographic variants were noted: (1) multiple discrete cysts of less than 10 mm characteristic of the classical description of PCOD were found in 39 percent of patients; (2) diffusely hypoechoic ovaries

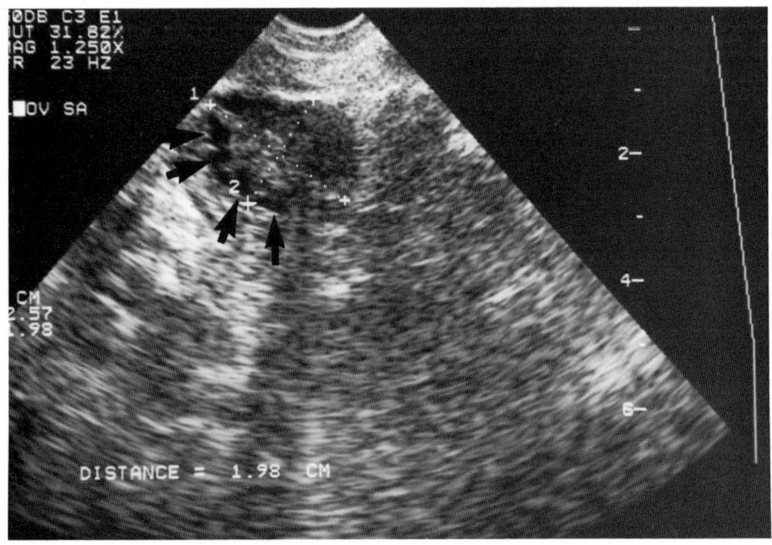

Fig. 18-9. A 23-year-old overweight (167 pounds) woman with a long history of anovulation. T-pelvic image of ovary (2.6 by 2.0 cm) on day 3 of her cycle showing multiple subcapsular follicles (arrows). The ovarian volume is upper limits of normal (7.9 cm^3). She ultimately achieved a pregnancy using Clomid.

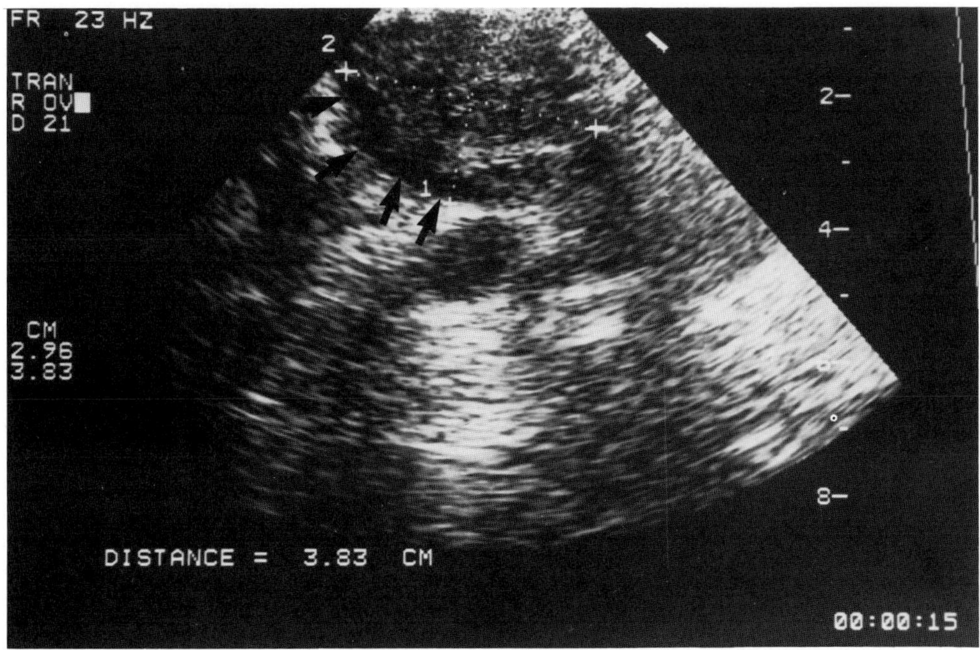

Fig. 18-10. Patient with obesity, hirsutism, amenorrhea, and infertility with LH of 7.0 mIU/ml, FSH of 2.3 mIU/ml, mildly elevated serum testosterone (85.6 ng/dl; normal, 20 to 80 ng/dl), enlarged ovary (17.5 cm^3), and small subcortical follicles (arrows). This patient fulfilled the clinical, chemical, and anatomic criteria for PCOD.

were noted in 25 percent of patients; and (3) in 7 percent, the ovaries were isoechoic compared with the uterus. In several surgical series, normal-sized ovaries were noted in 29 to 40 percent of patients with PCOD, which is consistent with the ultrasound imaging data.[27]

Some of the apparent discrepancies in the sonographic findings of PCOD revolve around the criteria used to make the diagnosis. The classic anatomic criteria are not present in all patients with clinical or endocrine findings suggestive of PCOD. Therefore, an ultrasound showing ovarian enlargement can help make the diagnosis, but a normal ultrasound examination with normal-sized ovaries does not rule out PCOD if the clinical or biochemical abnormalities characteristic of the syndrome are present. By confirming anovulation, ultrasound may also suggest the diagnosis of PCOD in a patient with normal-sized ovaries and the clinical and/or endocrine criteria of PCOD.

Treatment of PCOD depends on the desires of the patient. If the patient desires pregnancy, treatment of the anovulation with clomiphene citrate is frequently effective, but sometimes menotropins (human menopausal gonadotropins [hMG]) are necessary.

GnRH agonists have also been used in the treatment of PCOD. GnRH agonists down-regulate the pituitary gland, suppress gonadotropin release, and result in a hypoestrogenic state. With GnRH agonist treatment, the ovarian volume of PCOD patients has been noted to decrease markedly from 16.88 to 8.81 cm^3, and the microcysts disappeared.[24]

The patient who does not desire pregnancy but who complains of hirsutism and/or anovulation may be treated with oral contraceptives. Surgical wedge resection of the ovary should rarely be used, since medical therapy is generally effective. In addition, wedge resection of the ovaries has been associated with infertility secondary to pelvic adhesions. Buttram and Vaquero noted adhesions in 34 percent of patients after wedge resection.[28]

The occurrence of endometrial carcinoma in patients with PCOD should be kept in mind. Endometrial carcinoma has been reported even in young patients with PCOD. Jafari et al[29] reported six cases of adenocarcinoma of the endometrium in patients with PCOD. The average age of the patients was only 27.8 years, with a range from 23 to 33 years.[30] Therefore, the endometrium should be imaged carefully in the PCOD patient, and an endometrial biopsy should be

Table 18-5. Sonographic Findings in PCOD

Enlarged ovary[a] (> 8 cm) in two-thirds (may be hypoechoic or isoechoic)
Multiple small cysts (0.2-0.6 cm)
Anovulation (lack of follicular development)
Resting follicular or atypical hyperechoic (see Ch. 6 and 11) endometrium

[a] Note: A normal-sized ovary does not exclude the diagnosis of PCOD.

considered in the patient with irregular bleeding or abnormal endometrial findings (Table 18-5).

EMPTY FOLLICLE SYNDROME

Coulam et al[31] described an empty follicle syndrome in 1986 in which some aspirated follicles did not contain ova. The follicular fluid in patients with the empty follicle syndrome has an increased E_2-to-progesterone ratio and an increased androstenedione level, suggesting that the syndrome results from dysfunctional follicular development. Hilgers et al[32] reported on 87 infertility patients and was able to identify a cumulus within the follicle in 47 percent of cycles; they suggested that the remaining patients had the empty follicle syndrome. The empty follicle syndrome was more common in patients over the age of 30 (43 percent versus 53 percent), but did not correlate with gravidity. Most of the patients in these series had endometriosis. However, the cumulus oophorus was also reported to be absent in five of nine patients with pelvic adhesions without endometriosis.

Although there is some evidence of an empty follicle syndrome, this diagnosis remains controversial. It is not clear whether the nonvisualization of a cumulus complex by ultrasound results from the absence of the cumulus complex (empty follicle syndrome) or lack of localization of the cumulus or, as noted previously, whether the cumulus is actually being visualized. The empty follicle syndrome or at least the sonographic diagnosis of a cumulus within the follicle may be an artifact.[12] Additional data are needed to determine whether the empty follicle syndrome constitutes a real entity, whether it can be diagnosed by ultrasound, and whether it occurs in almost one-half of infertility patients.

LUTEINIZED UNRUPTURED FOLLICLE SYNDROME

The concept of pseudo-ovulation with luteinization of an unruptured follicle was first suggested in 1969 by Van Hall and Mastboom.[33] The term LUF was first used by Jewelewicz in 1975.[34] The absence of an ovulatory stigma at laparoscopy was used as the criterion to prove the existence of the LUF syndrome.[35,36] Kerin et al[37] detected the LUF syndrome in 4.9 percent of cycles in regularly menstruating women. Bateman et al[38] reported the recovery of an oocyte from a stigma-bearing follicle suggesting the failure of oocyte release; four additional oocytes were recovered from unruptured follicles in the luteal phase.[2] Luciano et al[39] noted a 6 percent (3/50) incidence of LUF among infertility patients. Two of three cases occurred in CC-stimulated cycles; however, these patients had follicular rupture in subsequent evaluations, indicating that LUF may not recur in later cycles. The LH surge, serum E_2, and progesterone concentrations were in the normal range during LUF cycles. Therefore, a normal midluteal phase progesterone does not necessarily confirm ovulation, but may be found in patients with LUF. The LUF syndrome can be suggested when a follicle persists for more than 2 days after the peak of the LH surge. Some follicles continue to increase in size, but most follicles in LUF cycles decrease 2 to 5 mm in diameter. The progressive increase in follicular size with disappearance of the follicle in midcycle indicates ovulation. The appearance of cul-de-sac fluid in the midluteal phase noted on serial ultrasound also suggests ovulation. Check et al[40] found the absence of cul-de-sac fluid in the midluteal phase to be unreliable for the diagnosis of LUF. Therefore, the absence of midcycle cul-de-sac fluid is consistent with but not diagnostic of LUF.

Using serial sonographic examinations, Liukkonen et al[41] suspected LUF syndrome in 57 of 100 cycles in 37 women with unexplained infertility. Laparoscopy confirmed LUF syndrome in 18 of 21 patients with a corpus luteum without an ovulatory stigma (86 percent). LUF syndrome seems to be relatively common in infertility patients and to occur in almost 1 in 20 cycles even in normally menstruating patients. There has been some suggestion that the incidence of LUF is increased in patients with endometriosis and idiopathic infertility and in patients undergoing ovulation induction with clomiphene citrate.[42] Since these follicles luteinize and produce progesterone but do not ovulate, they could be viewed as a variant of a corpus luteal cyst. Unless careful monitoring is done in the periovulatory period, the differentiation of LUF from a small corpus luteal cyst may be difficult.

I have had the experience of imaging a developing follicle during the follicular phase of a cycle that did not disappear. After reaching the size of a preovulatory follicle, the follicle remained the same size throughout the luteal phase of the cycle and was completely anechoic without the development of echoes within the follicle consistent with a corpus luteum. (A corpus luteum generally has a lacy pattern or hyperechoic area within the cyst, characteristic of blood [see Ch. 7]). Although a diagnosis of LUF could have been made, the patient became pregnant in that cycle, clearly ruling out the possibility of anovulation. Therefore, the persistence of what appears to be a follicle does not always rule out ovulation. Although these exceptions can be discouraging to the clinician and sonographer, the complexity of the biology and limitations of the tools used must be appreciated.

LUTEAL-PHASE DEFECT

Luteal-phase defect is a condition characterized by abnormal hormonal and/or endometrial histology in the luteal phase of the menstrual cycle. Luteal-phase deficiency is thought to result from abnormal corpus luteal function and/or an inadequate endometrial response. It is reported to be present in 3 to 5 percent of infertility couples and to be associated with recurrent abortions. The diagnosis is generally based on an endometrial biopsy that is histologically more than 3 days out of phase with the expected pattern or a persistent decreased midluteal phase progesterone below 10 pg/ml.[43]

Sonographic findings in luteal-phase defect are nonspecific. Check et al[44] reported immature follicles (less than 17 mm diameter) in 52 percent of patients with luteal-phase defect. LUF was noted in 8 percent of patients. They noted only two pregnancies in 500 treatment cycles when the developing preovulatory follicle was less than 17 mm in diameter.[44]

PREMATURE OVARIAN FAILURE, MENOPAUSE, RESISTANT OVARY SYNDROME, AND WHO TYPE I ANOVULATION

Infertility patients with premature ovarian failure or resistant ovarian syndrome (younger than 35 years of age) and the older infertility patient desiring pregnancy who is, in fact, perimenopausal with anovulation are generally suspected clinically by a history of amenorrhea or missed periods. The diagnosis is confirmed by an elevated FSH (greater than 50 mIU/ml), with low serum estradiol (hypergonadotrophic hypogonadism). Older patients are generally considered to be experiencing early menopause.

The distinction between premature ovarian failure and menopause (at least with our current level of understanding) is based on age. Some studies use age 35 as the criterion to separate the two conditions clinically, whereas others use age 40. However, menopause is a normal physiologic event, whereas premature menopause is suspected to have a pathologic etiology.

The pelvic ultrasonographic findings in a patient with premature ovarian failure may suggest abnormal ovarian and uterine functioning. The patient generally has a straight-line resting endometrium, and the uterus may be small consistent with low serum estrogen levels. The ovaries lack evidence of follicular development and ovulation (Fig. 18-8). Generally, even the small (less than 10 mm) nonovulatory (immature) follicles are decreased or absent. Mehta et al[45] noted immature follicles (small, less than 10 mm follicles that are generally present in normal ovulating patients) in only 5 percent of menopausal patients compared to 95 percent of patients with normal ovarian function on oral contraceptives. In patients with hypergonadotrophic hypogonadism, immature follicles were noted in 41 percent. However, Mehta et al[45] felt that those hypergonadotrophic hypogonadal patients with immature follicles noted on ultrasound had resistant ovary syndrome, whereas those patients without ultrasound evidence of immature follicles were experiencing premature ovarian failure. Generally, the differentiation of premature ovarian failure from resistant ovary syndrome has required laparoscopy or laparotomy with ovarian biopsy. The histologic presence of primordial or immature follicles is consistent with resistant ovary, whereas the absence of such follicles indicates premature ovarian failure. Patients

Table 18-6. Ultrasound Findings in Premature Ovarian Failure and Resistant Ovary Compared to Normal and Menopausal Patients

	Ovary Volume (ml)	*Immature Follicles*	*Endometrium*	*Uterus*
Normal	4-8	Yes	Varies with phase of cycle	4 cm thick 5 cm width
Menopausal	1.8	No	Thin single line 2.0 mm	Small
Premature ovarian failure	1.4	No	Thin single line 2.8 mm	Small
Resistant ovary	2.8	Yes	Thin single line 2.2 mm	Small

(Data from Mehta et al.[45])

with WHO type I anovulation with low endogenous estrogen production, patients with premature ovarian failure, and patients with resistant ovary syndrome will have similar sonographic findings consistent with anovulation and low estrogen, with the possible exception of the presence of immature follicles in patients with resistant ovary syndrome noted above (Table 18-6).

OVULATION INDUCTION

Ovulation can be achieved in 90 percent of anovulatory women using currently available ovulation induction techniques, and 50 to 70 percent of these women will eventually become pregnant. Ultrasound has become an important technique in monitoring responses to ovulation induction using Clomid or pulsatile GnRH and is imperative when using hMG therapy (Pergonal).

Clomiphene Citrate

Clomiphene citrate (CC) should be the initial drug of choice for induction of ovulation in the patient desiring pregnancy who has confirmed anovulation or infrequent or dysfunctional ovulation. Clomiphene citrate therapy is much less expensive and safer than hMG therapy.

CC is a weak estrogen with some structural similarities to diethylstilbestrol. It binds to estrogen receptors and reduces the replenishment of cytoplasmic estrogen receptors. With clomiphene citrate treatment, the hypothalamic-pituitary axis perceives the circulating estrogen level to be decreased and increases GnRH and gonadotropin (FSH, LH) secretion.

Only 10 percent of anovulatory patients with decreased endogenous estrogen who do not withdraw to progesterone (WHO type I) will ovulate when treated with clomiphene citrate.[46] Anovulation associated with thyroid disease or hyperprolactinemia should be evaluated and treated before initiating CC therapy. Elevated serum FSH (greater than 50 mIU/ml) can be helpful in the diagnosis of premature ovarian failure or menopause in the patient who does not menstruate after progesterone withdrawal. FSH and LH can also be useful in diagnosing PCOD. As noted above, a serum LH level three times as high as the FSH concentration is consistent with PCOD. Ultrasound can be helpful in the diagnosis of PCOD and at least suggestive in patients with premature ovarian failure, menopause, or WHO type I anovulation.

Since clomiphene citrate is a relatively safe drug, monitoring of ovarian response is not nearly as critical as with gonadotropic therapy (Pergonal). BBT measurements, LH kits, or midluteal phase serum progesterone determinations have all been used to monitor responses to CC. However, the use of serial transvaginal ultrasound has several advantages. Ultrasound monitoring allows visualization of the developing follicle with evaluation of adequate and progressive enlargement of the follicle and accurate confirmation that ovulation has occurred. Localization of the follicle (right or left side) may be important in patients with a unilateral salpingectomy or unilateral tubal obstruction or disease.

Ultrasound monitoring also allows fine tuning of CC dosing. Patients with multiple large follicles and especially those who develop ovarian hyperstimulation syndrome (OHSS) using clomiphene citrate should have the dosage lowered in the next cycle. Likewise, the patient who has poor follicular development should have the dose increased in subsequent cycles.

Transvaginal ultrasound also allows evaluation of the endometrial response to clomiphene citrate. A single-line (resting) endometrium suggests anovulation. This is particularly true if no developing follicle is noted during the follicular phase. Patients failing to ovulate may need their clomiphene citrate dose increased.

Clomiphene citrate is very effective in inducing ovulation in properly selected anovulatory patients. Ovulation is noted in 57 to 91 percent of patients. However, only 27 to 40 percent of these women will eventually become pregnant, and 25 percent of these patients will spontaneously abort.[42] Many of the pregnancies achieved in CC cycles result in unrecognized early pregnancy losses. In a study by Bateman et al,[47] there was a 13 percent clinical pregnancy rate in CC cycles; however there was also a 13 percent (per CC cycle) subclinical pregnancy loss. Fifty percent of CC-associated pregnancies resulted in subclinical losses compared to only 16.6 percent in normal control cycles.[47]

The low pregnancy rate compared to the ovulatory rate, and the high abortion rate have been attributed to the adverse effect of clomiphene citrate on the endometrium. CC has been reported to deplete estrogen receptors.[48] Yagel et al[49] noted a significant decrease in endometrial thickness and uterine volume by ultrasound in patients treated with CC compared to controls and patients treated with hMG.[49] These changes could be reversed with the addition of 20 μg/day of ethanol estradiol for 7 days beginning on day 10 of the cycle. Randall and Templeton noted thinner endometrial thickness by ultrasound before the LH surge in CC cycles, despite the fact that serum E_2 levels were higher in those cycles.[50] Gonen and Casper[51] also noted a significantly thinner endometrium in a comparison of CC only- and CC + hMG-stimulated cycles. In some CC-stimulated patients the endometrium may also be histologically out of phase.[52] Deichert et al[53] have reported a higher pregnancy rate in patients with a thicker endometrium. Gonen and Casper[51] have noted that implantation was unlikely if the endometrium was less than 6 mm thick 1 day after hCG administration. These studies tend to confirm that CC induces ovulation, but has a detrimental effect on the endometrium.

The diameters of the leading follicle may be large in CC cycles. Randall and Templeton[50] reported a mean diameter of 21.6 mm in spontaneous cycles compared to 27.2 mm in CC cycles at the onset of the LH surge.

Table 18-7. Advantages of Ultrasound Monitoring of Clomiphene Citrate Therapy

Better regulation of dosing
Diagnosis of functional cyst before initiating therapy
Localization of follicular development (right or left side)
Confirmation of ovulation
Evaluation of the endometrial response
Diagnosis of mild OHSS
Diagnosis of LUF syndrome
Diagnosis of dysfunctional ovarian cyst development

A sonographic evaluation before the initiation of a second treatment cycle is much more sensitive in detecting ovarian hyperstimulation with multiple follicles or a persistent corpus luteal cyst from a previous cycle than is the pelvic examination. Repeat CC cycles should not be done in the presence of OHSS or a large corpus luteal cyst. In patients with significant OHSS, the pelvic examination must be done very gently to avoid rupture of the ovary and bleeding. Other monitoring methods, such as BBT, serial urinary LH evaluations (LH kits), or serum progesterone determination, do not allow this fine tuning of clomiphene citrate dosing. Also, LUF syndrome or dysfunctional ovarian cyst syndrome can be diagnosed by transvaginal ultrasound, but not by more passive monitoring techniques (Table 18-7). However, ultrasound monitoring is more labor intensive and more expensive.

There are wide variations in the responses of PCOD patients to Clomid stimulation. Some patients with PCOD can be quite sensitive to clomiphene citrate therapy and require very minimal doses, such as 25 mg/day, for adequate stimulation. Other patients are very resistant and require high doses of up to 200 to 250 mg/day to induce ovulation. Some PCOD patients develop multiple small follicles during CC stimulation and are predisposed to developing OHSS with increased dosages. Patients with multiple small follicles and no dominant follicle will not ovulate. This type of response to clomiphene citrate will also not be diagnosed by BBT, LH kits, or midluteal phase progesterone determination. Although transvaginal ultrasound allows closer monitoring of clomiphene citrate therapy and better dose adjustment, there is currently no proof that the pregnancy rate is any higher or the complication rates are any lower with ultrasound monitoring than with other techniques.

A single folliculogram generally takes less than 10

minutes of actual imaging time. An initial folliculogram is generally done on day 3 to 5 of the menstrual cycle to ensure that the patient did not develop OHSS or a persistent corpus luteal cyst in a previous cycle. A repeat scan is done on day 12 or 13 and as needed thereafter to confirm ovulation and evaluate endometrial development.

hMG Therapy

Pelvic ultrasound plays a critical role in selecting patients for hMG therapy and monitoring their treatment. In fact, hMG therapy should generally not be administered unless ultrasound monitoring is available. Since clinicians competent in pelvic sonography are generally called on to monitor hMG therapy and potential complications, hMG therapy is reviewed in detail.

hMG is used as a form of replacement therapy in the treatment of infertility due to hypogonadotropic anovulation. It may also be used in the anovulatory patient who has either failed to ovulate or failed to achieve a pregnancy with clomiphene citrate therapy. In addition, hMG is used to superovulate patients with a normal ovulatory history for IVF or gamete intrafallopian transfer (GIFT) to allow multiple follicular development and the potential recovery of multiple oocytes.

More recently, hMG has also been used in combination with intrauterine insemination for the treatment of idiopathic infertility. Serhal et al[54] reported on 62 women with idiopathic infertility treated with hMG (Pergonal) superovulation plus intrauterine insemination (IUI). Patients treated with IUI alone achieved only a 6.7 percent pregnancy rate per couple with a 2.7 percent pregnancy rate per cycle. Patients treated with Pergonal without IUI had a 12 percent overall pregnancy rate, with a 6.1 percent pregnancy rate per treatment cycle. Pergonal combined with IUI resulted in 40 percent of couples achieving a pregnancy and a 31.5 percent pregnancy rate per treatment cycle.

The combination of gonadotropins and/or IUI in another larger study involving 991 cycles in 302 patient couples with a variety of infertility problems compared with 2,668 untreated cycles in 255 couples was not as successful.[54,55] However, only 25 couples in this series had idiopathic infertility.[55] The pregnancy rate per cycle with IUI plus hMG was 9.8 percent compared to 1.4 percent in untreated control patients (Table 18-8).[55]

Table 18-8. IUI Therapy

Treatment	*No. of Patients*	*% of Pregnancies/Cycle*
Untreated	255	1.4
hMG-IUI	45	9.8
Clomid-IUI	10	5.0
IUI only	11	3.4

(Modified from Corson et al,[55] with permission.)

IUI plus hMG resulted in a significant improvement in fecundity in anovulatory patients, but not in ovulatory patients. IUI plus hMG was helpful in patients with tubal disease not severe enough to preclude IUI, cervical factor infertility, and patients with a poor postcoital test. IUI alone or in combination with gonadotropin was not of benefit in patients with poor sperm motility, morphology, or oligospermia. However, in patients with a low sperm penetration assay (11 percent or less), IUI with or without hMG was of benefit. The addition of hCG to the IUI was not more beneficial in this group of patients than IUI alone.

Therefore, the result of the combination of hMG plus IUI varies considerably depending on the specific infertility problem and seems to be most beneficial in couples with idiopathic infertility; however, it may be useful in other clinical situations (Table 18-9).[55]

Clinically, hMG therapy should be used only after an adequate infertility evaluation confirms the absence of other infertility problems or after other infertility problems have been corrected and other simpler, safer, and less expensive methods, such as clomiphene citrate, have failed or are not indicated (Table 18-10). There should also be no contraindications to the use of hMG therapy.

Table 18-9. Use of IUI and Gonadotropins in Infertility

	hMG-IUI	*IUI*
Anovulation	+	−
Tubal factor[a]	+	−
Cervical factor	+	+
Poor postcoital test	+	+
↓Sperm motility	−	−
↓Sperm morphology	−	−
↓Sperm concentration	−	−
↓Sperm penetration assay	−	+

[a] Not severe enough to preclude IUI.
(Modified from Corson et al,[55] with permission.)

Table 18-10. Clinical Uses of hMG

Used for anovulation in
Hypogonadotropic hypogonadal patients (WHO type I)
Clomiphene failure patients
IVF/GIFT
Combined with IUI for:
Idiopathic infertility
Anovulation
Cervical factor/poor postcoital test
Tubal disease not severe enough to preclude IUI
Used after
An adequate infertility evaluation
Other infertility problems absent or corrected
No contraindications

A minimum evaluation before hMG therapy should include at least two semen analyses and confirmation of anovulation. The patient should have a normal endocrine profile and evaluation of ovarian competency before initiating hMG therapy. Tubal patency is generally evaluated by hysterosalpingography before the initiation of hMG therapy (Table 18-11).

Contraindications to hMG therapy should be excluded before initiating therapy. They include (1) premature ovarian failure, perimenopausal or postmenopausal with elevated gonadotropins or resistant ovary syndrome (Savage's syndrome); (2) pregnancy; (3) tubal obstruction; or (4) other causes of infertility before correction. Patients with elevated prolactins and pituitary microadenomas should be thoroughly evaluated and treated with bromocriptine before considering hMG therapy. Likewise, thyroid or other endocrine problems should be corrected before hMG therapy.

hMG is a potent therapy with a potential for serious complications. Therefore, it should not be utilized unless there are appropriate indications, an adequate infertility work-up has been completed, and there are no contraindications. In addition, the clinician should be familiar with this form of therapy and have had experience using gonadotropins. Adequate monitoring techniques, such as rapid serum 17-beta-estradiol evaluations with same day results and ultrasound, should be available.

Table 18-11. Evaluation before hMG Therapy

Normal semen analyses (two)
Evidence of anovulation: BBT, progesterone, folliculograms, etc.
Normal endocrine functions: prolactin, thyroid, etc.
Ovarian competency: gonadotropins normal or low
Normal tubes and genital tract: hysterosalpingogram, laparoscopy

Types of Therapy

hMG may be given singly or in combination with Clomid. If given with Clomid, hMG may be administered either sequentially or concomitantly. It may also be combined with FSH (Metrodin). hMG may be given by a fixed dose or a variable dose regimen. Fixed dose regimens, such as Pergonal administered on days 1, 3, and 5 of the menstrual cycle with hCG given on day 8, have been demonstrated to yield a lower pregnancy rate than variable dose regimens in which dosing is adjusted daily based on serial E_2 determinations and ultrasound folliculograms. Therefore, most clinicians have abandoned fixed dose regimens.

Initiation of Therapy

In the chronic anovulatory patient, hMG therapy may be initiated without a menstrual period or after menses following withdrawal of progesterone. In the hypoestrogenic patient, therapy may be initiated after a cycle in which the uterus and endometrium are primed with an estrogen-progesterone cycle followed by menses. Therapy may also be initiated in the hypoestrogenic patient without first inducing a period.

Estrogen and Ultrasound Monitoring with hMG

Although urinary or serum E_2 levels may be used to monitor hMG therapy, most physicians now use serum levels to adjust the daily dose of hMG. One reason for doing so is the correlation between serum E_2 levels and the incidence of OHSS. Serum E_2 levels are generally drawn in the morning, and the results should be available by late afternoon of the same day. hMG (Pergonal) may be given in the morning after drawing the serum E_2 or in the evening when results of the morning E_2 levels are available. It is important to recognize the difference in these two regimens. Serum E_2 will peak 8 to 10 hours after hMG administration; therefore, when hMG is given in the evening, the peak of E_2 activity will occur the following morning. The morning E_2 will therefore more accurately reflect the peak in serum E_2. However, when hMG is given in the morning and the serum E_2 determination is drawn during the same office visit (in the morning), the E_2 will not reflect peak levels, since the last dose of Pergonal was given the previous morning (24 hours). Using this technique, dosing is based on the previous day's E_2 level. However, the advantage of both drawing the serum and giving the hMG injection in the morning is that the patient only has to come to the office once each day.

Despite the convenience of both drawing E_2 and injecting Pergonal in the morning, I prefer to draw the serum in the morning and give the hMG injection in the evening when the serum E_2 levels are available. The patient's husband may be taught to administer the medication, or a visiting nurse can give the evening injection. When morning E_2 levels and morning Pergonal injections are given together, the peak E_2 levels should not be allowed to exceed 1,500 pg/ml to limit the incidence of severe OHSS. When the 8 a.m. E_2 level is utilized and hMG is administered in the evening, peak serum E_2 levels of 2,000 pg/ml are generally used as a maximal E_2 level in order to avoid severe OHSS, which can cause life-threatening complications. Mild OHSS can occur even with lower serum E_2 levels. In fact, mild OHSS is not uncommon even with careful monitoring of Pergonal therapy. However, serious complications with mild OHSS are uncommon.

In comparing ultrasound versus E_2 in hMG monitoring, Check et al[40] noted that the ultrasound scan agreed with serum E_2 measurements 57 percent of the time. However, 24 percent of patients had very high serum E_2 levels before the dominant follicle reached 17 mm or greater in size. In addition, 20 percent of patients had an ovulatory follicle of greater than 17 mm in size despite relatively low serum E_2 levels. In Check et al's study,[40] patients with either low E_2 or only small follicles noted on ultrasound were continued on hMG injections until *both* criteria (E_2 and follicular size) were judged adequate. Using this technique, all patients ovulated. There was a 39 percent pregnancy rate (in one stimulated cycle), which is an excellent result. There was a 3 percent incidence of mild OHSS and an 8 percent incidence of multiple gestations. Four of the five patients with multiple gestations and all of the patients with OHSS had serum E_2 levels above 2,000 pg/ml, suggesting that, if the more conservative E_2 criterion had been utilized, there would have been fewer complications of OHSS and multiple pregnancies. However, this study does illustrate the fact that some patients require aggressive hMG stimulation despite high E_2 levels to achieve adequate follicular development, and others need continued hMG therapy despite the presence of adequate follicular size on ultrasound to allow adequate endocrine (hormonal) development of the follicle. However, aggressive management results in more complications.

hMG and Follicular Growth

There is generally a good correlation between follicular diameter as measured by sonography and serum E_2 levels.[56] hMG-stimulated follicles are generally 2 to 4 mm larger than follicles in normally ovulating patients. In addition, hMG stimulated follicles are generally larger than follicles stimulated by clomiphene citrate for any given serum E_2 level (Fig. 18-11).[56]

Marrs et al[57] studied 70 hMG cycles in 25 anovulatory women. The mean maximum follicular diameter 6 days before administration of hCG was 11.3 ± 0.3 mm, which increased to 21.2 ± 0.6 mm with daily hMG administration (Fig. 18-12).[57] There was an excellent correlation ($R = 0.981$) between follicular size and serum E_2 levels (Fig. 18-13) and between total follicular volume and E_2 levels (Fig. 18-14).[57]

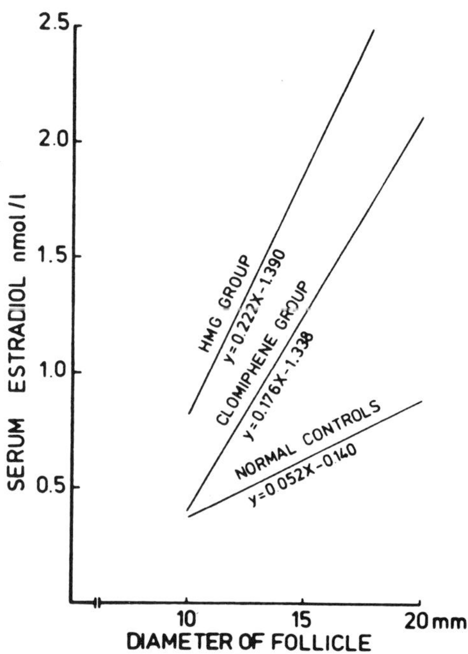

Fig. 18-11. Correlation of follicular diameter and serum E_2 in patients with normal cycles or receiving clomiphene citrate or hMG therapy. (From Ylostalo et al,[56] with permission.)

Fig. 18-12. Daily mean ± standard error of the mean of follicle diameter before hCG administration. (From Marrs et al,[57] with permission.)

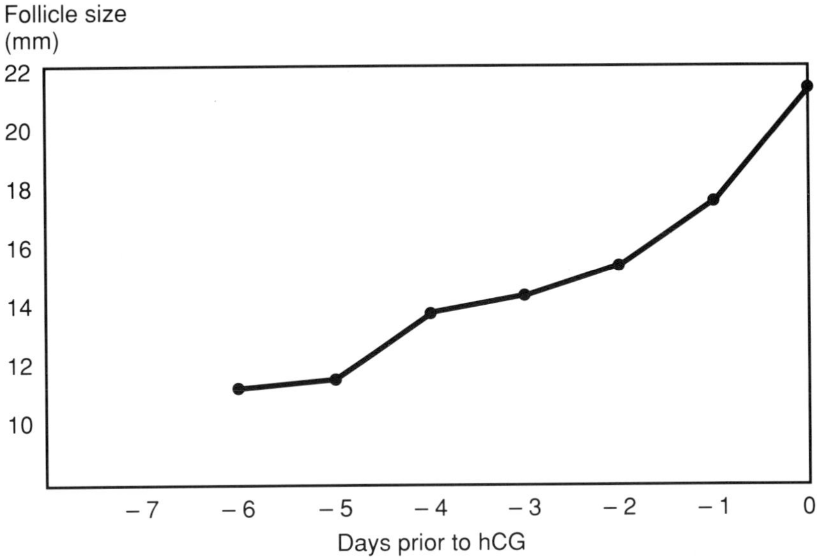

Timing of Human Chorionic Gonadotropin (hCG)

An LH surge and ovulation generally do not occur spontaneously with hMG therapy. Therefore, hCG must be added to achieve ovulation. hCG and LH have considerable molecular homology, and hCG may be used to trigger ovulation as a substitute for LH. hCG is much cheaper and more readily available than LH.

hCG is administered when at least one follicle of 18 to 20 mm is noted on ultrasound and the serum E_2 above 300 pg/ml indicates a mature follicle. If there are multiple follicles, serum E_2 should be 500 to 1,000 pg/ml (Fig. 18-15).

Success of hMG Therapy

From a summary of 13 different studies published between 1970 and 1982, a 43.9 percent pregnancy

Fig. 18-13. Correlation of mean E_2 level and follicle diameter. (From Marrs et al,[57] with permission.)

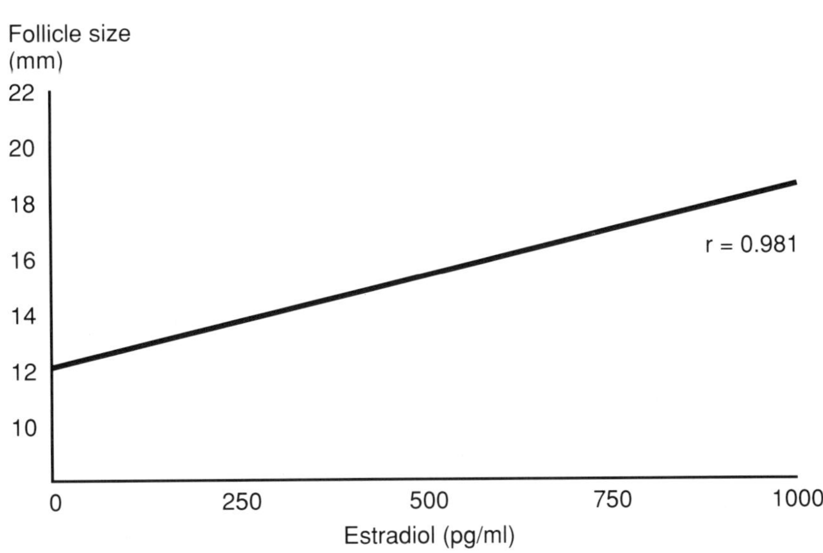

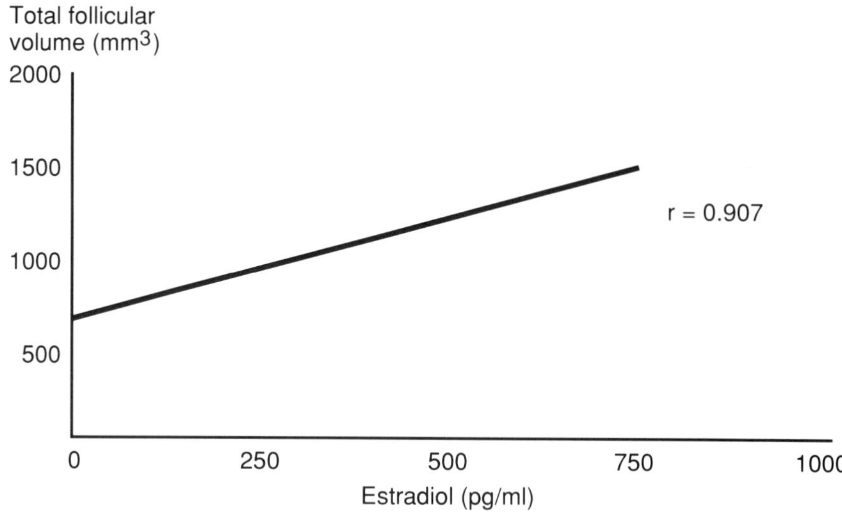

Fig. 18-14. Correlation of mean E_2 level and follicle volume. (From Marrs et al,[57] with permission.)

rate has been achieved using hMG.[58] These studies included 5,745 patients and 15,740 stimulated cycles (Table 18-12).[58]

Blankstein et al[58] noted a lower pregnancy rate with hMG therapy in patients with hypothalamic pituitary dysfunction (21.4 percent) compared with patients with hypogonadotropic anovulation (91.2 percent). Most pregnancies are achieved in the first five hMG cycles. A cumulative pregnancy rate of 94 percent in hypogonadotropic patients and a 93 percent pregnancy rate in normal gonadotropic patients were achieved by the fifth hMG cycle in those patients who ultimately achieved a pregnancy (Table 18-13).[58]

A pregnancy rate of between 28 and 57 percent per hMG cycle has been reported.[58] Continued hMG stimulation for more than five unsuccessful hMG cycles is generally unproductive. A patient who has failed five hMG cycles should be reevaluated and other forms of therapy considered.

A higher pregnancy rate has been reported with hMG therapy when a three-line endometrium is imaged by ultrasound.[59] A correlation between endometrial thickness and pregnancy has also been reported. Pregnancy is uncommon when the endometrium is less than 6 mm thick. Shoham et al[59] noted a significantly thicker endometrium in pregnant patients (10.4 mm) compared to nonpregnant patients (8.9 mm). The endometrial thickness was 13 mm in only 1.2 percent of nonpregnant patients compared to 42 percent of patients who achieved a pregnancy.[59]

Complications of hMG Therapy

Abortion. There is an increased abortion rate in hMG cycles of 20 to 25 percent compared with an expected incidence of 10 to 15 percent in unstimulated or natural cycles. Check et al[44] reported that progesterone supplementation (progesterone vaginal suppositories [50 mg/day] beginning 3 days after hCG) decreased the abortion rate in hMG-stimulated patients. Blankstein et al[58] have suggested that there is no increase in the abortion rate in a second hMG pregnancy after an initial abortion. Ultrasound can be useful in detecting early pregnancy and a blighted ovum or abnormal pregnancy that will eventually abort (see Ch. 13).

Multiple Pregnancies. Multiple gestations are noted in about 20 percent of hMG pregnancies. Twins account for about three-fourths of the multiple gestations, and triplets or higher multiples occur in the remaining one-fourth. The high rate of multiple pregnancies results from multiple ovulations. The multiple pregnancies are fraternal, rather than identical.

Ultrasound is an important tool in early diagnosis of multiple pregnancies. However, almost one-half of the twin pregnancies diagnosed before 10 weeks of gestation will be absorbed. The disappearance of a second twin has been termed the vanishing twin syndrome. Because of the high incidence of vanishing twins, it is important to rescan the patient after 10 weeks before concluding that the patient diagnosed as having twins in early pregnancy will actually deliver twins.

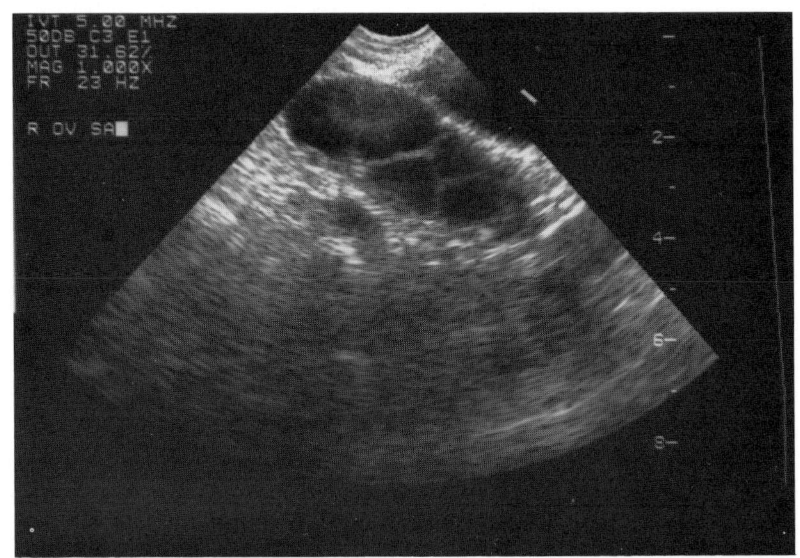

A

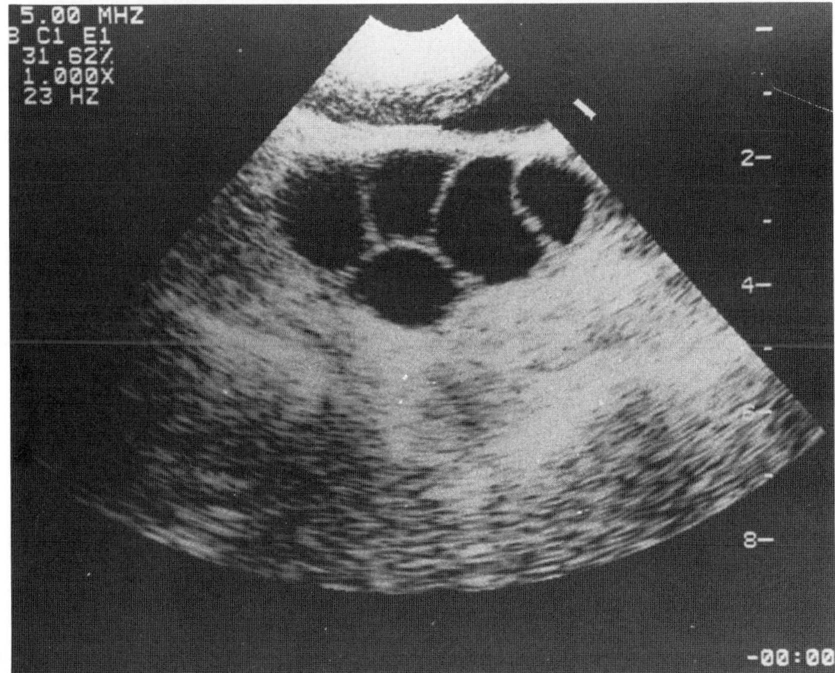

B

Fig. 18-15. (**A**) T-pelvic image of the ovary after hMG stimulation. The serum E_2 was 794 pg/ml. (**B**) T-pelvic image of the ovary during hMG stimulation. The serum E_2 was 791 pg/ml.

Table 18-12. Success Rate with hMG Therapy

	No. of Patients	*Cycles*	*Pregnancies*	*% Pregnant*
13 studies (1970-1982)	5,745	15,740	2,525	43.9

(Modified from Blankstein et al,[58] with permission.)

Ovarian Hyperstimulation Syndrome (OHSS). OHSS is a complication of hMG therapy characterized by ovarian enlargement secondary to the development of multiple luteal cysts. Based on the degree of ovarian enlargement and associated clinical findings, Jewelewicz et al[60] divided OHSS into mild, moderate, and severe categories (Table 18-14). The incidence of severe hyperstimulation from six reports involving 11,343 cases was 0.84 percent (Table 18-15).[58] However, these estimates were generally made using clinical criteria. Ultrasound allows a much more accurate assessment of ovarian size and aids in the diagnosis of OHSS.

Torsion, rupture, or hemorrhage of the ovary may result from the ovarian enlargement. Fluid shifts, including ascites and hydrothorax, are responsible for most of the problems associated with OHSS.

Mild and moderate OHSS is not uncommon. Fortunately, it is unusual for the patient to experience major complications with milder forms of ovarian hyperstimulation. The patient usually only experiences some mild to moderate abdominal pain, bloating, nausea, and/or mild ascites. In contrast, the patient with severe ovarian hyperstimulation can be quite ill and should be hospitalized and given supportive care.

Using transvaginal ultrasound, many if not most patients have some luteal cysts and mild OHSS after hMG therapy. However, careful monitoring during ovulation induction using ultrasound can generally limit the incidence of severe OHSS with the potential of serious complications to less than 1 percent.

Table 18-13. Cumulative Pregnancy Rate with hMG

	% Achieving Pregnancy	
Cycles	*Low Gonadotropins*	*Normal Gonadotropins*
1	47	39
2	71	57
3	84	75
4	90	86
5	94	93

(Modified from Blankstein et al,[58] with permission.)

Shoham et al[59] was able to limit the number of patients with severe OHSS to only one over a 6-year period, by limiting the number of dominant follicles to three. If there were more than three leading follicles hCG was withheld.

Complications of OHSS. In severe OHSS, massive fluid shifts and ascites are followed by hypovolemia and hemoconcentration. Fluid shifts result in an elevated hematocrit and increased serum osmolality and hypotension. The hypotension and hypovolemia result in decreased renal perfusion, oliguria, azotemia, and sometimes renal failure. Respiratory compromise can occur secondary to the ascites and hydrothorax. Thrombosis may result from the hemoconcentration. Congestive heart failure can occur when ascites fluid is reabsorbed into the vascular system.

The major complication from OHSS that is associated with the ovary is hemorrhage from rupture or torsion of the ovary. The patient should be hospitalized if severe OHSS occurs. Severe OHSS is characterized by weight gain greater than 10 pounds, a hematocrit over 50 percent, hypotension, oliguria, and dyspnea with ovarian enlargement greater than 10 cm in diameter. Ultrasound clearly reveals the massive ovarian enlargement and increased peritoneal fluid.

Treatment of OHSS. The treatment of OHSS is nonspecific and is directed toward correction of the physiologic changes. No pelvic examination should be done because of the risk of rupturing the enlarged ovaries. The patient should be monitored for the potential development of a twisted or torsed ovary characterized by fever, elevated leukocyte count, and abdominal pain and tenderness. Every effort should be made to avoid surgery, since spontaneous resolution will eventually occur. However, if ovarian torsion or uncontrolled hemorrhage from ovarian rupture occurs, surgery may be necessary.

The patient with severe OHSS should be placed at bed rest, and there should be careful monitoring and management of fluid therapy to maintain blood pressure and urinary output. Mannitol may be necessary.

Table 18-14. Classification of OHSS

Classification	*Ovarian Enlargement (cm)*	*Clinical Findings*
Mild	< 5	
Moderate	5-20	
Severe	> 10	Ascites, > 10 lb. weight gain

(Modified from Jewelewicz et al,[60] with permission.)

However, furosemide (Lasix) and other diuretics should be avoided because of the depleted intravascular volume. Hyperkalemia may have to be treated with potassium exchange resins.

In experimental animal systems, indomethacin and antihistamines have been helpful in treatment. However, their value in humans with OHSS has not been proved. (Table 18-16).

Spontaneous resolution will occur in 2 to 3 weeks in the nonpregnant patient. OHSS is generally more severe and lasts longer in the pregnant patient, and resolution may not occur for 4 to 8 weeks.

Transvaginal ultrasound-guided aspiration of ascitic fluid has been reported to produce a rapid and marked improvement of symptoms of OHSS. In a study of 21 cases of OHSS, the 11 patients treated with aspiration of ascitic fluid required only an average of 4 days of hospitalization compared to 11 days for patients treated conservatively.[61] Urinary output and electrolyte imbalance improved rapidly, and it was possible to discontinue IV therapy within 24 hours of aspiration. The fluid volume aspirated varied from 900 to 6100 ml and contained a high concentration of estradiol (average 6,500 pg/ml). Although this approach is preliminary and needs confirmation and additional study, aspiration may offer a real advancement in therapy since current treatment is almost exclusively supportive.

Congenital Malformations. Harlap[62] noted one major and five minor malformations in 66 infants born after hMG treatment (15.2 and 75.8/1,000, respectively). This incidence is close to the expected rate in the general population of 10.3 and 72.4/1,000, respectively. Other studies by Hack and Lunenfeld[63] and Caspi et al[64] also noted an incidence of congenital anomalies after hMG therapy similar to that of the general population (Table 18-17). Hendricks[65] reported that the congenital anomaly rate in twins was double the expected incidence in singleton pregnancies. Considering the 20 percent incidence of multiple pregnancies with hMG therapy, some increase in the congenital anomaly rate might be expected because of this factor alone. However, current data would indicate that there is little or no increase in the congenital anomaly rate with hMG therapy. Although level II ultrasound with a detailed review of fetal anatomy for congenital anomalies may be used in pregnancy and/or as an aid for correct needle placement for genetic amniocentesis, neither procedure is indicated based solely on a pregnancy resulting from hMG therapy.

Table 18-15. Incidence of OHSS with hMG

	No. of Treatment Cycles	*Mild*	*Severe*
Six reports	11,343	3.4%	0.84%

(Modified from Blankstein et al,[58] with permission.)

hMG Plus Clomiphene Citrate

hMG may be combined with clomiphene citrate in order to decrease the amount of hMG utilized. hMG is quite expensive, and combination therapy allows as

Table 18-16. Treatment of OHSS

Bed rest
No examinations
Strict fluid input and output monitoring
Fluid therapy
  Maintain urine output
  Maintain blood pressure
K^+ exchange resins
Mannitol
?Indomethacin
?Antihistamines

Table 18-17. Congenital Malformations[a]

	Major	*Minor*
Hack & Lunenfeld[63]	0	50.0
Caspi et al[64]	25.5	70.1
Harlap (per 1,000)[62]	15.2	75.8
Expected per 1,000	10.3	72.4

[a] Congenital anomalies in twins two times expected rate.[65]
(Data from Harlap,[62] Hack and Lunenfeld,[63] Caspi et al,[64] and Hendriks.[65])

much as a 50 percent reduction in the amount of hMG utilized. For example, in a comparison of hMG alone with hMG plus CC, the mean number of follicles and the serum E_2, were not significantly different despite a 36 percent decrease in the hMG used. However, the addition of CC may be associated with some of its deleterious effects on endometrial development and an increased subclinical abortion rate discussed above.[51]

REFERENCES

1. Quagliarello J, Arny M: Inaccuracy of basal body temperature charts in predicting urinary luteinizing hormone surges. Fertil Steril 45:334, 1986
2. Bomsel-Helmreich O, Gougeon A, Thebault A et al: Healthy and atretic human follicles in the preovulatory phase: differences in evolution of follicular morphology and steroid content of follicular fluid. J Clin Endocrinol Metab 48:686, 1979
3. Pache TD, Vladimiroff TW, Hop WC, Fauser BC: How to discriminate between normal and polycystic ovaries. Transvag Study Radiol 183:421, 1992
4. Hackeloer BJ, Fleming R, Robinson HP et al: Correlation of ultrasonic and endocrinologic assessment of human follicular development. Am J Obstet Gynecol 135:122, 1979
5. Hamilton CJCM, Evers JLH, Tan FES, Hoogland HJ: The reliability of ovulation prediction by a single ultrasonographic follicle measurement. Human Reprod 2:103, 1987
6. Forman RG, Robinson J, Yudkin P et al: What is the true follicular diameter: an assessment of the reproducibility of transvaginal ultrasound monitoring in stimulated cycles. Fertil Steril 56:989, 1991
7. Bonilla-Musoles F, Pardo G, Perez-Gil M et al: Abdominal ultrasonography versus transvaginal scanning: accuracy in follicular development evaluation and prediction of oocyte retrieval in stimulated cycles. J Clin Ultrasound 17:469, 1989
8. O'Herlihy C, de Crespigny LJ, Lopata A et al: Preovulatory follicular size: a comparison of ultrasound and laparoscopic measurements. Fertil Steril 34:24, 1980
9. Kerin JF, Edmonds DK, Warnes GM et al: Morphological and functional relations of graafian follicle growth to ovulation in women using ultrasonic, laparoscopic and biochemical measurements. Br J Obstet Gynaecol 88:81, 1981
10. Ritchie WGM: Sonographic evaluation of normal and induced ovulation. Radiology 161:1, 1986
11. Mendelson EB, Friedman H, Neiman HL et al: The role of imaging in infertility management. AJR 144:415, 1985
12. Zandt-Stastny D, Thorsen MK, Middleton WD et al: Inability of sonography to detect imminent ovulation. AJR 152:91, 1989
13. Picker RH, Smith DH, Tucker MH, Saunders DM: Ultrasonic signs of imminent ovulation. J Clin Ultrasound 11:1, 1983
14. Jaffe R, Ben-Aderet N: Ultrasonic screening in predicting the time of ovulation. Gynecol Obstet Invest 18:303, 1984
15. Jaffe R, Abramowicz J, Ben-Aderet N: Correlation between the endocrine profile of ovulation and the ultrasonically detected 'double contour' of the preovulatory follicle. Gynecol Obstet Invest 24:119, 1987
16. Bryce RL, Shuter B, Sinosich MJ et al: The value of ultrasound, gonadotropin, and estradiol measurements for precise ovulation prediction. Fertil Steril 37:42, 1982
17. Collins W, Jurkovic D, Bourne T et al: Ovarian morphology, endocrine function and intra-follicular blood flow during the peri-ovulatory period. Hum Reprod 6:319, 1991
18. Gonen Y, Casper RF, Jacobson W, Blankier J: Endometrial thickness and growth during ovarian stimulation: a possible predictor of implantation in in vitro fertilization. Fertil Steril 52:446, 1989
19. Hill LM, Coulam CB, Kislak SL, Peterson CS, Runco CJ. Sonographic evaluation of the cervix during ovulation induction. Am J Obstet Gynecol 157:1170, 1987
20. Ayers JWT, Knight L, Grady E, Peterson EP: Transvaginal sonographic endometrial morphology—the bioassay of ovarian steroidogenesis in spontaneous and induced cycles. Abstract P-123. p. S84. Abstracts of the 44th Annual Meeting of the American Fertility Society. Presented at The 44th Annual Meeting of the American Fertility Society, Atlanta, October 1988
21. Stein IF, Leventhal ML: Amenorrhea associated with bilateral polycystic ovaries. Am J Obstet Gynecol 29:181, 1935
22. Swanson M, Sauerbrei EE, Cooperberg PL: Medical implications of ultrasonically detected polycystic ovaries. J Clin Ultrasound 9:219, 1981

23. Sample WF, Lippe BM, Gyepes MT: Gray-scale ultrasonography of the normal female pelvis. Radiology 125:447, 1977
24. Jaffe R, Abramowicz J, Eckstein N et al: Sonographic monitoring of ovarian volume during LHRH analogue therapy in women with polycystic ovarian syndrome. J Ultrasound Med 7:203, 1988
25. el Tabbakh GH, Lotfy I, Azab I et al: Correlation of the ultrasonic appearance of the ovaries in polycystic ovarian disease and the clinical, hormonal, and laparoscopic findings. Am J Obstet Gynecol 154:892, 1986
26. Hann LE, Hall DA, McArdle CR, Seibel M: Polycystic ovarian disease: sonographic spectrum. Radiology 150:531, 1984
27. Hall DA: Sonographic appearance of the normal ovary, of polycystic ovary disease, and of functional ovarian cysts. Semin Ultrasound 4:149, 1983
28. Buttram VC, Vaquero C: Post-ovarian wedge resection adhesive disease. Fertil Steril 26:874, 1975
29. Jafari K, Javaheri G, Ruiz G: Endometrial adenocarcinoma and the Stein-Leventhal syndrome. Obstet Gynecol 51:97, 1978
30. Eddy WA: Endometrial carcinoma in Stein-Leventhal syndrome treated with hydroxyprogesterone caproate. Am J Obstet Gynecol 131:581, 1978
31. Coulam CB, Bustillo M, Schulman JD: Empty follicle syndrome. Fertil Steril 46:1153, 1986
32. Hilgers TW, Dvorak AD, Tamisiea DF et al: Sonographic definition of the empty follicle syndrome. J Ultrasound Med 8:411, 1989
33. Van Hall EV, Mastboom JL: Luteal phase insufficiency in patients treated with clomiphene. Am J Obstet Gynecol 103:165, 1969
34. Jewelewicz R: Management of infertility resulting from anovulation. Am J Obstet Gynecol 122:909, 1975
35. Koninckx PR, Heyns WJ, Corvelyn PA, Brosens IA: Delayed onset of luteinization as a cause of infertility. Fertil Steril 29:266, 1978
36. Marik J, Hulka J: Luteinized unruptured follicle syndrome: a subtle cause of infertility. Fertil Steril 29:270, 1978
37. Kerin JF, Kirby C, Morris D et al: Incidence of the luteinized unruptured follicle phenomenon in cycling women. Fertil Steril 40:620, 1983
38. Bateman BG, Kolp LA, Nunley WC et al: Oocyte retention after follicle luteinization. Fertil Steril 54:793, 1990
39. Luciano AA, Peluso J, Koch EI et al: Temporal relationship and reliability of the clinical, hormonal, and ultrasonographic indices of ovulation in infertile women. Obstet Gynecol 75:412, 1990
40. Check JH, Goldberg BB, Kurtz A et al: Serum estradiols versus pelvic sonography in monitoring hMG therapy. Int J Fertil 30:61, 1985
41. Liukkonen S, Koskimies AI, Tenhunen A, Ylostalo P: Diagnosis of luteinized unruptured follicle (LUF) syndrome by ultrasound. Fertil Steril 41:26, 1984
42. Garcia J, Jones GS, Wentz AC: The use of clomiphene citrate. Fertil Steril 28:707, 1977
43. March CM, Shoupe D: Luteal-phase defects. In Mishell DR, Davajon V, Lobo RA (eds): Infertility, Contraception and Reproductive Endocrinology. p. 793. Blackwell Scientific, Boston, 1991
44. Check JH, Rankin A, Teichman M: The risk of fetal anomalies as a result of progesterone therapy during pregnancy. Fertil Steril 45:575, 1986
45. Mehta AE, Matwijiw I, Lyons EA, Faiman C: Noninvasive diagnosis of resistant ovary syndrome by ultrasound. Fertil Steril 57:56, 1992
46. ACOG. Medical induction of ovulation. p. 1. ACOG Technical Bulletin 120, September 1988
47. Bateman BG, Kolp LA, Nunley WC et al: Subclinical pregnancy loss in clomiphene citrate-treated women. Fertil Steril 57:25, 1992
48. Clark JH, Peck EJ Jr, Anderson JN: Oestrogen receptors and antagonism of steroid hormone action. Nature 251:446, 1974
49. Yagel S, Ben-Chetrit A, Anteby E et al: The effect of ethinyl estradiol on endometrial thickness and uterine volume during ovulation induction by clomiphene citrate. Fertil Steril 57:33, 1992
50. Randall JM, Templeton A: Transvaginal sonographic assessment of follicular and endometrial growth in spontaneous and clomiphene citrate cycles. Fertil Steril 56:208, 1991
51. Gonen Y, Casper RF: Sonographic determination of a possible adverse effect of clomiphene citrate on endometrial growth. Hum Reprod 5:670, 1990
52. Yeko TR, Nicosia SM, Maroulis GB et al: Histology of midluteal corpus luteum and endometrium from clomiphene citrate-induced cycles. Fertil Steril 57:28, 1992
53. Deichert U, Hackeler BJ, Daume E: The sonographic and endocrinologic evaluation of the endometrium in the luteal phase. Hum Reprod 1:219, 1986
54. Serhal PF, Katz M, Little V, Woronowski H: Unexplained infertility—the value of Pergonal superovulation combined with intrauterine insemination. Fertil Steril 49:602, 1988
55. Corson SL, Batzer FR, Gocial B, Maislin G: Intrauterine insemination and ovulation stimulation as treatment of infertility. J Reprod Med 34:397, 1989
56. Ylostalo P, Ronnberg L, Jouppila P: Measurement of the ovarian follicle by ultrasound in ovulation induction. Fertil Steril 31:651, 1979
57. Marrs RP, Vargyas JM, March CM: Correlation of ultrasonic and endocrinologic measurements in human menopausal gonadotropin therapy. Am J Obstet Gynecol 145:417, 1983
58. Blankstein J, Mashiach S, Lunenfeld B: Ovulation Induction and In Vitro Fertilization. Year Book Medical Publishers, Chicago, 1986
59. Shoham Z, Di Carlo C, Patel A et al: Is it possible to run a successful ovulation induction program based solely on

ultrasound monitoring? The importance of endometrial measurements. Fertil Steril 56:836, 1991

60. Jewelewicz R, Dyrenfurth I, Warren MP, Vande Wiele RL: Ovarian hyperstimulation syndrome: relationship between pre-ovulatory estrogen levels and ovarian hyperstimulation in gonadotropin-treated patients. p. 235. In Rosenberg E (ed): Gonadotropin Therapy in Female Infertility. Exerpta Medica, Amsterdam, 1973
61. Aboulghar MA, Mansour RT, Serour GI, Amin Y: Ultrasonically guided vaginal aspiration of ascites in the treatment of severe ovarian hyperstimulation syndrome. Fertil Steril 53:933, 1990
62. Harlap S: Ovulation induction and congenital malformations. Lancet 2:961, 1976
63. Hack M, Lunenfeld B: The influence of hormone induction of ovulation on the fetus and newborn. Pediatr Adolesc Endocrinol 5:191, 1979
64. Caspi E, Ronen J, Schreyer P, Goldberg MD: The outcome of pregnancy after gonadotrophin therapy. Br J Obstet Gynaecol 83:967, 1976
65. Hendriks CH: Twinning in relation to birth weight, mortality, and congenital anomalies. Obstet Gynecol 27:47, 1966

19

Follicular Aspiration and In Vitro Fertilization

Gregory S. Neal
Zev Rosenwaks
Melvin G. Dodson

In vitro fertilization (IVF) has become an indispensable therapeutic modality in the treatment of infertility. Although IVF was initially utilized for treating patients with severely damaged fallopian tubes and/or pelvic adhesions, the list of indications has expanded to include patients with endometriosis or idiopathic infertility who have not achieved a pregnancy when treated by more conventional therapies, as well as male factor infertility when there is a significant decrease in sperm number, motility, and/or morphology. IVF is now also indicated for patients with immunologic infertility in an attempt to surmount any problem with fertilization that may be caused by antisperm antibodies. There are five basic steps followed in the IVF procedure: (1) a thorough infertility evaluation and patient selection, (2) ovulation induction and monitoring, (3) follicular aspiration, (4) in vitro fertilization, and (5) embryo transfer. Ultrasound has significant applicability in several of these areas.

Ultrasound is becoming an increasingly important tool in the basic infertility evaluation to diagnose anovulation, uterine fibroids, and congenital müllerian anomalies and may even suggest pelvic adhesions (see specific areas for discussion). Ultrasound is essential for monitoring ovulation induction in patients treated with human menopausal gonadotropins (hMG) and is an integral part of the follicular aspiration procedure. The Society of Assisted Reproductive Technology (SART) reported in 1987 that 57 percent of 8,725 IVF oocyte retrievals were done by ultrasound-guided aspiration, 1 percent by ultrasound and laparoscopy combined, and 41 percent by laparoscopy alone.[1] In contrast, data obtained from the 1990 SART Report disclose that, of 16,405 IVF oocyte retrievals, 95 percent were performed by ultrasound, 4 percent by laparoscopy, 0.5 percent by a combination of both, and 0.1 percent by laparotomy.[2] Coincident with the dominance obtained in oocyte retrievals, ultrasound has also been used during embryo transfer to determine proper placement of the embryo.

IVF OVULATION INDUCTION

Although the initial IVF success reported by Steptoe and Edwards, culminating in the birth of Louise Brown in 1978, utilized a natural menstrual cycle with laparoscopic follicular aspiration timed to the luteinizing hormone (LH) surge, almost all IVF programs today use some form of ovulation induction.[3]

The stimulation of multiple ovarian follicles during ovulation induction for IVF, which has also been termed controlled ovarian hyperstimulation, is necessary since it is acknowledged that the pregnancy rate from IVF increases with the number of embryos transferred.[4] Despite the genesis of multiple follicles providing multiple embryos for transfer, the IVF process is relatively inefficient in producing a pregnancy, as evidenced by the overall clinical pregnancy rate for IVF of 19 percent per retrieval in 1991.[5] Although some IVF clinics are currently achieving pregnancy rates greater than 30 percent per oocyte retrieval, these excellent results nevertheless require multiple follicles. Follicular stimulation can be achieved with clomiphene citrate (Clomid, Serophene), hMG (Pergonal), follicle stimulating hormone (Metrodin, FSH), or a combination of these drugs.[6] More recently, gonadotropin releasing hormone agonists (GnRH-a) have been added to improve follicular recruitment and to prevent a premature LH surge.[7] As yet, no single stimulatory regimen has been demonstrated to be clearly superior, although the most common protocol currently employed consists of a GnRH analog in combination with Metrodin and Pergonal. Patients are monitored by measurement of daily serum estradiol (E_2)levels and ultrasonographic determination of follicular size. The ovarian stimulation regimen is then individually tailored to the patient's response based on these two parameters.

Ultrasound monitoring may be done either transabdominally or transvaginally; however, most IVF programs utilize the transvaginal approach as it provides superior image quality of the ovaries and developing follicles.

OOCYTE RETRIEVAL

The original method for oocyte retrieval as described by Steptoe and Edwards involved laparoscopic follicle aspiration under general anesthesia. Although this method was relatively safe and effective, several disadvantages became quite apparent. Dodson et al[8] described a 7 percent incidence of failure to recover oocytes at the time of laparoscopy due to dense pelvic adhesions. Laparoscopy is a relatively invasive procedure with inherent surgical and general anesthesia risks and is not an ideal technique for the group of patients who require multiple attempts at IVF before conceiving. The general anesthesia required for laparoscopy is associated with an increased incidence of postoperative nausea and vomiting, which contributes to a longer recovery period. Another possible disadvantage of laparoscopic aspiration is that the oocytes are exposed to the CO_2 environment required to maintain a pneumoperitoneum. Mastroyannis et al[9] reported a toxic effect of exposure of oocytes to CO_2 secondary to the pneumoperitoneum used during laparoscopy. Daya et al[10] compared oocytes obtained under ultrasonic guidance to those obtained by laparoscopy to determine whether CO_2 exposure caused any adverse consequences. The results suggested that CO_2 exposure may indeed affect fertilization, but once it has occurred there is no influence on the rate of cleavage of the embryos. In contrast, Feichtinger et al[11] did not find any change in follicular fluid pH after aspiration performed by laparoscopy. Consequently, the importance of a CO_2 pneumoperitoneum on ovum viability remains controversial.

Refinements in ultrasound technology hastened the arrival of ultrasound-guided aspiration techniques as the preferred method of oocyte retrieval. Ultrasound assisted ovum aspiration may be performed with transabdominal or transvaginal ultrasound imaging in conjunction with various established modes of oocyte retrieval. Transabdominal sonography has been used with percutaneous-transvesicular, periurethral, and transvaginal needle aspiration, whereas transvaginal ultrasound has proven practical in transvaginal needle puncture. Transabdominal ultrasonography was the initial means available for oocyte retrieval, and the first application was reported by Lenz et al,[12] who suggested a percutaneous and transvesicular route of follicular puncture. The technique demands a full bladder to provide acoustic shadowing for image enhancement and requires use of a low frequency ultrasound probe that is capable of providing transmission to the relatively distant ovaries. Lenz and Lauritsen were also the first to propose the use of ultrasound-guided retrievals in cases of extreme pelvic adhesive disease.[12,13] Lewin et al[14] performed a prospective, randomized study comparing laparoscopic oocyte retrieval with ultrasonically guided percutaneous and transvesical retrieval using a single midline percutaneous puncture. Ultrasound aspiration was found to be as effective as laparoscopy in terms of oocyte retrieval and conception rates.

One of the first deviations from the transvesical approach was described by Gleicher et al[15] in a case of oocyte retrieval using transabdominal ultrasound imaging and transvaginal needle puncture. Dellenbach et al[16] reported the first large series using the same technique in an outpatient setting and successfully achieved five normal births.

The procedure requires two individuals; one performs the transvaginal needle puncture using a free-hand technique while the partner controls the ultrasound transducer. One of the early problems with the free-hand technique was the difficulty experienced with proper spatial orientation. If the needle is not in the path of the ultrasound beam, it is not visible, and control of needle movement can be compromised, which could lead either to procedure failure or increased complications. Consequently, abdominal and vaginal ultrasound transducers are fitted with fixed needle guides that directly couple the path of the needle to the plane of the ultrasound beam. Despite its early acceptance, the transvesical approach is more difficult, more invasive, and requires more analgesia than transvaginal aspiration; as a result, the transabdominally guided oocyte retrieval approach is probably now only of historical interest except for the occasional case when the ovaries are located very high in the pelvis.

Before transvaginal oocyte retrieval became the norm, Parsons et al[17] described a periurethral route of follicular puncture using transabdominal imaging of the ovaries. In this technique, the aspiration needle is advanced through the urethra by way of a urinary catheter. Once the follicle to be punctured was identified, the tip of the aspirating needle was guided to the bladder wall adjacent to the follicle, and the needle was then guided into the follicle. The use of periurethral oocyte retrieval was further validated by Wisanto et al[18] who demonstrated excellent recovery, fertilization, and pregnancy rates. However, this technique has been reported to be painful and more difficult to learn than simple transvaginal follicular puncture and is therefore rarely used today.

Studies using ultrasound instead of laparoscopy as the technique of choice for oocyte retrieval have demonstrated the value of the ultrasound approach. Ultrasound aspiration can be performed using sedation rather than general anesthesia and is a simpler, less invasive procedure than laparoscopy. The use of sedation, the lack of surgical incisions, and the absence of a CO_2 pneumoperitoneum produce less postaspiration pain and discomfort while providing a more rapid patient recovery than that noted with laparoscopy. The follicle aspiration procedure can be less expensive when done in an ambulatory surgical center without the need for hospitalization or general anesthesia. Furthermore, use of the sonographic technique gives the physician a better appreciation of the number of follicles and their relative positions within the ovary. Indeed, sonographic visualization of follicles, particularly those deeper in the ovary, is actually better than direct laparoscopic visualization of the ovaries. Stimulated ovaries are heavier than usual and are situated deep in the pouch of Douglas close to the vaginal fornix. This location permits close proximity between the vaginal transducer and the ovaries and allows use of a higher frequency transducer (5-7 MHz), which generally provides improved image quality. The need for a full bladder for acoustic enhancement is not necessary, and bladder puncture is avoided with transvaginal sonography. The main disadvantages of ultrasound-guided needle puncture revolve around the fact that it is a blind procedure and the pelvic organs are not visualized directly.

Of the various available modalities, transvaginal ultrasound with transvaginal oocyte retrieval is currently the method of choice in most IVF programs. As the transition developed from abdominal ultrasound techniques to transvaginal ones, many uncontrolled studies were published espousing the merits of transvaginal ultrasound-guided oocyte retrieval.[19-23] Other studies compared laparoscopic retrieval to transvaginal retrieval and found transvaginal oocyte retrieval to be equal or superior to laparoscopy with respect to every parameter evaluated.[24-27] Several investigators compared multiple methods of oocyte retrieval to the transvaginal technique and reached the same conclusions promoting the superiority of the transvaginal method.[28,29] Despite the uncontrolled nature of many of these studies, the mean number of oocytes recovered per patient and per follicle, the fertilization rate, and the clinical pregnancy rate were found to be comparable to results previously obtained using either the laparoscopic, transvesical, or periurethral techniques. Janssen-Caspers et al[30] compared percutaneous-transvesical retrieval (using transabdominal ultrasound) to transvaginal ultrasound-guided oocyte retrieval in a prospective, randomized study involving 47 patients. A significantly greater number of oocytes were obtained using the transvaginal procedure, whereas the fertilization rate, number of embryos transferred, and pregnancy rate were not statistically different. Flood et al[31] compared cycles of transvaginal retrieval to laparoscopic cycles in the same patient using the same gonadotropin stimulation protocol to eliminate individual patient and stimulation variability between methods of retrieval. The total number of follicles aspirated per cycle, the number of oocytes with fractured zonae, and the fertilization rate were not statistically different between the two procedures. These data overwhelmingly validate the efficacy of the transvaginal retrieval technique and demonstrate some of the advantages of this technique over those previously described.

The technique for endovaginal oocyte retrieval varies somewhat among IVF programs. At Cornell the retrievals are performed with a 7.0-MHz endovaginal probe that has a focal range of 50 mm starting 10 mm from the tip of the probe. The transducer is draped with a sterile plastic sleeve, and sterile Aquasonics (Parker Laboratories, Inc., Orange, NJ) coupling jelly is applied liberally to the probe tip before a sterile, nonlubricated latex condom is placed over the transducer. It is important that all materials utilized are not toxic to embryos, and testing in a mouse zygote culture system should be done routinely to ensure compliance with this edict. A sterile needle guide is placed over the condom, and its alignment is carefully assessed for proper orientation, as a misshapen or misaligned needle guide can cause serious complications. The needle guide permits the introduction of an aspiration needle into the field of view parallel to the longitudinal axis of the transducer and is demonstrated visually on the ultrasound monitor as a broken line superimposed onto the ultrasound image on the screen. The surgeon's gloves and the ultrasound probe are irrigated with an abundant amount of sterile water to remove any talc, and the probe is then covered with sterile mineral oil (E.R. Squibb & Sons, Inc., Princeton, NJ) before placement in the vagina. The choice of an external condom coupling agent is quite important as some gels have been shown to be embryotoxic[32]; however, the mineral oil used at Cornell is the same oil used in our microdroplet culture system and is not toxic to embryos. After adequate analgesia is obtained, the patient is placed in the dorsolithotomy position, and the vagina and perineum are prepped with providone-iodine that is subsequently vigorously irrigated by rinsing with sterile water. The patient is then draped in a sterile fashion, and the ultrasound probe with attached needle guide is placed in the posterior vaginal fornix to visualize the stimulated ovaries. A single lumen needle is attached to tubing connected to a two-hole rubber stopper that has previously been placed in a clear plastic, sterile embryo collection tube (Fig. 19-1). This collection tube is placed in a 37°C warming block and is connected to low wall suction at 100 mmHg. The transducer position is adjusted so that the programmed puncturing line on the monitor screen crosses the follicle to be punctured (Fig. 19-2). The aspiration needle is placed within the needle guide and is advanced quickly through the vaginal wall into the follicle (Fig. 19-3). Once the needle is visualized within the follicle (Fig. 19-4A), gentle suction is applied by pressing the foot pedal to remit the required 100 mmHg suction pressure. As the fluid is removed and the follicle collapses, the needle is rotated slowly to ensure complete emptying of the follicle. When the follicle is collapsed fully, the needle tip can still be visualized (Fig. 19-4B) and is withdrawn slowly and advanced into the next follicle where the procedure is duplicated. The process is repeated until all follicles of both ovaries have been aspirated. Each collection tube should be filled no higher than halfway and then handed to an embryologist who carefully searches through the follicular fluid to identify the oocytes, which are then judiciously transferred to fresh culture medium. At the end of the retrieval, the pelvis should be sonographically visualized to check for excess culde-sac fluid that could indicate the inadvertent puncture of a pelvic blood vessel. The endovaginal probe is then removed, and a speculum is placed into the vagina to evaluate for hemostasis. If bleeding is noted from a puncture site(s), pressure should be diligently applied; this maneuver is sufficient in over 95 percent of cases for achieving hemostasis. In the

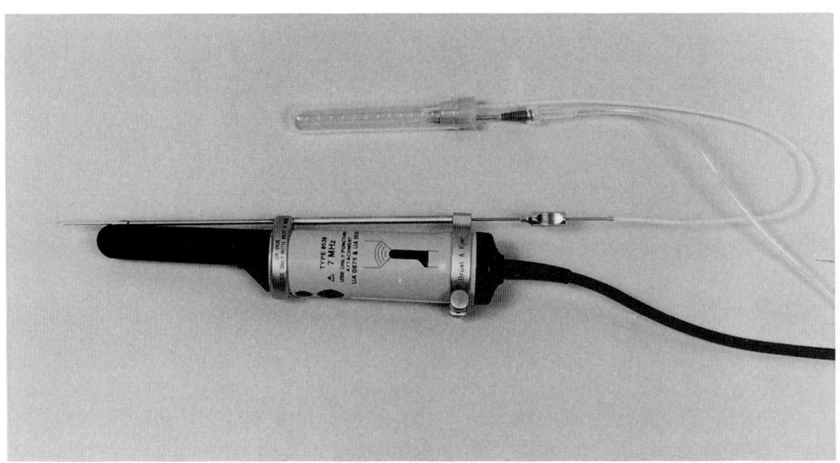

Fig. 19-1. Transvaginal ultrasound transducer with attached needle guide and aspiration needle. The aspiration needle is attached to an embryo collection tube that is connected to wall suction at 100 mmHg. The transducer is draped with a sterile plastic sleeve and condom before oocyte retrieval.

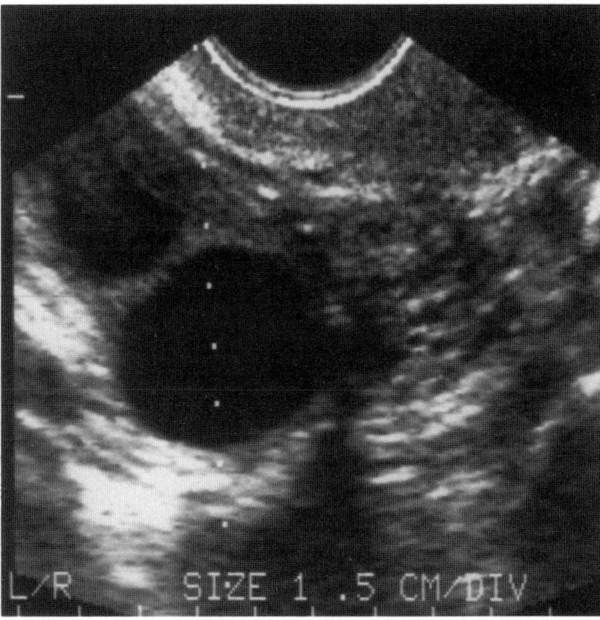

Fig. 19-2. Transvaginal ultrasound image demonstrating the programmed puncturing line that is aligned with the longitudinal axis of the transducer needle guide. This puncturing line ensures accurate placement of the aspiration needle.

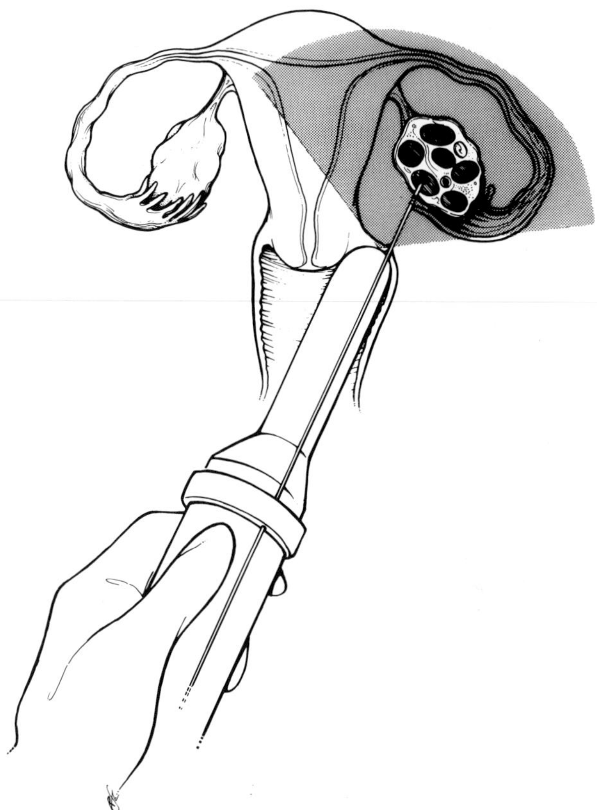

Fig. 19-3. Schematic image of transvaginal ultrasound-guided follicle aspiration. The transvaginal probe with attached needle guide is placed into the posterior vaginal fornix, and the aspiration needle is advanced through the vaginal wall into the follicle.

rare case of persistent vaginal bleeding from a puncture site, a figure of eight suture can be incorporated as needed.

The needle used for oocyte retrieval is an important part of the equipment needed to perform a successful procedure. The needle should be exceedingly sharp in order to puncture the vaginal and ovarian follicle walls easily. The inner diameter is also critical since damage to the oocyte can occur if the diameter is too small. However, too large a diameter causes unnecessary trauma to the patient, potentially resulting in increased pain and complications. Lewin et al[33] reported on the use of a 1.6-mm ID (internal diameter) needle and summarized the literature relating needle size and oocyte recovery rates. The literature review suggested an increase in the number of oocytes recovered as the needle diameter increased. Aziz et al[34] in a prospective, randomized study evaluated the effect of needle caliber on IVF outcome. The two needles used in the study were standard 16- and 18-gauge single channel aspiration needles with internal diameters of 1.19 mm and 0.84 mm, respectively. Immediately before starting the oocyte retrieval, the surgeon randomly picked "right or left" ovary and "small or large" needle. Thus, each patient served as her own control for each parameter considered. Using the smaller diameter needle had no significant effect upon the number of oocytes collected per follicle aspirated or on the fertilization rate. With the smaller needle there was also no increased incidence of fractured zonae, and there was indeed a significant reduction in pain as perceived by the patient. Scott et al[35] compared single and double lumen aspiration needles in a prospective, randomized study to determine if the potential advantage of a second channel to allow follicle flushing would in fact increase oocyte yield at retrieval. No differences in the number or quality of oocytes provided for IVF were noted, and

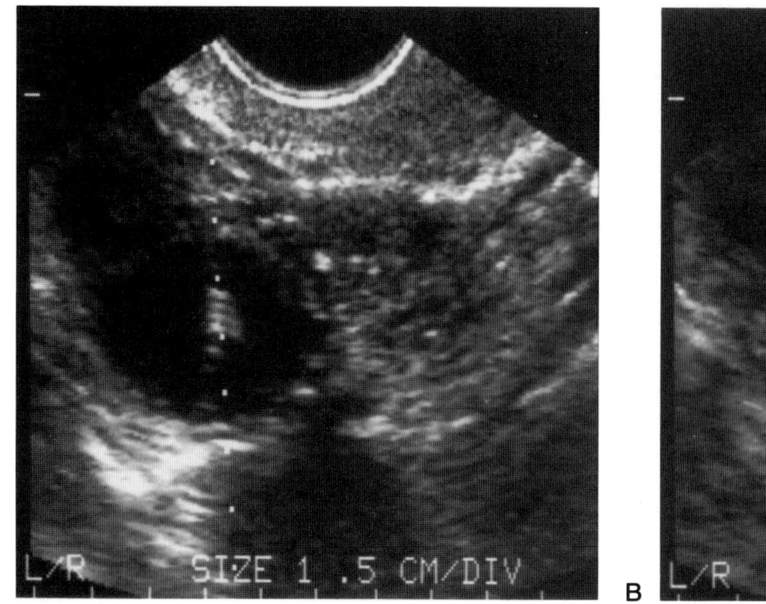

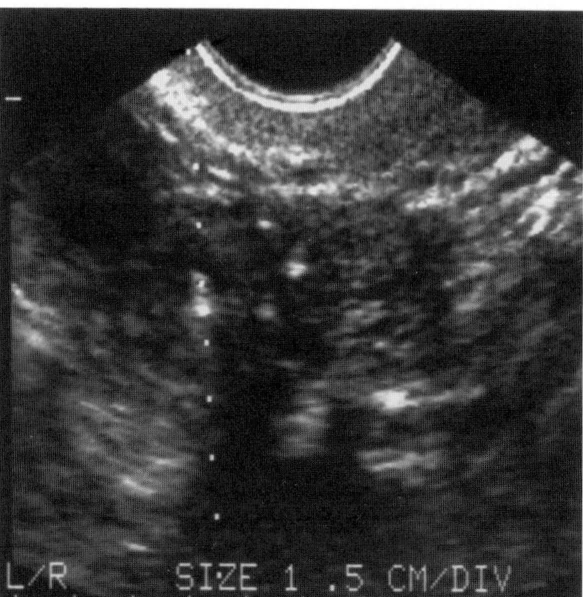

Fig. 19-4. **(A)** Transvaginal ultrasound image of a follicle with a clearly visible needle tip in the center of the follicle. **(B)** Transvaginal ultrasound image of the same follicle completely emptied. Note that the needle tip is still visible.

the single lumen needle proved to be technically easier to use, as the double lumen needle frequently deviated from the intended path. A single channel aspiration needle is used at Cornell (Swemed Lab AB, Västra Frölunda, Sweden) with an outer diameter of 1.6 mm, an inner diameter of 1.0 mm, and a length of 250 mm. The needle has shallow grooves near the tip that enhance the echoes from this part of the needle (Fig 19-5). Some programs manually score needles with a triangular file to provide echogenicity superior to that of commercially scored needles. Use of a scored needle is essential because it is important to see the needle tip at all times not only for successful aspiration of oocytes but also to prevent vascular injury since the hypogastric vein and artery lie immediately adjacent to the stimulated ovary.

Anesthesia requirements vary depending upon the specific method utilized for oocyte retrieval. Whereas laparoscopy requires general anesthesia, the ultrasound-guided techniques are generally performed with intravenous sedation, local infiltration, or a combination of both. Initial attempts at transabdominal ultrasound imaging for oocyte retrieval often utilized a transvesical approach that was usually quite painful and occasionally required general anesthesia. This approach is currently employed infrequently, except in cases where the ovaries are inadequately visualized by transvaginal ultrasound; regional anes-

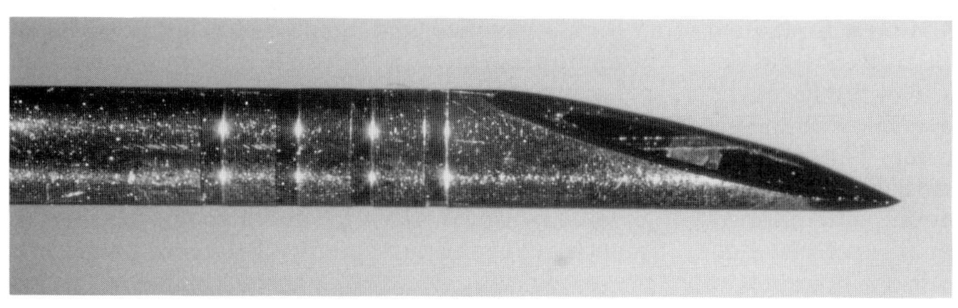

Fig. 19-5. The aspiration needle has shallow grooves near the tip which enhance echogenicity.

thesia may also be a reasonable alternative in these instances.[36]

Today, the majority of oocyte retrievals are performed transvaginally under ultrasonographic guidance which requires sedation or local anesthesia. For the extreme case of natural-cycle IVF where a single dominant follicle is aspirated, Ramsewak et al[37] concluded that follicle aspiration can be performed without analgesia. Notwithstanding, Dellenbach et al[16] used atropine (0.5 mg), pethidine (100 mg), and flunitrazepam (0.2 mg/10 kg) for premedication along with lidocaine injected locally at the puncture site(s). Feichtinger and Kemeter[21] employed atropine (0.25 mg), haloperidol (2.5 mg), flunitrazepam (2 mg), and pentazocine (30 mg) intravenously and did not consider local analgesia necessary. Evers et al[22] reported on analgesia consisting of diazepam (10 mg) and meperidine (50 mg) intravenously plus 5 ml of 2 percent lidocaine injected into the vaginal wall.

These methods all provide adequate analgesia, but the long half-life of diazepam and the occasional nausea from the narcotics have resulted in the frequent use of propofol as the anesthetic agent of choice for oocyte retrieval in many programs. Propofol (2,6-diisopropylphenol, Diprivan, Stuart Pharmaceuticals, Wilmington, DE) is an intravenous sedative hypnotic agent with a rapid onset, a rapid termination of sedation, and minimal associated nausea. It provides a fairly deep level of sedation that ensures that the patient does not move during periods of discomfort while also providing a fast, alert return to wakefulness, enabling the patient to be discharged as quickly as possible. Sedation is initiated with fentanyl (50–100 μg), and a propofol drip (50 to 100 mg) is titrated to patient response. Propofol boluses are given before the start of the procedure and when puncture of the second ovary is initiated; the drip is discontinued 5 minutes before the end of the procedure.

Coetsier et al[38] observed that, after a large number of oocytes were harvested, the fertilization rates for oocytes retrieved at the end of the procedure were lower than those obtained at the beginning. Indeed, a previous study had suggested that propofol added to culture medium reduced the rate of fertilization in mouse oocytes. Therefore, Coetsier et al[38] obtained follicular fluid at the time of oocyte retrieval and determined that propofol does steadily increase in the follicular fluid in a dose and time dependent manner; however, these investigators had used propofol for 3 years before the study with respectable fertilization and pregnancy rates so it is unlikely that propofol exerts any unfavorable effects in an IVF setting. Furthermore, Sia-Kho et al[39] compared IVF pregnancy rates in protocols using propofol and midazolam during transvaginal oocyte retrieval and noted excellent fertilization and pregnancy rates that were well above the national averages in the propofol group. Consequently, propofol is the drug of choice for transvaginal oocyte retrieval.

Complications following transvaginal ultrasound-directed oocyte retrieval are rare, but must be recognized early in order to avoid more serious sequelae. Baber et al[40] reported on 600 transvaginal retrievals and noted three pelvic abscesses, three pelvic hematomas, five cases of sustained vaginal bleeding requiring a vaginal pack, and one case of vaginal bleeding necessitating a vaginal suture—an overall significant complication rate of 2 percent. Evers et al[22] described 181 transvaginal sector scan-guided follicle aspirations with no major complications and with bleeding from puncture sites noted in only 44 (24 percent) cases. The bleeding stopped spontaneously in 42 cases, whereas two cases required application of pressure at the bleeding site. Flood et al[31] recorded two cases of pyosalpinx requiring hospitalization and intravenous antibiotic therapy several days after transvaginal drainage of a hydrosalpinx. It is recommended that aspiration of these structures should be avoided; however, if inadvertently punctured, intravenous antibiotic prophylaxis should be administered immediately. Bennett et al[41] monitored complications of 2,670 transvaginal follicle aspirations in a prospective manner during a 4-year study period. Vaginal bleeding was the most frequently encountered problem, occurring in 229 (8.6 percent) cases. In most cases the blood loss was minor, and only one case required a suture to control the hemorrhage. Two cases of ovarian bleeding were noted, one of which was self-limiting, but the other required an emergency laparotomy to oversew bleeding sites on the ovary. Minor pelvic infection requiring antibiotic therapy was noted in nine cases (0.3 percent), whereas nine other cases (0.3 percent) of severe pelvic infection led to pelvic abscess formation. Eight of the latter cases required either laparotomy or colpotomy for abscess drainage. Bennett et al[41] acknowledged that a preoperative vaginal cleansing preparation is useful and suggested that it is prudent to avoid unnecessary needling of hydrosalpinges, cysts, and endometriomas during oocyte retrieval. Although routine antibiotic prophylaxis is recommended by some investigators,[42] Bennett et al[41] felt that data supporting routine prophylaxis are currently not available. In another series, Dicker et al[43] reported on 3,656 oocyte retrievals occurring during a 5-year period; 14 patients presented with an acute abdomen after the procedure. Nine of these patients (0.25 percent) developed tubo-ovarian or pelvic abscesses that required laparotomy and adnexectomy in three cases and abscess drainage by culdocentesis in six cases. Three patients had significant hemorrhage that required surgical intervention, and two cases of ruptured endometriomas were detected, also terminating in laparotomy. At Cornell antibiotic prophylaxis is used for transvaginal oocyte retrieval in patients who have a history of pelvic infection or a history of tubal disease, as this cohort has the highest incidence of infection in our IVF patient population.[44] Although severe complications after transvaginal oocyte retrieval are rare, prompt diagnosis and timely intervention are crucial in order to manage these cases effectively.

EMBRYO TRANSFER

In IVF centers that employ assisted hatching,[45] embryo transfer is performed 72 hours after oocyte retrieval, at which time embryos have developed to the four- to eight-cell stage. However, many programs still prefer embryo transfer to be performed 48 hours after follicular aspiration when the embryos are at the two- to four-cell stage. The embryo transfer technique is envisioned by many as a simple technique, but it requires precision and patience in order to be executed effectively. The patient is placed in a dorsolithotomy with slight Trendelenburg position on an exam table that is located adjacent to the embryology suite. A speculum is placed in the vagina, the cervix is identified, any excess cervical mucus is aspirated, and the cervix is then cleansed gently with sterile gauze that has been moistened with culture medium. An empty transfer catheter (Wallace catheter, Marlow Surgical Technologies, Inc., Essex, UK) is carefully passed through the cervical canal and into the uterine cavity as a mock transfer in order to verify the correct placement before the actual transfer. The Wallace catheter is quite pliable and has a calibrated, firm outer sheath that can be placed in the proximal cervical canal to aid in passage if resistance is encountered during the transfer (Fig. 19-6). On occasion, however, the pliable Wallace catheter is unable to negotiate the correct path to the uterine cavity, and a catheter with more memory, such as the Tom Cat catheter (Sherwood Medical, St. Louis, MO) must be substituted. In the markedly retroverted or anteverted uterus a tenaculum may be applied to the cervix with traction in order to straighten out the cervicouterine axis and allow smooth passage of the catheter. Many commercially available embryo transfer catheters have a stopper consisting of a ring to limit insertion of the catheter to a depth of 3 to 4 cm, whereas others have graduated markings to allow for proper placement.

After correct catheter placement is verified, a tu-

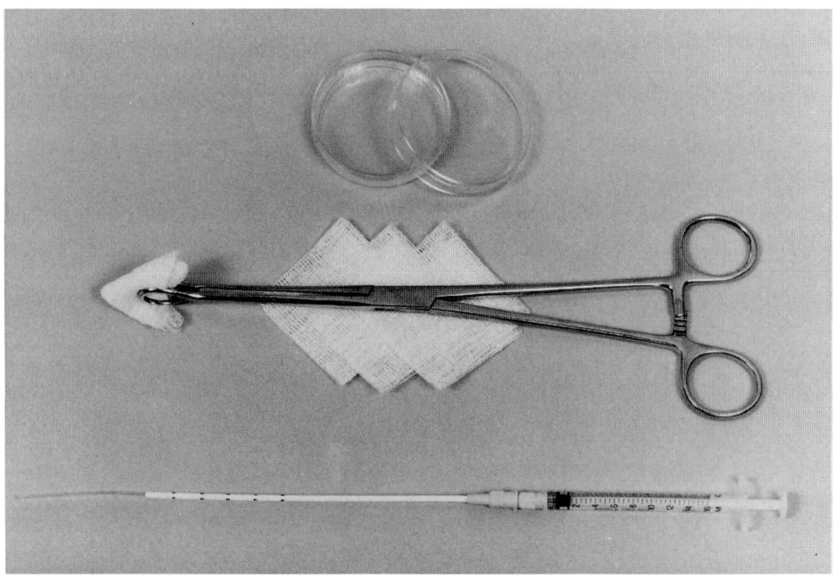

Fig. 19-6. Embryo transfer set: sponge stick and embryo culture media to cleanse the cervix; a tuberculin syringe attached to a Wallace catheter illustrating the soft internal catheter and the firmer, scored outer sheath.

berculin syringe is attached to the proximal end of the catheter and is used by the embryologist to load the embryos into the distal end of the catheter in as small a volume of medium as possible (generally 20 to 30 μl). The catheter is placed carefully through the cervical canal and into the uterine cavity at a depth of 5.5 to 6.5 cm, and the syringe plunger is pushed gently to expel the embryos. After injection of the embryos a momentary pause is warranted before the catheter is removed slowly and handed to the embryologist who judiciously flushes it to ensure that all embryos were indeed transferred. Although many physicians involved in IVF have their personal technique when performing an embryo transfer—whether withdrawing slowly or rapidly or waiting a certain interval between embryo injection and catheter withdrawal—no one technique has been demonstrated to be superior.

Although the embryo transfer is seemingly the simplest of the IVF procedures, it is also quite critical and seems to be the least efficient step in IVF. Despite high fertilization and cleavage rates in many IVF programs, the overall national clinical pregnancy rate remains relatively low.[5] However, it is not clear whether the low pregnancy rate is reflective of poor embryo quality, a poor hormonal milieu, an endometrial factor, or a problem in the embryo transfer technique. Various aspects of the embryo transfer technique have been proposed to influence IVF outcome. One is the choice of transfer catheter.[46-48] An acceptable catheter for human embryo transfer should (1) be easy to use, (2) ensure proper placement in the uterus, and (3) be made of a nontoxic material. A mouse zygote culture system is routinely used in many centers to verify that a given catheter is not embryotoxic. Wisanto et al[48] compared the performance of the Frydman, TDT, and Wallace catheters and reported a significantly higher pregnancy rate with the Frydman catheter; however, the highest frequency of difficult transfers was also noted with this catheter. On the other hand, Al-Shawah et al[46] found no difference in pregnancy outcome between the Wallace and Frydman catheters, whereas Gonen et al[47] found that the Tom Cat catheter yielded a significantly higher pregnancy rate than the Frydman catheter. The Wallace catheter used at Cornell has afforded excellent success, although the Tom Cat catheter is also employed when the Wallace catheter does not easily negotiate the cervical canal. The need for multiple attempts to accomplish the embryo transfer is also a poor prognostic variable. Visser et al[49] reported that retention of embryos in the transfer catheter significantly reduced the pregnancy rate from 20.3 percent per transfer to 3.0 percent, whereas the immediate retransfer of retained embryos did not improve outcome. A third factor potentially affecting IVF outcome is contamination of the transfer catheter with blood. Leonard et al[50] reported a significantly lower pregnancy rate in cases where there was contamination of the transfer catheter with blood. Wisanto et al[48] noted a pregnancy rate of 7.7 percent in cases where cervical bleeding had occurred compared to 21.3 percent when no bleeding was noted. These comments on possible causes of failure in IVF related to embryo transfer reinforce the notion that the embryo transfer procedure is critical, requires significant skill and deliberation, and should be performed as atraumatically as possible.

Ultrasound in Embryo Transfer

Although most physicians performing embryo transfer (ET) still prefer the standard transcervical route of replacement using a blind approach, others are evaluating the incorporation of ultrasound-assisted transfer. Some investigators feel that embryo transfer under ultrasound guidance could improve the results of in vitro fertilization-embryo transfer (IVF-ET), especially when used in conjunction with an echogenic catheter that enhances the proper positioning of the catheter near the uterine fundus. Ultrasound may also be useful in guiding the catheter in cases of uterine malformations. Strickler et al[51] reported the use of transabdominal ultrasound to guide catheter placement during embryo transfer in 16 cases compared with 12 transfers guided by "clinical feel." Under real-time ultrasound guidance the catheter guide was inserted into the internal cervical os, and the catheter was advanced to the fundus until it was noted to curl against the endometrium. It was then withdrawn slightly, and the embryo transfer was performed. A 0.1-ml bolus of air was used to flush the catheter; both the transfer medium containing the embryos and the bolus of air were recognized ultrasonically. These researchers noted that sonographically guided embryo placement was less difficult and the position of the catheter was more accurately determined than blind catheter placement. Wisanto et al,[48] in their study of different embryo transfer catheters, found transabdominal ultrasonography helpful when used with the TDT catheter. Al-Shawaf et al[46] prospectively evaluated pregnancy outcome after embryo transfer with and without abdominal ultrasound assistance and found that ultrasound did not influence the pregnancy or implantation rates. Hurley et al[52] studied the use of transvaginal ultrasound-guided embryo transfer in a controlled trial. Pregnancy rates in 94 patients using ultrasound-guided transfer were increased over a control group of 246 patients, although statistical significance was achieved only in the subgroup of single embryo transfers. Embryo transfer was confirmed by direct visualization of the catheter within the uterus, by noting identification of air bubbles purposefully inserted with the embryos, and by verifying that the flushed catheter no longer contained the embryo(s).

In the cow and the horse, surgical embryo transfer through the uterine wall using a flank incision has been more successful than transcervical embryo transfer. Surgical embryo transfer was attempted by Lenz et al[53] using transfundal transfer of embryos under transabdominal ultrasound guidance. None of the 10 patients in the study became pregnant, and there seems to be no indication for this semi-invasive technique that requires either general anesthesia or heavy sedation. Parsons et al[54] reported two pregnancies after ultrasound-guided transfers; one involved transabdominal ultrasound imaging with periurethral placement of a 14-gauge catheter guide through the anterior myometrium into the endometrial cavity, whereas the other utilized a transvaginal surgical embryo transfer route. These techniques were attempted in patients with a history of previous difficult transcervical embryo transfers; however, no other pregnancies have been reported, and these procedures are rarely used today.

Jansen et al[55] recently introduced a novel transcervical ultrasonographic-guided intrafallopian tube transfer technique. The procedure used a series of sliding catheters to cannulate the tubal ostium, permitting embryo transfer at the ampullary-isthmic junction; placement of the cannula and transfer catheter was verified by transvaginal ultrasonography. The injection of embryos was carried out when coronal ultrasound scanning detected movement of air bubbles through the adnexa, confirming the absence of tubal obstruction. One to three embryos were transferred into each tube for a maximum of four with one ongoing pregnancy recorded. Scholtes et al[56] evaluated essentially the same procedure in a group of 38 patients with idiopathic infertility. Transvaginal ultrasound scanning was used before starting the procedure to define the position of the uterus, and abdominal sonography was effective at the time of transfer in delineating intratubal catheter placement. A maximum of four embryos were transferred to one tube. Difficulty in cannulating one tube was evidenced on ultrasound by curling of the catheter in the uterine cavity. Transcervical intrafallopian transfer was accomplished in 25 patients, with eight clinical pregnancies and five ongoing pregnancies for a clinical and ongoing pregnancy rate per transfer of 32 percent and 20 percent, respectively. A control group of randomly selected patients with nontubal factor infertility undergoing standard IVF-ET at the same time had similar pregnancy rates, although no statistical analysis was performed in this small study. Diedrich et al[57] selected 113 patients with male factor infertility and evaluated the efficacy of transvaginal tubal transfer. In instances when tubal transfer could not technically be performed, standard intrauterine embryo transfer was undertaken. One of 18 (5.6 percent) intrauterine transfers resulted in pregnancy, whereas 29 pregnancies (31 percent) were achieved in the transcervical tubal transfer group. Scholtes et al[58] performed the first prospective, randomized study comparing transcervical intrafallopian transfer with intrauterine transfer. Transfer of up to four embryos was performed under abdominal ultrasonographic guidance. These authors note that ultrasound permits assessment of aberrant cannulation, kinking, or folding of the catheter. A significantly higher pregnancy rate was observed in the group who underwent intrauterine embryo transfer than in the tubal transfer group. These investigators concluded that transcervical intrafallopian transfer did not seem to have a place in assisted conception, in spite of the theoretical advantages known to be associated with tubal transfers.

Another embryo transfer technique using ultrasound guidance has been termed the "Towako method" and entails a transvaginal-guided transmyometrial transfer with intraendometrial placement of embryos.[59] This method has been used in 698 cases thus far and is reserved for those patients with repeated unsuccessful conventional transcervical embryo transfer, as well as for those with difficult transcervical transfers. The overall clinical pregnancy rate of 26.8 percent is encouraging, and 75 babies have already been delivered. Finally, Werner-von der Burg[60] has reported the first pregnancy following intrafollicular gamete transfer. In this case, the patient had standard ovulation induction and oocyte retrieval of all follicles except for the lead follicle. Two oocytes were drawn up into an embryo transfer catheter in which there was already 0.5 ml of a previously prepared semen suspension. After a targeted puncture of the leading follicle, the transfer catheter was threaded through the aspiration needle, and the gametes were transferred to the follicle under transvaginal ultrasound monitoring. The flow into the follicle was easily identified ultrasonically, and no obvious leakage of fluid was noted. The patient was monitored carefully to rule out an ovarian or tubal pregnancy, and the pregnancy was ongoing at the time of publication. Although we can speculate whether this approach has any usefulness in our treatment armamentarium, further randomized studies are needed to demonstrate its safety and efficacy.

SUMMARY

Transvaginal ultrasound-guided follicle aspiration was a major developmental step in the evolution of contemporary IVF practice. Not only has it made IVF aspiration more efficient but it also allowed this procedure to be performed under local anesthesia or intravenous sedation. The usefulness of novel ultrasound techniques in surgical and nonsurgical intrauterine transfers, although of major scientific interest, remains to be demonstrated.

REFERENCES

1. SART: In vitro fertilization/embryo transfer in the United States: 1987 results from the National IVF-ET Registry. Fertil Steril 51:13, 1989
2. SART: In vitro fertilization-embryo transfer (IVF-ET) in the United States: 1990 resultes from the IVF-ET Registry. Fertil Steril 57:15, 1992
3. Steptoe PC, Edwards RG, Purdy JM: Clinical aspects of pregnancies established with cleavage embryos grown in vitro. Br J Obstet 87:757, 1980
4. Rosenwaks Z, Muasher SJ, Acosta AA: Use of hMG and/or FSH for multiple follicle development. Clin Obstet Gynecol 29:148, 1986
5. SART: Assisted reproductive technology in the United States and Canada: 1991 results from the Society for Assisted Reproductive Technology generated from the American Fertility Society Registry. Fertil Steril 59:956, 1993
6. Scott RT, Rosenwaks Z: Ovulation induction for assisted reproduction. J Reprod Med 34:108, 1989
7. Meldrum DR, Wisot A, Hamilton F, Gutlay AL et al: Routine pituitary suppression with leuprolide before ovarian stimulation for oocyte retrieval. Fertil Steril 51:455, 1989
8. Dodson MG, Young RL, Poindexter AN et al: A detailed program view of in vitro fertilization with a discussion and comparison of alternative approaches. Surg Gynecol Obstet 162:89, 1986
9. Mastroyannis C, Hosoi Y, Yoshimura Y et al: The effect of a carbon dioxide pneumoperitoneum on rabbit follicular oocytes and early embryonic development. p. 38. No. 377. Program Supplement of the Conjoint Annual Meeting of the American Fertility Society and The Canadian Fertility and Andrology Society, Toronto, Canada, September-October, 1986
10. Daya S, Wikland M, Nilsson L, Enk L: Effect on fertilization of intra-peritoneal exposure of oocytes to carbon dioxide. Hum Reprod 2:603, 1987
11. Feichtinger W, Kemeter P, Szalay S: The Vienna program of in vitro fertilization and embryo-transfer—a successful clinical treatment. Europ J Obstet Gynecol Reprod Biol 15:63, 1983
12. Lenz S, Lauritsen JG, Kjellow M: Collection of human oocytes for in vitro fertilization by ultrasonically guided follicular puncture. Lancet 1:1163, 1981
13. Lenz S, Lauritsen JG: Ultrasonically guided percutaneous aspiration of human follicles under local anesthesia: a new method of collecting oocytes for in-vitro fertilization. Fertil Steril 38:673, 1982
14. Lewin A, Laufner N, Rabinowitz R et al: Ultrasonically guided oocyte collection under local anesthesia: the first choice method for in-vitro fertilization—a comparative study with laparoscopy. Fertil Steril 46:257, 1986
15. Gleicher N, Friberg J, Fullan N et al: Egg retrieval for in vitro fertilization sonographically by controlled vaginal culdocentesis. Lancet 2:508, 1983
16. Dellenbach P, Nisand I, Moreau L et al: Transvaginal sonographically controlled follicle puncture for oocyte retrieval. Fertil Steril 44:656, 1985
17. Parsons J, Riddle A, Booker M et al: Oocyte retrieval for in vitro fertilization by ultrasonically guided needle aspiration via the urethra. Lancet 2:1076, 1985
18. Wisanto A, Braeckman P, Camus M et al. Perurethral ultrasound-guided ovum pickup. J In Vitro Fert Embryo Transf 5:107, 1988
19. Wikland M, Enk L, Hammarberg K, Nilsson L: Use of vaginal transducer for oocyte retrieval in an IVF/ET program. J Clin Ultrasound 15:245, 1987
20. Baber R, Porter R, Picker R et al: Transvaginal ultrasound directed oocyte collection for in vitro fertilization: successes and complications. J Ultrasound Med 7:377, 1988
21. Feichtinger W, Kemeter P: Transvaginal sector scan sonography for needle guided transvaginal follicle aspiration and other applications in gynecologic routine and research. Fertil Steril 45:722, 1986
22. Evers JLH, Larsen JF, Gnany GG, Sieck UV: Complications and problems in transvaginal sector scan-guided follicle aspiration. Fertil Steril 49:278, 1988
23. Katayama KP, Roesler M, Gunnarson C et al: Ultra-

sound-guided transvaginal needle aspiration of follicles for in vitro fertilization. Obstet Gynecol 72:271, 1988

24. Gonen Y, Blanker J, Casper RF: Transvaginal ultrasonically guided follicular aspiration: a comparative study with laparoscopically guided follicular aspiration. J Clin Ultrasound 18:257, 1990
25. Brinsmead M, Stanger J, Oliver M et al: A randomized trial of laparoscopy and transvaginal ultrasound-directed oocyte pickup for in vitro fertilization. J In Vitro Fert Embryo Transf 6:149, 1989
26. Lavy G, Restrepo-Candelo H, Diamond M et al: Laparoscopic and transvaginal ova recovery: the effect on ova quality. Fertil Steril 49:1002, 1988
27. Deutinger J, Reinthaller A, Csaicsich P et al: Follicular aspiration for in vitro fertilization: sonographically guided transvaginal versus laparoscopic approach. Eur J Obstet Gynecol Reprod Biol 26:127, 1987
28. Seifer DB, Collins RL, Paushter DM et al: Follicular aspiration: a comparison of an ultrasonic endovaginal transducer with fixed needle guide and other retrieval methods. Fertil Steril 49:462, 1988
29. Wiseman DA, Short WB, Pattinson HA et al: Oocyte retrieval in an in vitro fertilization-embryo transfer program: comparison of four methods. Radiology 173:99, 1989
30. Janssen-Caspers HA, Wladimiroff JW, van Gent I et al: Ultrasonically guided percutaneous and transvaginal follicle aspiration; a comparative study. Hum Reprod 3:337, 1988
31. Flood JT, Muasher SJ, Simonetti S, Kreiner D et al: Comparison between laparoscopically and ultrasonographically guided transvaginal follicular aspiration methods in an in vitro fertilization program in the same patients using the same stimulation protocol. J In Vitro Fert Embryo Transf 6:180, 1989
32. Carver-Ward JA, DeVol EB, Evers JL: A method to prevent arrest of embryo development by ultrasound coupling gels after transvaginal ultrasound-guided oocyte retrieval. Hum Reprod 2:611, 1987
33. Lewin A, Laufner N, Rabinowitz R, Schenker JG: Ultrasonically guided oocyte recovery for in vitro fertilization: an improved method. J In Vitro Fert Embryo Transfer 3:370, 1986
34. Aziz N, Biljan MM, Taylor CT et al: Effect of aspirating needle calibre on outcome of in-vitro fertilization. Hum Reprod 8:1098, 1993
35. Scott RT, Hofmann GE, Muasher SJ et al: A prospective randomized comparison of single- and double-luman needles for transvaginal follicular aspiration. J In Vitro Fert Embryo Transf 6:98, 1989
36. Kogosowski A, Lessing JB, Amit A et al: Epidural block: a preferred method of anesthesia for ultrasonically guided oocyte retrieval. Fertil Steril 47:166, 1987
37. Ramsewak SS, Kumar A, Welsby R et al: Is analgesia required for transvaginal single-follicle aspiration in in vitro fertilization? A double-blind study. J In Vitro Fert Embryo Transf 7:103, 1990
38. Coetsier T, Dhont M, De Sutter P et al: Propofol anaesthesia for ultrasound guided oocyte retrieval: accumulation of the anesthetic agent in follicular fluid. Hum Reprod 7:1422, 1992
39. Sia-Kho E, Grifo J, Liermann A, Mills A, Rosenwaks Z: Comparison of pregnancy rates between propofol and midazolam in IVF-vaginal retrieval of oocytes. Anesthesiology 79(3a), A1012, 1993
40. Baber R, Porter R, Picker R et al: Transvaginal ultrasound directed oocyte collection for in vitro fertilization: successes and complications. J Ultrasound Med 7:377, 1988
41. Bennett SJ, Waterhouse JJ, Cheng WC, Parsons J: Complications of transvaginal ultrasound-directed follicle aspiration: a review of 2670 consecutive procedures. J Assist Reprod Genet 10:72, 1993
42. Meldrum DR, Wisot A, Hamilton F, Gutlay AL et al: Routine pituitary suppression with leuprolide before ovarian stimulation for oocyte retrieval. Fertil Steril 51:455, 1989
43. Dicker D, Ashkenazi J, Feldberg D, Levy T et al: Severe abdominal complications after transvaginal ultrasonographically guided retrieval of oocytes for in vitro fertilization and embryo transfer. Fertil Steril 59:1313, 1993
44. Sultan KM, Neal GS, Grifo JA et al: Incidence of pelvic infection following transvaginal oocyte aspiration for in vitro fertilization and embryo transfers. J Assist Reprod Genet 10:PP189, 1993
45. Cohen J: Assisted hatching of human embryos. J In Vitro Fert Embryo Transf 8:179, 1991
46. Al-Shawaf T, Dave R, Harper J et al: Transfer of embryos into the uterus: how much do technical errors affect pregnancy rates? J Assist Reprod Genet 10:31, 1993
47. Gonen Y, Dirnfeld M, Goldman S, Koifman M, Abramovici H: Does the choice of catheter for embryo transfer influence the success rate of in-vitro fertilization? Hum Reprod 6:1092, 1991
48. Wisanto A, Janssens R, Deschacht J et al: Performance of different embryo transfer catheters in a human in vitro fertilization program. Fertil Steril 52:79, 1989
49. Visser DS, Fourie FL, Kruger HF: Multiple attempts at embryo transfer: effect on pregnancy outcome in an in vitro fertilization and embryo transfer program. J Assist Reprod Genet 10:37, 1993
50. Leonard G, Berkeley A, Alikani M et al: Difficulty of embryo transfer and IVF pregnancy outcome. Hum Reprod P268, 1991
51. Strickler RC, Christianson C, Crane JP et al: Ultrasound guidance for human embryo transfer. Fertil Steril 43:54, 1985
52. Hurley VA, Osborn JC, Leoni MA, Leeton J: Ultrasound-guided embryo transfer: a controlled trial. Fertil Steril 55:559, 1991
53. Lenz S, Leeton J, Rogers P, Trounson A: Transfundal transfer of embryos using ultrasound. J In Vitro Fert Embryo Transf 4:13, 1987
54. Parsons JH, Bolton VN, Wilson L, Campbell S: Preg-

nancies following in vitro fertilization and ultrasound-directed surgical embryo transfer by periurethral and transvaginal techniques. Fertil Steril 48:691, 1987

55. Jansen R, Anderson JC, Sutherland PD: Nonoperative embryo transfer to the fallopian tube. New Engl J Med 319:288, 1988
56. Scholtes MCW, Roozenberg BJ, Alberda AT, Zeilmaker GH: Transcervical intrafallopian transfer of zygotes. Fertil Steril 54:283, 1990
57. Diedrich K, Bauer O, Werner A et al: Transvaginal intratubal embryo transfer: a new treatment for male infertility. Hum Reprod 6:672, 1991
58. Scholtes MC, Roozenburg BJ, Verhoeff A, Zeilmaker GH: A randomized study of transcervical intrafallopian transfer of pronucleate embryos controlled by ultrasound versus intrauterine transfer of four- to eight-cell embryos. Fertil Steril 61:102, 1994
59. Kato O: New technique on implantation: transmyometrial embryo transfer intraendometrium: "the Towako Method." J Assist Reprod Genet 10:S-4, 1993
60. Werner-von der Burg W, Coordes I, Hatzmann W: Pregnancy following intrafollicular gamete transfer. Hum Reprod 8:771, 1993

20

Transvaginal Color Doppler

Asim Kurjak Sanja Kupesic
Ivica Zalud Mladen Predanic

Assessment of the female pelvis is greatly facilitated by color Doppler imaging that allows for simultaneous overlayed display of anatomic (gray-scale) and flow (color) information. Two primary colors are used to differentiate flow direction. Typically, blood flow toward the transducer is displayed in red, whereas blood flowing away from the transducer is displayed in blue. It is important to remember that color selection is completely arbitrary and on most machines can be changed by the operator. Color Doppler imaging presents flow information simultaneously across an entire region of interest, superimposing it on the gray-scale image. Therefore, display permits rapid identification of vascular structures, both large and small, and typically results in reduced examination times.

There are many different designs of transvaginal probes. However, probes capable of color Doppler imaging usually use phased-array technology. The purpose of this chapter is to provide an overview of transvaginal color Doppler in obstetrics and gynecology.

EXAMINATION TECHNIQUE

Normal menstruating women are best scanned during days 1 to 10 of the cycle to exclude changes in intraovarian blood flow that are known to occur during the formation of the corpus luteum.[1] After visualization of pelvic anatomy by B-mode, color Doppler sonography is used to locate blood flow in normal or newly formed pelvic vessels. Subsequently, structures of particular interest are examined for prominent areas of vascularization, probably reflecting neovascularization. These vessels usually appear as continuously fluctuating color, rather than the pulsate color seen with normal arteries. A color flow of interest could be explored with Doppler sample volume until the typical spectral waveform is seen. The angle of the transducer should be moved to obtain the maximum waveform amplitude and clarity. Quantification of color flow can be done by pulsed Doppler waveform analysis. The peak systolic (A) and end diastolic (B) Doppler shift frequency can be recorded, and A/B ratio, the Pourcelot resistance index, or the pulsatility index may be calculated.[2]

The Pourcelot resistance index (RI) is a useful way of expressing blood flow impedance distal to the point of sampling.[3] Each separate parameter is angle dependent. Once they are in proper relation, the resistance indexes become independent of the angle between the investigated vessels and the emitted ultrasound beam. The increased value of RI is believed to result from increased peripheral vascular resistance.[4]

NORMAL PELVIC BLOOD FLOW

The newly developed color Doppler modality and pulsed wave Doppler provide a unique noninvasive method for evaluating normal and abnormal conditions in the female pelvis.[5] Transvaginal ultrasound displays uterine, iliac, and ovarian blood flow in pregnant and nongravid women and identifies physiologic flow patterns (Plates 1–4). The transvaginal transducer clearly displays the entire vessel coursing from the sides of the cervix, up to the lateral wall of the uterus, along the fallopian tube, and terminating above the ovaries. The uterine artery spectral Doppler waveform, in both nongravid and first trimester women, has high impedance (low diastolic flow) with a characteristic hump during diastole. At about 14 to 18 weeks of pregnancy, this high impedance flow changes to low impedance with copious diastolic flow. Uterine flow states can be determined easily by the Doppler spectrum.

The iliac vein is most commonly seen immediately below the ovary. The ability to view iliac veins is an excellent way to document patency or thrombosis. The iliac arteries at the bifurcation have characteristic waveforms. The common and external iliac arteries that are part of the aorto-femoral segment show plug flow, a window under the waveform, and a reversed component during diastole. The internal iliac artery, in contrast, has parabolic flow with an even disturbation of velocities within the waveform.

The functional ovary has cyclical changes. The dominant follicle develops a low impedance shunt, probably due to neovascularization of the follicle and ensuing corpus luteum. The dominant follicle in the ovary is detected easily with color Doppler. With pulsed Doppler, it displays high diastolic flow (Plate 5). This low impedance, intraovarian vascularity increases with both ovulation and corpus luteum development and usually resolves by the 24th day of the menstrual cycle (Plate 6). If pregnancy occurs, the low impedance luteal activity persists throughout the first trimester. Absence of luteal flow is believed to be incompatible with a viable pregnancy, either intrauterine or extrauterine. Correlation between vascular flow and ovarian hormonal response is probable, but requires further evaluation.

EARLY PREGNANCY

Transvaginal color Doppler enables a close look at early embryonic development and blood flow studies in embryonal and fetal vessels (Plates 7 and 8). Some recent studies showed promising results in imaging and analyzing of the blood flow in the spiral artery, umbilical cord, fetal aorta, and intracranial circulation.[6-9] Since the process of placentation in the uterus or in the tube is the same, the vascular changes and flow patterns that occur during placentation localize the products of conception. Vascular changes associated with placentation are currently detectable before 40 days of menstrual age.

The characteristics of the spiral artery blood flow are high velocity and low impedance. The high velocity probably results from the large pressure gradient between the maternal arteries and the intervillous space. The signal characteristics of the spiral artery flow reflect the hemodynamics of early placentation and correlate with the histologic examination of products of conception.[10]

Lacunar spaces, which are the precursors of the intervillous space, are present within the developing placenta 10 days after conception. The lacunar and intervillous spaces offer little resistance to blood flow and thus produce signals with a large diastolic component. The high systolic velocity reflects the large pressure gradient that exists between the maternal circulation and the developing placenta. At less than 22 days after conception, only low systolic velocities can be detected transvaginally (versus 26 days transabdominally). Dillon proposed that, as the placenta develops, larger and higher pressure maternal blood vessels are invaded, and a larger volume of blood flow enters the intervillous space.[11] This development produces signals with higher velocity and larger amplitude.

We performed a study to investigate the clinical usefulness of transvaginal color Doppler in the abnormal early pregnancy (Plates 9–11).[12] The study groups comprised 61 pregnant women whose gestational age ranged from 7 to 12 weeks from the last menstrual period. All patients apparently had a normal developing pregnancy; there were no clinical symptoms of pathology, e.g., bleeding in early pregnancy. The diagnosis of early pregnancy failure was made by conventional ultrasound. Eighty-two patients with clinically and ultrasonographically normal pregnancy whose gestational age ranged from 7 to 12 weeks served as a control group. Color signals from both uterine arteries could be seen easily. Location was lateral to the cervix. There was no statistically significant difference between the RI in the left or right uterine artery and among investigated groups of patients. A color signal seen within the echoic area in proximity to the intrauterine gestational sac was considered to be blood flow in the spiral arteries. The visualization rate and the mean RI values in all cases are shown in Table 20-1. It should be pointed that in nine (31 percent) cases of blighted ovum and in five (26 percent) cases of missed abortion, spiral artery blood flow could not be detected. In the control group, spiral artery blood flow was always visualized.

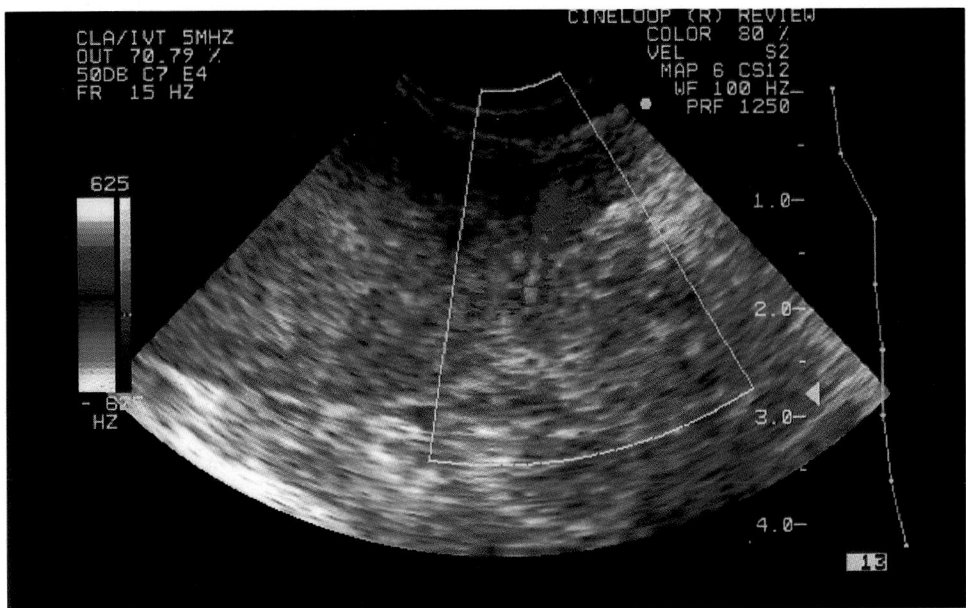

Plate 20-1.

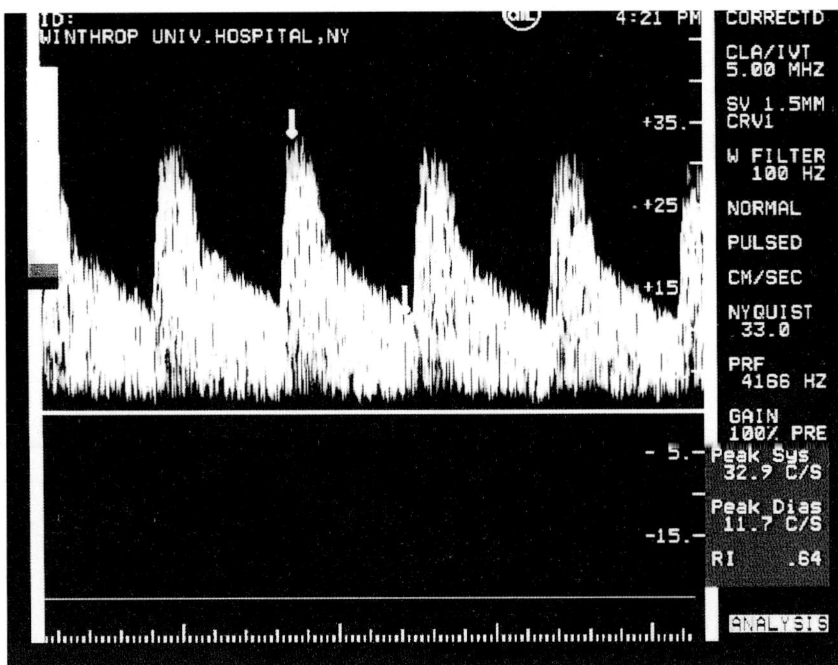

Plate 20-2.

Plate 20-1. The left uterine artery and vein visualized by transvaginal color Doppler.

Plate 20-2. Doppler waveform extracted from the uterine artery. Note high velocity and high resistance to blood flow.

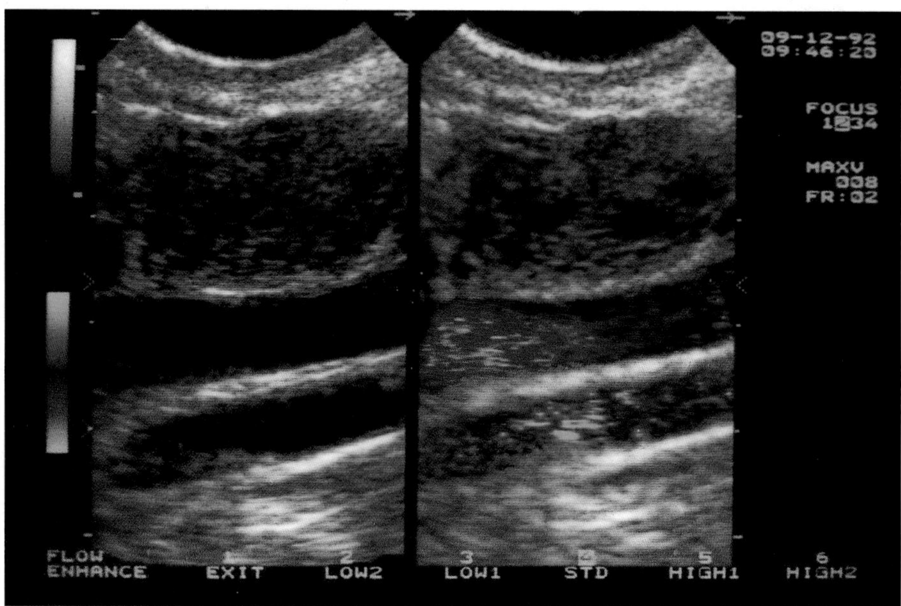

Plate 20-3.

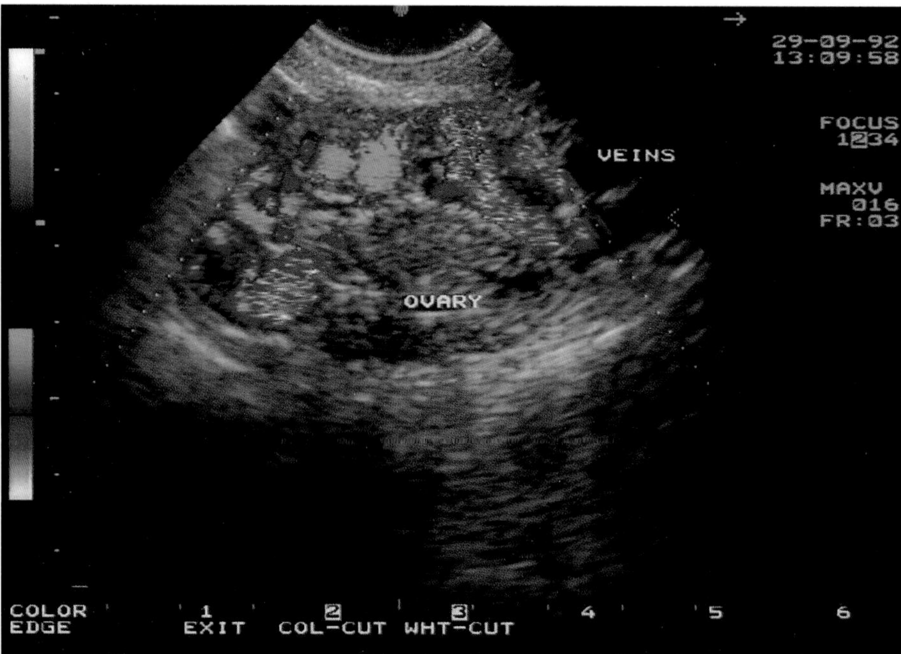

Plate 20-4.

Plate 20-3. Internal iliac vessels visualized by B-mode ultrasound **(left)** and color Doppler **(right)**. Note high intensity of red color due to high velocity of blood flow in the internal iliac artery. Blue color is not prominent, because of low velocity of blood flow in the internal iliac vein.

Plate 20-4. Dilated uterine veins in postmenopausal woman. Tortuous vessel is reason for mixture of red and blue color. Doppler analysis might be of help to easily distinguish this condition from adnexal mass.

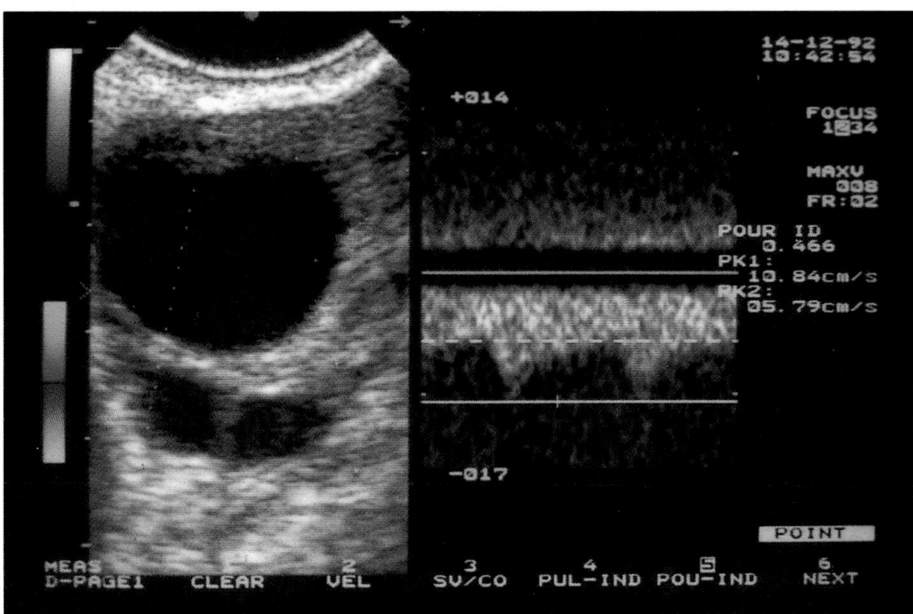

Plate 20-5.

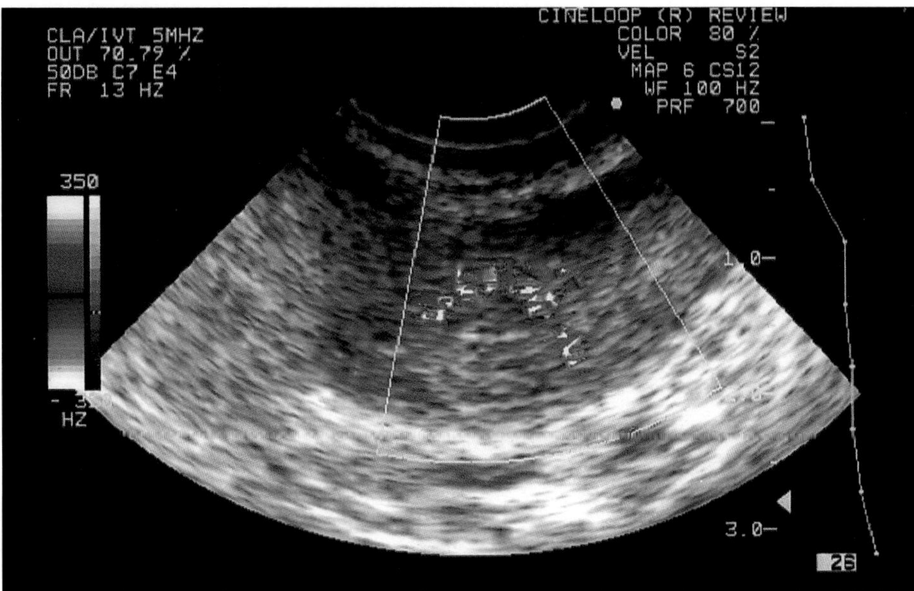

Plate 20-6.

Plate 20-5. Mature preovulatory follicle. Follicular blood flow was detected by color Doppler. Pulsed Doppler analysis **(right)** showed increased diastolic blood flow and moderate resistance index (RI=0.466).

Plate 20-6. Corpus luteum neovascularization. Semilunar color flow is almost typical for this condition, Very small, newly formed vessels are the reasons for a variety of color. Randomly dispersed vessels can also be present.

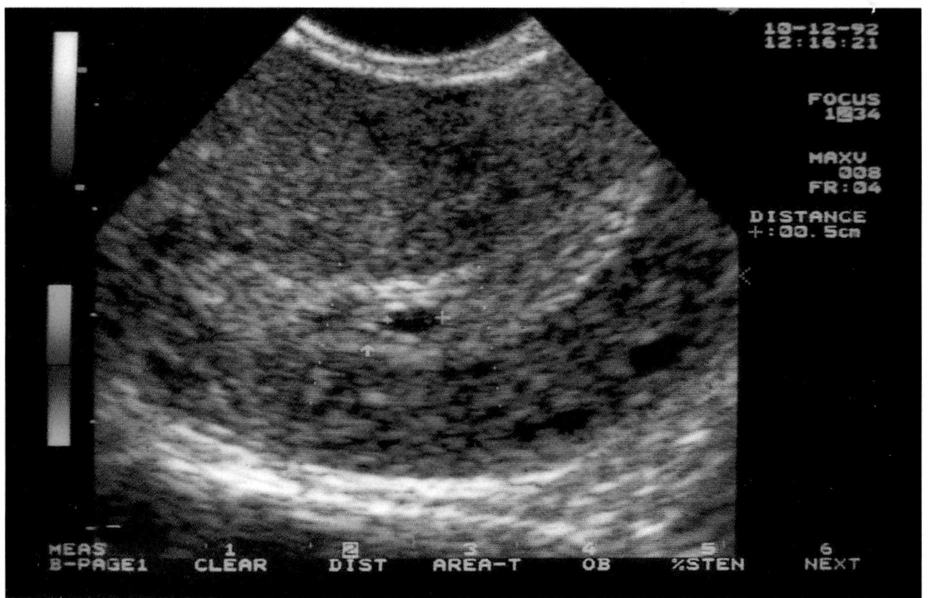

Plate 20-7.

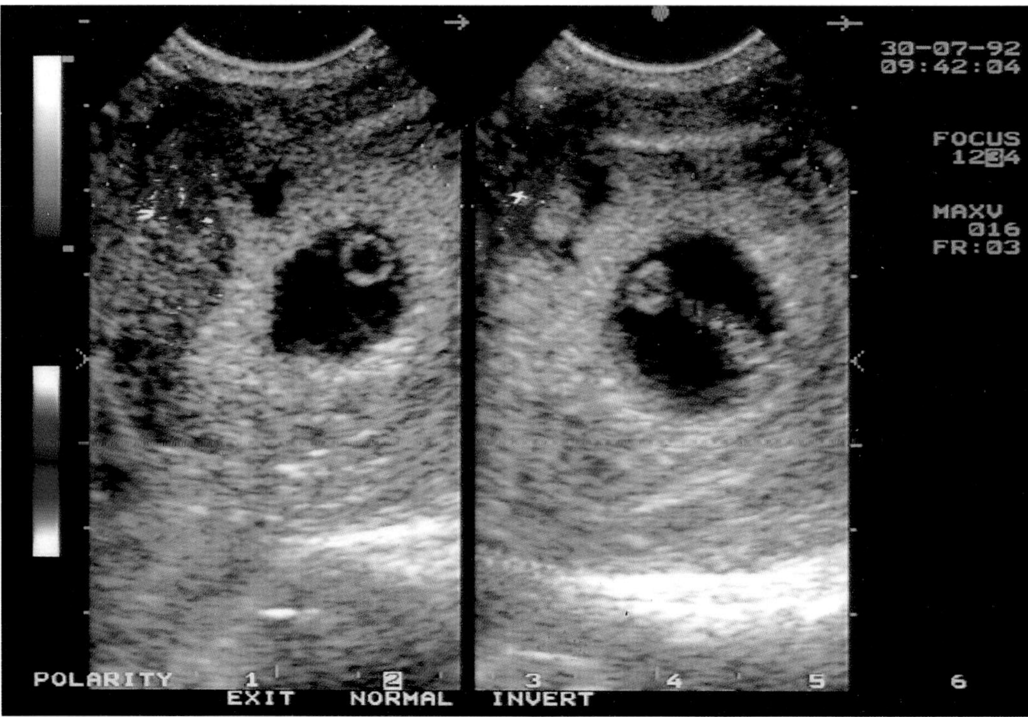

Plate 20-8.

Plate 20-7. Early intrauterine pregnancy detected by transvaginal ultrasound at 4 weeks and 3 days of amenorrhea. Blood flow *(arrow)* was visualized at the periphery of gestational sac. This is the first visible sign of trophoblast activity.

Plate 20-8. Spiral artery blood flow was detected by color Doppler at the proximity of intrauterine gestational sac at 6 weeks of gestation **(left)**. Yolk sac is also visualized. Umbilical blood flow is coded in color **(right)**.

Table 20-1. Visualization Rate and the RI Values of Intervillous Blood Flow

Patients	*Number*	*Visualization rate*	*RI*	*SD*
Molar pregnancy	13	13 (100%)	0.38	0.03
Blighted ovum	29	20 (69%)	0.43	0.03
Missed abortion	19	14 (74%)	0.43	0.02
Control group	82	82 (100%)	0.45	0.04

RI, resistance index; SD, standard deviation.

Statistical analysis showed a significantly higher RI in the control group in comparison with other groups of patients ($P < 0.01$) and a significantly lower RI in molar pregnancy in comparison with other groups of patients ($P < 0.01$). There was no difference in the RI between blighted ovum and missed abortion. Some of the blighted ova were richly vascularized. However, the RI values were almost the same, whether the spiral arteries were full of color or not.

One could speculate that the intensity of color flow corresponds to trophoblast activity. Abundant color flow may indicate which blighted ovum will undergo molar changes. If so, color might play an important role in the early detection of molar pregnancy. Furthermore, different patterns of blood flow (intensity of color, number of vessels, velocity, and RI) might reflect the level of molar tissue invasion. Although no typical ultrasound feature can be used for differentiation between choriocarcinoma and molar pregnancy, color Doppler characterization could be of diagnostic value.

Several authors have analyzed blood flow in the uterine circulation.[13–19] Brosens et al[20] described morphologic changes in the uterine circulation during early pregnancy. Stabile and colleagues[21] demonstrated a falling trend in RI values in the subplacental vessels just within the myometrium, whether the pregnancy was complicated or not. The resistance index was compared with the values obtained from 73 uncomplicated pregnancies and 38 women with threatened miscarriage and normal outcome. There was no apparent difference in the values for RI in the ten patients whose pregnancies had failed, although three live ectopic pregnancies studied had higher values. Jurkovic et al[22] from our group studied the blood flow in the main uterine artery and the radial and spiral arteries. Characteristic flow velocity waveforms were obtained in more than 90 percent of cases. The incidence of impedance to flow decreased with gestation, and there was a progressive fall in these indices from the uterine artery, through the radial, to the spiral artery. Blood velocity in the uterine artery, in this study, increased exponentially with gestation.

ECTOPIC PREGNANCY

Ectopic pregnancy is a potentially lethal condition that has increased dramatically in incidence in recent years. The location of pregnancy, whether intra- or extrauterine, can often be established with ultrasound techniques. Imaging is most useful when an intrauterine gestation is not seen. Transabdominal imaging may yield only nonspecific findings, such as the presence of an adnexal mass or an intrauterine sac-like structure.[23–26] Imaging alone, however, provides only anatomic information that may permit differentiation between an extrauterine gestational sac and some other adnexal mass, or between a very early pregnancy and a pseudogestational sac. Doppler evaluation, which has recently been used to supplement ultrasound imaging in cases of suspected ectopic pregnancy, adds physiologic information to the anatomic detail provided by imaging (Plate 12). Taylor et al[27] identified a characteristic pattern of flow around extrauterine gestational sacs. High velocity (Doppler shift of up to 5 kHz at an insonating frequency of 3 MHz) and low impedance (Pourcelot index of 0.385 ± 0.02) flow was seen in 38 (54 percent) of 70 ectopic pregnancies. The corpus luteum had a similar but lower velocity (less than 2.1 kHz) and statistically higher impedance (Pourcelot index of 0.504 ± 0.2).

Our group was interested to see whether transvaginal color Doppler could provide an earlier and more accurate diagnosis of ectopic pregnancy.[28] A vaginal ultrasound and color Doppler were done, and blood was drawn for a quantitative beta-hCG in 184 amenorrhoic women. Suspected adnexal masses were carefully examined for color flow, and if found, a resistance index calculation was done. Ectopic pregnancy was defined as ectopic color flow, usually very prominent and randomly dispersed inside the solid part of the adnexal mass and clearly separated from ovarian tissue and corpus luteum. Pulsed Doppler waveform analysis showed a very low impedance signal, and the calculated RI was below 0.40 due to increased end diastolic flow. Among the 184 patients, 6 had a normal intrauterine pregnancy, 103 had an ectopic gestation, and 75 were not pregnant. Of the 103 ectopic pregnancies, 18 had adnexal cystic structures suggestive of a gestational sac, with 7 having live embryos. Of the remaining patients, 85 had solid, cystic, or complex adnexal masses. Color flow was seen in 95 patients. It should be noted that there were no cases in which the RI was higher than 0.40. Based upon this data a cut-off point of 0.40 or less has been selected as that which discriminates a potential ectopic from other types of vascular structures that might be present in the adnexa, such as with inflammatory disease or benign ovarian tumors. The fact that the intervillous space lacks muscle layer could explain the low resistance blood flow. The brightness of color is usually high, indicating high velocity of ectopic flow. Adnexal color flow patterns with a RI of 0.40 or less were seen in 92 documented ectopic masses and 3 nonectopic masses. Eleven ectopic masses showed no color flow, and there were 75 women who were not pregnant and had no color flow. Therefore, high predictive values, sensitivity, specificity, and accuracy of this diagnostic method have been obtained.

The results obtained by transvaginal color Doppler diagnosis of ectopic pregnancy have been good enough to encourage its clinical application. We suggest that the current policy would be to delay surgical management if there is no ectopic blood flow outside the empty uterus in amenorrhoic patients. On the contrary, if there is color flow in the adnexal region with a resistance index of 0.40, the patient should be scheduled for laparoscopy. The hypothesis is that the absence of color flow from the ectopic pregnancy and corpus luteum may indicate that the ectopic pregnancy is no longer viable. There is no doubt that some ectopic embryos die and are resorbed. Color Doppler signals might then prove helpful in predicting which ectopic embryos could be treated expectantly.

PROCESS OF ANGIOGENESIS AND NEOVASCULARIZATION

Angiogenesis is the process of generating capillary blood vessels that leads to neovascularization. It occurs during embryonic development and during several physiologic and pathologic conditions in adult life. For example, ovulation and wound healing could not take place without angiogenesis. Angiogenesis is also associated with chronic inflammation and with certain immune reactions. For example, the angiogenesis associated with retrolental fibroplasia or with diabetic retinopathy may lead to blindness in both cases. New capillaries may invade the joints in arthritis. In physiologic situations, as in the development of the corpus luteum or in ovulation, angiogenesis subsides or is turned off once the process is completed. In certain processes, angiogenesis is abnormally prolonged, although still self-limited, as in pyogeneic granuloma or keloid formation.

However, many malignant diseases of unknown cause are dominated by angiogenesis, mostly in solid tumors. The process of angiogenesis developed within a tumor is called neo-angiogenesis or neovascularization. Tumor neovascularization differs, at least in a temporal way, from the other types of angiogenesis in the physiologic or pathophysiologic conditions described above. Tumor neovascularization is not self-limiting. Once tumor-induced angiogenesis starts, it continues indefinitely until the host dies or the tumor is eradicated.[29,30]

Recent evidence suggests that the development of metastases also depends on angiogenesis. Before tumors are generally able to shed cells into the circulation, tumor cells must gain access to the vasculature in the primary tumor, survive in the circulation, arrest in the microvasculature of the target organ,[31,32] exit from this vasculature,[33] grow in the target organ, and induce angiogenesis.[34] Angiogenesis is necessary both at the beginning and at the end of this cascade of events. Tumor cells can enter the circulation by penetrating through proliferating capillaries. Growing capillaries have fragmented basement membranes and are leaky.[35]

Tumor-induced vessels are often dilated and saccular and may even contain tumor cells within the endothelial lining.[36] Tumor vasculature does not conform to the vasculature of normal tissues, e.g., artery to arteriole to capillary to postcapillary venule to venule to vein.[36] Tumors may contain giant capillaries and arteriovenous shunts without intervening capillaries. Newly formed vessels contain no smooth muscle in their wall, but instead only some fibrous connective tissues.[37] Quantitative morphometric studies in induced animal tumors show that vascular volume, length, and surface area increase during the early stages of tumor growth and then decrease after the onset of necrosis. The number of large diameter vessels increases in the later stages of growth.[38]

New blood vessels and vascular channels in a tumor arise from existing vessels. Tumor vessels contain a relative paucity of smooth muscle in their walls in comparison to their caliber. Since most resistance to flow occurs at the level of the muscular arterioles, vessels deficient in these muscular elements offer reduced resistance to blood flow and transmit larger volume flow than vessels with high resistance. Indeed, the evidence for the regulator role of angiogenesis in tumor growth is strong, but it is still not clear what part this phenomenon plays in the process of cancer metastasis.[39-41]

The field of angiogenesis research, which began as an inquiry into the mechanisms by which tumors induce a new blood supply, has now broadened to include a diverse group of scientists who are addressing central questions. It is of particular interest to gynecologists that clinical application of transvaginal color and pulsed Doppler technique has opened up new frontiers in the study of pelvic tumor vascularity.

PELVIC PATHOLOGY

Uterine Tumors

The vascularity of uterine masses has been studied intensively by our group and others.[42-44] Benign uterine masses are less vascularized than malignant ones. Of 291 benign uterine masses, 157 were vascularized.[42] The vascularization of uterine fibroids is supported by the already existing vessels, the normal myometrial vessels originating from terminal branches of the uterine artery. In our recent report,[45] fibroid arterial supply and uterine blood flow were studied. A group of 161 women — 101 patients with palpable uterine fibroids and 60 normal women as controls — was evaluated. There was an increase in blood velocity and a decrease in impedance in both uterine arteries in patients with uterine fibroids. Furthermore, a diastolic flow was always present in the main arteries supplying these leiomyomas. The mean Pourcelot resistance index (RI) of myometrial blood flow was 0.54, whereas the mean pulsatility index (PI) was 0.89. The vascularization of the benign uterine mass was largely dependent on the tumor size, its position, and the extent of secondary degenerative changes. Large and laterally positioned fibroids, especially those with necrotic, degenerative, and inflammatory changes, usually showed increased diastolic flow and lower resistance index. Uterine blood flow had a RI of 0.84 in control group, whereas a lower RI of 0.74 was noted in patients with uterine fibroids. The difference between patients with fibroids and healthy volunteers is statistically significant and may have predictable value in growth rate evaluation of the benign uterine mass.

Hata et al[16] studied 10 women with normal uteri and 21 with uterine myomas by measuring the resistance index in the arcuate artery. The mean RI was 0.768 ± 0.;75 in normal uteri and 0.679 ± 0.131 in patients with uterine myomas. The authors' observations were similar to ours.[45] It is worthy to mention here that sometimes uterine leimyomas with secondary changes exhibit important alterations in their vascular characteristics (Plate 13). A marked reduction in blood flow impedances was noticed, resulting in an overlap with the values for malignant conditions. These observations are still under extensive study in our institute as we work to develop a method for discriminating myomas with secondary changes from other conditions.

Several studies[42,46,47-50] have proved that color flow and pulsed Doppler seem to increase the ability to diagnose the endometrial carcinoma accurately. It was found that arteries that supply endometrial cancer have abnormal blood flow with low vascular impedance.[51-54] In our recent study,[49] of 750 postmenopausal women hysterectomized for different gynecologic indications, 35 had endometrial carcinoma. Endometrial blood flow was absent in normal, atrophic, and most cases of hyperplastic endometria. Ninety-one percent of cases of endometrial carcinoma displayed intratumoral and/or peritumoral abnormal blood flow with low impedance to blood flow 0.42 ± 0.02. Areas of neovascularization were demonstrated in detected cases of endometrial carcinoma. The newly formed vessels were categorized as intratumoral (displaying colored zones within the endometrial echo) or peritumoral (displaying colored zones very close to the endometrial echo). The intratumoral blood vessels displayed lower velocity than peritumoral blood vessels. The mean RI in tumoral blood vessels in cases with endometrial carcinoma was significantly lower than in endometrial hyperplasia.

Bourne et al[47] have studied the impedance to blood flow in uterine arteries of women with endometrial carcinoma (n = 17), in women with no apparent endometrial pathology (n = 85), and those taking hormone replacement therapy (n = 35). They used an arbitrary cut-off value of a PI less than 1.5 as a basis of a positive test result. They concluded that in postmenopausal women who had bleeding the predictive value of a positive test result would be 94 percent and a negative result 91 percent. However, one might expect better predictive values if more specific vessels had been selected; namely, intratumoral and peritumoral vessels.[48-50] Furthermore, the use of the PI as a parameter of impedance to blood flow seems to be less sensitive and less specific in studying tumor angiogenesis when compared to RI. Hata et al[46] measured the resistance index in the arcuate artery of ten cases with endometrial carcinoma and found a significantly low RI (0.535 ± 0.158) compared to that of normal uterus ($RI = 0.767 \pm 0.75$). The RI in the series of Hata et al is higher than ours, as they measured it in the arcuate artery instead of the spiral artery in our series and they only had ten cases of endometrial carcinoma. Merce and co-workers[55] found a significant decrease in the RI of the uterine and intramyometrial arteries in women with endometrial abnormalities, including two cases with endometrial carcinoma, compared with normal histology. The authors concluded that the RI of intramyometrial (arcuate and radial) arteries was highly accurate in predicting positive findings in comparison with the RI of uterine arteries, which was less accurate and less specific in predicting endometrial pathology.

Uterine sarcomas are well vascularized tumors. In our last study, eight patients with uterine sarcoma were recently examined, and data were analyzed.[56] There was no statistical difference between the RIs in the right and left uterine arteries in each group separately; however, a decline in the RI was noticed in each artery when compared with the corresponding one in normal, myomatous, and sarcomatous uteri, respectively. Abnormal blood vessels were seen in all cases with sarcoma (100 percent), whereas 30 percent of myomas revealed tumoral blood flow. There was a decline in the resistance index (RI) from normal, myomatous, through sarcomatous uteri. The mean RI in cases with sarcoma was 0.37 ± 0.03. The peak systolic velocity also showed a decline from normal, myomatous, through sarcomatous uteri, with the lowest peak systolic velocities (Ps) recorded in cases with sarcomas ($Ps = 16.8 \pm 6.4$ cm/s). In the same study, we investigated tumoral blood flow both in benign (myomas) and malignant (sarcomas) uterine lesions in order to assess the criteria for detecting uterine sarcoma and to improve the accuracy of ultrasound in the differentiation between the tumors. The typical finding for sarcoma was the presence of irregular, thin, randomly dispersed vessels with low impedance, as well as low velocity of the intra- and peritumoral blood flow. Both uterine arteries in cases with uterine sarcoma also had a low RI low and low peak systolic velocity in comparison to that of normal or myomatous uteri in women matched for age and parity. From our study, it seems that transvaginal color Doppler can differentiate with reliability myomas from sarcomas.

In an unpublished study, the blood flow characteristics in the descending branch of the uterine artery in cases of *cervical carcinoma* were studied. This work included 89 patients with histologically proved cervical carcinoma and 24 healthy women as a control group. The descending branch of the uterine artery was not visualized in 18 percent (16/89) of cases with cervical cancer and in 17 percent (4/24) in the control group. The RI in patients with cancer cervix was significantly lower than that of healthy women. The PI in the cancer group was lower than that of the control group, but at the border of significance. It seems that the new Doppler technique is not as useful in cervical carcinoma as in the detection of ovarian malignancy. However, we expect that color Doppler may become a useful tool in the follow-up of patients treated from cervical cancer.

Adnexal Masses

From a diagnostic point of view, tumors of the ovary include "swellings" of all kinds that involve the ovary. However, adnexal tumors may represent neoplasms, functional cysts, inflammatory masses, endometriosis, ectopic pregnancy, as well as intraligamentory fibroids or pathology of the fallopian tubes. Ovarian tumors are of great concern because of their malignant potential and our limited ability to distinguish between benign and malignant neoplasms accurately before surgery. Ovarian malignant neoplasms cause more deaths than any other female genital tract malignancy.[57] Due to a paucity of early and specific symptoms, the disease had spread beyond the ovaries in 70 to 90 percent of the cases when detected.[58–60]

Transvaginal sonography has already established a high detection rate of ovarian tumors.[61–63] An effort has been made to predict malignant tumors by describing a sonographic score based on several morphologic characteristics.[62,63] The advantages of this technique have been first demonstrated by the Zagreb and London scientific groups. The Zagreb group [43] has studied pelvic masses and observed low impedance in intratumoral blood flow (RI below 0.41) in malignant ovarian lesions. One false-positive result (a granulosa cell tumor) among 15 benign cystic masses was found. In benign ovarian masses the RI was always above 0.40. The London group[64] supported these results in 18 women with ovarian tumors, 8 of which were malignant. Pulsatility index (PI) values were below 1.0. One false-positive (a dermoid cyst) and one false-negative result (a borderline serous cystadenoma) were obtained. Both groups agree that this technique can detect ovarian cancer at

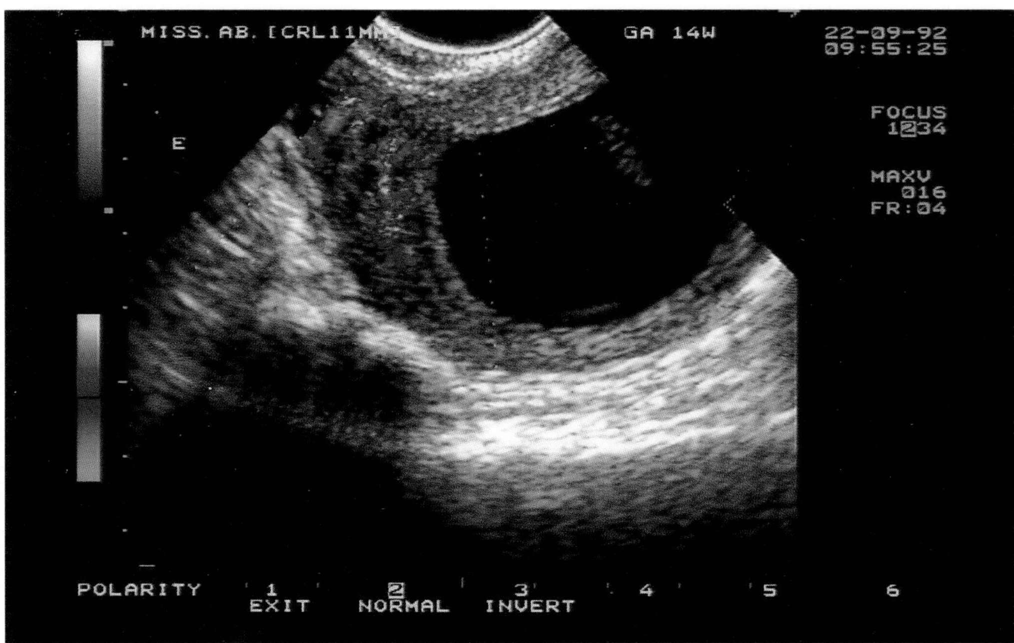

Plate 20-9.

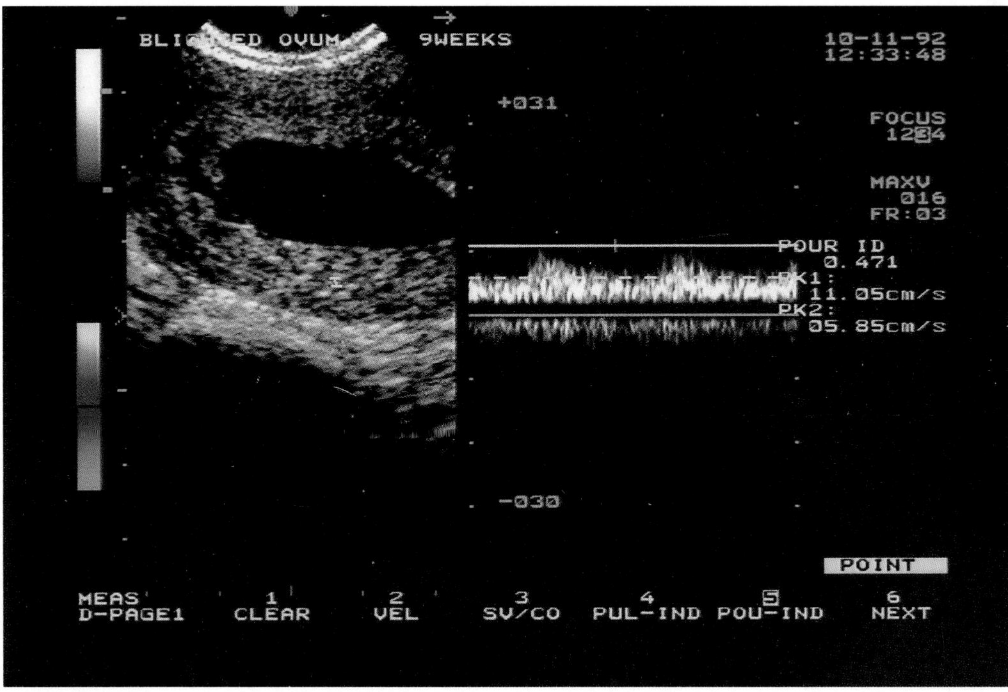

Plate 20-10.

Plate 20-9. An example of missed abortion. Intensive color flow is noted on maternal side of maternal-fetal circulation. There is no blood flow and therefore no color on visualized embryo.

Plate 20-10. Purely vascularized blightened ovum visualized by transvaginal color Doppler.

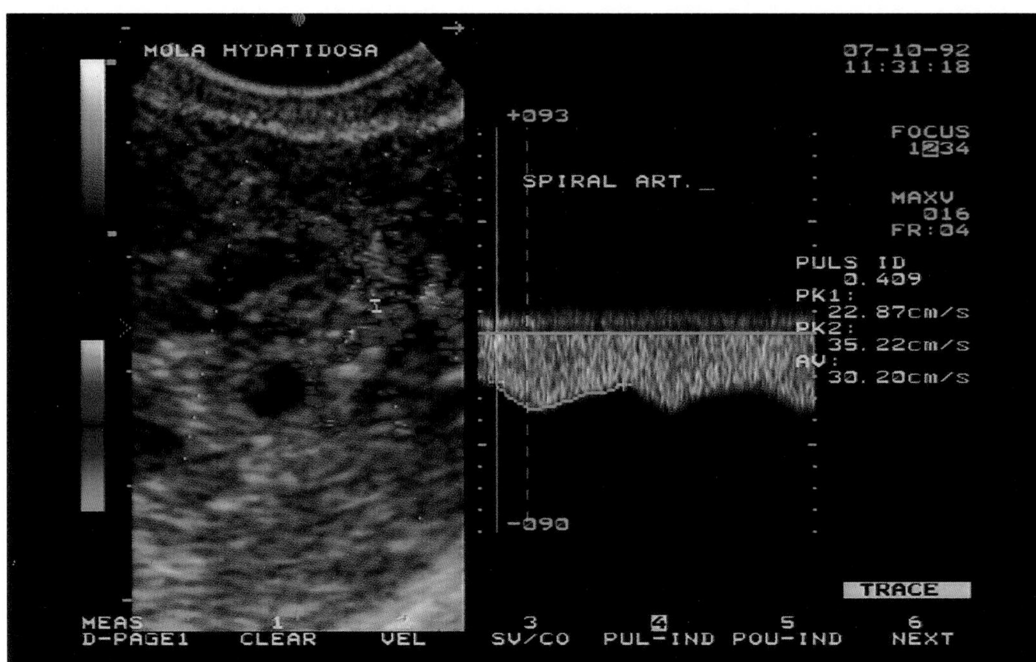

Plate 20-11

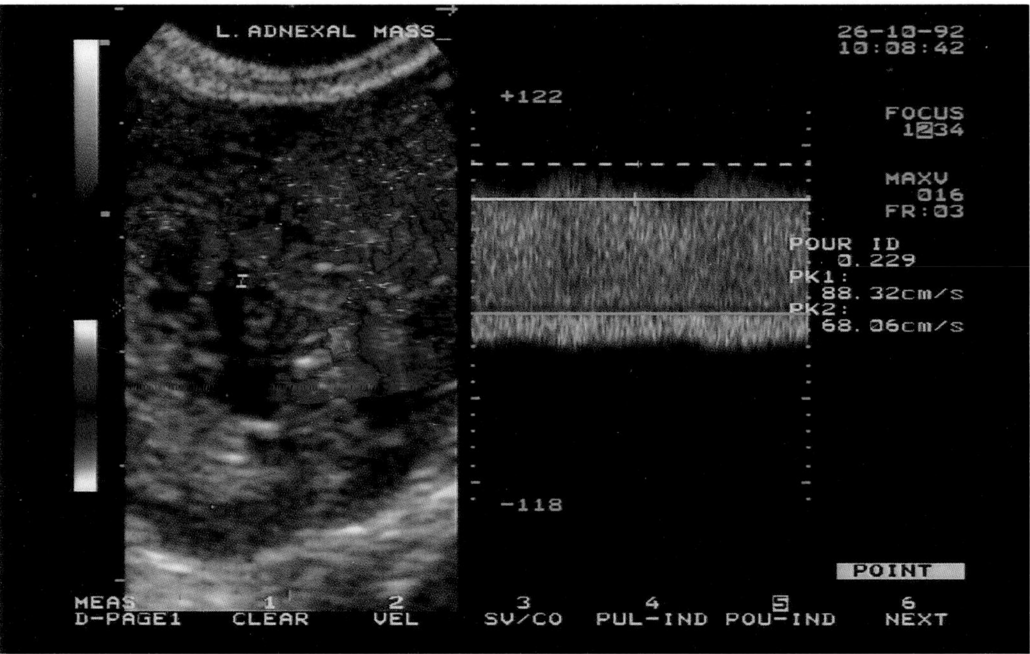

Plate 20-12.

Plate 20-11. Molar pregnancy is usually richly vascularized, presenting abundant color flow. Resistance to blood flow is very low.

Plate 20-12. Complex adnexal mass presented in an amenorrhoic patient with vaginal bleeding. Color and pulsed Doppler were indicative for ectopic pregnancy. Diagnosis was confirmed on surgery.

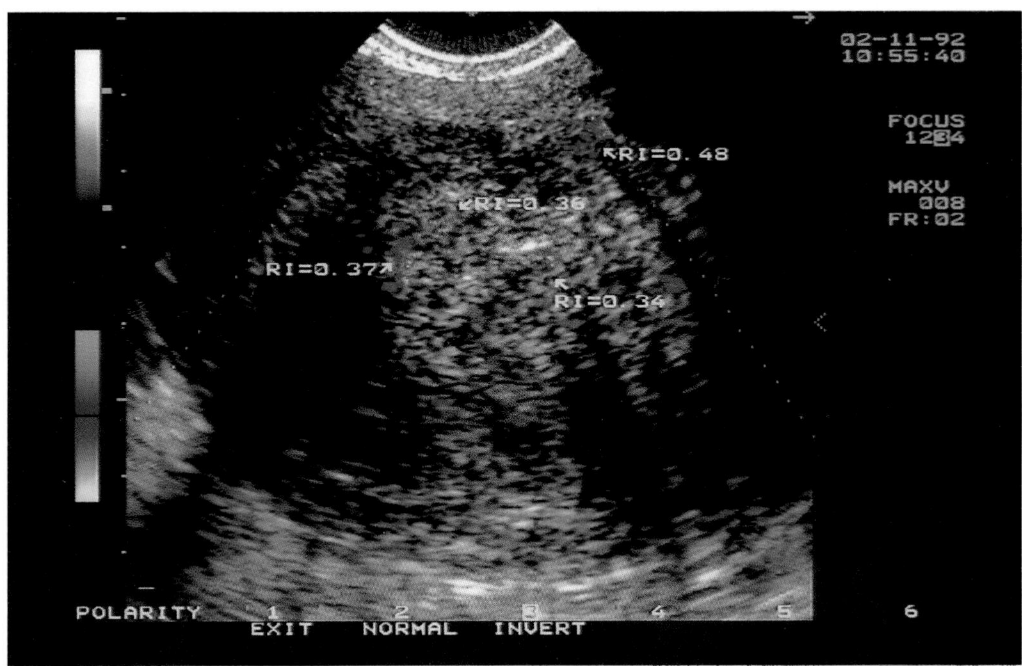

Plate 20-13.

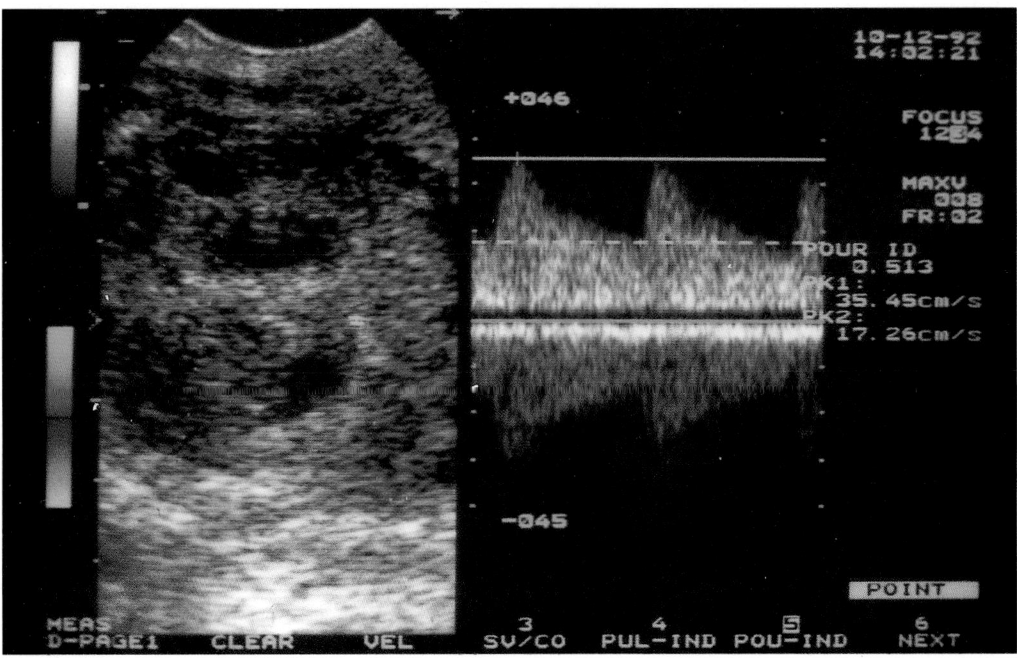

Plate 20-14.

Plate 20-13. Variety of tumor vessels with different resistance to blood flow detected in tumor. Degenerating pedunculated myoma was diagnosed on surgery.

Plate 20-14. Complex ovarian mass. Color Doppler indicated tumor feeding vessels. Pulsed Doppler **(right)** showed moderate resistance to blood flow. Benign nature of the mass was proved on surgery.

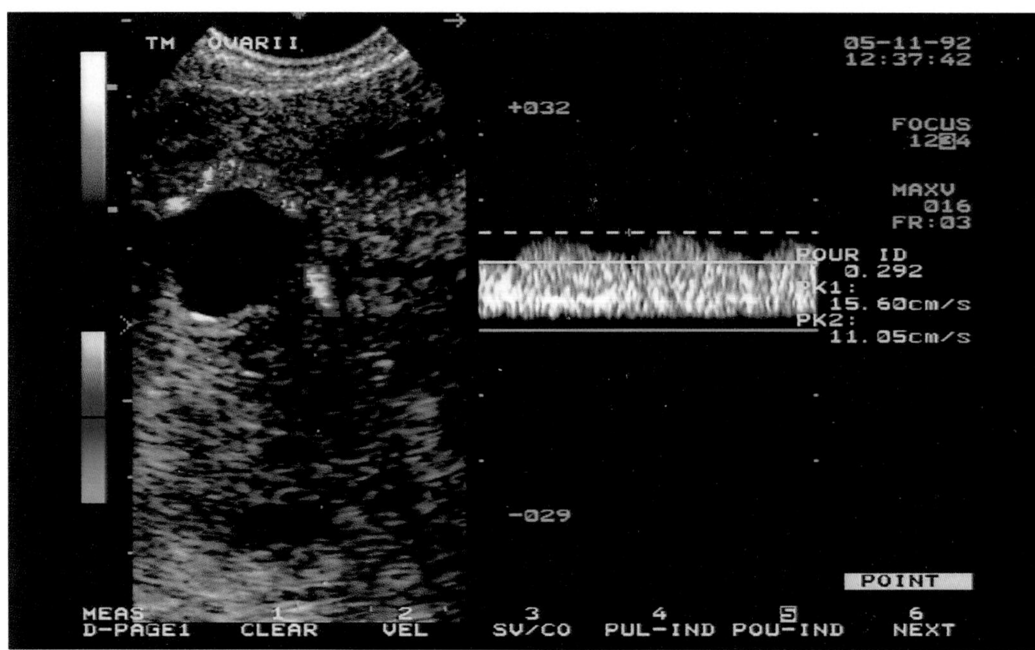

Plate 20-15.

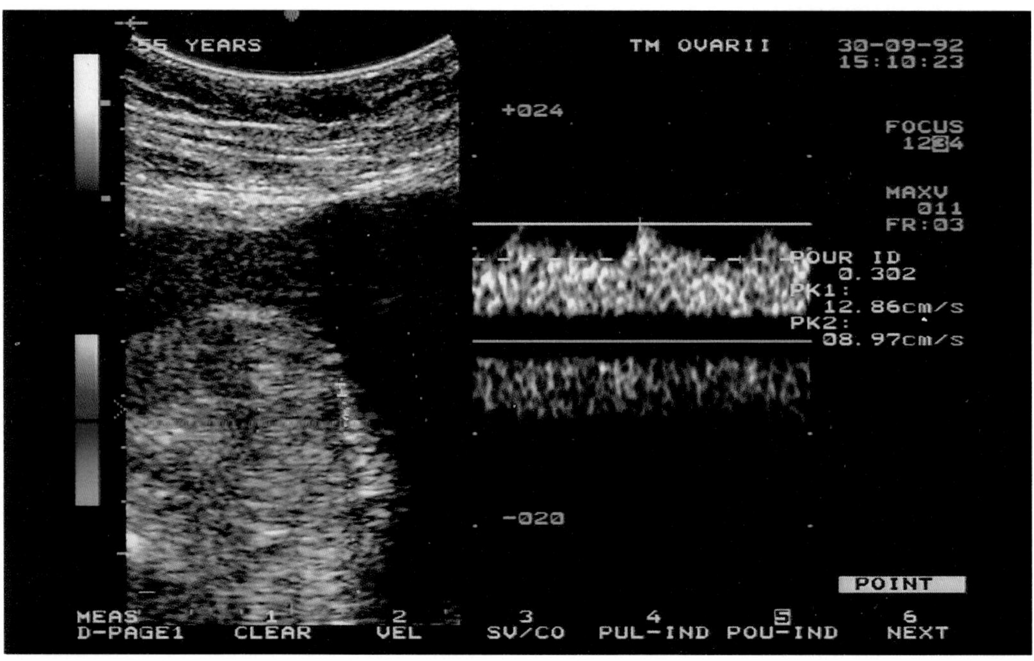

Plate 20-16.

Plate 20-15. Adnexal tumor with some cystic components was seen on transvaginal ultrasound. Color Doppler showed numerous intratumoral vessels. Pulsed Doppler **(right)** showed very low resistance to flow (RI=0.292). Ovarian cystadenocarcinoma (FIGO II) was diagnosed on histopathology.

Plate 20-16. Solid adnexal lesion floating in pelvic-free fluid. Vascular network was seen by color Doppler. Pulsed Doppler **(right)** was suggestive for malignancy. Metastatic ovarian carcinoma was confirmed on pathology.

its earliest stages. A high RI to blood flow can be used to exclude the presence of invasive primary ovarian cancer.[65,66] At the same time, color flow mapping could be used to identify potentially malignant ovarian masses and help elucidate the early stages of tumorigenesis. In our study,[65] a larger group of patients were examined. Among 680 histologically proved pelvic masses, 624 benign and 56 malignant adnexal lesions were found. In every benign lesion except one the RI was above 0.40, whereas in 54 of 56 malignant lesions RI was below or equal to .40. Seven primary and nine secondary ovarian carcinomas were discovered. Each of these tumors except one (stage Ia missed with color Doppler) showed areas of neovascularization. A cut-off point of 0.40 for RI and 1.00 for PI were established and used.[43,64–68] Although these cut-off values were criticized,[51,54] they have value for distinguishing benign from malignant vascularization.[69]

Blood flow characteristics may change with the metastatic potential of the tumor or stage of the disease. Hata et al[51] found low impedance blood flow in eight cases of ovarian cancer (mean RI = 0.50), as well as in four benign lesions. The mean RI values in malignant vessels were much higher in comparison with ours.[43,64,65] An overlap in results was probably caused by their inability to discriminate blood flow in endometrioid ovarian cysts and corpus luteum cysts from that of carcinoma. In addition, in one case the authors misinterpreted internal iliac artery Doppler signals as those within the ovary. The same authors[70] published a mean RI value of 0.88 ± 0.2 for the same benign ovarian tumors and 0.50 ± 0.1 for malignant ones. These results were obtained from 20 ovarian tumors—12 benign and 8 malignant. The possible differences in RI values between these and our results should be sought in way of pulsed Doppler signal assessment. Abnormal signals represent reduced vascular impedance to blood flow due to tumoral neovascularization. Hence, the smallest index value should be considered a reference value for abnormal angiogenesis and possible malignancy.

Fleischer and co-workers[68] described significant differences between PI values of 32 benign lesions (1.8 ± 0.8) and 11 malignant ones (0.8 ± 0.6). However, the range of benign (4.0 to 0.7) and malignant (1.5 to 0.4) masses did overlap. The overlap in results occurred at low PI values (> 1.0) obtained from benign lesions (dermoid cyst, cystadenoma containing a dermoid cyst, endometrioma, benign sclerosing stromal tumor, and thecoma). The flow velocity parameters published in this paper allowed us to calculate the RIs for these lesions. For benign sclerosing stromal tumor and luteinized thecoma, RI values of 0.50 and 0.60, respectively, were calculated. According to our cutoff value of 0.40, these tumors would be assessed as benign ovarian masses,[71] rather than malignant. In another study, published by the same group,[66] similar results were found. Three relatively vascular benign lesions (one immature teratoma, one cystadenoma containing a dermoid cyst, and one endometrioma) caused an overlap between the PI values of benign and malignant masses. On the contrary, Weiner et al[72] found the PI of the intraovarian or intratumoral blood vessels to be greater than 1.0 in 35 of the 26 benign tumors and less than 1.0 in all 16 malignant cases. A recent report from Timor-Tritsch et al[73] demonstrated mean PI values for benign lesions of 1.15 and of 0.45 for malignant ones. These values are much lower than in previous papers. According to these results, it seems that the PI cut-off value should be significantly reduced. At the same time, Kawai and colleagues[74] have suggested a PI cut-off value of 1.25! This surprising statement was suggested after the comparison of results from 12 benign and 11 malignant lesions. Indeed, Japanese authors[51,54,74] have significantly higher PI and RI values for adnexal lesions than their European and American colleagues.[61,65–68,72,73]

A recent publication[75] suggested that a practical cut-off value for either pulsatility or resistance indices that could assist in differentiating between malignant or benign lesions does not exist! In the group of 72 patients authors found 61 benign, 8 malignant, and 3 borderline adnexal tumors. The mean PI of tumor blood vessels was 1.2 in benign, 0.7 in malignant, and 0.6 in borderline neoplasms. The corresponding mean RI values were 0.6, 0.5, and 0.5. The differences were not significant, and the overlap between the malignant and the benign lesions was large. However, this paper contained several misinterpretations.[76] The authors failed to report in which phase of the menstrual cycle the examination had taken place, and they had not used the lowest RI or PI value as the representative value for assessed adnexal mass.

Although there are different opinions about cut-off values, all authors agree that recognition of angiogenesis as a reference point for malignant changes within the ovary has proved to be a highly sensitive parameter. Given that neovascularization is an obligate event in malignant change, this recognition may enable us to observe the earliest stages in ovarian oncogenesis.

Considering the vascularization of adnexal masses, the neovascularization detection rate for benign lesions is four times lower than for malignant tumors.[77] In a group with benign adnexal masses (n = 428), neovascularization was found in 99 cases (22%), whereas in 69 (99%) of 70 malignant adnexal neoplasms neovascularization were demonstrated (Plates 14-16). The difference between benign and malignant tumor vascularization in terms of vascular impedance to blood flow is obvious. However, the location of vascularization is another important parameter in reducing the overlap between benign and malignant tumors. Fleischer and colleagues[68] suggested that, macroscopically, tumor vasculature can be categorized as peripheral and central. Although this classification is not appropriate and is anatomically incorrect, it may help in the location of ultrasonically detectable vessels within a tumor. The authors reported that in benign masses, peripheral arteries had an average PI of 2.4 (range, 0.7–4.0), central arteries averaged a PI of 0.9, and septal arteries a mean PI of 0.7 (range, 0.7 to 0.9). The peripheral arteries of malignant masses had a mean PI of 1.1 (range, 0.4 to 2.0), central vessels a mean PI of 0.6 (range, 0.5 to 0.9), and septal arteries a mean PI of 0.5. It is proposed that peripheral vessels within tumor tissue originate from pre-existing host vasculature, whereas central vessels develop as a response to tumor cells angiogenic activity and/or due to necrotic processes. Vessels displayed within septa or papillae represent specific intratumoral branches. Very similarly to Fleischer and colleagues, our group classified tumoral vessel location as central, peripheral, pericystic, within papillary projections, and septal.[77,78] Our results showed that benign adnexal masses are mostly vascularized as pericystic and peripheral, whereas in malignant tumors central and septal vascularization with low RI values are more frequent. Significant differences between the RIs of benign and malignant ovarian lesions occur between vessels located in the central part, papillary projections, and septa in comparison with pericystically and peripherally located vessels ($P < 0.005 - 0.001$).

Another important parameter in the assessment of tumor blood vessels is their arrangement.[79,80] Vessels have been categorized as no vessel seen, single vessel, and diffuse vessels. In our recent retrospective study,[78] it was found that benign adnexal masses were mostly peripherally vascularized by regularly separated vessels (91.8 percent) recruited from the preexisting host vascular network. In malignant tumors, diffuse vessels were more common (28 percent) than in benign adnexal lesions. Vessels located within the central solid part of tumors showed this vascular arrangement presentation four times higher than regularly separated vessels. It is likely that wherever the diffuse vessel arrangement is present, high angiogenic activity exists. Information about vessel location, arrangement, and Doppler characteristics were used to produce a new scoring system.[81] High specificity and sensitivity have been achieved. Morphologic and blood flow characteristics had been evaluated separately, and final assessment was done using the combination of these two scoring systems.

Few authors have documented the presence of abnormal flow spectra around the periphery of malignant tumors.[82–84] High velocity signals in breast cancers established the hypothesis that such signals resulted from arteriovenous anastomosis.[82] These results were confirmed by several groups.[85–87] Fleischer et al[68] could not confirm these findings, however;[68] they found that the mean blood flow velocities in peripheral arteries of the malignant tumors were around 21 cm/s, whereas in central arteries they were 11 cm/s. Peak systolic velocities obtained from benign and malignant tumor vessels[78] did not exceed 40 cm/s, which has been established as a cut-off point for distinguishing benign from malignant tumors by Dock et al.[88] Furthermore, there was no significant difference between benign and malignant adnexal tumors. Consequently, measuring blood flow velocities could be omitted in further studies due to the lack of significant differences between malignant and benign ovarian masses.

In the future postmenopausal women will constitute an increased proportion of the gynecological patient population. The predominant issues of the past relating to obstetrics, family planning and contraception will be replaced by preventive medicine and caring for the elderly. Our group examined 1,000 postmenopausal women with transvaginal color and pulsed Doppler ultrasound.[79] Seventy-four percent were asymptomatic; the others were referred or self-referred for symptoms. There were 83 women with findings that resulted in surgery. Separation of the groups into those with benign and malignant lesions did not reveal significant differences in age, duration of menopause, or symptomatology. Thirty tumors were malignant, a prevalence rate of 36 percent. An ultrasound score was used to analyze the morphology of all tumors. The score was successful in separating benign from malignant with all indices of normality 90 percent or greater. Color flow was identified in 29 of 30 malignant tumors and in 64 percent of benign masses. An RI cut-off value of 0.40 in the feeder vessels had a sensitivity of 93 percent and a specificity of 98 percent for separating benign from malignant. Positive and negative predictive values were 97 and 96 percent. If others can confirm our good results, we believe that the accuracy of new modalities fulfill the criteria for a sensitive laboratory screening test.[89,90] Furthermore, knowing that a tumor is benign allows for conservative management or a simple surgical approach, such as laparoscopy.

Kurjak and colleagues have suggested that the demonstration of areas of angiogenesis with abnormal flow could be used for early ovarian carcinoma detection.[65,91] Two of 18 stage I ovarian cancer cases were discovered only due to the presence of abnormal blood flow in normal-sized ovaries.[92] Bourne et al[64] reported seven cases of primary ovarian carcinoma. In six cases areas of neovascularization and low PI values were found. The false-negative result was obtained from an early borderline serous cystdenocarcinoma. The overall detection rate was 85.7 percent. The same authors were unable to define a cut-off value to separate the RI and PI of early ovarian cancers, corpora lutea, and preovulatory follicles.[54,69] However, luteal and follicular blood flow could be excluded with examination in the proliferative menstrual phase, from the 3rd to the 10th menstrual day.

In the literature, fallopian tube carcinoma by B-mode vaginal sonography is described[93]. Our group recently presented a case of primary adenocarcinoma of the fallopian tube (stage I FIGO) detected by transvaginal color Doppler[94]. The patient was referred for ultrasonic examination as her gynecologist suspected an adnexal mass. A complex mass with solid parts was seen separate from the uterus, as well as the ovary of the same side. Color Doppler analysis showed highly vascularized areas in the solid part with a low resistance index (RI = 0.35). The diagnosis was suspected on the basis of clinical and sonographic evaluations; namely, the areas of neovascularization presented by the colored zone, and by the low RI detected by Doppler waveform analysis. These findings were documented at laparotomy and histology.

INFERTILITY

Transvaginal ultrasound—color flow Doppler is a dramatic tool for the investigator to study and observe the female reproductive system and vascular changes within the pelvis. The follicle and corpus luteum of the ovary and endometrium are the only areas in the normal adult body where angiogenesis occurs[95,96]. Uterine artery waveform analysis shows high to moderate flow velocity. The RI depends on age, phase of the menstrual cycle, and special conditions, such as pregnancy, uterine tumors, etc.

Transvaginal color Doppler can be used to obtain flow velocity waveforms from the uterine arteries at any time during the menstrual cycle (Fig. 20-1).[95] It is apparent that there are complex relationships between the concentration of ovarian hormones in peripheral venous plasma and uterine artery blood flow parameters.[97,98] In most women, there is a small amount of end diastolic flow in the uterine arteries in the proliferative phase. Collins and co-workers[99] reported that diastolic flow in the uterine arteries disappeared during the day of ovulation. Goswamy et al[97] found an increasing RI and systolic/diastolic ratio during the postovulatory drop in the serum estradiol concentration. Steer et al[100] reported increased uterine artery impedance 3 days after the LH peak. Sholtes and colleagues[101] recorded the highest pulsatility index (PI) value in the uterine arteries on cycle day 16. These findings may be explained by increased uterine contractility[102] and compression of the vessels transversing the uterine wall that decrease their diameter and cause consequently higher resistance to flow.

During the normal menstrual cycle there is a sharp increase in end diastolic velocities between the proliferative and secretory phase of the menstrual cycle. It is particularly interesting that the lowest blood flow impedance occurs during the time of peak luteal function, during which time implantation is most likely to occur. It is logical that blood supply to the uterus should be high in the late luteal phase as reported by Kurjak et al,[95] Goswamy et al,[97,98] Battaglia,[103] and Steer et al.[100] In anovulatory cycles these changes are not present, and continuous increase in the resistance index is not seen. In some infertile patients the end diastolic flow is not present.[98] There are no data yet to speculate whether absent diastolic flow is associated with infertility or poor reproductive performance. It seems that transvaginal color Doppler may be used as a noninvasive assay of uterine receptivity that would enable clinicians to cryopreserve the embryos if uterine conditions are adverse, and to reduce the number of transferred embryos when conditions are optimal. Uterine artery blood flow could be used to predict a hostile uterine environment before embryo transfer.[100] Those women with poor uterine perfusion could then be advised that pregnancy is unlikely in their current treatment cycle and to have their embryos cryopreserved for transfer at a later date.

One of the major problems associated with current IVF practice is the need to use multiple embryo transfers to increase the pregnancy rate, which results

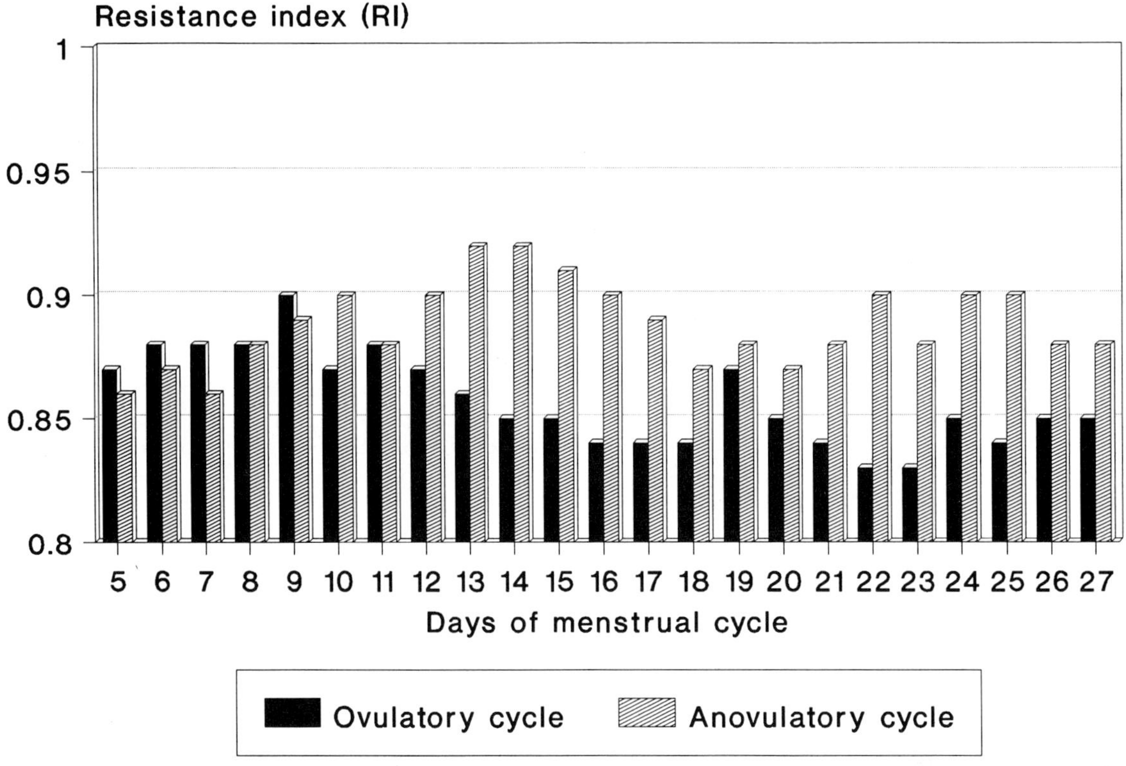

Fig. 20-1. Uterine artery flow velocity during the menstrual cycle (72 ovulatory and 28 anovulatory); $P < 0.05$.

in an increased incidence of multiple pregnancy. This increased incidence may contribute to increased obstetric risk and diminished perinatal outcome when compared to singleton pregnancies. It is well known that the probability of pregnancy is strongly related to embryo quality and uterine receptivity. Instead of doing an endometrial biopsy, which may cause trauma and bleeding at the implantation site, uterine receptivity could be assessed by color Doppler ultrasound. This noninvasive procedure is rapid, easy to perform, and may predict the likelihood of implantation, minimizing the risk of multiple pregnancy. Circulatory changes similar to those observed in the main uterine arteries are seen in the minute arteries (radial and spiral arteries). The endometrium has an exceptional capacity to undergo changes in structure and function during the menstrual cycle. The histologic changes include the striking development of blood vessels, the spiral arteries becoming more developed during the menstrual cycle. The increased endometrial vascularity during the menstrual cycle depends on the changes in the uterine, arcuate, and radial artery blood flow. Blood flow velocity waveforms changes in spiral arteries during normal ovulatory cycles have been described for the first time using transvaginal color Doppler.[104] Endometrial perfusion may be used to predict implantation success rate and to reveal unexplained infertility problems.

Using the same method it becomes possible to assess intraovarian blood flow during the ovarian cycle (Figs. 20-2 and 20-3).[95] Color Doppler facilitates the detection of small vascular areas in the ovarian stroma and follicular rim.[95] Blood flow velocity waveforms from the follicle can be seen when the follicle reaches 10 to 12 mm in its diameter and may be a hemodynamics parameter of its growth, maturation, and ovulation. The RI is approximately 0.54 ± 0.04 until ovulation approaches. A decline begins 2 days before ovulation and reaches its nadir at ovulation, 0.44 ± 0.04. At the time of presumed ovulation there is increased vascularity on the inner wall of the follicle and a coincident surge in a blood velocity just before eruption. These changes may represent the dilatation of new vessels that have developed between the relatively vascular theca-cell layer and the normally hypoxic granulosa-cell layer of the follicle.[105] These vas-

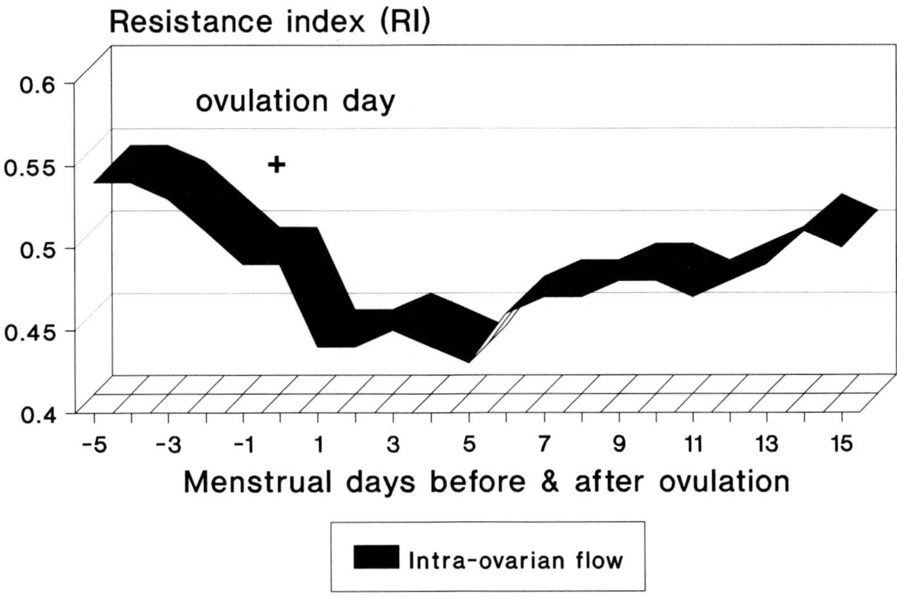

Fig. 20-2. Intraovarian mean resistance index during the menstrual cycle. The day before ovulation there is significant drop in the resistance index, and it remains lower for the remainder of the cycle.

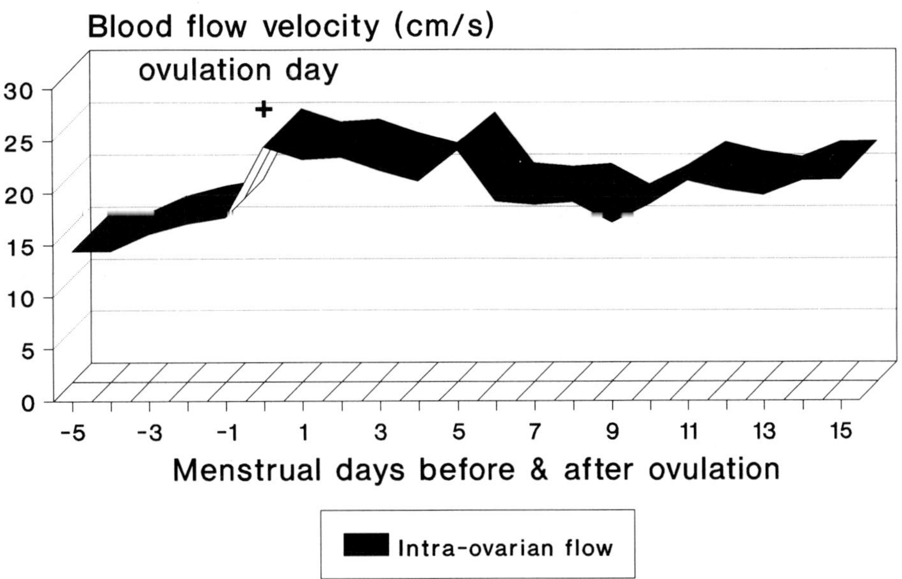

Fig. 20-3. Intraovarian blood flow velocity during the menstrual cycle. There is a marked increase in Doppler flow velocity on the day of ovulation, and it remains at that level for the rest of the cycle.

cular changes compound the effects of the oxygen concentration across the follicular epithelium. Immediately after follicular rupture, there is a further dramatic increase in the velocity of blood flow to the early corpus luteum. The RI remains at that level for 4 to 5 days and then gradually climbs to a level of 0.50 ± 0.04, which is still lower than that seen in the proliferative phase. Collins et al[99] found that the changes in PI observed from the wall of the dominant follicle and corpus luteum were less marked than the changes in blood velocity. Merce and co-workers[106] were obtaining Doppler shift waveforms from the parenchyma of the nondominant ovary and from the parenchyma adjacent to the dominant follicle or corpus luteum in the dominant ovary. Like Kurjak and coworkers,[95] Merce et al[106] detected lower blood flow velocity waveform index in the dominant ovary during the luteal than in follicular phase. Increased resistance to blood flow was observed in the late luteal phase. These blood flow changes reflect changes in vascularization and function of the corpus luteum. Increased blood supply to the ovary containing the dominant follicle and corpus luteum is necessary for delivery of steroid precursors to the ovary and removal of progesterone. Therefore, in both uterine and ovarian vessels changes in flow velocity occur before ovulation, implying that these changes are complex and, not purely secondary to progesterone action. Undoubtedly, many other vasoactive compounds, such as prostaglandins, are involved in the regulation of the vasculature.

CONCLUSIONS

The color Doppler modality is now a valuable approach to the pathology of female reproductive organs. Its validity for the delineation of morphologic characteristics of pelvic abnormalities has been widely tested, and results are promising. At the same time, the opportunities to investigate all vascular hemodynamic changes in vivo permits a better understanding of physiologic and pathophysiologic events in fertility, postmenopause, normal and abnormal intrauterine pregnancy, and ectopic gestation. Still, many unanswered questions remain, and new ones arise. More experience is required until transvaginal color Doppler is proved beneficial for routine clinical use.

REFERENCES

1. Zalud I, Kurjak A: The assessment of luteal blood flow in pregnant and nonpregnant women by transvaginal color Doppler. J Perinat Med 18:215, 1990
2. Thompson RS, Trudinger BJ, Cook CM: Doppler ultrasound waveforms indices: A/B ratio, pulsatility index and Pourcelot ratio. Br J Obstet Gynaecol 95:581, 1988
3. Pourcelot L: Applications clinique de l'examen Doppler transcutane. In Peronneau P (ed): Velocimetre ultrasonore Doppler. Vol. 34. Inserm, Paris, 1974
4. Kurjak A, Alfirevic Z, Miljan M: Conventional and color Doppler in the assessment of fetal and maternal circulation. Ultrasound Med Biol 14:337, 1988
5. Kurjak A: Transvaginal color Doppler. Parthenon Publishing, Carnfoth, NJ, 1990
6. Jaffe R, Warsof SL: Transvaginal color Doppler imaging in the assessment of utero-placental blood flow in the normal first trimester pregnancy. Am J Obstet Gynecol 164:781, 1991
7. Arduini D, Rizzo G, Boccolini MR, Romanini C, Mancuso S: Functional assessment of utero-placental and fetal circulations by means of color Doppler ultrasonography. J Ultrasound Med 9:249, 1990
8. Kurjak A, Miljan M, Zalud I: Transabdominal and transvaginal color Doppler in the assessment of feto-maternal circulation during all three trimesters of pregnancy. Eur J Obstet Gynecol Reprod Med 36:240, 1990
9. Kurjak A, Predanic M, Kupesic-Urek S, Funduk-Kurjak B, Demarin V, Salihagic S: Transvaginal color Doppler study of middle cerebral artery blood flow in early normal and abnormal pregnancy. Ultrasound Obstet Gynecol 2:424, 1992
10. Taylor KJW, Meyer WR: New techniques in the diagnosis of ectopic pregnancy. Obstet Gynecol Clin North Am 18:39, 1991
11. Dillon EH, Feyock AI, Taylor KJW: Pseudogestational sacs: Doppler US differentiation from normal and abnormal intrauterine pregnancies. Radiology 76:539, 1990
12. Kurjak A, Zalud I, Crvenkovic G, Salihagic A, Matijevic R: Transvaginal color Doppler in the assessment of abnormal early pregnancy. J Perinat Med 19:155, 1991
13. Alfirevic Z, Kurjak A: Transvaginal colour Doppler in normal and abnormal early pregnancy. J Perinat Med 18:173, 1990
14. Dautinger J, Rudelstdorfer R, Bernarschek G: Vaginosonographic velocimetry of both main uterine arteries by visual vessel recognition and pulsed Doppler method during pregnancy. Am J Obstet Gynecol 159:1072, 1988
15. Jauniaux E, Jurkovic D, Kurjak A, Hustin J: Assess-

ment of placental development and function. p. 68. In Kurjak A (ed): Transvaginal Color Doppler. p. 68. Parthenon Publishing, Carnfoth NJ, 1990
16. Schulman H, Fleischer AC, Farmakides G et al: Development of uterine artery compliance in pregnancy as detected by Doppler ultrasound. J Obstet Gynecol 155:103, 1986
17. Steer CV, Campbell S, Pampiglione JS et al: Transvaginal color flow imaging of the uterine arteries during the ovarian and menstrual cycles. Hum Reprod 5:391, 1990
18. Schulman H: The clinical implication of Doppler ultrasound analysis of uterine and umbilical arteries. Am J Obstet Gynecol 156:889, 1987
19. Stabile I, Bilardo C, Patella N: Doppler measurement of uterine blood flow in the first trimester of normal and complicated pregnancies. Trophoblast 3:301, 1988
20. Brosens I, Robertson WB, Dixon HG: The physiological response of the vessels of the placental bed to normal pregnancy. J Pathol Bact 93:569, 1967
21. Stabile I, Grudizinskas J, Campbell S: Doppler ultrasonographic evaluation of abnormal pregnancies in first trimester. J Clin Ultrasound 18:365, 1990
22. Jurkovic D, Jauniaux E, Kurjak A et al: Transvaginal color Doppler assessment of utero-placental circulation in early pregnancy. Obstet Gynecol 77:365, 1991
23. Kadar N, Taylor KJW, Rosenfield AT, Romero R: Combined use of serum hCG and sonography in the diagnosis of ectopic pregnancy. Am J Radiol 141:609,1983
24. Romero R, Kadar N, Castro D et al: The value of adnexal sonographic findings in the diagnosis of ectopic pregnancy. Am J Obstet Gynecol 158:52, 1988
25. Emerson DS, Cartier MS, Altieri LA et al: Diagnostic efficacy of endovaginal color Doppler flow imaging in an ectopic pregnancy screening program. Radiology 183:413, 1992
26. Pellerito JS, Taylor KJW, Quedens-Case C et al: Ectopic pregnancy: evaluation with endovaginal color flow imaging. Radiology 183:407, 1992
27. Taylor KJW, Ramos IN, Feyock AL et al: Ectopic pregnancy: duplex Doppler evaluation. Radiology 173:93, 1990
28. Kurjak A, Zalud I, Schulman H: Ectopic pregnancy: transvaginal color Doppler of trophoblastic flow in questionable adnexa. J Ultrasound Med 10:685, 1991
29. Folkman J, Long D, Becker F: Growth and metastasis of tumor in organ culture. Tumor Res 16:453, 1963
30. Folkman J: The intestine as an organ culture. p. 113. In Burdette J (ed): Carcinoma of the Colon and Antecedent Epithelium. Springfield, IL: Charles C Thomas, 1970
31. Folkman J, Shing Y: Angiogenesis—minireview. J Biol Chem 267:10931, 1992
32. Nicholson GL: Organ specificity of tumor metastasis : role of preferential adhesion, invasion and growth of malignant cells at specific secondary sites. Cancer Metast Rev, 7:143, 1988
33. Boxberger HJ, Pawelety N, Speiss E, Kniehuber R: An in vitro model study of BS p 73 rat tumor cell invasion into endothelial monolayer. Anticancer Res 9:1777, 1989
34. Weidner N, Semple JP, Welch WR, Folkman J: Tumor angiogenesis and metastasis—correlation in invasive breast carcinoma. N Engl J Med 324:1, 1991
35. Dvorak HF, Nagy JA, Dvorak JT, Dvorak AM: Identification and characterization of the blood vessels of solid tumors that are leaky to circulating macromolecules. Am J Pathol 133:95, 1988
36. Jain RK: Determinants of tumor blood flow. Cancer Res 48:2641, 1988
37. Gammill SL, Shipkey FH, Himmelfarb EH, Parvey LS, Rabinoowitz JG: Roentgenology—pathology correlation study of neovascularization. Am J Radiol 126:376, 1976
38. Jain RK, Ward-Hartley KA: Dynamics of cancer cell interaction with microvasculature and interstitium. Biorheology 24:117, 1987
39. Folkman J: Tumor angiogenesis. Adv Cancer Res 43:175, 1988
40. Furcht LT: Critical factors controlling angiogenesis products, cells matrix and growth factors. Lab Invest 55:505, 1986
41. Mahdevan V, Hart IR: Angiogenesis and metastasis. Eur J Cancer 27:679, 1991
42. Kurjak A, Zalud I: The characterization of uterine tumors by transvaginal color Doppler. Ultrasound Obstet Gynecol 1:50–1991
43. Kurjak A, Zalud I, Jurkovic D, Alfirevic Z, Miljan M: Transvaginal color Doppler for the assessment of pelvic circulation. Acta Obstet Gynecol Scand 68:131, 1989
44. Kurjak A, Jurkovic D, Alfirevic Z, Zalud I: Transvaginal color Doppler imaging. J Clin Ultrasound 18:227, 1990
45. Kurjak A, Kupesic-Urek S, Miric D: The assessment of benign uterine tumor vascularization by transvaginal color Doppler. Ultrasound Med Biol 18:645, 1992
46. Hata K, Makihara K, Hata T et al: Transvaginal color Doppler imaging for hemodynamic assessment of reproductive tract tumors. Jpn Int J Obstet Gynecol 36:301, 1991
47. Bourne TH, Campbell S, Steer CV, Royston P, Whitehead MI, Collins WP: Detection of endometrial cancer by transvaginal ultrasonography with color flow imaging and blood flow analysis: a preliminary report. Gynecol Oncol 40:253, 1991
48. Kupesic-Urek S, Shalan H, Kurjak A: Early detection of endometrial cancer by transvaginal color Doppler. Eur J Obstet Gynecol (in press).
49. Kurjak A, Shalan H, Sosic A, Benic S, Zudenigo D, Kupesic, S: Endometrial carcinoma in postmenopausal women: evaluation by transvaginal color Doppler so-

nography. Am J Obstet Gynecol (submitted for publication).
50. Shalan H, Kurjak A, Sosic A: Endometrial carcinoma in postmenopausal women and transvaginal color and pulsed Doppler sonography. Ultrasound Obstet Gynecol, suppl. 2:160, 1992
51. Hata T, Hata K, Senoh D, Makihara K, Aoki S, Takamiya O, Kitao M: Doppler ultrasound assessment of tumor vascularity in gynecologic disorders. J Ultrasound Med 8:309, 1989
52. Bourne TH, Reynold KMM, Campbell S: Screening for ovarian and uterine carcinoma. p. 267. In Nyberg DA, Hill LM, Bohm-Velez M, Mendelson EB (eds): Transvaginal Ultrasound. Mosby Year Book, St. Louis, 1992
53. Bourne TH, Campbell S, Whitehead MI et al: Detection of endometrial cancer in postmenopausal women by transvaginal ultrasonography and colour flow imaging. Br Med J 299:369, 1990
54. Bourne TH: Transvaginal color Doppler in gynecology. Ultrasound Obstet Gynecol 1:359, 1991
55. Merce LT, Garica L, De La Fuente F: Doppler ultrasound assessment of endometrial pathology. Acta Obstet Gynecol Scand 70:525, 1991
56. Kurjak A, Shalan H, Kupesic S, Sosic A: Uterine sarcoma: a report of 8 cases studied by transvaginal color and pulsed Doppler sonography. J Ultrasound Med (submitted for publication).
57. Boring C, Squires T, Tang T: Cancer statistics 1991. CA 41:19, 1991
58. Sigurdsson K, Aim P, Gulldberg B: Prognostic factors in malignant epithelial ovarian tumors. Gynecol Oncol 15:370, 1983
59. Einhorn N, Nilsson B, Sjovall K: Factors influencing survival in carcinomas of the ovary. Cancer 55:2019, 1985
60. Yancik R, Gloeckler RL, Yates JW: Ovarian cancer in the elderly: an analysis of surveillance, epidemiology, and end results program data. Am J Obstet Gynecol 154:639, 1986
61. Rottem S, Levit N, Thaler I, Yoffe N et al: Classification of ovarian lesions by high frequency transvaginal sonography. J Clin Ultrasound 18:359, 1990
62. Granberg S, Nosrom A, Wikland M: Tumors in the lower pelvis as imaged by vaginal sonography. Gynecol Oncol 37:224, 1990
63. Sassone AM, Timor-Tritsch IE, Artner A, Carolyn W, Warren WB: Transvaginal sonographic characterization of ovarian disease: evaluation of a new scoring system to predict ovarian malignancy. Obstet Gynecol 78:70, 1991
64. Bourne T, Campbell S, Steer C, Whitehead MI, Collins WP: Transvaginal color flow imaging: a possible new screening technique for ovarian cancer. Br Med J 299:1367, 1989
65. Kurjak A, Zalud I, Alfirevic A: Evaluation of adnexal masses with transvaginal color ultrasound. J Ultrasound Med 10:295, 1991
66. Fleischer AC, Rogers WH, Rao BK, Keppler DM, Jones HW: Transvaginal color Doppler sonography of ovarian masses with pathological correlation. Ultrasound Obstet Gynecol 1:275, 1991
67. Kurjak A: Screening for ovarian malignancy by transvaginal color flow mapping. Ultrasound Obstet Gynecol, suppl. 1. 1:85, 1991
68. Fleischer AC, Rodgers WH, Rao BK, Keppler DM, Worrel JA, Williams L, Howard WJ: Assessment of ovarian tumor vascularity with transvaginal color Doppler sonography. J Ultrasound Med 10:563, 1991
69. Campbell S, Bourne TH, Reynolds K, Hampson J, Royston P, Whitehead MI, Collins WP: Role of colour Doppler in an ultrasound-based screening programme. p. 237. In Sharp F, Mason WP, Creasman W (eds): Ovarian Cancer. 2: Biology, Diagnosis and Management. Chamman Hall Medical, London, 1992
70. Hata K, Makihara K, Hata T et al: Transvaginal color Doppler imaging for hemodynamic assessment of reproductive tract tumors. Int J Gynecol Obstet, 36:301, 1991
71. Kurjak A, Predanic M, Shalan H: Resistance versus pulsatility index. J Ultrasound Med (in press).
72. Weiner Z, Thaler I, Beck D, Rottem S, Deutchs M, Brandes JM: Differentiating malignant from benign ovarian tumors with transvaginal color flow imaging. Obstet Gynecol 79:159, 1992
73. Timor-Tritsch IE, Lerner J, Monteagudo A, Santos R: Transvaginal sonographic characterization of ovarian masses using color-flow directed Doppler measurements. Ultrasound Obstet Gynecol suppl. 1. 2:171, 1992
74. Kawai M, Kano T, Kikkawa F, Maeda O, Oguchi H, Tomoda Y: Transvaginal Doppler ultrasound with color flow imaging in the diagnosis of ovarian cancer. Obstet Gynecol 79:163, 1992
75. Tekay A, Jouppila P: Validity of pulsatility and resistance indices in classification of adnexal tumors with transvaginal color Doppler ultrasound. Ultrasound Obstet Gynecol 2:338, 1992
76. Shalan H, Predanic M: Discrimination between benign and malignant adnexal tumors letter. Ultrasound Obstet Gynecol 2:447, 1993
77. Kurjak A, Kupesic-Urek S: Transvaginal color Doppler in early detection of ovarian cancer. J Eur Med Ultrasound 12:15, 1992
78. Kurjak A, Zalud I, Schulman H: Adnexal masses. p. 93. In Kurjak A (ed): Transvaginal Color Doppler Sonography. Parthenon Publishing Group, Lanks, United Kingdom, 1990
79. Kurjak A, Schulman H, Sosic A, Zalud I, Shalan H: Transvaginal ultrasound, color flow, and Doppler waveform of the postmenopausal adnexal mass. Obstet Gynecol, (in press).
80. Kurjak A, Predanic M, Kupesic-Urek S: Transvaginal color and pulsed Doppler assessment of adnexal tumors vascularity. Gynecol Oncol (submitted for publication).
81. Kurjak A, Predanic M: New scoring system for predic-

tion of ovarian malignancy based on transvaginal color Doppler. J Ultrasound Med (in press).
82. Wells PNT, Halliwell M, Skidmore R, Webb AJ, Woodcock JP: Tumor detection by ultrasonic Doppler blood flow signals. Ultrasonics 15:231, 1977
83. Burns PN, Halliwell M, Wells PNT, Webb AJ: Ultrasonic Doppler studies of the breast. Ultrasound Med Biol 8:127, 1982
84. Minasian M, Bamber JC: A Preliminary assessment of an ultrasonic Doppler method for the study of blood flow in human breast cancer. Ultrasound Med Biol 8: 357, 1982
85. Jellins J, Kossoff G, Boyd J, Reeve TS: The complementary role of Doppler to the B-mode examination of the breast. J Ultrasound Med 59:89, 1983
86. Taylor KJW, Ramos I, Carter D, Morse SS, Snower D, Fortune K: Correlation of Doppler ultrasound tumor signals with neovascular morphologic features. Radiology 166:57, 1988
87. Hata H, Hata K, Yamane Y, Kitao M: Real-time two-dimensional and pulsed Doppler ultrasound detection of intrapelvic neoplastic tumor and abnormal pathogenic changes: preliminary report. J Cardiovasc Ultrasonog 7:135, 1988
88. Dock W, Grabanwoger F, Metz V, Elbenberger K, Farres M: Tumor vascularization: assessment with duplex sonography. Radiology 181:241, 1991
89. Kurjak A: Ultrasound and ovarian cancer, editorial. Ultrasound Obstet Gynecol 1:231, 1992
90. Kurjak A, Salihagic A, Kupesic-Urek S, Predanic A: Clinical value of the assessment of gynecological tumor angiogenesis by transvaginal color Doppler. Ann Med 24:97, 1992
91. Kurjak A, Shalan H, Matijevic R, Predanic M: Stage I ovarian cancer by transvaginal color Doppler sonography: a report of 18 cases. Ultrasound Obstet Gynecol (submitted for publication).
92. Kurjak A, Shalan H, Matijevic R: Early stage of ovarian cancer: diagnostic potential of transvaginal color Doppler imaging, abstracted. Ultrasound Obstet Gynecol 2:100, 1992
93. Timor-Tritsch IE, Rottem S, Lewit N: The fallopian tubes. p. 131. In Timor-Tritsch IE, Rottem S: (eds): Transvaginal Sonography. 2nd Ed. Elsevier, New York, 1991
94. Shalan H, Sosic A, Kurjak A: Fallopian tube carcinoma: recent diagnostic approach by color Doppler imaging. Ultrasound Obstet Gynecol 2:297, 1992
95. Kurjak A, Kupesic-Urek S, Schulman H: Transvaginal color Doppler in the assessment of ovarian and uterine blood flow in infertile women. Fertil Steril 56:870, 1991
96. Findlay JK: Angiogenesis in reproductive tissues. J Endocrinol 111:357, 1986
97. Goswamy RK, Williams G, Streptoe PC: Decreased uterine perfusion: a cause of infertility. Hum Reprod 3:955, 1988
98. Goswamy RK, Streptoe PC: Doppler ultrasound study of uterine artery in spontaneous ovarian cycles. Hum Reprod 3:721, 1988
99. Collins W, Jurkovic D, Bourne T, Kurjak A, Campbell S: Ovarian morphology, endocrine function and intrafollicular blood flow during the peri-ovulatory period. Hum Reprod 3:319, 1991
100. Steer CV, Mills CV, Campbell S: Vaginal color Doppler assessment on the day of embryo transfer (ET) accurately predicts patients in an in vitro fertilization programme with suboptimal uterine perfusion who fail to be pregnant. Ultrasound Obstet Gynecol 1:79, 1991
101. Scholtes MCW, Wladimiroff JW, van Rijen HJM, Hop WCJ: Uterine and ovarian flow velocity waveforms in the normal menstrual cycle: a transvaginal study. Fertil Steril 52:981, 1989
102. Hauksson A, Akerlund M, Melin P: Uterine blood flow and myometrial activity at menstruation, and the action of vasopressin and a synthetic antagonist. Br J Obstet Gynaecol 95:898, 1988
103. Battaglia C, Larocca E, Lanzani A, Valentini M, Genazzani AR: Doppler ultrasound studies of the uterine arteries in spontaneous and IVF cycles. Gynecol Endocrinol 4:245, 1990
104. Kupesic S, Kurjak A: Uterine and ovarian perfusion during the preovulatory period assisted by transvaginal color Doppler. Fertil Steril (in press).
105. Merce LT, Garces D, Barco MJ, de la Fuente F: Intraovarian Doppler velocimetry in ovulatory, disovulatory and anovulatory cycles. Ultrasound Obstet Gynaecol 2:197, 1992

Index

Page numbers followed by *f* indicate figures; those followed by *t* indicate tables.

A

Abdominal ultrasonography. *See also* Transabdominal ultrasonography.
  imaging of fetal heart by, 224
  of ovaries, postmenopausal, 121
  visualization of fetal head by, 231, 231f
Abortion, spontaneous
  confirmation of, 2–3
  hMG-related, 304
  incomplete, ultrasound in, 212, 212t
  inevitable
    diagnosis of, 210, 211t
    differentiated from developing pregnancy, 192
    presumptive signs of, 193
  leiomyoma-related, 158
  vaginal bleeding and, 169, 170t, 205, 206
Abscess
  diverticular, 138, 148
  pelvic, 318
  tubo-ovarian, 149, 318
    drainage of, transvaginal ultrasound for, 149, 150f, 151, 151f, 152f–154f, 154, 155f
Acardia, 232, 234f
Acoustic impedance, 46–47
Acute abdomen, oocyte retrieval-related, 317
Adenomyosis
  diagnosis of, 172
  uterine, 52
    symptoms of, 56, 60
    transvaginal ultrasonography of, 56, 60, 60t
Adhesions, 162
  ovarian, 105, 106f
  pelvic, 40, 195
Adnexa
  in endometriosis, 162
  evaluation of, in infertility, 158
  left, visualization of, 138
Adnexal masses
  cyst. *See* Cysts, adnexal.
  identification of, in ectopic pregnancy, 200, 241, 242, 242f, 243, 243f, 246f
  imaging of, transvaginal ultrasound compared with transabdominal ultrasound, 10
  observation of, 124
  sonographic findings in, 127
  transvaginal color Doppler evaluation of, 330–333
    in differentiation of benign and malignant disease, 331–332
Age. *See also* Conceptual age; Gestational age.
  ovarian volume and diameter related to, 109, 110f, 111t, 120, 121
Amenorrhea
  etiology of, 163, 167f
    anatomic, 163, 164
    endocrine abnormalities, 164, 167, 168, 168f
    ovarian failure, 164
  hypoestrogenic, 167
  normal endometrial pattern in, 91
  normoestrogenic, 167
  withdrawal to progesterone challenge in, 293, 293f
Amnion, in early pregnancy, 193, 196, 198f
Amniotic cavity, formation of, 188
Ampicillin, 274
Amplifier, of ultrasound machine, 19, 21f
Amplitude mode (A-mode), 19
Amplitude of sound, 17–18, 18f
Analgesia, in oocyte retrieval, 317
Anechoic echogenicity, 41
  defined, 41t
Anechoic pattern
  endometrial, 74, 75f, 88, 89, 90f
    in postmenopausal women, 97
  ovarian
    anovulation cycle and, 292
    in postmenopausal women, 121
  ovarian cyst and, 123f, 124, 125f
Anemia, hydatiform mole-related, 179
Anencephalus, 222
Anesthesia requirements, for oocyte retrieval, 316, 317
Aneuploidy, autosomal, 230
Angiogenesis, 328–329
Anosigmoidoscopy, 145
Anovulation. *See also* Ovulation, induction of.
  diagnosis of, 279, 280
  ultrasound evaluation of
    endometrial hyperechoic echo in, 87, 88
    in infertility, 159–160, 160t, 161
  WHO classification of, 290, 293, 298
Anovulatory cycles
  endometrium in, 293, 293f, 294
  ovary in, 290, 291f, 292, 292f, 293
Anterior posterior pelvic (AP-pelvic) plane
  description of, 12, 14f
  endometrial measurement in, 94
  imaging of ovaries in, 105, 106f, 108f, 135f
    of cysts, 127f
  imaging of uterus in, 26, 52, 135f
    for showing single-line endometrium, 117f
Antibiotics
  for pelvic inflammatory disease, 151
  prophylactic, use of
    in invasive techniques, 273

Antibiotics *(Continued)*
in ultrasound-guided oocyte retrieval, 317
Anticoagulants, menometorrhagia from, 169t, 170
AP-pelvic plane. *See* Anterior posterior pelvic plane.
Appendicitis, 133
diagnosis of, 138–140, 139f–140f
differentiated from pelvic inflammatory disease, 148
Arcuate vessels
calcification of, 67
imaging of, 33, 33f, 34f
Artifacts, acoustic
causes of, 43
comet tail, 46, 47, 48f
in endometrial ultrasound, 79
mirror image, 61
reverberation, 43, 46–47, 44f–48f
ring-down, 47, 47f
shadows. *See* Shadowing.
side-lobe, 48
slice-thickness, 48–49
split image, 47–48
Artificial insemination, timing of, 281, 284, 286t
Ascites, in ovarian cancer, 127
Ascitic fluid, aspiration of, in ovarian hyperstimulation syndrome, 307
Asherman's syndrome, 85
amenorrhea related to, 163
causes of, 174
diagnosis of, 163, 185
Assisted hatching, 318
Assisted reproductive technologies. *See also* In vitro fertilization.
aspiration of ovarian follicle for, 276–277
Athletic women, transverse ultrasonography in, 6
Atresia, cervical, 61, 61f, 64
Attenuation, 19
Autopsy data, as reference for normal uterine size, 51
Axial resolution, 1–2, 21

B

Basal body temperature
confirmation of ovulation by, 111, 117
diagnosis of anovulation by, 279
Bel, defined, 18
Beta-human chorionic gonadotropin (β-hCG), 149, 184, 188
in amenorrheic women, 327
levels
in ectopic pregnancy, 238
gestational sac imaging and, 199, 200, 200f
Biological effects of sound, 22, 23, 23t, 24
Biopsy, endometrial
in dysfunctional uterine bleeding, 174, 176
ultrasound in guiding of, 70
Biparietal diameter (BPD), 205
Birth control pills. *See* Oral contraceptives.
Bladder, urinary, 229
evaluation of, 31–33, 31f–32f
neurogenic, 263
polyps, diagnosis of, 4, 74
small bowel in relation to, 134f
ultrasound of, 249, 251f–252f
of carcinoma, 253, 255f, 256
of content, 253
of volume, 249, 250, 253f–254f
unstable, 262, 263
Bladder neck
hypermobility of, 249
ultrasound of, in stress incontinence, 262, 264f–267f, 270
Bladder wall
imaging of, as part of uterus, 52
thickened, 250, 252f, 256
thickness of, 249
Blastocyst, 188
Bleeding
breakthrough, 83, 85, 169
first trimester
with live fetus, 207, 208, 208t
management of, ultrasound in, 205–211, 211t
outcome of, 205, 205t
following ultrasound-guided oocyte retrieval, 317, 318
hydatiform mole-related, 179, 184
postmenopausal
in endometrial carcinoma, 102
endometrium in, 98–99
etiology of, 4, 5f
transvaginal ultrasound screening in, 11, 12
subchorionic, 208
uterine. *See* Dysfunctional uterine bleeding.
vaginal, abnormal. *See* Menometorrhagia.
Blood, in bladder, 253
Blood clot, 119
pelvic, visualization of, 38
retroplacental, 208
in ruptured ectopic pregnancy, 245
Blood flow
in embryonic and fetal vessels, 326, 327, 327t
pelvic, normal, evaluation by transvaginal color Doppler, 325–326
Bowel, 151. *See also* Rectum; Sigmoid colon; Small bowel.
gas in, artifacts caused by, 43, 44f
herniation of, 228, 229
into umbilical cord, 213, 213f, 214f
hyperechoic, fetal, 229
BPD (biparietal diameter), 205
Bradycardia, fetal, 206
Brain, sonoembryology of, 219, 220f, 223f
Breast
cancer of, high velocity signals in, 332
development of, premature, 185
Brightness mode (B-mode), 21
Broad ligament
dilated veins in, 64, 65f
imaging of, 33, 33f, 34f

C

CA-125, in endometriosis, 162
Calcification
in adenomyosis, 60
arcuate artery, 67
Calculi, acoustic shadows distal to, 43, 44f
Cancer. *See also* Carcinoma; *specific body area; specific type of cancer.*
angiogenesis in, 328
breast, 332
rectal, 140–145, 141f–144f
Candida albicans cystitis, 253
Cannula, Schultze, 273
Cannulization, tubal, 271, 273–274, 274t
Carcinoma
of bladder, 253, 255f, 256
endometrial. *See* Endometrium, carcinoma of.
ovarian, 126, 127, 127f, 128f, 129, 130f
anechoic, 128
detection of, 126–127
families at high risk for, 129
screening for, 128, 129–130, 130t
survival rates for, 120
Cardiac activity, fetal. *See* Fetus, cardiac activity of.
Catheter, for embryo transfer, 320–321
contamination of, 319
Frydman, 319
placement of, 318f, 319
Tom Cat, 318, 319
Wallace, 318, 318f, 319
Catheterization. *See also* Cannulization.
tubal, ultrasound-guided, 271, 273–274, 274t
Cathode ray tube, 19
Cavitation, 22

Central nervous system. *See also* Brain.
congenital anomalies of, transvaginal ultrasound in diagnosis of, 222, 223, 223t, 225f–226f
fetal, imaging of, 220
Cerclage, cervical. *See* Cervical cerclage.
Cervical atresia, ultrasound diagnosis of, 61, 61f, 64
Cervical carcinoma, 89
transvaginal color Doppler evaluation of, 330
Cervical cerclage, transvaginal ultrasound before, 233, 233t, 234f, 235t
Cervical-fundal length, measurement of, 30
Cervical incompetence, ultrasonic features of, 179, 180f
Cervical os, internal, 33, 34f, 179
large veins at level of, 67
Cervical stenosis, 89
Cervix, visualization of, 30–31, 31f
Cesarean section
scar, ultrasound imaging of, 69–70
vaginal delivery following, 70
Children
ovarian volume in, 109, 112
sexual disorders in, ultrasonography of, 185
uterine size and shape in, 53, 53t
Chlamydia trachomatis, 147, 161
Chorioadenoma destruens, 179
Choriocarcinoma, 179, 327
Chorionic cavity, imaging of, 188, 189f
Choroid plexus, cysts, congenital, 222
Chromosomal abnormalities, in cystic hygroma, 230
Cisterna magna, 222
Cleft lip and palate, 235
Clomid. *See* Clomiphene citrate.
Clomiphene citrate (Clomid), ovulation induction with, 298, 299t, 299–300
hMG combined with, 301, 307, 308
ultrasound monitoring during administration, 299, 299t
Clot. *See* Blood clot.
CO_2, oocytes exposed to, 312
Color Doppler imaging, transvaginal, 24, 325
in early pregnancy, 326, 327, 327t
in ectopic pregnancy, 327–328
examination techniques, 325
in infertility, 333, 334, 334f
normal pelvic blood flow evaluation by, 325–326
of pelvic pathology. *See* Pelvic pathology.
in process of angiogenesis and neovascularization, 328–329
Computed tomography, of pelvic thrombophlebitis, 131
"Concave sign," 159
Conceptual age (ovulation age), assignment of, 187
Condom, use of, 25
Condom coupling agent, external, 314
Confinement, expected date of, 187
Congenital anomalies, 219. *See also specific anomaly.*
diagnosis of, 4, 5f
hMG therapy-related, 307
role of transvaginal ultrasound in, 222, 235
in cardiac system anomalies, 224, 227, 227f, 227t–228t, 228
in central nervous system anomalies, 222, 223, 223t, 225f–226f
in evaluation of multiple pregnancy, 231, 232, 232f, 233f, 234f
in external body defects, nuchal translucency, 229, 229f, 230, 230t
in gastrointestinal tract anomalies, 222f, 228–229
in history of major congenital anomaly, 222
poor visualization of fetal head, 231, 231f–232f
before pregnancy reduction or cervical cerclage, 233, 233t, 234f, 235t
in pulmonary system anomalies, 228
reasons for not using, 220
in renal anomalies, 224t, 229
sonoembryology of, 219, 220, 220f, 221f, 221t
uterine, ultrasound diagnosis of, 60–64, 61f–63f
Contrast media, sonographic, 272
in endometrial cavity evaluation, 273
SH U 454. *See* SH U 454.
Coronal plane of pelvis, 12, 13f
Corpus hemorrhagicum, 112
Corpus luteum
after ovulation, 292
blood flow in, 336
in ectopic pregnancy, 237
formation of, 117
hemorrhagic, 119, 121
formation of, 287, 289f
Cost factors. *See* Economics.
Critical angle phenomenon, 43, 45f
Crohn's disease, 133
Crown-rump length (CRL)
determination of, 219
estimation of fetal size using, 188, 191
fetal cardiac activity related to, 206
fetal loss and, 208
related to sonographic dating of gestation, 203, 203f–204f, 203t, 205, 205t
relationship with gestational sac diameter, in oligohydramnios, 212
Crystal transducer, 19, 22
Cul-de-sac fluid, 11
in ectopic pregnancy, 245, 246, 246t
ovulation prediction by, 287
related to corpus luteum cysts, 119, 119f
visualization of, 36, 38, 38f
Culdocentesis, ectopic pregnancy diagnosis by, 238, 245, 246
Cumulus oophorous
in follicle, 281, 282f–283f
imaging of, 111
Cyst, ovarian, 9, 123f
abnormal uterine bleeding related to, 171
adnexal, 11
anechoic, 9, 121f, 122f
aspiration of, 271, 274–276
benign, 126, 128
choroid plexus, congenital, 222
corpus luteal, 107, 117, 117f, 119
diagnosis of, 92
in ectopic pregnancy, 243, 245
formation of, 121
hemorrhagic, 124, 171
imaging of, 119, 119f
management of, 126
missed menses related to, 167, 168, 168f
in pregnancy, 126
cytology of, 275–276
definition of, 275
diagnosis of, 92, 121, 124
differential, 121, 121t
differentiated from
endometrioma, 162
hydatiform mole, 185
para-ovarian cyst, 159
pelvic inflammatory disease, 149
follicular, 124, 124f
formation of, 121
imaging of, 171
management of, 126
infertility related to, 161
ultrasound findings in, 159, 159t
malignant character of, accuracy of sonography in predicting, 276
pathologic, 126–127
pelvic ultrasound of, 9
persistence of, 172
small, detection of, 128
surgery for, 129
theca-lutein, 184
Cystadenoma, ovarian, 125

Cystadenomatoid malformation (CAM), of lungs, 228
Cystic dilatation, ureterocele, 259, 262f
Cystitis, 250
bullous, 253
Candida albicans, 253
chronic, 253
Cystourethrography, voiding, 259
Cytologic evaluation, of ovarian cysts, 275–276
Cytomegalovirus infection, 212

D

Dandy-Walker malformation, diagnosis of, by transvaginal ultrasound, 222, 224, 226f
Decibel, defined, 18
Decidua capsularis, 192, 193
Decidua parietalis, 192, 193
Decidua-trophoblast reaction, as indicator of developmental potential of pregnancy, 192, 193, 193f, 194f
Deflections, 19
Diaphragmatic hernia, 235
Dilatation and curettage (D&C), 98
in dysfunctional uterine bleeding, 174
real-time transabdominal ultrasound during, 70
Diverticula
bladder, 250
urethral, 259, 260f–261f
Diverticular abscess, 138
differentiated from pelvic inflammatory disease, 148
Documentation, of ultrasound examination, 41–42
Doppler ultrasound, 24
B-mode scanning, 272
color. *See* Color Doppler imaging, transvaginal.
of corpus luteal cysts, 172
of ovarian artery, for follicular development determination, 111
waveform analysis, 325
Double contour sign, 281
Double decidual sign (DDS), 192, 193, 193f
absence of, 192
in ectopic pregnancy, 246t
Double wall sign, 159
Doxycycline, 274
Drugs, nonhormonal, menometorrhagia from, 169t, 170
Dysfunctional uterine bleeding (DUB), 173–174, 174t
anovulatory, 176, 177
with atypical poorly developed ultrasound endometrial pattern, 176f, 176–177, 177f
diagnosis of, 173
by transvaginal ultrasound, 173, 174, 174t
with hyperechoic ultrasound endometrial pattern, 177
PCOD in, 177
with single-line ultrasound endometrial pattern, 174, 175, 175f
with three-line ultrasound endometrial pattern, 175, 175f, 176
Dysmenorrhea, 161

E

E_2. *See* Estradiol.
E. coli, 154
Echoes, 18
Echogenicity, gain setting and, 40, 41t
Economics, related to transvaginal ultrasonography, 2–3
in screening, 11, 12
Ectopic pregnancy
adnexal mass related to, 200
diagnosis of, 3, 237, 238, 239f, 246f
culdocentesis, 245, 246
human chorionic gonadotropin levels, 238, 240
laparoscopy, 246
serum progesterone levels, 245, 246t
by transvaginal color Doppler, 327–328
ultrasound, 240, 241, 241f, 242, 242f, 243, 243f, 244f, 245
differentiated from
developing pregnancy, 192
normal pregnancy, 199
endometrial sonographic pattern in, 91
incidence of, 237
menometorrhagia in, 169
predisposing factors for, 237
rupture of, 240, 245
significant symptoms of, 237–238
vaginal bleeding in, 205
Ellipsoid, calculation of ovarian volume by, 105
Embryo(s), 188, 219
cryopreservation of, 333
development of
variations in rate of, 188
yolk sac in, 193
multiple, for in vitro fertilization, 311
Embryo collection tube, 314, 314f
Embryo transfer, 318, 319
equipment for, 318, 318f, 319
ultrasound in, 319–320
Empty bladder technique, in transvaginal ultrasound, 2
Endocrine abnormalities, amenorrhea-related to, 164, 167, 168, 168f
Endometrial biopsy. *See* Biopsy, endometrial.
Endometrial cavity
obliteration of, by embryo, 192
sonographic evaluation of, 273, 273t
Endometrial hyperplasia, 293
menometorrhagia from, 172
in postmenopausal women, 102
Endometrial lesions, menometorrhagia from, 172
Endometrial-myometrial junction, 77
Endometrioma, 99, 161
sonographic findings in, 162
Endometriosis
differentiated from pelvic inflammatory disease, 149
infertility related to, 161, 161f, 162
Endometrium, 73
abnormal sonographic patterns, 84, 85, 86f, 86t
absence of echo, 86f, 89, 89f, 91t. *See also* Anechoic pattern.
after ovulation, 290
in amenorrhea, 163, 164
in anovulatory cycles, 293, 293f, 294
atrophic, 97, 97f, 98, 164
atypical sonographic patterns, 85, 86t, 86–89, 89f, 91t, 165t
in dysfunctional uterine bleeding, 176f, 176–177, 177f
BCP, 165t
blood flow, transvaginal color Doppler evaluation of, 329, 334
carcinoma of, 99, 99t, 100, 100f, 101, 101f, 102, 102f, 103
menometorrhagia from, 172
in PCOD, 295, 296
postmenopausal bleeding in, 98–99
ultrasound of, 99, 99t, 100, 100f, 101f, 101–102, 103, 103f
in children, 53
consistency of pattern, 92
cystic hyperplasia of, 4, 64
development of, 73
in dysfunctional uterine bleeding, 173
sonographic evaluation of, 174, 174t, 175, 175f, 176, 176f, 177, 177f
during early proliferative phase, 74, 77
during follicular development, 287, 290
during follicular phase, 74, 74t, 77f, 77–79, 79f, 82t

hyperechoic. *See* Hyperechoic pattern, endometrial.
imaging of, for ovulation confirmation, 112
in infertility, 160
interface with myometrium, 77, 78f
late menstrual, 167
during late proliferative phase, 77, 79, 79f
layered pattern, 77
luteal phase, 79, 80, 80f, 81f, 82t, 292
missed menses in, 168, 168f
in menometorrhagia, 92–94, 93f, 94f, 95f
evaluation of, 172–173
during menses, 73–74, 74t, 75f–76f, 82t
mixed pattern, 88–89, 89f
motion of, 73, 96, 97f
normal patterns associated with clinical abnormalities, 89, 91–92, 92t
in PCOD, 160
in postmenopausal bleeding, 98–99
premenstrual, 80, 82, 82f, 83f
resting, 112, 117f
secretory, 88
single-line, 80, 84f, 117f, 135f, 165f, 165t
in amenorrhea, 167, 168f
in dysfunctional uterine bleeding, 174, 175, 175f,
during menstrual cycle, 74, 75f
in menstrual dys-synchrony, 89, 91
thickened, 82, 83, 83f
sonographic patterns in users of birth control pills, 82, 83, 83f, 84, 84f
thickened, 82, 83f, 84f
in pregnancy, 304
thickness of, 79, 80, 88
in amenorrhea, 167
in endometrial carcinoma, 98
measurement, 94, 96, 96t
in postmenopausal women, 52, 97, 98, 98f
pregnancy achievement and, 290
three-line, 77, 78f, 79, 165t, 166f
in dysfunctional uterine bleeding, 175, 175f, 176
follicular, 112
hMG therapy and, 304
in late luteal phase, 88
in menstrual dys-synchrony, 89, 91
transitional, 165t, 166f
ultrasound-imaged, 164f
classification of, 165t
visualization of, 30
Endovaginal probe, 5-MHz, for ovarian examination, 33
Endovaginal ultrasonography
of adenomyosis, 60
for evaluation of ovarian morphology, 12
in uterine congenital anomalies, 64
Enhancement, 48
Enteritis, regional, 135f
Equipment. *See* Ultrasound equipment.
Estradiol (E_2)
follicular development and, 281
levels
correlation with endometrial thickness, 96, 287, 290
ovulation confirmation by, 111
ovulation prediction by, 284, 286, 287
in PCOD, 160
use in hMG therapy, 301
Estrogen
endometrial effects, 97, 102
levels, in dysfunctional uterine bleeding, 174, 175
menometorrhagia and, 92, 93f
production of, 112
use in hMG therapy, 301–302
Exencephalus, 222, 225f
External body defects, nuchal translucence, 219, 229, 229f, 230, 230t

F

Face, frog-eye appearance of, 222, 225f
Fallopian tube
carcinoma of, 333
catheterization and recannulization of, 271, 273–274, 274t
evaluation of, in infertility, 158
obstruction of, 273
patency, evaluation of
by hysterosalpingography, 271
sonographic, 272–273
visualization of, 36, 37f
False-negative rate, in ultrasonography, 9
False-positive rate, in ultrasonography, 9
Families, risk for ovarian cancer in, 129
Fertilization. *See also* In vitro fertilization.
variability in timing of, 187–188
Fetal pole, visualization of, 196, 197f
Fetus, 219
cardiac activity of, 193, 213, 219
detection of, 196, 196f, 206, 206f
gestational sac size related to, 202, 202f, 203
development of, early, 204f, 212t, 213, 213f, 214f, 215f
head of
poor visualization of, 231, 231f, 232f
size of, 219
transvaginal scan of, 223f
limb buds of, 213
normal, hydatiform mole in, 184f, 185
Fibroids, uterine, 328
Fingers, fetal, visualization of, 219
Fistula, genitourinary, 263
Fluid, cul-de-sac. *See* Cul-de-sac fluid.
Follicle, ovarian, 35, 36
aspiration of, 271
in assisted reproductive technologies, 276–277
in in vitro fertilization, 313, 314, 315f, 316f, 317
Bomsel-Helmreich, 119
collapse of, 112, 117
development of, 73, 111, 113f, 280f, 280–281
in anovulatory patient, 160
endometrium during, 287, 290
hMG effects on, 302, 302f, 303f, 304f, 305f
monitoring of, 279
disappearance of, 159
distinguished from cyst, 275
dominant, 111, 112, 112f, 119, 281
development of, oral contraceptives effects on, 119, 120
transvaginal color Doppler evaluation of, 326
"double contour" sign, 281
empty follicle syndrome, infertility and, 296
enlarged, 124
immature, in ovarian failure, 164
luteinized but unruptured follicle syndrome (LUF), 112, 160, 161
diagnosis of, 279
infertility related to, 296–297
multiple, 112, 124
stimulation of, in in vitro fertilization, 311, 312
nonovulatory, 280, 280f
persistence of, 176
in postmenopausal women, 121
in premature ovarian failure, 207
immature, 109, 111, 119
in dysfunctional uterine bleeding, 176
size of, 287
in clomiphene citrate cycles, 299
ovulation prediction by, 281, 284, 285f, 286f, 286t, 287, 288f–289f
transvaginal ultrasound of, transabdominal ultrasound compared with, 11
volume of, 33, 35, 35f
calculation of, 280
Follicle stimulating hormone (FSH), 280
anovulation diagnosis with, 298
hMG use with, 301
levels, ovulation prediction by, 284, 286
Follicular phase of menstrual cycle, endometrium during, 73, 74, 74t, 77f, 77–79, 79f, 82f

Folliculogram, 279
during anovulatory cycle, 292
in clomiphene citrate therapy, 299–300
limitations of, 287
Foot, rocker bottom, 235
Frequency used in ultrasound, 17, 17f
Full bladder technique, 250
in transabdominal ultrasonography, accuracy of, 9
Fundus. *See* Uterine fundus.

G

Gain. *See also* Time-gain compensation.
settings
for bladder evaluation, 30
echogenicity and, 40, 41t
Gas, acoustic artifacts related to, 43, 44f
Gas bubbles, enlargement of, 22
Gas interface, distance from transducer, 44f, 45f–47f, 46
Gastrointestinal tract. *See also* specific organ.
congenital anomalies of, transvaginal ultrasound in diagnosis of, 222f, 228–229
Genitalia, fetal, 219
Gestation. *See* Pregnancy.
Gestational age
assignment of, 187
dating of, by crown-rump length. *See* Crown-rump length.
visualization of fetal anatomic structures and, 224, 224t
Gestational blind spot, 245
Gestational sac, 169, 193
distorted, 169
eccentric placement of, 61
empty, 206, 207f, 208
failure in visualization of, 199
rate of growth of, 191, 192, 192t
size of, 188, 200
correlation with last menstrual period, 191f
fetal cardiac activity related to, 202, 202f, 203
human chorionic gonadotropin levels and, 200, 201, 201f, 208, 209f, 210, 210t, 211, 211t
relationship with crown-rump length, 212
visualization of, 188–189, 189f–190f, 191, 191f, 191t, 192, 192t
in ectopic pregnancy, 240
hCG levels for, 199, 200, 200f, 201t
volume of, 191
Gestational trophoblastic disease, features of, 179, 183f, 184–185
Glove, 25
Gonadotropin(s). *See also* Human chorionic gonadotropin; Human menopausal gonadotropin.
in infertility, 300, 300t
Gonadotropin releasing hormone (GnRH) agonists, for PCOD, 295
Graded compression ultrasound, in appendicitis, 139
Granulosa cells, follicular development and, 280, 281
Gynecology. *See also* Pelvic examination.
transvaginal ultrasonography uses in, 2, 3t, 4

H

Halo, surrounding endometrium, 77, 78f, 79
in endometrial carcinoma, 101
Hard copy documentation, 40
Hematoma
intrauterine, 208
subchorionic, 208
Hematometrium, 4, 5f, 89
Hernia
bowel. *See* Bowel, herniation of.
diaphragmatic, 235
midgut, 219, 222f
Hertz, 17, 18f
High flow area, in hydatiform mole, 184
Histological samples, in postmenopausal bleeding, 98
History, 6
Holoprosencephaly, 222, 235
Honeycomb pattern, in adenomyosis, 60
Hormones
effect on uterine size, 52
menometorrhagia related to, 170
Human chorionic gonadotropin (hCG). *See also* Beta-human chorionic gonadotropin.
added to hMG for ovulation induction, 303, 395f
as adjunct to early pregnancy imaging, 197, 198
discriminatory zone, 199, 200, 200f, 201t
gestational sac size and, 200, 201, 201f
standards for, 198, 199, 199t
doubling time, 188
endometrial effects, 96, 299
levels
in ectopic pregnancy, 238, 240
gestational dating by, 188, 191t, 245
gestational sac size and, 208, 209f, 210, 210t, 211, 211t
in incomplete abortion, 212
titers, in ectopic adnexal mass, 242
Human menopausal gonadotropin (hMG)
endometrial thickness effects, 96
ovulation induction by, 300
clinical uses, 300, 301t
combined with clomiphene citrate, 307, 308
complications related to, 304, 306, 307, 307t, 308t
contraindications to, 301
estrogen and ultrasound monitoring with, 301–302
evaluation before, 301, 301t
follicular growth and, 302, 302f, 303f, 304f, 305f
human chorionic gonadotropin combined with, 303, 305f
induction of therapy, 301
intrauterine insemination with, 300, 300t
success of, 300, 300t, 303, 304, 306t
types of therapy, 301
Hydatiform mole, 179, 184
partial or incomplete, 184
sonographic findings in, 179, 183f, 184–185
vaginal bleeding in, 205
Hydranencephaly, 235
Hydrocephalus, 222, 223f
Hydropic changes, of placenta, differentiated from hydatiform mole, 184, 185
Hydrops, fetal, 232
transvaginal ultrasound in diagnosis of, 228, 230, 232
Hydrosalpinx
in endometriosis, 162
fallopian tube, ultrasound findings in, 159, 159t
following ultrasound-guided oocyte retrieval, 317
ovarian, 271
Hygroma, cystic, fetal, 229, 229f, 230t, 230
Hymen, imperforate, 64
Hyperechoic echogenicity, 40
defined, 41t
Hyperechoic material, in pelvic inflammatory disease, 148
Hyperechoic pattern
bowel, fetal, 229
endometrial, 88, 89, 89f, 165t, 166f
in dysfunctional uterine bleeding, 176, 177
as indication of pathology, 84, 85
poorly developed, 86, 87f, 87–88
thickened, 85, 86, 87f

of sigmoid colon, 138
Hypergonadotrophic hypogonadal patient, immature follicle in, 297
Hypermenorrhagia, 172
Hypoechoic echogenicity, 40
defined, 41t
Hypoechoic pattern, endometrial, 74, 75f, 77, 79, 82, 88, 89f
as indication of pathology, 84, 85
Hypogastric vein, identification of, 35, 36
Hypogonadotropic hypogonadic patient, 290
Hysterectomy specimens, as reference for normal uterine size, 51
Hysterosalpingography (HSG)
application of, 271, 272, 273
in Asherman's syndrome, 163
in diagnosis of unicornuate uterus, 63f, 64
disadvantages of, 271
Hysteroscopy, use in endometrial cavity evaluation, 273

I

Iliac arteries, blood flow, transvaginal color Doppler evaluation of, 326
Iliac vein, internal, imaging of, 35f, 36, 36f
Image, ultrasound, 3
display orientation, 14, 15f
quality of, transvaginal ultrasound compared with transabdominal ultrasound, 10
resolution of, 21–22, 22f
Imaging routine, in pelvic examination, 28
Incidence, angle of, 18, 18f, 19
Incontinence. *See* Stress incontinence.
Infection, related to invasive techniques, 273
Infertility, 157
confirmation of ovulation in, 111–112, 113f–117f, 117, 118f, 119
endometriosis in, 161, 161f, 162
history of, ectopic pregnancy related to, 237
initial evaluation of
of fallopian tubes and adnexa, 158–159, 159t
of ovaries, 159–160, 160t, 161
of uterus, 157, 158
transvaginal color Doppler in evaluation of, 333, 334, 334f
tubal factor in, 273
ultrasound evaluation of, 311
Infundibulopelvic ligament, 33, 33f
Intensity of sound. *See* Sound intensity.
Internal echo pattern, in hemorrhagic corpus luteal cysts, 171
International Reference Preparation (IRP) for human chorionic gonadotropin, 199, 199t, 238
Intervillous spaces, transvaginal color Doppler evaluation of, 326, 327t
Intrafallopian tube transfer technique, 320
Intrauterine device (IUD), 201
imaging of, within endometrial cavity, 73
localization and/or perforation of, 179, 181f–182f
Intrauterine insemination, hMG used with, 300, 300t
Invasive techniques, sonographic, 271, 272t
contrast media used in, 272
endometrial cavity evaluation, 273, 275t
infection and antibiotic prophylaxis related to, 273
ovarian cyst aspiration, 274–276
ovarian follicle aspiration in assisted reproductive technologies, 276–277
sonosalpingography, 271, 272
tubal catheterization and recannulization, 273–274, 274t
tubal patency evaluation, 272–273
In vitro fertilization (IVF), 161, 311. *See also* Assisted reproductive technologies.
embryo transfer in, 318, 318f, 319–321
heterotopic pregnancy rate in, 240
natural cycle, 317
oocyte retrieval in. *See* Oocyte retrieval.
ovulation induction in, 311 312
pregnancy rates following, 311–312
use of transvaginal color Doppler in, 333, 334
vanishing twin syndrome associated with, 211, 212
Isoechoic echogenicity, 40, 41f, 41t

K

Keyboard sign, 133
Kidney, pelvic, imaging of, 259, 263f

L

Lacunar spaces, transvaginal color Doppler evaluation of, 326
Laparoscopy, 272
advantages and disadvantages of, 271
in appendicitis, 138
ectopic pregnancy diagnosis by, 238, 246
in endometriosis, 162
in oocyte retrieval, 312, 313
in ovarian enlargement, 107
Laparotomy, in ovarian enlargement, 107
Last menstrual period (LMP), 73, 187, 188
correlation with gestational sac diameter, 191f
crown-rump length plotted against, 205
dating of pregnancy by, 188
discrepancy between crown-rump length and fetal age by, 208
gestational age from, 191t
Lateral resolution, 21, 22, 22f
Leiomyoma, uterine, 51, 201
bleeding from, 172
blood flow in, transvaginal color Doppler evaluation of, 329
calcification associated with, 67
differential diagnosis of, 60
endometrial, 84
infertility related to, 157, 158
malignant degeneration of, 67, 69
measurement of, 12
transvaginal ultrasonography of, 55, 55f, 56, 56t, 57f–59f
compared with transabdominal ultrasonography, 11
LH. *See* Luteinizing hormone.
Linear regression relationship, bladder volume calculation by, 250, 253f
Luteal phase of menstrual cycle
defects in, infertility related to, 297
endometrium during, 73, 79, 80, 80f, 81f, 82t, 87, 88
menometorrhagia and, 93, 94, 94f
Luteinized but unruptured follicle syndrome. *See* under Follicle, ovarian.
Luteinizing hormone (LH), levels
anovulation diagnosis with, 279, 298
ovulation prediction by, 284, 286
peak, 281
surge in, ovulation confirmation by, 111, 112, 112f, 113f, 114f, 279

M

Mechanical distortion, 22
Medium, sound wave travel through, 18
Medroxyprogesterone acetate, for menometorrhagia, 173
Megahertz (MHZ), 17
Menometorrhagia, 169
drug-related, 169t, 170
endometrial imaging in, 92, 93f, 94, 94f, 95f
etiology of, 169t
hyperechoic endometrial pattern in, 88
in nonpregnant patients, causes of, 170–171

Menometorrhagia *(Continued)*
anatomic pelvic pathology, 171–173, 173t
dysfunctional uterine bleeding, 172–174, 174t
PCOD-related, 177
postmenopausal, 169
pregnancy-related, 169, 169t, 170t
in ectopic pregnancy, 169
in systemic disease, 170
Menopause
beginning of, 293f
premature ovarian failure distinguished from, 297, 298t
Menses. *See also* Menstrual cycle.
endometrium during, 73, 74, 74t, 75f–76f, 82f
effect of birth control pills on, 82, 83
Menstrual cycle
dys-synchrony, normal endometrial patterns associated with, 89, 91–92, 92t
follicular phase of. *See* Follicular phase of menstrual cycle.
history, anovulation cycle and, 292
length of, timing of ovulation by, 202
luteal phase of. *See* Luteal phase of menstrual cycle.
ovarian blood flow during, transvaginal color Doppler evaluation of, 334–336, 335f
ovarian volume during, 107
proliferative phase. *See* Proliferative phase of menstrual cycle.
Menstrual weeks, expressing uterine size by palpation in terms of, 52
Metrodin, 312
Microbubble contrast media, 272
Microcephalus, 222
Midgut hernia, 219, 222f
Mineral oil, 314
Monosomy X, 230
Mucosal folds, of small bowel, 133
Mucus, cervical, in ovulation induction cycles, 290
Müllerian anomalies
infertility related to, 158
ultrasound diagnosis of, 61, 61f, 64
Myoma, uterine, blood flow in, 329
Myomectomy, in infertility, 157
Myometrium
in children, 53
echogenicity of, 40
in endometriosis, 162
hysterosalpingographic evaluation of, 272
interface with endometrium, 77, 78f
invasion of, by endometrial carcinoma, 101, 101f
size of, 52
thickness of, in postmenopausal women, 52
transvaginal ultrasound of, 28, 30
veins of, visualization of, 64, 65f

N

Needle, aspiration, in oocyte retrieval, 313, 314, 315, 315f, 316, 316f
Needle guide, for oocyte retrieval, 314
Needle puncture, in oocyte retrieval, 312–313
Neisseria gonorrhea, 147, 161
Neovascularization
in adnexal masses, 331, 332
in endometrial carcinoma, 329
study of, application of transvaginal color Doppler to, 328–329
Nodularity, in endometriosis, 161
Nodules, ovarian tumors with, 127
Nuchal translucency, 219
transvaginal ultrasound in diagnosis of, 229, 229f, 230, 230t
Nuclear magnetic resonance imaging
endometrial thickness measurement by, 96
of pelvic thrombophlebitis, 131

O

Obese patient, evaluation of, 7, 8f, 11
Oblique plane, endometrial measurement in, 94
Obstetrics, transvaginal ultrasound uses in, 1, 2
Office equipment, ultrasonographic, 2
OHSS. *See* Ovarian hyperstimulation syndrome.
Oligohydramnios, in early pregnancy, 212
Omphalocele, formation of, 222f, 228–229
Oocyte, 287
in luteinized unruptured follicle syndrome, 296
Oocyte retrieval, 205, 311
laparoscopic, 312, 313
ultrasound-guided, 312
advantages of, 313
anesthesia requirements for, 316, 317
aspiration needle for, 313, 315, 316, 316f
complications of, 317–318
endovaginal, 313–314
free-hand technique, 312–313
periurethral, 313
pregnancy rates following, 317
procedure for, 314, 315
sedation for, 313
transabdominal approach in, 312, 313, 314
transvaginal approach in, 312, 313, 314, 314f, 315f, 317
transvesical approach in, 313, 314
Oral contraceptives
breakthrough bleeding associated with, 83, 85, 169
effects of
on endometrial image, 73, 82, 83
on ovarian image, 119, 120
Ovarian artery, Doppler ultrasound of, for follicular development determination, 111
Ovarian failure
amenorrhea related to, 164
diagnosis of, 164
premature, 160, 298
infertility in, 297, 298, 298t
ultrasound findings in, 298t
Ovarian hyperstimulation syndrome (OHSS)
clomiphene citrate in, 298, 299
complications of, 306
controlled, 311
estrogen-related, 301, 302
hMG-related, 306, 307, 307t
treatment of, 306, 307, 307t
Ovarian stroma, echogenicity of, 33, 35
Ovarian vein, thrombosis of, 130–131
Ovary(ies)
anechoic pattern. *See* under Anechoic pattern.
in anovulatory cycles, 290, 291f, 292, 292f, 293
blood flow, during menstrual cycle, transvaginal color Doppler evaluation of, 334–336, 335f
cancer of. *See also* Carcinoma, ovarian.
screening for, 11–12
transvaginal color Doppler evaluation of, 333
corpus luteum. *See* Corpus luteum.
cysts of. *See* Cysts, ovarian.
enlargement of, in PCOD, 171
follicles of. *See* Follicle, ovarian.
imaging of, 105, 105f, 107f, 108f
of carcinoma, 126, 127, 127f, 128, 128f, 129, 130f. *See also* Carcinoma, ovarian.
in children, 109, 111t
for confirmation of ovulation, 111–112, 113f–117f, 117, 118f, 119
of diameter and volume, 105, 107, 109, 109f, 110f
of enlargement, 107, 121, 121t, 122f–124f, 125f, 125–126

in infertility, 159–160, 160t, 161
of oral contraceptive effects on, 119, 120
of ovarian vein thrombosis, 130–131
in postmenopausal women, 120, 121, 121f
transvaginal ultrasound compared with transabdominal ultrasound, 11
masses, ultrasound-detected, management of, 126
pathologic evaluation of, accuracy of transvaginal ultrasound measurement in, 12
postmenopausal, localization of, 35
relationship to uterus, in pelvic adhesions, 185
resistant ovary syndrome, 160, 297, 298t
size and volume of
age effects on, 120, 121
in children, 109, 110f, 111t
in PCOD, 294
wedge resection of, for PCOD, 295
Ovulation. *See also* Anovulation.
confirmation of, 111–112, 113f–117f, 117, 118f, 119, 287, 288f–290f
endometrium after, 290
endometrium during, 73
induction of, 279, 298
with clomiphene citrate, 298, 299t, 299–300
in empty follicle syndrome, 296
endometrium in, 287, 290
follicular development, 280f, 280–281
with hMG therapy. *See* Human menopausal gonadotropin.
in in vitro fertilization, 311 312
in luteal phase defect, 297
in luteinized unruptured follicle syndrome, 296–297
in PCOD, 294, 294f–295f, 295, 296, 296t
in premature ovarian failure, menopause, resistant ovary syndrome, and WHO type I anovulation, 297, 298, 298t
late, diagnosis of, 88
predicting of, 281–282, 282f–286f
timing of, 187–188
ultrasound examination for, 92
in infertility, 159–160, 160t, 161
Ovulation age. *See* Conceptual age.
Ovum
aspiration of, ultrasound-assisted, 312
transmigration of, in ectopic pregnancy, 237

P

PCOD. *See* Polycystic ovarian disease.
Pelvic anatomy, transvaginal ultrasound examination of, using transvaginal probe, 28, 28t
of adhesions, 40
of bladder, 31–33, 31f–32f
of blood clots, 38
of broad ligament and arcuate vessels, 33, 33f, 34f
of cervix, 30–31, 31f
of cul-de-sac, 36, 38, 38f
of endometrium, 30
of fallopian tubes, 36, 37f
of ovary, 33, 35, 35f, 36, 36f
of pelvic muscle and pelvic sidewall, 38, 39f, 40f
of sigmoid colon and small bowel, 38, 40f, 41f
of uterus, 28–30, 29f, 30f, 33f
Pelvic examination. *See also* specific structure.
contrast sonosalpingography, 271
by transvaginal color Doppler, 325–326
transvaginal ultrasound in, 1, 3, 4, 6–9, 25, 84
accuracy of measurements, 12
documentation of, 41–42
gain setting, 40, 41, 41t
for ovarian pathology, 125–126
of pelvic anatomy. *See* Pelvic anatomy, transvaginal ultrasound examination of.
in pelvic inflammatory disease, 149
of pelvic planes, 12, 13f–14f, 14
real-time, 10
sonic coupling and prevention of probe contamination, 25–27, 26f, 27f
time-gain compensation in, 41
Pelvic fluid, increased, etiology of, 138t
Pelvic inflammatory disease (PID), 4, 7f
acute, 147
differential diagnosis of, 148, 149, 150f, 151t
pelvic abscess drainage, transvaginal ultrasound in, 149, 150f, 151f, 152f–154f, 154, 155f
ultrasound in, 147, 148, 148t, 149f
differentiated from endometriosis, 161
imaging of, transvaginal ultrasound compared with transabdominal ultrasound, 10
Pelvic pathology
abnormal endometrial patterns in, 84
organic, menometorrhagia in, 170, 171–173, 173t
transvaginal color Doppler in evaluation of
of adnexal masses, 330–333
of uterine tumors, 329–330
transvaginal ultrasound compared with transabdominal ultrasound in evaluation of, 11
Perforation, uterine, 69–70
Pergonal, 312
Period of wound wave, 17, 18f
Peritoneum, ovarian, visualization of, 35, 35f, 36, 36f
Periurethral route, in oocyte retrieval, 313
Photographs, 10
Physician training, for transvaginal ultrasonography, 3
Piezoelectric effect, 19
Placenta, hydropic changes in, differentiated from hydatiform mole, 184, 185, 186
Placentation, transvaginal color Doppler evaluation of, 326
Polycystic ovarian disease (PCOD)
amenorrhea in, 167
anovulatory patients with, 290
characteristics of, 294
diagnosis of, 160, 294, 298
endometrial carcinoma in, 295, 296
endometrial hyperechoic area in, 87
immature follicles in, 164
menometorrhagia and, 170–171, 177
ovarian size in, 107
ovulation induction in, 294, 294f, 295, 295f, 296, 296t
response to clomiphene citrate, 299
treatment of, 295
Polyp
bladder, diagnosis of, 4, 7f
endometrial, 84
intracervical, 4, 6f
Postcoital tests, timing of, 284, 286t
Postmenopausal women
adnexal tumors in, transvaginal color Doppler evaluation of, 332–333
endometrium in, 96, 97, 97f, 98, 98f
menometorrhagia in, 170
ovarian volume and diameter in, 107, 109f, 120, 121, 121f
Pregnancy
cervical shortening and dilatation in, 179
corpus luteal cysts in, 126
early, 187, 197t
adjuncts to imaging, human chorionic gonadotropin. *See* Human chorionic gonadotropin.
amnion in, 196, 198f
crown-rump length and sonographic dating of, 203, 203f–204f, 203t, 205, 205t

Pregnancy *(Continued)*
decidua-trophoblastic reaction, 192, 193, 193f, 194f
developmental landmarks, gestational age, and last menstrual period, 188
early fetal development, 204f, 212t, 213, 213f, 214f, 215f
fetus and fetal cardiac activity, 196, 197f, 197t
first trimester bleeding, ultrasound in management of, 205–211, 211t
incomplete abortion, 212, 212t
oligohydramnios in, 212
ovulation and variability in timing of fertilization, 187–188
role of yolk sac in sonography, 193, 195f–196f, 196, 197t
routine sonography in, 214, 215, 215t
sac size, fetal cardiac activity and, 202, 202f, 203
transvaginal color Doppler evaluation of, 326, 327, 327t
vanished twin syndrome, 211–212
visualization of gestational sac, 188–189, 189f–190f, 191, 191f, 191t, 192, 192t
ectopic. *See* Ectopic pregnancy.
extrauterine, 199
heterotopic, 240
intrauterine
coexistence with ectopic pregnancy, 240
imaging of, 240
lack of confirmation of, 245
vaginal bleeding in, 169, 169t, 170t
molar, transvaginal color Doppler in evaluation of, 327
multiple, 214. *See also* Twin pregnancy.
evaluation of, by transvaginal ultrasound, 231, 232, 232f, 233f, 234f
hMG-related, 304
IVF-related, 334
normal, hCG levels in, 240
reduction, transvaginal ultrasound before, 233, 233t, 234f, 235t
safety of ultrasound examination in, 24
uterine volume in, 52
Pregnancy rate
after embryo transfer, 319–320
after hMG therapy, 303, 304, 306t
decrease in, 80
improvement of, 287
in vitro fertilization-related, 311–312
Pregnancy tests, ectopic pregnancy diagnosis by, 238
Premenstrual phase, endometrium during, 80, 82, 82f, 83f
Probe. *See* Endovaginal probe; Transvaginal probe.
Progestational agents, for menometorrhagia, 173
Progesterone
for dysfunctional uterine bleeding, 174, 175
endometrial effects, 80, 96, 102
levels
in diagnosis of impending abortion, 211
in ectopic pregnancy, 245
production of, 112
Progesterone challenge
in amenorrhea, 167
anovulatory cycles and, 293
withdrawal bleeding in, 167
Proliferative phase of menstrual cycle, 92
early, endometrium during, 74, 77
late, endometrium during, 77, 79, 79f
Propofol, 317
Pseudogestational sac, in ectopic pregnancy, 240, 241f
Puberty, precocious, 185
Pubic symphysis, bladder neck in relation to, in stress incontinence, 262, 267f–269f
Pulmonary system, congenital anomalies of, transvaginal ultrasound in diagnosis of, 228
Pulsatility index (PI)
in adnexal masses, 330, 331
mean, in uterine tumors, 329
Pulse generator, 19
Pulse length, relation to axial resolution, 21
Pyometrium, 99
Pyosalpinx, 4, 7f
following ultrasound-guided oocyte retrieval, 317

R

Radiation torque, 22
Radiographs, 9
RAYL, 18
Real-time sonography
description of, 9–10
in embryo transfer, 319
transabdominal. *See under* Transabdominal ultrasonography.
transvaginal. *See under* Transvaginal ultrasonography.
Recannulization, tubal, ultrasound guided, 273–274, 274t
Rectovaginal septum, tubo-ovarian abscess in relation to, 151
Rectum, cancer of, 140–145. 141f–144f
recurrence rates, 143f, 144f, 145
Reflection, 19
assumptions related to, 43
property of, 18
Refraction, Snell's law of, 46f
Renal anomalies, diagnosis of, transvaginal ultrasound for, 224t, 229
Resistance index (RI)
in abnormal early pregnancy, 326, 327, 327t
in adnexal masses, 330, 331
in ectopic pregnancy, 328
in infertility, 333
of ovarian blood flow, 336
Pourcelot, of myometrial blood flow, 329
Resistant ovary syndrome, 160, 297, 298t
Resolution, image, 21–22, 22f
Retroperitoneal nodes, tumor involvement in, 127
RI. *See* Resistance index.
Ringer's solution, 158
Rupture, uterine, 69–70

S

Sacral agenesis, 235
Sagittal plane of pelvis, 12, 13f
Saline, 158, 273
Sarcoma, uterine, 67
transvaginal color Doppler evaluation of, 330
Scatter, 19
Screening tool, ultrasound as
in ovarian cancer, 128, 129–130, 130t
transvaginal ultrasound, 11–12
Second International Standard (2IS) for human chorionic gonadotropin, 199, 199t, 238
Septa, thickness of, ovarian malignancy related to, 127
Sexual development, disorders of, ultrasonography of, 185
Sexual differentiation, disorders of, 163, 164
Shadowing, shadows, 43, 44f
in adenomyosis, 60
clean, 43
critical angle phenomenon, 43, 45f
dirty, 43
edge, 43
in endometrial ultrasound, 79
refraction, 43, 44f–46f
reverberation artifacts in association with, 46, 44f–47f
SH U 454
in hysterosalpingography, 272
in infertility evaluation, 158
in tubal patency evaluation, 272

Sigmoid colon, ultrasound imaging of, 138f, 138–140
Sliding organ sign, 158
Small bowel
  obstruction of, 133
  sonographic evaluation of, 133, 134f–137f, 138t
Snell's law, 18–19, 46f
Solid objects, acoustic shadows distal to, 43, 44f
Sonic coupling, in pelvic examination, 25–27, 26f, 27f
Sonoembryology
  at eight to ten weeks' gestation, 219, 220f, 221f, 221t
  at fourteen to sixteen weeks' gestation, 220, 224t
  at ten to twelve weeks' gestation, 219, 223f
  at twelve to fourteen weeks' gestation, 219, 220t, 224t
Sonosalpingography
  application of, 271, 272
  in endometrial cavity evaluation, 273
Sound
  absorption of, 21
  audible, 17
  biological effects of, 22, 23, 23t, 24
  physics of, 2, 17, 18, 18f, 19
  reflection of, multiple, 46
  spatial peak intensity of, 18
  speed of, 17
  temporal peak energy of, 18
  velocity of, 17, 43
Sound beam
  diameter of, 21, 22, 22f
  effect on tissues, 22
Sound intensity, 18
  defined, 22, 23, 23t
Sound pulse, 19
Sound wave, 17
  characteristics of, 18
  generation of, 19
  intensity of, 18, 19
  refracted or bent, 18–19
  travel of, 43
Speckling, acoustic, 48
Spina bifida, diagnosis of, by transvaginal ultrasound, 224, 226f
Spine, fetal, visualization of, 224, 226f
Spiral artery, blood flow, transvaginal color Doppler evaluation of, 326
Standard deviation (SD), in congenital anomalies, uterine, 61
Stool, 138
Stress incontinence, transvaginal ultrasound in, 262, 264f–267f, 270
Surgery
  embryo transfer, 320
  for leiomyoma, 157, 158
  for ovarian cysts, 129
  pelvic ultrasound prior to, 6
  for stress incontinence, 263
Systemic disease, menometorrhagia in, 169t, 170

T

Temperature. *See* Basal body temperature.
Theca tissue, 281
Thecoma, luteinized, 331
Thelarche, idiopathic premature, 185
Third International Standard (3IS) for human chorionic gonadotropin, 199, 199t
Third-party payers, 41
Thrombophlebitis, pelvic, 131
Thrombosis, ovarian vein, 130–131
Time considerations, related to transvaginal ultrasonography, 2
  transabdominal ultrasonography compared with, 10
Time-gain compensation (TMG), 41
Towako method for embryo transfer, 320–321
T-pelvic plane. *See* Trans-pelvic plane.
Training, physician, for transvaginal ultrasonography, 3
Transabdominal ultrasonography
  in appendicitis, 138, 138f
  ectopic pregnancy diagnosis by, 238
  in embryo transfer, 319
  in endometrial biopsy, 70
  full bladder technique. *See* Full bladder technique.
  in oocyte retrieval, 312, 313
  for ovarian cancer detection, 127
  real-time
    of endometrial carcinoma, 101
    use during dilatation and curettage or suction curettage, 70
  safety of, 23
  technical advantages of, 2
  versus transvaginal ultrasound imaging, 10–11
  of uterine congenital anomalies, 61
Transcervical ultrasonography, embryo transfer guided by, 320
Transducer, ultrasound. *See* Ultrasound transducer.
Transmission, angle of, 19
Trans-pelvic (T-pelvic) plane
  description of, 12, 13f, 14
  endometrial measurement in, 94
  image display orientation and, 14
  imaging of ovaries in, 26, 105, 108f, 115f–116f
  imaging of uterus in, 26, 51, 52
Transrectal ultrasound, in cancer, 140
  in recurrence, 145
Transvaginal color Doppler. *See* Color Doppler imaging, transvaginal.
Transvaginal probe
  contamination, prevention of, 25–27, 27f
  fallopian tube visualization by, 36
  finger, 26–27, 27f
  5-MHz, 2
  lower frequency, 9
  pelvic anatomy visualization by. *See* Pelvic anatomy, transvaginal ultrasound examination of.
  in pelvic inflammatory disease diagnosis, 147
  7.5-MHz, 2, 3
  technical advantages of, 2
  uterine position using, 55
  in uterus examination, 28
Transvaginal ultrasonography
  clinical indications for, 1, 3t, 4
  economics of, 2–3
  high frequency, technical advantages of, 1–2
  image display orientation in, 14, 15f
  measurements, accuracy of, 12
  of ovaries. *See* Ovaries.
  in pelvic examination. *See* Pelvic anatomy; Pelvic examination.
  pelvic planes imaged by, 12, 13f–14f, 14
  physician training for, 3
  real-time, 3, 9–10
    gestational sac visualization by, 201
  safety of, 23
  as screening tool, 11–12
  transabdominal ultrasound imaging versus, 10–11
  of uterus. *See* Uterus.
Transverse plane, of pelvis, 12, 13f
Transvesical route, in oocyte retrieval, 313
Trophoblast, 188, 327. *See also* Gestational trophoblastic disease.
Trophoblastic reaction, as indicator of developmental potential of pregnancy, 192, 193, 193f, 194f
Trophoblastic shell, imaging of, 188, 189f
Tubo-ovarian abscess. *See* Abscess, tubo-ovarian.
Tumor
  hemorrhagic corpus luteal cyst differentiation from, 171–172
  metastasis, by angiogenesis, 328
  neovascularization. *See* Neovascularization.
Twin(s), congenital anomalies in, hMG-related, 307
Twinning, conjoined, transvaginal ultrasound in diagnosis of, 232, 233

Twin pregnancy
hMG-related, 304
vanishing twin syndrome, 208, 211–212
Twin reversed arterial perfusion (TRAP) syndrome, 232

U

Ultrasonography
artifacts in. *See* Artifacts.
three-dimensional, 2
transabdominal. *See* Transabdominal ultrasonography.
transvaginal. *See* Transvaginal ultrasonography.
Ultrasound equipment, assumptions in processing acoustic data, artifacts related to, 43
Ultrasound image. *See* Image.
Ultrasound machine, description of, 19, 21, 21f
Ultrasound transducer
1.6, 9
3.5-MHz, 9
5-MHz
abdominal, in ovarian vein thrombosis, 130–131
in appendicitis, 138
7.5-MHz, in appendicitis, 138
description of, 19, 20f
discomfort related to, 10
distance from gas interface, 44f, 45f–47f, 46
fixed focal point of, 22
frequency of, 21, 22
high frequency, 1, 2
intensity of, characterization of, 22, 23, 23t
linear array, in pelvic inflammatory disease, 148, 150f
in oocyte retrieval, 313–314, 314, 314f
piezoelectric element of, 19
pelvic plane imaging and, 12
range of motion of, 12
side-lobe beams, artifacts resulting from, 48
transabdominal, 22
in uterus examination, 28
vaginal, 22
Umbilical cord, herniation of bowel into, 213, 213f, 214f
Ureter
ectopic, 263
imaging of, 32, 32f, 33f, 249, 250f
technique for, 256, 256f, 257f–258f
Ureterocele, imaging of, 259, 262f
Urethra
dysfunction of, incontinence due to, 268f
imaging of, 32, 32f, 249
technique for, 256, 259, 259f
lead pipe or drainpipe, 263
localization of, in stress incontinence, 262
Urethra-vesical angle obstruction, 263
Urethrography, double-balloon, 259
Urethroscopy, 259
Urinary tract, congenital anomalies of, 64
Urine
"jet" of turbulence, 252f, 256
volume, estimation of, 250
of residual volume, 250
Urodynamics, sonographic, 262–270, 264f–269f
Urogram, excretory, 253
Urogynecology
pelvic kidney, 259, 263f
sonographic urodynamics, 262–270, 264f–269f
ureters, 256, 259, 259f, 260f–262f
urinary bladder. *See* Bladder, urinary.
Uterine artery
blood flow
impedance to, 329
transvaginal color Doppler evaluation of, 326
calcification of, 67
flow velocity waveforms from, 333, 334f
Uterine bleeding, dysfunctional. *See* Dysfunctional uterine bleeding.
Uterine cavity
fluid distension of, 99
hydatiform moles in, 179
Uterine fundus
in children, 53
width and thickness of, 51
Uterine horn, rudimentary, 64
Uterine vessels, transvaginal ultrasound of, 64–67, 65f–67f
Uterus
bicornuate, 4, 5f
ultrasound diagnosis of, 61, 62f, 63f
blood supply to, 333, 334f
circulation in, transvaginal color Doppler evaluation of, 327
didelphys, ultrasound diagnosis of, 61, 62f, 64
evaluation of, in infertility, 157, 158
lateral deviation of, 53, 55
leiomyoma of. *See* Leiomyoma, uterine.
relationship to ovary, in pelvic adhesions, 185
retroverted, 70
septate, ultrasound diagnosis of, 61, 62f, 63f, 64, 158
size and shape, normal limits of, 51
small, 70
transvaginal ultrasound of, 28, 29f–30f, 30, 33, 51
of adenomyosis, 56, 60, 60t
of arcuate artery calcification, 67
in children, 53
of congenital anomalies, 60–61, 61f, 62f–63f, 64
in diagnosis and prevention of uterine perforation or rupture, 69–70
of leiomyomas, 55, 56f, 56t, 59f
of position, 53–55, 54f
of postmenopausal uterus, 52–53, 53t
of size and shape, 51–52, 52t
of tumors and cysts, 67, 68f, 69, 69f
of uterine vessels, 64–67, 65f–67f
tumors of, transvaginal color Doppler in evaluation of, 329–330
unicornuate
subclasses or variations in, 64
ultrasound diagnosis of, 61, 62f, 64, 158
version of, 54f, 55
volume of, calculation of, 52, 52t

V

Vaginal imaging, fetal heart motion detection by, 202
Valvulae conniventes, sonographic image of, 133
Vanishing twin syndrome, 208, 211–212
Vascular shock, in ectopic pregnancy, 238
Vasculature, tumor, 328–329
Vibrations, 19
Videotapes, 42
Vitelline duct, 193, 195f

W

Water enema, 138
Wavelength of sound, 17, 18f
axial resolution and, 21
World Health Organization (WHO), classification of anovulation, 290, 293, 298

Y

Yolk sac
distorted, 169
presence of, exclusion of ectopic pregnancy by, 240
role in early pregnancy sonography, 193, 195f–196f, 196, 196t
visibility of, 219

Z

Zona pellucida, 188
Zygote, 188

About the Editor

Melvin G. Dodson received his undergraduate degree from the University of Florida and his Doctor of Medicine degree from the University of Miami School of Medicine. He completed his internship and residency in obstetrics and gynecology at the Jackson Memorial Hospital and the University of Miami School of Medicine and received his Doctor of Philosophy degree in Microbiology and Immunology from Loyola University of Chicago Stritch School of Medicine. Dr. Dodson has served on the faculty at the medical school at Loyola of Chicago and at the Baylor College of Medicine, in Houston. He was Professor and Chairman of the Department of Obstetrics and Gyncecology and Professor of Microbiology at East Tennessee State University and The Nicholas J. Thompson Professor and Chairman of the Department of Obstetrics and Gynecology and Professor of Microbiology at Wright State University School of Medicine, in Dayton, Ohio. He has published over 135 scientific articles and abstracts and was a co-author of a prize paper for Current Clinical and Basic Investigation at the American College of Obstetrics and Gynecology Annual Meeting in 1983, 1987, and 1988. In 1993, Dr. Dodson returned to Florida after 18 years in academic medicine and is now in private practice in obstetrics and gynecology.